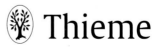

Color Atlas of Neurology

Reinhard Rohkamm, M.D.

Professor
Neurological Clinic
Nordwest-Krankenhaus Sanderbusch
Sande, Germany

172 illustrations by Manfred Güther

Translation revised by Ethan Taub, M.D.

Thieme
Stuttgart · New York

Library of Congress Cataloging-in-Publication Data is available from the publisher.

This book is an authorized translation of the 2nd German edition published and copyrighted 2003 by Georg Thieme Verlag, Stuttgart, Germany. Title of the German edition: Taschenatlas Neurologie

Original translator: Suzyon O'Neal Wandrey, Berlin, Germany

Translator/editor: Ethan Taub, M.D., Zürich, Switzerland

© 2004 Georg Thieme Verlag,
Rüdigerstrasse 14, 70469 Stuttgart, Germany
http://www.thieme.de
Thieme New York, 333 Seventh Avenue,
New York, NY 10001 USA
http://www.thieme.com

Cover design: Cyclus, Stuttgart
Typesetting by primustype R. Hurler GmbH, Notzingen
Printed in Germany by Grammlich, Pliezhausen

ISBN 3-13-130931-8 (GTV)
ISBN 1-58890-191-2 (TNY)   1 2 3 4 5

Preface

The nervous system and the muscles are the seat of many primary diseases and are affected secondarily by many others.

This pocket atlas is intended as an aid to the detection and diagnosis of the symptoms and signs of neurological disease. The text and illustrations are printed on facing pages, to facilitate learning of the points presented in each.

The book begins with a summary of the fundamentals of neuroanatomy in Chapter 1. Chapter 2 concerns the functions of the nervous system and the commonly encountered syndromes in clinical neurology. Individual neurological diseases are discussed in Chapter 3. The clinical neurological examination is best understood once the material of the first three chapters is mastered; it is therefore presented in the last chapter, Chapter 4.

The choice of topics for discussion is directed toward questions that frequently arise in clinical practice. Some of the illustrations have been reproduced from previous works by other authors, because they seemed to us to be optimal solutions to the problem of visually depicting a difficult subject. In particular, we would like to pay tribute here to the graphic originality of the late Dr. Frank H. Netter.

Many people have lent us a hand in the creation of this book. Our colleagues at the Sanderbusch Neurological Clinic were always ready to help us face the difficult task of getting the book written while meeting the constant demands of patient care. I (R.R.) would particularly like to thank our Oberärzte (Senior Registrars), Drs. Helga Best and Robert Schumann, for their skillful cooperation and support over several years of work. Thanks are also due to the radiologists, Drs. Benno Wördehoff and Ditmar Schönfeld, for providing images to be used in the illustrations. This book would never have come about without the fascination for neurology that was instilled in me in all the stages of my clinical training; I look back with special fondness on the time I spent as a Resident in the Department of Neurology at the University of New Mexico (Albuquerque). Above all, I thank the many patients, past and present, who have entrusted me with their care.

Finally, cordial thanks are due to the publishers, Georg Thieme Verlag, for their benevolent and surefooted assistance throughout the development of this book, and for the outstanding quality of its production. Among the many members of the staff to whom we are grateful, we would like to single out Dr. Thomas Scherb, with whom we were able to develop our initial ideas about the format of the book, as well as Dr. Clifford Bergman and Gabriele Kuhn, who saw this edition through to production with assurance, expertise, and the necessary dose of humor.

We dedicate this book to our families: Christina, Claire, and Ben (R.R.) and Birgit, Jonas, and Lukas (M.G.).

Reinhard Rohkamm, Sande
Manfred Güther, Bermatingen
Autumn 2003

Contents

1 Fundamentals   1

Overview 2
Skull 4
Meninges 6
Cerebrospinal Fluid 8

Blood Vessels 10
Carotid Arteries 11
Anterior Circulation of the Brain 12
Vertebral and Basilar Arteries 14
Posterior Circulation of the Brain 16
Intracranial Veins 18
Extracranial Veins 20
Spinal Circulation 22

Central Nervous Sysstem 24
Anatomical and Functional Organization . 25
Brain Stem 26
Cranial Nerves 28
Spine and Spinal Cord 30

Peripheral Nervous System 32
Dermatomes and Myotomes 33
Brachial Plexus 34
Nerves of the Upper Limb 35
Lumbar Plexus 36
Nerves of the Lower Limb 37

2 Normal and Abnormal Function of the Nervous System   39

Motor Function 40
Reflexes 41
Motor Control 42
Motor Execution 44
Central Paralysis 46
Peripheral Paralysis 50
Cerebellum 54
Vestibular System 56
Vertigo 58
Gait Disturbances 60
Tremor 62
Dystonia 64
Chorea, Ballism, Dyskinesia, Myoclonus .. 66
Myoclonus, Tics 68

Brain Stem Syndromes 70
Midbrain Syndromes 71
Pontine Syndromes 72
Medullary Syndromes 73

Cranial Nerves 74
Skull Base Syndromes 75
Smell 76
Taste 78
Visual pathway 80
Visual Field Defects 82
Oculomotor Function 84
Oculomotor Disturbances 86
Nystagmus 88
Pupillomotor Function 90
Pupillary Dysfunction 92
Trigeminal Nerve 94
Facial Nerve 96
Facial Nerve Lesions 98
Hearing 100
Disturbances of Deglutition 102

Sensation 104
Sensory Disturbances 106

Contents

Pain 108

Sleep 112
Normal Sleep 113
Sleep Disorders 114

Disturbances of Consciousness 116
Acute Disturbances of Consciousness 116
Coma 118
Comalike Syndromes, Death 120

Behavioral Manifestations of Neurological
Disease 122
Language 124
Aphasia 126
Agraphia, Alexia, Acalculia, Apraxia 128
Speech Disorders 130

Disturbances of Orientation 132
Disturbances of Memory 134
Dementia 136
Pseudo-neurological Disorders 138

Autonomic Nervous System (ANS) 140
Organization 141
Hypothalamus 142
Limbic System and Peripheral ANS 144
Heart and Circulation 148
Respiration 150
Thermoregulation 152
Gastrointestinal Function 154
Bladder Function, Sexual Function 156

Intracranial Pressure 158

3 Neurological Syndromes 165

Central Nervous System 166
Stroke 167
Headache 182
Epilepsy: Seizure Types 192
Epilepsy: Classification 196
Epilepsy: Pathogenesis and Treatment . . . 198
Nonepileptic Seizures 200
Parkinson Disease: Clinical Features 206
Parkinson Disease: Pathogenesis 210
Parkinson Disease: Treatment 212
Multiple Sclerosis 214
CNS Infections 222
Brain Tumors 254

Metastases 262
Trauma 266
Cerebellar Diseases 276
Myelopathies 282
Malformations and Developmental
Anomalies 288
Neurodegenerative Diseases 296
Encephalopathies 306

Peripheral Nerve and Muscle 316
Peripheral Neuropathies 316
Myopathies 334
Neuromuscular Disorders 346

4 Diagnostic Evaluation 349

Diagnostic Evaluation 350
History and Physical Examination 350
Neurophysiological and Neuro-
psychological Tests 352

Cerebrovascular Ultrasonography,
Diagnostic Imaging, and Biopsy
Procedures 353

5 Appendix 355

References 409

Index 415

1 Fundamentals

- Anatomy
- Physiology

Neurology is the branch of medicine dealing with diseases of the central, peripheral, and autonomic nervous systems, including the skeletal musculature.

Central Nervous System (CNS)

■ Brain

The **forebrain** or prosencephalon (supratentorial portion of the brain) comprises the telencephalon (the two cerebral hemispheres and the midline structures connecting them) and the diencephalon.

The **midbrain** or mesencephalon lies between the fore brain and the hind brain. It passes through the tentorium cerebelli.

The **hindbrain** or rhombencephalon (infratentorial portion of the brain) comprises the pons, the medulla oblongata (almost always called "medulla" for short), and the cerebellum. The mid brain, pons, and medulla together make up the **brain stem**.

■ Spinal cord

The spinal cord is approximately 45 cm long in adults. Its upper end is continuous with the medulla; the transition is defined to occur just above the level of exit of the first pair of cervical nerves. Its tapering lower end, the *conus medullaris*, terminates at the level of the L3 vertebra in neonates, and at the level of the L1–2 intervertebral disk in adults. Thus, lumbar puncture should always be performed at or below L3–4. The conus medullaris is continuous at its lower end with the threadlike *filum terminale*, composed mainly of glial and connective tissue, which, in turn, runs through the lumbar sac amidst the dorsal and ventral roots of the spinal nerves, collectively called the *cauda equina* ("horse's tail"), and then attaches to the dorsal surface of the coccyx. The cervical, thoracic, lumbar, and sacral portions of the spinal cord are defined according to the segmental division of the vertebral column and spinal nerves.

Peripheral Nervous System (PNS)

The peripheral nervous system connects the central nervous system with the rest of the body. All motor, sensory and autonomic nerve cells and fibers outside the CNS are generally considered part of the PNS. Specifically, the PNS comprises the ventral (motor) nerve roots, dorsal (sensory) nerve roots, spinal ganglia, and spinal and peripheral nerves, and their endings, as well as a major portion of the autonomic nervous system (sympathetic trunk). The first two cranial nerves (the olfactory and optic nerves) belong to the CNS, but the remainder belong to the PNS.

Peripheral nerves may be purely motor or sensory but are usually mixed, containing variable fractions of motor, sensory, and autonomic nerve fibers (axons). A peripheral nerve is made up of multiple bundles of axons, called *fascicles*, each of which is covered by a connective tissue sheath (*perineurium*). The connective tissue lying between axons within a fascicle is called *endoneurium*, and that between fascicles is called *epineurium*. Fascicles contain myelinated and unmyelinated axons, endoneurium, and capillaries. Individual axons are surrounded by supportive cells called *Schwann cells*. A single Schwann cell surrounds several axons of unmyelinated type. Tight winding of the Schwann cell membrane around the axon produces the myelin sheath that covers myelinated axons. The Schwann cells of a myelinated axon are spaced a small distance from one another; the intervals between them are called *nodes of Ranvier*. The nerve conduction velocity increases with the thickness of the myelin sheath. The specialized contact zone between a motor nerve fiber and the muscle it supplies is called the *neuromuscular junction* or *motor end plate*. Impulses arising in the *sensory receptors* of the skin, fascia, muscles, joints, internal organs, and other parts of the body travel centrally through the sensory (afferent) nerve fibers. These fibers have their cell bodies in the dorsal root ganglia (pseudounipolar cells) and reach the spinal cord by way of the dorsal roots.

Autonomic Nervous System (ANS)

The autonomic nervous system regulates the function of the internal organs in response to the changing internal and external environment. It contains both central (p. 140 ff) and peripheral portions (p. 146ff).

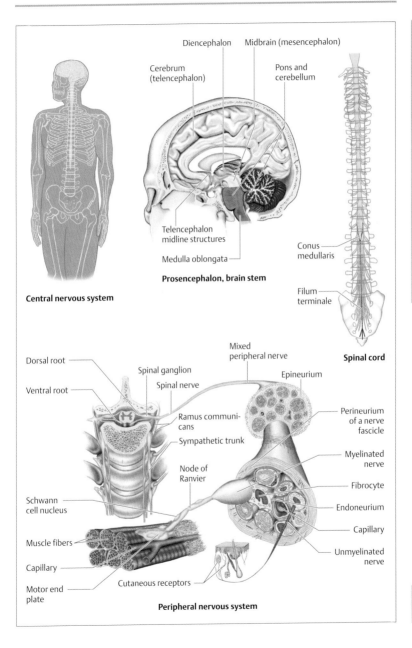

Diencephalon
Midbrain (mesencephalon)

Cerebrum
(telencephalon)

Pons and
cerebellum

Telencephalon
midline structures

Medulla oblongata

Conus
medullaris

Filum
terminale

Prosencephalon, brain stem

Central nervous system

Spinal cord

Mixed
peripheral nerve

Dorsal root

Spinal ganglion

Epineurium

Ventral root

Spinal nerve

Ramus communi-
cans

Perineurium
of a nerve
fascicle

Sympathetic trunk

Myelinated
nerve

Node of
Ranvier

Fibrocyte

Schwann
cell nucleus

Endoneurium

Capillary

Muscle fibers

Unmyelinated
nerve

Capillary

Motor end
plate

Cutaneous receptors

Peripheral nervous system

Overview

3

The skull (cranium) determines the shape of the head; it is easily palpated through the thin layers of muscle and connective tissue that cover it. It is of variable thickness, being thicker and sturdier in areas of greater mechanical stress. The thinner bone in temporal and orbital portions of the cranium provides the so-called *bone windows* through which the basal cerebral arteries can be examined by ultrasound. Thinner portions of the skull are more vulnerable to traumatic fracture. The only joints in the skull are those between the auditory ossicles and the *temporomandibular joints* linking the skull to the jaw.

Neurocranium

The neurocranium encloses the brain, labyrinth, and middle ear. The outer and inner tables of the skull are connected by cancellous bone and marrow spaces (*diploë*). The bones of the *roof of the cranium* (calvaria) of adolescents and adults are rigidly connected by sutures and cartilage (synchondroses). The *coronal suture* extends across the frontal third of the cranial roof. The *sagittal suture* lies in the midline, extending backward from the coronal suture and bifurcating over the occiput to form the *lambdoid suture.* The area of junction of the frontal, parietal, temporal, and sphenoid bones is called the *pterion*; below the pterion lies the bifurcation of the middle meningeal artery.

The *inner skull base* forms the floor of the cranial cavity, which is divided into anterior, middle, and posterior cranial fossae. The *anterior fossa* lodges the olfactory tracts and the basal surface of the frontal lobes; the *middle fossa*, the basal surface of the temporal lobes, hypothalamus, and pituitary gland; the *posterior fossa*, the cerebellum, pons, and medulla. The anterior and middle fossae are demarcated from each other laterally by the posterior edge of the (lesser) wing of the sphenoid bone, and medially by the *jugum sphenoidale.* The middle and posterior fossae are demarcated from each other laterally by the upper rim of the petrous pyramid, and medially by the dorsum sellae.

Scalp

The layers of the scalp are the skin (including epidermis, dermis, and hair), the subcuticular connective tissue, the fascial *galea aponeurotica*, subaponeurotic loose connective tissue, and the cranial periosteum (*pericranium*). The hair of the scalp grows approximately 1 cm per month. The connection between the galea and the pericranium is mobile except at the upper rim of the orbits, the zygomatic arches, and the external occipital protuberance. Scalp injuries superficial to the galea do not cause large hematomas, and the skin edges usually remain approximated. Wounds involving the galea may gape; scalping injuries are those in which the galea is torn away from the periosteum. Subgaleal hemorrhages spread over the surface of the skull.

Viscerocranium

The viscerocranium comprises the bones of the orbit, nose, and paranasal sinuses. The superior margin of the *orbit* is formed by the frontal bone, its inferior margin by the maxilla and zygomatic bone. The frontal sinus lies superior to the roof of the orbit, the maxillary sinus inferior to its floor. The *nasal cavity* extends from the anterior openings of the nose (nostrils) to its posterior openings (choanae) and communicates with the *paranasal sinuses*—maxillary, frontal, sphenoid, and ethmoid. The infraorbital canal, which transmits the infraorbital vessels and nerve, is located in the superior (orbital) wall of the maxillary sinus. The portion of the sphenoid bone covering the sphenoid sinus forms, on its outer surface, the bony margins of the optic canals, prechiasmatic sulci, and pituitary fossa.

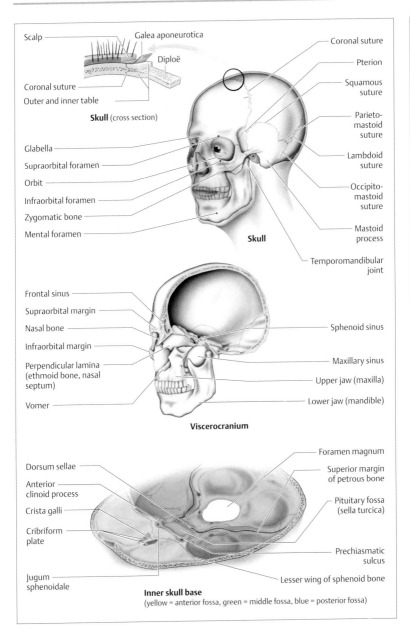

Scalp
Galea aponeurotica
Diploë
Coronal suture
Outer and inner table

Skull (cross section)

Coronal suture
Pterion
Squamous suture
Parieto-mastoid suture
Lambdoid suture
Occipito-mastoid suture
Mastoid process

Glabella
Supraorbital foramen
Orbit
Infraorbital foramen
Zygomatic bone
Mental foramen

Skull

Temporomandibular joint

Frontal sinus
Supraorbital margin
Nasal bone
Infraorbital margin
Perpendicular lamina (ethmoid bone, nasal septum)
Vomer

Sphenoid sinus
Maxillary sinus
Upper jaw (maxilla)
Lower jaw (mandible)

Viscerocranium

Dorsum sellae
Anterior clinoid process
Crista galli
Cribriform plate
Jugum sphenoidale

Foramen magnum
Superior margin of petrous bone
Pituitary fossa (sella turcica)
Prechiasmatic sulcus
Lesser wing of sphenoid bone

Inner skull base
(yellow = anterior fossa, green = middle fossa, blue = posterior fossa)

The *meninges* lie immediately deep to the inner surface of the skull and constitute the membranous covering of the brain. The pericranium of the inner surface of the skull and the dura mater are collectively termed the *pachymeninges*, while the pia mater and arachnoid membrane are the *leptomeninges*.

Pachymeninges

The pericranium contains the meningeal arteries, which supply both the dura mater and the bone marrow of the cranial vault. The pericranium is fused to the dura mater, except where they separate to form the dural venous sinuses. The virtual space between the pericranium and the dura mater—the *epidural space*—may be forced apart by a pathological process, such as an epidural hematoma. Immediately beneath the dura mater, but not fused to it, is the arachnoid membrane; the intervening virtual space—the *subdural space*—contains capillaries and transmits bridging veins, which, if injured, can give rise to a subdural hematoma. The *falx cerebri* separates the two cerebral hemispheres and is bordered above and below by the superior and inferior sagittal sinuses. It attaches anteriorly to the crista galli, and bifurcates posteriorly to form the tentorium cerebelli, with the straight sinus occupying the space between the falx and the two halves of the tentorium. The much smaller *falx cerebelli* separates the two cerebellar hemispheres; it encloses the occipital sinus and is attached posteriorly to the occipital bone.

The *tentorium cerebelli* separates the superior aspect of the cerebellum from the inferior aspect of the occipital lobe. It rises toward the midline, taking the shape of a tent. The opening between the two halves of the tentorium, known as the tentorial *notch* or *incisura*, is traversed by the midbrain; the medial edge of the tentorium is adjacent to the midbrain on either side. The tentorium attaches posteriorly to the sulcus of the transverse sinus, laterally to the superior rim of the pyramid of the temporal bone, and anteriorly to the anterior and posterior clinoid processes. The tentorium divides the cranial cavity into the *supratentorial* and *infratentorial spaces*.

The pituitary stalk, or infundibulum, accompanied by its enveloping arachnoid membrane, passes through an aperture in the posterior portion of the *diaphragma sellae* (diaphragm of the sella turcica), a horizontal sheet of dura mater lying between the anterior and posterior clinoid processes. The pituitary gland itself sits in the sella turcica, below the diaphragm.

The meningeal branches of the three divisions of the *trigeminal nerve* (pp. 28 and 94) provide sensory innervation to the dura mater of the cranial roof, anterior cranial fossa, and middle cranial fossa. The meningeal branch of the *vagus nerve* (p. 29), which arises from its superior ganglion, provides sensory innervation to the dura mater of the posterior fossa. Pain can thus be felt in response to noxious stimulation of the dura mater, while the cerebral parenchyma is insensitive. Some of the cranial nerves, and some of the blood vessels that supply the brain, traverse the dura at a distance from their entry into the skull, and thereby possess an *intracranial extradural segment*, of a characteristic length for each structure. Thus the rootlets of the trigeminal nerve, for instance, can be approached surgically without incising the dura mater.

Pia Mater

The cranial pia mater is closely apposed to the brain surface and follows all of its gyri and sulci. The cerebral blood vessels enter the brain from its surface by perforating the pia mater. Except for the capillaries, all such vessels are accompanied for a short distance by a pial sheath, and thereafter by a glial membrane that separates them from the neuropil. The perivascular space enclosed by this membrane (*Virchow–Robin space*) contains cerebrospinal fluid. The *choroid plexus* of the cerebral ventricles, which secretes the cerebrospinal fluid, is formed by an infolding of pial blood vessels (*tela choroidea*) covered by a layer of ventricular epithelium (*ependyma*).

Arachnoid Membrane

The dura mater is closely apposed to the arachnoid membrane; the virtual space between them (subdural space) contains capillaries and bridging veins. Between the arachnoid membrane and the pia mater lies the *subarachnoid space*, which is filled with cerebrospinal fluid and is spanned by a network of delicate trabecular fibers.

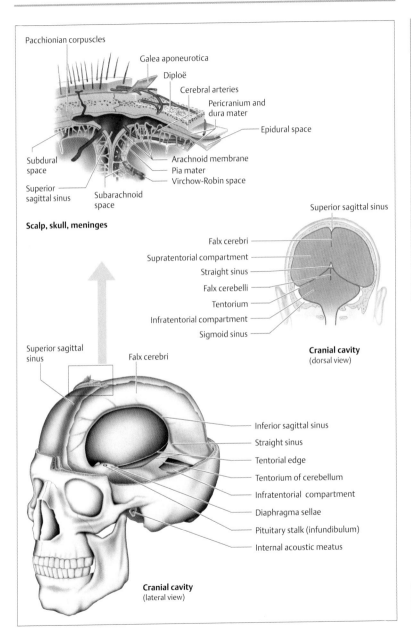

Pacchionian corpuscles
Galea aponeurotica
Diploë
Cerebral arteries
Pericranium and dura mater
Epidural space
Subdural space
Arachnoid membrane
Pia mater
Virchow-Robin space
Superior sagittal sinus
Subarachnoid space

Scalp, skull, meninges

Superior sagittal sinus
Falx cerebri
Supratentorial compartment
Straight sinus
Falx cerebelli
Tentorium
Infratentorial compartment
Sigmoid sinus

Cranial cavity
(dorsal view)

Superior sagittal sinus
Falx cerebri
Inferior sagittal sinus
Straight sinus
Tentorial edge
Tentorium of cerebellum
Infratentorial compartment
Diaphragma sellae
Pituitary stalk (infundibulum)
Internal acoustic meatus

Cranial cavity
(lateral view)

Meninges

Cerebral Ventricles and Cisterns

The fluid-filled *cerebral ventricles* constitute the inner CSF space. Each of the two lateral ventricles communicates with the third ventricle through the *interventricular foramen of Monro* (one on each side). Fluid passes from the third ventricle through the *cerebral aqueduct* (of *Sylvius*) into the fourth ventricle, and thence through the single midline foramen (of *Magendie*) and paired lateral foramina (of *Luschka*) into the *subarachnoid space* (outer CSF space). Dilatations of the subarachnoid space are called *cisterns*. The *cerebellomedullary cistern (cisterna magna)* lies between the posterior surface of the medulla and the undersurface of the cerebellum. The *cerebellopontine cistern* occupies the cerebellopontine angle. The *ambient cistern* lies lateral to the cerebral peduncle and contains the posterior cerebral and superior cerebellar arteries, the basal vein, and the trochlear nerve. The *interpeduncular cistern* lies in the midline between the cerebral peduncles and contains the oculomotor nerves, the bifurcation of the basilar artery, and the origins of the superior cerebellar and posterior cerebral arteries; anterior to it is the *chiasmatic cistern*, which surrounds the optic chiasm and the pituitary stalk. The portion of the subarachnoid space extending from the foramen magnum to the dorsum sellae is collectively termed the *posterior cistern*.

Cerebrospinal Fluid (CSF)

The CSF, a clear and colorless ultrafiltrate of blood plasma, is mainly produced in the choroid plexus of the cerebral ventricles and in the capillaries of the brain. It normally contains no red blood cells and at most 4 white blood cells/μl. Its functions are both *physical* (compensation for volume changes, buffering and equal distribution of intracranial pressure despite variation in venous and arterial blood pressure) and *metabolic* (transport of nutrients and hormones into the brain, and of waste products out of it). The total CSF volume in the adult is ca. 150 ml, of which ca. 30 ml is in the spinal subarachnoid space. Some 500 ml of cerebrospinal fluid is produced per day, corresponding to a flow of ca. 20 ml/h. The normal pulsation of CSF reflects brain pulsation due to changes in cerebral venous and arterial volume, respiration, and head movements. A Valsalva maneuver increases the CSF pressure.

CSF circulation. CSF formed in the choroid plexus flows through the ventricular system and through the foramina of Magendie and Luschka into the basal cisterns. It then circulates further into the spinal subarachnoid space, over the surfaces of the cerebellum and cerebrum, eventually reaching the sites of CSF absorption. It is mainly absorbed through the *arachnoid villi* (arachnoid granulations, pacchionian corpuscles), which are most abundant along the superior sagittal sinus but are also found at spinal levels. CSF drains through the arachnoid villi in one direction, from the subarachnoid space to the venous compartment, by a valve mechanism. This so-called *bulk flow* is apparently achieved with the aid of pinocytotic vacuoles that transport the CSF, and all substances dissolved in it, in ladlelike fashion. At the same time, CSF diffuses into the brain tissue adjacent to the CSF space and is absorbed by the capillaries.

The Blood–CSF and Blood–Brain Barriers

These "barriers" are not to be conceived of as impenetrable; under normal conditions, all plasma proteins pass into the CSF. The larger the protein molecule, however, the longer it takes to reach the CSF, and the steeper the plasma/CSF concentration gradient. The term *blood–brain barrier* (BBB) is a collective term for all barriers lying between the plasma and the neuropil, one of which is the *blood–CSF barrier* (BCB). Disease processes often alter the permeability of the BBB, but very rarely that of the BCB.

Morphologically, the BCB is formed by the choroid epithelium, while the BBB is formed by the tight junction (zonula occludens) of capillary endothelial cells. Up to half of all cerebral capillaries have a tubular structure, i.e., they have no connecting interstices. *Physiologically*, the system of barriers enables the regulation of the osmolarity of brain tissue and CSF and, thereby, the intracranial pressure and volume. *Biochemically*, the BCB is permeable to water-soluble substances (e.g., plasma proteins) but not to liposoluble substances such as anesthetics, psychoactive drugs, and analgesics. The BBB, on the other hand, is generally permeable to liposoluble substances (of molecular weight less than 500 daltons) but not to water-soluble substances.

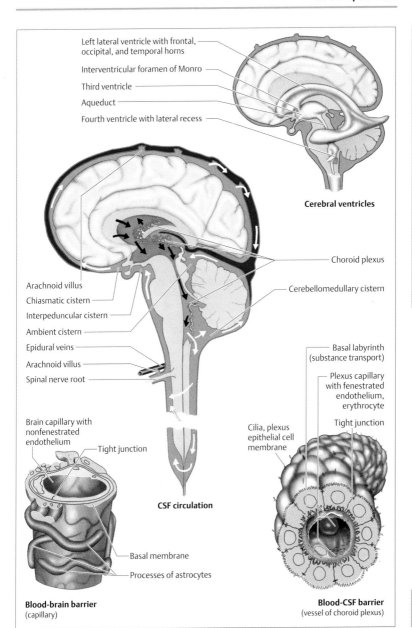

Left lateral ventricle with frontal, occipital, and temporal horns

Interventricular foramen of Monro

Third ventricle

Aqueduct

Fourth ventricle with lateral recess

Cerebral ventricles

Choroid plexus

Cerebellomedullary cistern

Arachnoid villus
Chiasmatic cistern
Interpeduncular cistern
Ambient cistern

Epidural veins
Arachnoid villus
Spinal nerve root

Basal labyrinth (substance transport)

Plexus capillary with fenestrated endothelium, erythrocyte

Tight junction

Cilia, plexus epithelial cell membrane

Brain capillary with nonfenestrated endothelium
Tight junction

CSF circulation

Basal membrane

Processes of astrocytes

Blood–brain barrier
(capillary)

Blood–CSF barrier
(vessel of choroid plexus)

Cerebrospinal Fluid

9

Blood is pumped from the left ventricle of the heart to the aortic arch and thence to the common carotid arteries and anterior circulation of the brain (internal carotid, middle cerebral, and anterior cerebral arteries), and to the subclavian arteries and posterior circulation of the brain (vertebral, basilar, and posterior cerebral arteries). The *anterior circulation* supplies the eyes, basal ganglia, part of the hypothalamus, the frontal and parietal lobes, and a large portion of the temporal lobes, while the *posterior circulation* supplies the brain stem, cerebellum, inner ear, occipital lobes, the thalamus, part of the hypothalamus, and a smaller portion of the temporal lobes.

Venous blood from the *superficial and deep cerebral veins* (p. 18 ff) drains via the dural venous sinuses into the internal jugular veins and thence into the the the superior vena cava and right atrium. The *extracranial and intracranial portions* of the blood supply of the brain as well as that of the spinal cord will be detailed further in the following paragraphs.

Carotid Arteries: Extracranial Portion

The brachiocephalic trunk arises from the aortic arch behind the manubrium of the sternum and bifurcates at the level of the sternoclavicular joint to form the right subclavian and common carotid arteries. The left common carotid artery (usually adjacent to the brachiocephalic trunk) and subclavian artery arise directly from the aortic arch. The common carotid artery on either side bifurcates at the level of the thyroid cartilage to form the internal and external carotid arteries; these arteries lie parallel and adjacent to each other after the bifurcation, with the external carotid artery lying medial. A dilatation of the common carotid artery at its bifurcation is called the *carotid sinus*.

The *external carotid artery* gives off the superior thyroid, lingual, facial, and maxillary arteries anteriorly, the ascending pharyngeal artery medially, and the occipital and posterior auricular arteries posteriorly. The maxillary and superficial temporal arteries are its terminal branches. The *middle meningeal artery* is an important branch of the maxillary artery.

The *internal carotid artery* gives off no extracranial branches. Its cervical portion runs lateral or dorsolateral to the external carotid artery, then dorsomedially along the wall of the pharynx (parapharyngeal space) in front of the transverse processes of the first three cervical vertebrae, and finally curves medially toward the carotid foramen.

Carotid Arteries: Intracranial Portion

The internal carotid artery (ICA) passes through the base of the skull in the carotid canal, which lies within the petrous part of the temporal bone. It runs upward about 1 cm, then turns anteromedially and courses toward the petrous apex, where it emerges from the temporal bone to enter the cavernous sinus. Within the sinus, the ICA runs along the lateral surface of the body of the sphenoid bone (C5 segment of the ICA), then turns anteriorly and passes lateral to the sella turcica along the lateral wall of the sphenoid bone (segment C4). It then bends sharply back on itself under the root of the anterior clinoid process, so that it points posteriorly (segment C3, carotid bend). After emerging from the cavernous sinus, it penetrates the dura mater medial to the anterior clinoid process and passes under the optic nerve (*cisternal segment*, segment C2). It then ascends in the subarachnoid space (segment C1) till it reaches the *circle of Willis*, the site of its terminal bifurcation. Segments C3, C4, and C5 of the ICA constitute its *infraclinoid segment*, segments C1 and C2 its *supraclinoid segment*. Segments C2, C3, and C4 together make up the carotid siphon.

The *ophthalmic artery* arises from the carotid bend and runs in the optic canal inferior to the optic nerve. One of its ocular branches, the *central retinal artery*, passes together with the optic nerve to the retina, where it can be seen by ophthalmoscopy.

Medial to the clinoid process, the *posterior communicating artery* arises from the posterior wall of the internal carotid artery, passes posteriorly in proximity to the oculomotor nerve, and then joins the posterior cerebral artery.

The *anterior choroidal artery* usually arises from the ICA and rarely from the middle cerebral artery. It crosses under the optic tract, passes laterally to the crus cerebri and lateral geniculate body, and enters the inferior horn of the lateral ventricle, where it joins the tela choroidea.

Cerebral Circulation

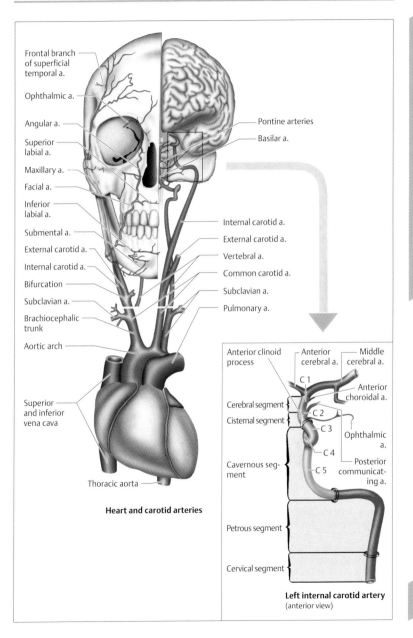

Frontal branch of superficial temporal a.

Ophthalmic a.

Angular a.

Superior labial a.

Maxillary a.

Facial a.

Inferior labial a.

Submental a.

External carotid a.

Internal carotid a.

Bifurcation

Subclavian a.

Brachiocephalic trunk

Aortic arch

Superior and inferior vena cava

Thoracic aorta

Pontine arteries

Basilar a.

Internal carotid a.

External carotid a.

Vertebral a.

Common carotid a.

Subclavian a.

Pulmonary a.

Heart and carotid arteries

Anterior clinoid process

Anterior cerebral a.

Middle cerebral a.

C 1

Anterior choroidal a.

Cerebral segment

C 2

Cisternal segment

C 3

Ophthalmic a.

C 4

Cavernous segment

C 5

Posterior communicating a.

Petrous segment

Cervical segment

Left internal carotid artery
(anterior view)

11

Cerebral Circulation

The anterior and middle cerebral arteries are the terminal branches of the internal carotid artery. They originate at the ICA bifurcation, located in the circle of Willis at the level of the anterior clinoid process, between the optic chiasm and the temporal pole.

Anterior Cerebral Artery (ACA)

The ACA is the more medial of the two arteries arising from the ICA bifurcation. It ascends lateral to the anterior clinoid process and past the the optic nerve and optic chiasm, giving off a small branch, the anterior communicating artery (ACommA), which crosses the midline to join the contralateral ACA. The segment of ACA proximal to the origin of the ACommA is its *precommunicating segment* (segment A1). The A1 segments on either side and the ACommA together form the anterior half of the circle of Willis. Segment A1 gives off an average of eight basal perforating arteries that enter the brain through the anterior perforated substance. The *recurrent artery of Heubner* arises from the ACA near the origin of the ACommA, either from the distal part of A1 or from the proximal part of A2.

The *postcommunicating segment* of the ACA (segments A2 to A5) ascends between the frontal lobes and runs toward the occiput in the interhemispheric fissure, along the corpus callosum and below the free border of the falx cerebri, as the *pericallosal artery*. Segment A2, which usually gives off the *frontopolar artery*, ends where the artery turns forward to become apposed to the genu of the corpus callosum; segment A3 is the frontally convex arch of the vessel along the genu. The A4 and A5 segments run roughly horizontally over the callosal surface and give off supracallosal branches that run in a posterior direction.

Distribution. The basal perforating arteries arising from A1 supply the ventral hypothalamus and a portion of the pituitary stalk. Heubner's artery supplies the head of the caudate nucleus, the rostral four-fifths of the putamen, the globus pallidus, and the internal capsule. The blood supply of the inferior portion of the genu of the corpus callosum, and of the olfactory bulb, tract, and trigone, is variable.

The ACommA gives off a few small branches (anteromedial central branches) to the hypothalamus.

Branches from the postcommunicating segment of the ACA supply the inferior surface of the frontal lobe (frontobasilar artery), the medial and parasagittal surfaces of the frontal lobe (callosomarginal artery), the paracentral lobule (paracentral artery), the medial and parasagittal surfaces of the parietal lobe (precuneal artery), and the cortex in the region of the parieto-occipital sulcus (parieto-occipital artery).

Middle Cerebral Artery (MCA)

The MCA is the more lateral of the two arteries arising from the ICA bifurcation. Its first segment (M1, sphenoidal segment) follows the anterior clinoid process for a distance of 1 to 2 cm. The MCA then turns laterally to enter the depths of the Sylvian fissure (i.e., the Sylvian cistern), where it lies on the surface of the insula and gives off branches to it (M2, insular segment). It bends back sharply to travel along the surface of the operculum (M3, opercular segment) and then finally emerges through the Sylvian fissure onto the lateral convexity of the brain (M4 and M5, terminal segments).

Distribution. Small branches of M1 (the thalamostriate and lenticulostriate arteries) supply the basal ganglia, the claustrum, and the internal, external, and extreme capsules. M2 and M3 branches supply the insula (insular arteries), lateral portions of the orbital and inferior frontal gyri (frontobasal artery), and the temporal operculum, including the transverse gyrus of Heschl (temporal arteries). M4 and M5 branches supply most of the cortex of the lateral cerebral convexity, including portions of the frontal lobe (arteries of the precentral and triangular sulci), the parietal lobe (anterior and posterior parietal arteries), and the temporal lobe (arteries of central and postcentral sulci). In particular, important cortical areas supplied by M4 and M5 branches include the primary motor and sensory areas (precentral and postcentral gyri) and the language areas of Broca and Wernicke.

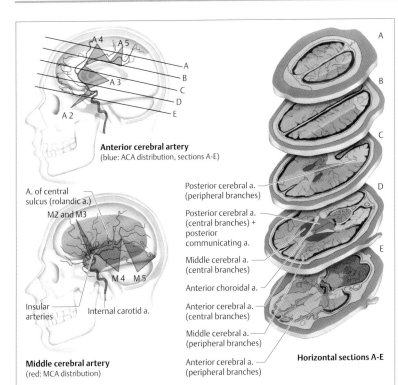

Anterior cerebral artery
(blue: ACA distribution, sections A-E)

A. of central
sulcus (rolandic a.)
M2 and M3
M 4   M 5
Insular
arteries
Internal carotid a.

Middle cerebral artery
(red: MCA distribution)

A 4 A 5
A 3
A 2

Posterior cerebral a.
(peripheral branches)

Posterior cerebral a.
(central branches) +
posterior
communicating a.

Middle cerebral a.
(central branches)

Anterior choroidal a.

Anterior cerebral a.
(central branches)

Middle cerebral a.
(peripheral branches)

Anterior cerebral a.
(peripheral branches)

Horizontal sections A-E

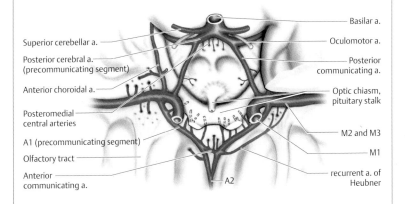

Superior cerebellar a.

Posterior cerebral a.
(precommunicating segment)

Anterior choroidal a.

Posteromedial
central arteries

A1 (precommunicating segment)

Olfactory tract

Anterior
communicating a.

Basilar a.

Oculomotor a.

Posterior
communicating a.

Optic chiasm,
pituitary stalk

M2 and M3

M1

recurrent a. of
Heubner

A2

Circle of Willis

Extracranial Portion

The vertebral artery arises from the arch of the subclavian artery at a point designated V0. The prevertebral or V1 segment extends from V0 to the foramen transversarium of the transverse process of C6. The transversarial or V2 segment passes vertically through the foramina transversaria of C6 through C2, accompanied by venous plexuses and sympathetic nerves derived from the cervical ganglia. It gives off branches to the cervical nerves, vertebrae and intervertebral joints, neck muscles, and cervical spinal cord. Often, a prominent branch at the C5 level anastomoses with the anterior spinal artery. The V3 segment, also called the atlas (C1) loop, runs laterally and then vertically to the foramen transversarium of C1, which it passes through, winds medially along the lateral mass of C1, pierces the posterior atlanto-occipital membrane behind the atlanto-occipital joint, and then enters the dura mater and arachnoid membrane at the level of the foramen magnum. The two vertebral arteries are unequal in size in about 75 % of persons, and one of them is extremely narrow (hypoplastic) in about 10 %, usually on the right side.

Intracranial Portion

The V4 segment of the vertebral artery lies entirely within the subarachnoid space. It terminates at the junction of the two vertebral arteries to form the basilar artery, at the level of the lower border of the pons. Proximal to the junction, each vertebral artery gives off a mediobasal branch; these two branches run for ca. 2 cm and then unite in the midline to form a single *anterior spinal artery*, which descends along the anterior surface of the medulla and spinal cord (see p. 23). The *posterior inferior cerebellar artery* (PICA), which originates from the V4 segment at a highly variable level, curves around the inferior olive and extends dorsally through the root filaments of the accessory nerve. It then ascends behind the fibers of the hypoglossus and vagus nerves, forms a loop on the posterior wall of the fourth ventricle, and gives off terminal branches to the inferior surface of the cerebellar hemisphere, the tonsils, and the vermis. It provides most of the blood supply to the dorsolateral medulla and the posteroinferior surface of the cerebellum. The *posterior spinal artery* (there is one on each side) arises from either the vertebral artery or the PICA.

The *basilar artery* runs in the prepontine cistern along the entire length of the pons and then bifurcates to form the posterior cerebral arteries. Its inferior portion is closely related to the abducens nerves, its superior portion to the oculomotor nerves. Its paramedian, short circumferential, and long circumferential branches supply the pons and the superior and middle cerebellar peduncles.

The *anterior inferior cerebellar artery* (AICA) arises from the lower third of the basilar artery. It runs laterally and caudally toward the cerebellopontine angle, passes near the internal acoustic meatus, and reaches the flocculus, where it gives off terminal branches that supply the anteroinferior portion of the cerebellar cortex and part of the cerebellar nuclei. The AICA lies basal to the abducens nerve and ventromedial to the facial and auditory nerves in the cerebellopontine cistern. It often gives rise to a labyrinthine branch that enters the internal acoustic meatus.

The *superior cerebellar arteries* (SCA) of both sides originate from the basilar trunk just below its bifurcation. Each SCA travels through the perimesencephalic cistern dorsal to the oculomotor nerve, curves around the cerebral peduncle caudal and medial to the trochlear nerve, and then enters the ambient cistern, where it gives off its terminal branches. The SCA supplies the upper pons, part of the mid brain, the upper surface of the cerebellar hemispheres, the upper portion of the vermis, and the cerebellar nuclei.

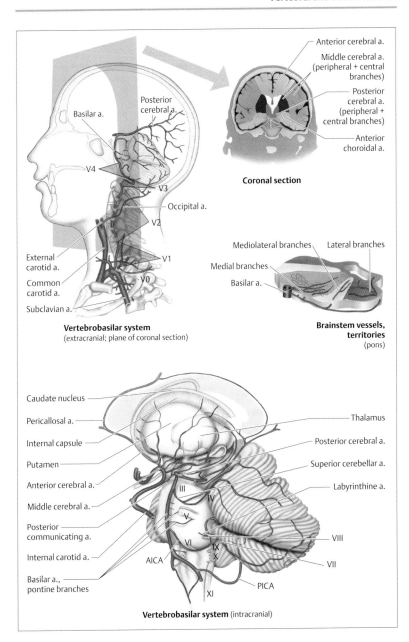

Anterior cerebral a.

Middle cerebral a. (peripheral + central branches)

Posterior cerebral a. (peripheral + central branches)

Anterior choroidal a.

Coronal section

Posterior cerebral a.

Basilar a.

V4

V3

Occipital a.

V2

External carotid a.

V1

V0

Common carotid a.

Subclavian a.

Vertebrobasilar system
(extracranial; plane of coronal section)

Mediolateral branches   Lateral branches

Medial branches

Basilar a.

Brainstem vessels, territories
(pons)

Caudate nucleus

Pericallosal a.

Internal capsule

Putamen

Anterior cerebral a.

Middle cerebral a.

Posterior communicating a.

Internal carotid a.

Basilar a., pontine branches

Thalamus

Posterior cerebral a.

Superior cerebellar a.

Labyrinthine a.

III

IV

V

VI

IX

X

AICA

XI

VIII

VII

PICA

Vertebrobasilar system (intracranial)

Cerebral Circulation

15

Posterior Cerebral Artery (PCA)

The *precommunicating segment* of the PCA (P1) extends from the basilar bifurcation to the origin of the *posterior communicating artery* (PCommA). Its course lies within the interpeduncular cistern, which is demarcated by the clivus and the two cerebral peduncles. The oculomotor nerve, after its emergence from the brain stem, runs between the PCA and the superior cerebellar artery. The *postcommunicating segment* (P2) curves laterally and backward around the crus cerebri and reaches the posterior surface of the midbrain at an intercollicular level.

The precommunicating and postcommunicating segments are together referred to as the *pars circularis* of the PCA. (Alternatively, the pars circularis may be divided into three segments—interpeduncular, ambient, and quadrigeminal—named after the cisterns they traverse.)

Distal to the pars circularis of the PCA is the *pars terminalis*, which divides above the tentorium and caudal to the lateral geniculate body to form its terminal branches, the *medial and lateral occipital arteries*.

Pars circularis. The *precommunicating segment* gives off fine branches (posteromedial central arteries) that pierce the interpeduncular perforated substance to supply the anterior thalamus, the wall of the third ventricle, and the globus pallidus. The *postcommunicating segment* gives off fine branches (posterolateral central arteries) to the cerebral peduncles, the posterior portion of the thalamus, the colliculi of the mid brain, the medial geniculate body, and the pineal body. Further branches supply the posterior portion of the thalamus (thalamic branches), the cerebral peduncle (peduncular branches), and the lateral geniculate body and choroid plexus of the third and lateral ventricles (posterior choroidal branches).

Pars terminalis. Of the two terminal branches of this terminal portion of the PCA, the lateral occipital artery (together with its temporal branches) supplies the uncus, the hippocampal gyrus, and the undersurface of the occipital lobe. The medial occipital artery passes under the splenium of the corpus callosum, giving off branches that supply it (dorsal branch to the corpus callosum) as well as the cuneus and pre-cuneus (parieto-occipital branch), the striate cortex (calcarine branch), and the medial surfaces of the occipital and temporal lobes (occipitotemporal and temporal banches), including the parasagittal portion of the occipital lobe.

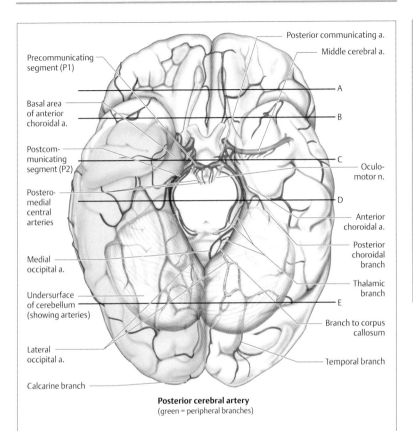

Posterior communicating a.

Middle cerebral a.

Precommunicating segment (P1)

A

Basal area of anterior choroidal a.

B

Postcommunicating segment (P2)

C

Oculomotor n.

Posteromedial central arteries

D

Anterior choroidal a.

Medial occipital a.

Posterior choroidal branch

Thalamic branch

Undersurface of cerebellum (showing arteries)

E

Branch to corpus callosum

Lateral occipital a.

Temporal branch

Calcarine branch

Posterior cerebral artery
(green = peripheral branches)

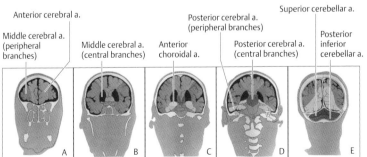

Anterior cerebral a.

Middle cerebral a. (peripheral branches)

Middle cerebral a. (central branches)

Anterior choroidal a.

Posterior cerebral a. (peripheral branches)

Posterior cerebral a. (central branches)

Superior cerebellar a.

Posterior inferior cerebellar a.

A   B   C   D   E

Regional arterial blood flow (frontal and coronal planes A-E)

17

Cerebral Circulation

Cerebral Veins

The *superficial cerebral veins* (cortical veins) carry blood from the outer 1–2 cm of the brain surface to large drainage channels such as the superior and inferior sagittal sinuses, the great cerebral vein of Galen, the straight sinus, and the tentorial veins. Thus, the cerebellar veins drain blood from the cerebellar surface into the superior vermian vein and thence into the great cerebral vein, straight sinus, and transverse sinuses. The *deep cerebral veins* (central veins) drain blood from the inner regions of the brain (hemispheric white matter, basal ganglia, corpus callosum, choroid plexus) and from a few cortical areas as well.

Superficial cerebral veins (cortical veins). The superficial cerebral veins are classified by their location as prefrontal, frontal, parietal, and occipital. Except for the *occipital veins*, which empty into the transverse sinus, these veins all travel over the cerebral convexity to join the superior sagittal sinus. They are termed *bridging veins* at their distal end, where they pierce the arachnoid membrane and bridge the subarachnoid space to join the sinus. The *superficial middle cerebral vein* (not shown) usually follows the posterior ramus of the Sylvian fissure and the fissure itself to the cavernous sinus. The *inferior cerebral veins* drain into the cavernous sinus, superior petrosal sinus, and transverse sinus. The *superior cerebral veins* drain into the superior sagittal sinus.

Deep cerebral veins (central veins). The *internal cerebral vein* arises bilaterally at the level of the interventricular foramen (of Monro). It traverses the transverse cerebral fissure to a point just inferior to the splenium of the corpus callosum. The *venous angle* at its junction with the superior thalamostriate vein can be seen in a laterally projected angiogram. The two internal cerebral veins join under the splenium to form the *great cerebral vein* (of Galen), which receives the basal vein (of Rosenthal) and then empties into the straight sinus at the anterior tentorial edge at the level of the quadrigeminal plate. The basal vein of Rosenthal is formed by the union of the anterior cerebral vein, the deep middle cerebral vein, and the striate veins. It passes posteromedial to the optic tract, curves around the cerebral peduncle, and empties into the internal vein or the great cerebral vein posterior to the brain stem.

Posterior fossa. The anterior, middle, and posterior veins of the posterior fossa drain into the great cerebral vein, the petrosal vein, and the tentorial and straight sinuses, respectively.

Extracerebral Veins

The extracerebral veins—most prominently, the dural venous sinuses—drain venous blood from the brain into the sigmoid sinuses and jugular veins.

The *diploic veins* drain into the extracranial veins of the scalp and the intracranial veins (dural venous sinuses).

The *emissary veins* connect the sinuses, diploic veins, and superficial veins of the skull. Infections sometimes travel along the emissary veins from the extracranial to the intracranial compartment.

The veins of the brain empty into the superior and inferior groups of dural venous sinuses. The sinuses of the superior group (the superior and inferior sagittal, straight, and occipital sinuses) join at the confluence of the sinuses (*torcular Herophili*), which drains into both transverse sinuses and thence into the sigmoid sinuses and internal jugular veins. The sinuses of the inferior group (superior and inferior petrosal sinuses) join at the cavernous sinus, which drains into the sigmoid sinus and internal jugular vein via the inferior petrosal sinus, or into the internal vertebral plexus via the basilar plexus.

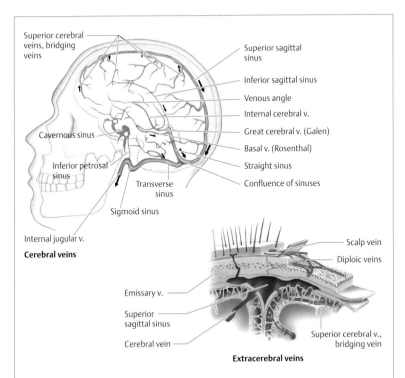

Superior cerebral veins, bridging veins

Superior sagittal sinus

Inferior sagittal sinus

Venous angle

Internal cerebral v.

Cavernous sinus

Great cerebral v. (Galen)

Basal v. (Rosenthal)

Inferior petrosal sinus

Straight sinus

Confluence of sinuses

Transverse sinus

Sigmoid sinus

Internal jugular v.

Cerebral veins

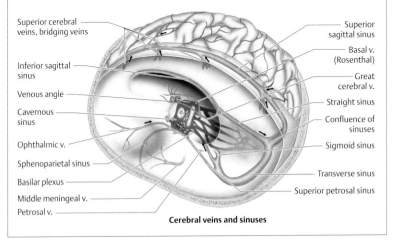

Scalp vein

Diploic veins

Emissary v.

Superior sagittal sinus

Cerebral vein

Superior cerebral v., bridging vein

Extracerebral veins

Superior cerebral veins, bridging veins

Superior sagittal sinus

Basal v. (Rosenthal)

Inferior sagittal sinus

Great cerebral v.

Venous angle

Straight sinus

Cavernous sinus

Confluence of sinuses

Ophthalmic v.

Sigmoid sinus

Sphenoparietal sinus

Transverse sinus

Basilar plexus

Superior petrosal sinus

Middle meningeal v.

Petrosal v.

Cerebral veins and sinuses

Cerebral Circulation

19

Craniocervical Veins

Anastomotic channels connect the cutaneous veins of the two sides of the head. Venous blood from the facial, temporal, and frontal regions drains into the facial and retromandibular veins and thence into the internal jugular vein. Some blood from the forehead drains via the naso-frontal, angular, and superior ophthalmic veins into the cavernous sinus. The occipital vein carries blood from the posterior portion of the scalp into the deep cervical vein and thence into the external jugular vein. Blood from the jugular veins continues to the brachiocephalic vein, superior vena cava, and right atrium. The venous channels in the spinal canal and the transcranial emissary veins play no more than a minor role in venous drainage. The pterygoid plexus links the cavernous sinus, the facial vein, and the internal jugular vein.

The numerous anastomoses between the extracranial and intracranial venous systems provide a pathway for the spread of infection from the scalp or face to the intracranial compartment. For example, periorbital infection may extend inward and produce septic thrombosis of the cavernous sinus.

Cranial Veins

The *facial vein* drains the venous blood from the face and anterior portion of the scalp. It begins at the inner canthus as the angular vein and communicates with the cavernous sinus via the superior ophthalmic vein. Below the angle of the mandible, it merges with the retromandibular vein and branches of the superior thyroid and superior laryngeal veins. It then drains into the internal jugular vein in the carotid triangle. The veins of the temporal region, external ear, temporomandibular joint, and lateral aspect of the face join in front of the ear to form the *retromandibular vein*, which either joins the facial vein or drains directly into the internal jugular vein. Its upper portion gives off a prominent dorsocaudal branch that joins the posterior auricular vein over the sternocleidomastoid muscle to communicate with the external jugular vein. Venous blood from the posterior portion of the scalp and the mastoid and occipital emissary veins drains into the *occipital vein*, which anastomoses with the occipital venous plexus and finally drains into the external jugular vein.

The *pterygoid plexus* lies between the temporalis, medial pterygoid, and lateral pterygoid muscles and receives blood from deep portions of the face, the external ear, the parotid gland, and the cavernous sinus, which it carries by way of the maxillary and retromandibular veins to the internal jugular vein.

Cervical Veins

The *deep cervical vein* originates from the occipital vein and suboccipital plexus. It follows the course of the deep cervical artery and vertebral artery to arrive at the brachiocephalic vein, which it joins.

The *vertebral vein*, which also originates from the occipital vein and suboccipital plexus, envelops the vertebral artery like a net and accompanies it through the foramina transversaria of the cervical vertebrae, collecting blood along the way from the cervical spinal cord, meninges, and deep neck muscles through the vertebral venous plexus, and finally joining the brachio-cephalic vein.

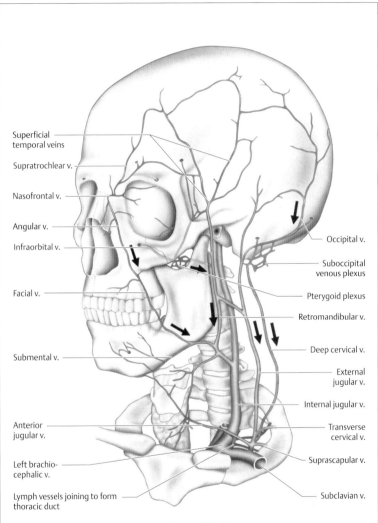

Superficial temporal veins

Supratrochlear v.

Nasofrontal v.

Angular v.

Infraorbital v.

Facial v.

Submental v.

Anterior jugular v.

Left brachio-cephalic v.

Lymph vessels joining to form thoracic duct

Occipital v.

Suboccipital venous plexus

Pterygoid plexus

Retromandibular v.

Deep cervical v.

External jugular v.

Internal jugular v.

Transverse cervical v.

Suprascapular v.

Subclavian v.

Extracranial veins

Arteries

Most of the blood supply of the spinal cord is supplied by the segmental spinal arteries, while relatively little comes from the vertebral arteries via the anterior and posterior spinal arteries. The segmental and spinal arteries are linked by numerous anastomoses.

Segmental arteries. The vertebral, ascending cervical, and deep cervical arteries give off cervical segmental branches; the thoracic and abdominal aorta give off thoracolumbar segmental branches via the posterior intercostal and lumbar arteries.

The segmental arteries give off radicular branches that enter the intervertebral foramen and supply the anterior and posterior roots and spinal ganglion of the corresponding level. The spinal cord itself is supplied by unpaired medullary arteries that originate from segmental arteries. The anatomy of these medullary arteries is variable; they usually have 5 to 8 larger ventral and dorsal branches that join up with the anterior and posterior spinal arteries. Often there is a single large radicular branch on one side, the *great radicular artery* (of Adamkiewicz), that supplies the entire lower two-thirds of the spinal cord. It usually enters the spinal canal in the lower thoracic region on the left side.

Spinal arteries. The spinal arteries run longitudinally down the spinal cord and arise from the vertebral artery (p. 14). The unpaired *anterior spinal artery* lies in the anterior median fissure of the spinal cord and supplies blood to the anterior two-thirds of the cord. The artery's diameter steadily increases below the T2 level. The two *posterior spinal arteries* supply the dorsal columns and all but the base of the dorsal horns bilaterally. Numerous anastomoses of the spinal arteries produce a *vasocorona* around the spinal cord. The depth of the spinal cord is supplied by these arteries penetrating it from its outer surface and by branches of the anterior spinal artery penetrating it from the anterior median fissure (sulcocommissural arteries).

Spinal Veins

Blood from within the spinal cord travels through the intramedullary veins, whose anat-

omy is variable, to the *anterior and posterior spinal veins*, which form a reticulated network in the pia mater around the circumference of the cord and down its length. The anterior spinal vein drains the anterior two-thirds of the gray matter, while the posterior and lateral spinal veins drain the rest of the spinal cord. These vessels empty by way of the *radicular veins* into the *external and internal vertebral venous plexuses*, groups of valveless veins that extend from the coccyx to the base of the skull and communicate with the dural venous sinuses via the suboccipital veins. Venous blood from the *cervical spine* drains by way of the vertebral and deep cervical veins into the superior vena cava; from the *thoracic and lumbar spine*, by way of the posterior intercostal and lumbar veins into the azygos and hemiazygos veins; from the *sacrum*, by way of the median and lateral sacral veins into the common iliac vein.

Watershed Zones

Because blood can flow either upward or downward in the anterior and posterior spinal arteries, the tissue at greatest risk of hypoperfusion is that located at a border zone between the distributions of two adjacent supplying arteries ("watershed zone"). Such vulnerable zones are found in the cervical, upper thoracic, and lower thoracic regions (ca. C4, T3–T4, and T8–T9).

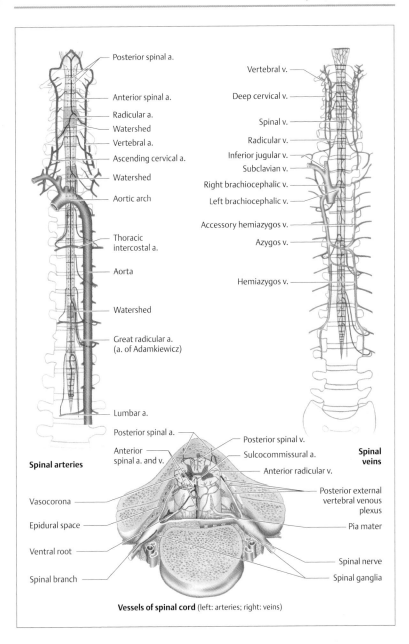

Posterior spinal a.

Anterior spinal a.

Radicular a.

Watershed

Vertebral a.

Ascending cervical a.

Watershed

Aortic arch

Thoracic intercostal a.

Aorta

Watershed

Great radicular a. (a. of Adamkiewicz)

Lumbar a.

Spinal arteries

Vertebral v.

Deep cervical v.

Spinal v.

Radicular v.

Inferior jugular v.

Subclavian v.

Right brachiocephalic v.

Left brachiocephalic v.

Accessory hemiazygos v.

Azygos v.

Hemiazygos v.

Posterior spinal a.

Anterior spinal a. and v.

Posterior spinal v.

Sulcocommissural a.

Anterior radicular v.

Spinal veins

Vasocorona

Epidural space

Ventral root

Spinal branch

Posterior external vertebral venous plexus

Pia mater

Spinal nerve

Spinal ganglia

Vessels of spinal cord (left: arteries; right: veins)

Cortical Structures

Different areas of the *cerebral cortex* (neocortex) may be distinguished from one another by their histological features and neuroanatomical connections. *Brodmann's* numbering scheme for cortical areas has been used for many years and will be introduced in this section.

Projection areas. By following the course of axons entering and leaving a given cortical area, one may determine the other structures to which it is connected by afferent and efferent pathways. The *primary projection areas* are those that receive most of their sensory impulses directly from the thalamic relay nuclei (primary somatosensory cortex, Brodman areas 1, 2, 3), the visual (area 17), or the auditory (areas 41, 42) pathways. The primary motor cortex (area 4) sends motor impulses directly down the pyramidal pathway to somatic motor neurons within brainstem and the spinal cord. The primary projection areas are somatotopically organized and serve the contralateral half of the body. Proceeding outward along the cortical surface from the primary projection areas, one encounters the *secondary projection areas* (motor, areas 6, 8, 44; sensory, areas 5, 7a, 40; visual, area 18; auditory, area 42), which subserve higher functions of coordination and information processing, and the *tertiary projection areas* (motor, areas 9, 10, 11; sensory, areas 7b, 39; visual, areas 19, 20, 21; auditory, area 22), which are responsible for complex functions such as voluntary movement, spatial organization of sensory input, cognition, memory, language, and emotion. The two hemispheres are connected by *commissural fibers*, which enable bihemispheric coordination of function. The most important commissural tract is the *corpus callosum*; because many tasks are performed primarily by one of the two hemispheres (cerebral dominance), interruption of the corpus callosum can produce various *disconnection syndromes*. Total callosal transection causes *split-brain syndrome*, in which the patient cannot name an object felt by the left hand when the eyes are closed, or one seen in the left visual hemifield (tactile and optic anomia), and cannot read words projected into the left visual hemifield (left hemialexia), write with the left hand (left hemiagraphia), or make pantomimic move-

ments with the left hand (left hemiapraxia). Anterior callosal lesions cause *alien hand syndrome* (diagonistic apraxia), in which the patient cannot coordinate the movements of the two hands. Disconnection syndromes are usually not seen in persons with congenital absence (agenesis) of the corpus callosum.

Cytoarchitecture. Most of the cerebral cortex consists of *isocortex*, which has six distinct cytoarchitectural layers. The Brodmann classification of cortical areas is based on distinguishing histological features of adjacent areas of isocortex.

Functional areas. The functional organization of the cerebral cortex can be studied with various techniques: direct electrical stimulation of the cortex during neurosurgical procedures, measurement of cortical electrical cortical activity (electroencephalography and evoked potentials), and measurement of regional cerebral blood flow and metabolic activity. Highly specialized areas for particular functions are found in many different parts of the brain. A lesion in one such area may produce a severe functional deficit, though partial or total recovery often occurs because adjacent uninjured areas may take over some of the function of the lost brain tissue. (The extent to which actual brain regeneration may aid functional recovery is currently unclear.) The specific anatomic patterns of functional localization in the brain are the key to understanding much of clinical neurology.

Subcortical Structures

The subcortical structures include the basal ganglia, thalamus, subthalamic nucleus, hypothalamus, red nucleus, substantia nigra, cerebellum, and brain stem, and their nerve pathways. These structures perform many different kinds of complex information processing and are anatomically and functionally interconnected with the cerebral cortex. Subcortical lesions may produce symptoms and signs resembling those of cortical lesions; special diagnostic studies may be needed for their precise localization.

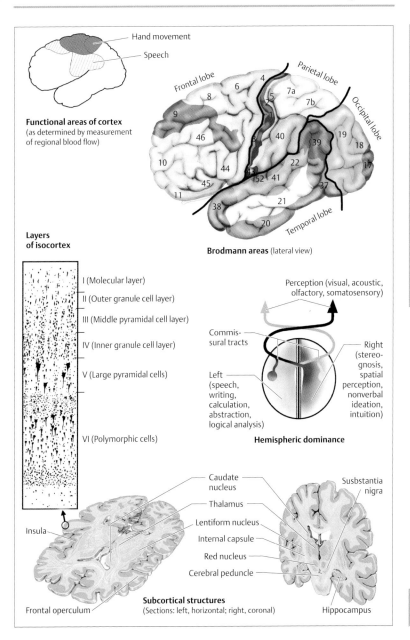

Hand movement
Speech

Functional areas of cortex
(as determined by measurement
of regional blood flow)

Frontal lobe
Parietal lobe
Occipital lobe
Temporal lobe

6 4
8 5 7a
9 7b
46 1
40 19
10 3 18
44 39 17
45 43 52 41 22 37
11 21
38 20

Brodmann areas (lateral view)

**Layers
of isocortex**

I (Molecular layer)
II (Outer granule cell layer)
III (Middle pyramidal cell layer)
IV (Inner granule cell layer)
V (Large pyramidal cells)
VI (Polymorphic cells)

Perception (visual, acoustic,
olfactory, somatosensory)

Commis-
sural tracts

Left
(speech,
writing,
calculation,
abstraction,
logical analysis)

Right
(stereo-
gnosis,
spatial
perception,
nonverbal
ideation,
intuition)

Hemispheric dominance

Caudate
nucleus
Thalamus
Lentiform nucleus
Internal capsule
Red nucleus
Cerebral peduncle

Susbstantia
nigra

Insula

Frontal operculum

Hippocampus

Subcortical structures
(Sections: left, horizontal; right, coronal)

The brain stem consists of the midbrain (mesencephalon), pons, and medulla. It contains the nuclei of the cranial nerves and ascending and descending tracts running to and from the brain, cerebellum, and spinal cord. It also contains autonomic centers that regulate cardiovascular function, breathing, and eating behavior as well as acoustic and vestibular relay nuclei. The flow of information along afferent and efferent pathways is regulated by reflex systems.

Nerve Pathways

All motor (p. 44) and sensory projection systems (p. 104) pass through the brain stem and communicate with its intrinsic structures at various sites. The central sympathetic pathway (p. 90) originates in the hypothalamus.

Reticular Formation

The reticular formation (RF) is a network of nuclei and interconnecting fibers that is anatomically intertwined with the cranial nerve nuclei and other fiber tracts of the brain stem. Different parts of the reticular formation perform different functions. The *reticular activating system* (RAS) provides the anatomical and physiological basis for wakeful consciousness (p. 116). The *medullary RF* contains the vital centers controlling the heartbeat, breathing, and circulation as well as reflex centers for swallowing and vomiting. The *pontine RF* contains centers for coordination of acoustic, vestibular, respiratory, and cardiovascular processes. The *midbrain RF* contains centers subserving visuospatial orientation and eating behavior (chewing, sucking, licking).

Reflex Systems (pp. 118ff)

Pupillary light reflex. The Edinger–Westphal nucleus in the midbrain, which is adjacent to the oculomotor nucleus, provides the efferent arm of the reflex loop (p. 90; examination, p. 92.)

Vestibulo-ocular reflex (VOR, p. 84). The vestibular nuclei receive their main input from the labyrinthine semicircular canals and collateral input from the cerebellar nuclei; their output is conveyed to the extraocular muscles through the medial longitudinal fasciculus, and to the spinal cord through the vestibulospinal tract. *Examination*: Suppression of visual fixation: the subject extends his arms and stares at his thumbs while spinning on a swivel chair. Nystagmus does not occur in normal subjects. *Oculocephalic reflex* (doll's eyes phenomenon): Horizontal or vertical passive rotation of the subject's head causes the eyes to rotate in the opposite direction; normally suppressible by awake persons, this reflex is seen in patients with impaired consciousness but preserved vestibular function. *Caloric testing*: The examiner first confirms that the patient's eardrums are intact, then instills cold water in the external auditory canal with the head elevated at a 30° angle (which inactivates the ipsilateral horizontal semicircular canal). This normally causes nystagmus in the contralateral direction, i.e., slow ipsilateral conjugate deviation of the eyes, followed by a quick jerk to the other side.

Corneal reflex. *Afferent arm*, CN V/1; *efferent arm*, CN VII, which innervates the orbicularis oculi muscle. *Examination*: Touching the cornea from the side while the subject looks forward evokes blinking. The reflex can also be assessed by electromyography (EMG).

Pharyngeal (gag) reflex. *Afferent arm*, mainly CN IX, X, and V/2; *efferent arm*, CN IX and X. The gag reflex may be absent in normal persons. *Examination*: Touching the soft palate or back of the pharynx evokes pharyngeal muscle contraction.

Cough reflex. *Afferent arm*, CN IX and X; *efferent arm*, via the solitary tract to the diaphragm and other participating muscle groups. *Examination*: Tested in intubated patients with endotracheal suction (tracheal reflex).

Masseter (jaw jerk) reflex. *Afferent arm*, probably CN V/3; *efferent arm*, CN V. *Examination*: Tapping the chin evokes jaw closure.

Acoustic reflex (p. 68). *Afferent arm*, projections of the cochlear nuclei to the RAS. *Examination*: Sudden, intense acoustic stimuli evoke a fright reaction including lid closure, startle, turning of the head, and increased alertness.

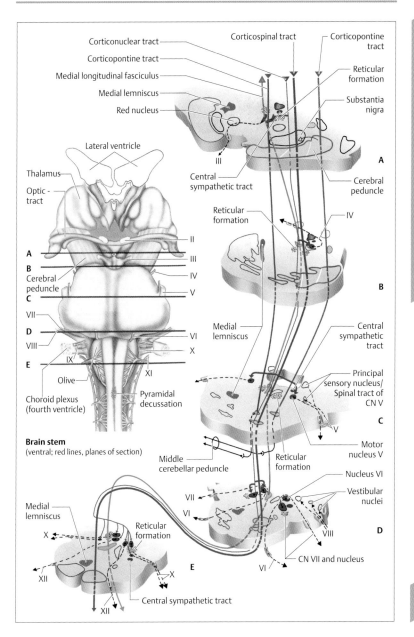

Corticonuclear tract
Corticopontine tract
Medial longitudinal fasciculus
Medial lemniscus
Red nucleus

Corticospinal tract
Corticopontine tract
Reticular formation
Substantia nigra

III
Central sympathetic tract
Cerebral peduncle

A

Lateral ventricle
Thalamus
Optic tract

II
A
III
B
IV
Cerebral peduncle
C
VII
D
VIII
E
IX
Olive
V
VI
X
XI

Choroid plexus (fourth ventricle)
Pyramidal decussation

Reticular formation
IV

B

Medial lemniscus
Central sympathetic tract

Principal sensory nucleus/ Spinal tract of CN V

V
Motor nucleus V

C

Brain stem
(ventral; red lines, planes of section)

Middle cerebellar peduncle
Reticular formation

Nucleus VI
Vestibular nuclei

VII
VI
VIII

Medial lemniscus
Reticular formation

CN VII and nucleus
VI

D

X
XII
X
XII
E
Central sympathetic tract

Cranial Nerve Pathways

Cranial Nerve	Origin/Course (see also pp. 70ff. and 74 ff)
I	Olfactory nerves ⇨ cribriform plate ⇨ olfactory bulb ⇨ olfactory tract ⇨ anterior perforated substance ⇨ lateral olfactory stria (⇨ parahippocampal gyrus) and medial olfactory stria (⇨ limbic system)
II	Retinal ganglion cells ⇨ optic disk ⇨ optic nerve ⇨ orbit ⇨ optic canal ⇨ optic chiasm ⇨ optic tract ⇨ lateral geniculate body (⇨ optic radiation ⇨ occipital lobe) and superior colliculi (⇨ pretectal area)
III	Midbrain ⇨ interpeduncular fossa ⇨ between superior cerebellar artery and posterior cerebral artery ⇨ tentorial edge ⇨ cavernous sinus ⇨ medial orbital fissure ⇨ oculomotor nerve, superior division (levator palpebrae and superior rectus muscles) and inferior division (medial and inferior rectus and inferior oblique muscles) or parasympathetic fibers ⇨ ciliary ganglion
IV	Midbrain ⇨ dorsal brainstem below the inferior colliculi ⇨ around the cerebral peduncle ⇨ lateral wall of the cavernous sinus ⇨ orbital fissure ⇨ superior oblique muscle
V	Pons ⇨ ca. 50 root filaments (sensory root = portio major; motor root = portio minor) ⇨ petrous apex ⇨ through the dura mater ⇨ trigeminal ganglion (V/1 ⇨ orbital fissure; V/2 ⇨ foramen rotundum, V/3 + portio minor ⇨ foramen ovale)
VI	Posterior margin of pons ⇨ up the clivus ⇨ through the dura mater ⇨ petrous apex ⇨ lateral to internal carotid artery in the cavernous sinus ⇨ orbital fissure ⇨ lateral rectus muscle
VII	Pons (cerebellopontine angle) above the olive ⇨ internal acoustic meatus ⇨ petrous pyramid (canal of facial nerve) ⇨ geniculum of facial nerve (⇨ nervus intermedius/greater petrosal nerve ⇨ gustatory fibers) ⇨ medial wall of the tympanic cavity ⇨ stylomastoid foramen ⇨ muscles of facial expression
VIII	Lateral to CN VII ⇨ vestibular nerve, cochlear nerve
IX	Medulla ⇨ jugular foramen ⇨ between carotid artery and internal jugular vein ⇨ root of the tongue
X	Posterolateral sulcus of medulla ⇨ jugular foramen ⇨ internal organs
XI	Cranial and spinal roots ⇨ trunk of accessory nerve ⇨ jugular foramen ⇨ muscles
XII	Medulla ⇨ hypoglossal canal ⇨ tongue muscles

CN = cranial nerve.

See Table 1, p. 356, for the functions of the cranial nerves.

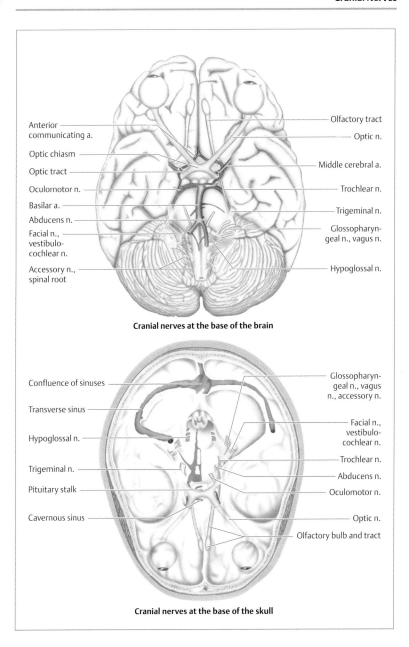

Anterior communicating a.

Optic chiasm

Optic tract

Oculomotor n.

Basilar a.

Abducens n.

Facial n., vestibulocochlear n.

Accessory n., spinal root

Olfactory tract

Optic n.

Middle cerebral a.

Trochlear n.

Trigeminal n.

Glossopharyngeal n., vagus n.

Hypoglossal n.

Cranial nerves at the base of the brain

Confluence of sinuses

Transverse sinus

Hypoglossal n.

Trigeminal n.

Pituitary stalk

Cavernous sinus

Glossopharyngeal n., vagus n., accessory n.

Facial n., vestibulocochlear n.

Trochlear n.

Abducens n.

Oculomotor n.

Optic n.

Olfactory bulb and tract

Cranial nerves at the base of the skull

Spine

The spine (vertebral column) bears the weight of the head, neck, trunk and upper extremities. Its flexibility is greatest in the cervical region, intermediate in the lumbar region, and lowest in the thoracic region. Its uppermost vertebrae (atlas and axis) articulate with the head, and its lowermost portion, the sacrum (which consists of 5 vertebrae fused together), articulates with the pelvis. There are 7 *cervical*, 12 *thoracic* (in British usage *dorsal*), and 5 *lumbar vertebrae*, making a total of 24 above the sacrum. Below the sacrum, the coccyx is composed of 3 to 6 *coccygeal vertebrae*.

Intervertebral Disks

Each pair of adjacent vertebrae is separated by an intervertebral disk. From the third decade of life onward, each disk progressively diminishes in water content, and therefore also in height. Its tensile, fibrous outer ring (*annulus fibrosus*) connects it with the vertebrae above and below and is held taut by the pressure in the central *nucleus pulposus*, which varies as a function of the momentary position of the body. The pressure that obtains in the sitting position is double the pressure when the patient stands, but that found in the recumbent position is only one-third as great. The interior of the disk has no nociceptive innervation, in contrast to the periosteum of the vertebral bodies, which is innervated by the meningeal branch of the segmental spinal nerve, as are the intervertebral joint capsules, the posterior longitudinal ligament, the dorsal portion of the annulus fibrosus, the dura mater, and the blood vessels.

Spinal Canal

The spinal canal is a tube formed by the *vertebral foramina* of the vertebral bodies stacked one on top of another; it is bounded anteriorly by the vertebral bodies and posteriorly by the vertebral arches (laminae). Its walls are reinforced by the intervertebral disks and the anterior and posterior longitudinal ligaments. It contains the spinal cord and its meninges, the surrounding fatty and connective tissues, blood vessels, and spinal nerve roots. Its normal sagittal diameter ranges

from 12 to 22 mm in the cervical region and from 22 to 25 mm in the lumbar region.

Spinal Cord

Like the brain, the spinal cord is intimately enveloped by the *pia mater*, which contains numerous nerves and blood vessels; the pia mater merges with the endoneurium of the spinal nerve rootlets and also continues below the spinal cord as the *filum terminale internum*. The weblike spinal *arachnoid membrane* contains only a few capillaries and no nerves. The *denticulate ligament* runs between the pia mater and the dura mater and anchors the spinal cord to the dura mater. In lumbar puncture, cerebrospinal fluid is withdrawn from the space between the arachnoid membrane and pia mater (*spinal subarachnoid space*), which communicates with the subarachnoid space of the brain. The spinal *dura mater* originates at the edge of the foramen magnum and descends from it to form a tubular covering around the spinal cord. Its lumen ends at the S1–S2 level, where it continues as the *filum terminale externum*, which attaches to the sacrum, thus anchoring the dura mater inferiorly. The dura mater forms sleeves around the anterior and posterior spinal nerve roots which continue distally, together with the arachnoid membrane, to form the epineurium and perineurium of the spinal nerves. Unlike the cranial dura mater, the spinal dura mater is not directly apposed to the periosteum of the surrounding bone (i.e., the vertebral canal) but is separated from it by the *epidural space*, which contains fat, loose connective tissue, and valveless venous plexuses (p. 22).

The *root filaments* (rootlets) that come together to form the ventral and dorsal spinal nerve roots are arranged in longitudinal rows on the lateral surface of the spinal cord on both sides. The *ventral root* carries only motor fibers, while the *dorsal root* carries only sensory fibers. (This so-called "law of Bell and Magendie" is actually not wholly true; the ventral root is now known to carry a small number of sensory fibers as well.) The cell bodies of the pseudounipolar sensory neurons are contained in the dorsal root ganglion, a swelling on the dorsal root just proximal to its junction with the ventral root to form the segmental spinal nerve.

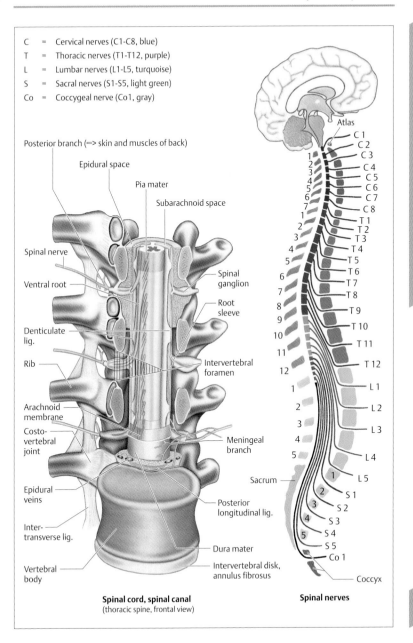

C = Cervical nerves (C1-C8, blue)
T = Thoracic nerves (T1-T12, purple)
L = Lumbar nerves (L1-L5, turquoise)
S = Sacral nerves (S1-S5, light green)
Co = Coccygeal nerve (Co1, gray)

Posterior branch (=> skin and muscles of back)

Epidural space

Pia mater

Subarachnoid space

Spinal nerve

Ventral root

Denticulate lig.

Rib

Arachnoid membrane

Costo-vertebral joint

Epidural veins

Inter-transverse lig.

Vertebral body

Spinal ganglion

Root sleeve

Intervertebral foramen

Meningeal branch

Posterior longitudinal lig.

Dura mater

Intervertebral disk, annulus fibrosus

Atlas

C 1
C 2
C 3
C 4
C 5
C 6
C 7
C 8
T 1
T 2
T 3
T 4
T 5
T 6
T 7
T 8
T 9
T 10
T 11
T 12
L 1
L 2
L 3
L 4
L 5
S 1
S 2
S 3
S 4
S 5
Co 1

Sacrum

Coccyx

Spinal cord, spinal canal
(thoracic spine, frontal view)

Spinal nerves

The precise region of impaired sensation to light touch and noxious stimuli is an important clue for the clinical localization of spinal cord and peripheral nerve lesions. Reflex abnormalities and autonomic dysfunction are further ones, as discussed below (p. 40, p. 110).

Dermatomes (pp. 34, 36)

A dermatome is defined as the cutaneous area whose sensory innervation is derived from a single spinal nerve (i.e., dorsal root). The division of the skin into dermatomes reflects the segmental organization of the spinal cord and its associated nerves. Pain dermatomes are narrower, and overlap with each other less, than touch dermatomes (p. 104); thus, the level of a spinal cord lesion causing sensory impairment is easier to determine by pinprick testing than by light touch. (The opposite is true of peripheral nerve lesions.) *Radicular pain* is pain in the distribution of a spinal nerve root, i.e., in a dermatome; *pseudoradicular pain* may occupy a bandlike area but cannot be assigned to any particular dermatome. Pseudoradicular pain can be caused by tendomyosis (pain in the muscles that move a particular joint), generalized tendomyopathy or fibromyalgia, facet syndrome (inflammation of the intervertebral joints), myelogelosis (persistent muscle spasm resulting from overexertion), and other conditions. For mnemonic purposes, it is useful to know that the C2 dermatome begins in front of the ear and ends at the occipital hairline; the T1 dermatome comes to the midline of the forearm; the T4 dermatome is at the level of the nipples (which, however, belong to T5); the T10 dermatome includes the navel; the L1 dermatome is in the groin; and the S1 dermatome is at the outer edge of the foot and heel.

Myotomes

A myotome is defined as the muscular distribution of a single spinal nerve (i.e., ventral root), and is thus the muscular analogue of a cutaneous dermatome. Many muscles are innervated by multiple spinal nerves; only in the paravertebral musculature of the back (erector spinae muscle) is the myotomal pattern clearly segmental (p. 31); the nerve supply here is

through the dorsal branches of the spinal nerves. Knowledge of the myotomes of each spinal nerve, and of the *segment-indicating muscles* (Table 2, p. 357) in particular, enables the clinical and electromyographic localization of radicular lesions causing motor dysfunction. The segment-indicating muscles are usually innervated by a single spinal nerve, or by two, though there is anatomic variation.

Plexuses (pp. 34, 36) and Peripheral Nerves (pp. 35, 37)

The ventral branches of spinal nerves supplying the limbs join together to form the cervical (C1–C4), brachial (C5–T1), lumbar (T12–L4), and sacral plexuses (L4–S4). The *brachial plexus* begins as three *trunks*, the upper (derived from the C5 and C6 roots), middle (C7), and lower (C8, T1). These trunks split into *divisions*, which recombine to form the lateral (C5–C7), posterior (C5–C8), and medial (C8 and T1) *cords* (named by their relation to the axillary artery). The cords of the brachial plexus branch into the nerves of the upper limb (p. 35). The nerves of the anterior portion of the lower limb are derived from the *lumbar plexus*, which lies behind and within the psoas major muscle (p. 37); those of the posterior portion of the lower limb from the *sacral plexus*. The coccygeal nerve (the last spinal nerve to emerge from the sacral hiatus) joins with the S3–S5 nerves to form the *coccygeal plexus*, which innervates the coccygeus and the skin over the coccyx and anus (mediates the pain of coccygodynia).

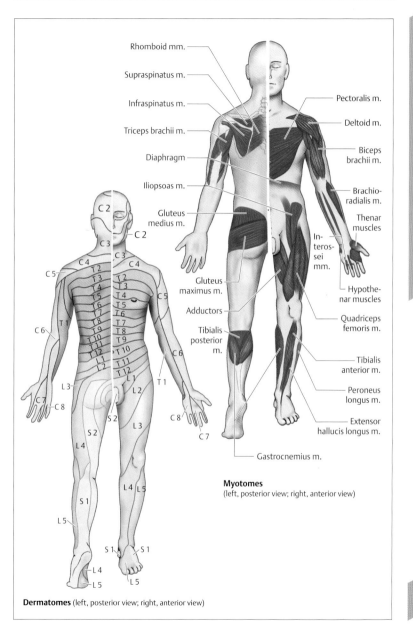

Rhomboid mm.

Supraspinatus m.

Infraspinatus m.

Triceps brachii m.

Diaphragm

Iliopsoas m.

Gluteus medius m.

Gluteus maximus m.

Adductors

Tibialis posterior m.

Pectoralis m.

Deltoid m.

Biceps brachii m.

Brachio-radialis m.

Thenar muscles

Interos-sei mm.

Hypothe-nar muscles

Quadriceps femoris m.

Tibialis anterior m.

Peroneus longus m.

Extensor hallucis longus m.

Gastrocnemius m.

C 2

C 2

C 3

C 3

C 4

C 4

C 5

C 5

C 6

C 6

C 7

C 7

C 8

C 8

T 1

T 1

T 2

T 3

T 4

T 5

T 6

T 7

T 8

T 9

T 10

T 11

T 12

T 2

T 3

T 4

T 5

T 6

T 7

T 8

T 9

T 10

T 11

T 12

L 1

L 2

L 3

L 2

L 3

L 4

L 4

L 5

L 5

S 1

S 1

S 1

S 1

S 2

S 2

L 4

L 5

Myotomes
(left, posterior view; right, anterior view)

Dermatomes (left, posterior view; right, anterior view)

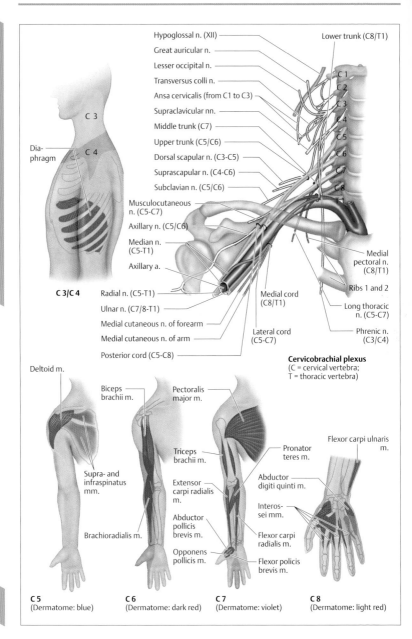

Hypoglossal n. (XII)
Great auricular n.
Lesser occipital n.
Transversus colli n.
Ansa cervicalis (from C1 to C3)
Supraclavicular nn.
Middle trunk (C7)
Upper trunk (C5/C6)
Dorsal scapular n. (C3-C5)
Suprascapular n. (C4-C6)
Subclavian n. (C5/C6)

Lower trunk (C8/T1)
C 1
C 2
C 3
C 4
C 5
C 6
C 7
C 8
T 1

C 3
C 4
Dia-
phragm

Musculocutaneous
n. (C5-C7)
Axillary n. (C5/C6)
Median n.
(C5-T1)
Axillary a.

Medial
pectoral n.
(C8/T1)
Ribs 1 and 2

C 3/C 4

Radial n. (C5-T1)
Ulnar n. (C7/8-T1)
Medial cutaneous n. of forearm
Medial cutaneous n. of arm
Posterior cord (C5-C8)

Medial cord
(C8/T1)

Lateral cord
(C5-C7)

Long thoracic
n. (C5-C7)
Phrenic n.
(C3/C4)

Cervicobrachial plexus
(C = cervical vertebra;
T = thoracic vertebra)

Deltoid m.

Biceps
brachii m.
Pectoralis
major m.

Triceps
brachii m.

Extensor
carpi radialis
m.

Abductor
pollicis m.

Brachioradialis m.

Supra- and
infraspinatus
mm.

Opponens
pollicis m.

Pronator
teres m.

Abductor
digiti quinti m.

Interos-
sei mm.

Flexor carpi
radialis m.

Flexor policis
brevis m.

Flexor carpi ulnaris
m.

C 5
(Dermatome: blue)

C 6
(Dermatome: dark red)

C 7
(Dermatome: violet)

C 8
(Dermatome: light red)

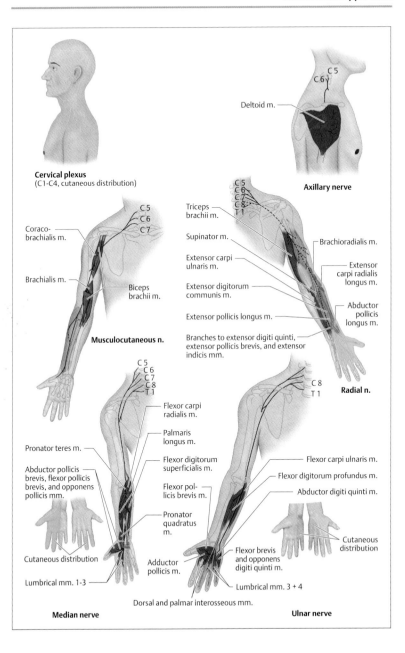

Cervical plexus
(C1–C4, cutaneous distribution)

Deltoid m.

C 5
C 6

Axillary nerve

Coraco-
brachialis m.

C 5
C 6
C 7

Brachialis m.

Biceps
brachii m.

Musculocutaneous n.

Triceps
brachii m.

C 5
C 6
C 7
C 8
T 1

Supinator m.

Extensor carpi
ulnaris m.

Extensor digitorum
communis m.

Extensor pollicis longus m.

Branches to extensor digiti quinti,
extensor pollicis brevis, and extensor
indicis mm.

Brachioradialis m.

Extensor
carpi radialis
longus m.

Abductor
pollicis
longus m.

C 8
T 1

Radial n.

C 5
C 6
C 7
C 8
T 1

Flexor carpi
radialis m.

Palmaris
longus m.

Flexor digitorum
superficialis m.

Flexor pol-
licis brevis m.

Pronator
quadratus
m.

Pronator teres m.

Abductor pollicis
brevis, flexor pollicis
brevis, and opponens
pollicis mm.

Cutaneous distribution

Lumbrical mm. 1–3

Adductor
pollicis m.

Flexor carpi ulnaris m.

Flexor digitorum profundus m.

Abductor digiti quinti m.

Flexor brevis
and opponens
digiti quinti m.

Lumbrical mm. 3 + 4

Dorsal and palmar interosseous mm.

Cutaneous
distribution

Median nerve

Ulnar nerve

Peripheral Nervous System

35

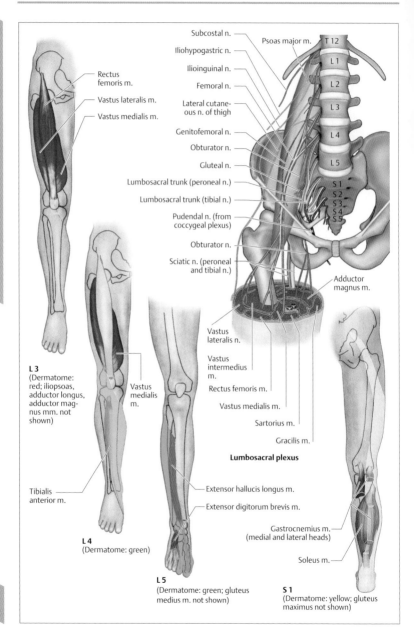

Rectus femoris m.

Vastus lateralis m.

Vastus medialis m.

Subcostal n.

Psoas major m.

T 12

Iliohypogastric n.

Ilioinguinal n.

L 1

Femoral n.

L 2

Lateral cutaneous n. of thigh

L 3

Genitofemoral n.

L 4

Obturator n.

L 5

Gluteal n.

Lumbosacral trunk (peroneal n.)

S 1
S 2
S 3
S 4
S 5

Lumbosacral trunk (tibial n.)

Pudendal n. (from coccygeal plexus)

Obturator n.

Sciatic n. (peroneal and tibial n.)

Adductor magnus m.

Vastus lateralis n.

Vastus intermedius m.

Rectus femoris m.

Vastus medialis m.

Sartorius m.

Gracilis m.

Lumbosacral plexus

L 3
(Dermatome: red; iliopsoas, adductor longus, adductor magnus mm. not shown)

Vastus medialis m.

Extensor hallucis longus m.

Extensor digitorum brevis m.

Gastrocnemius m. (medial and lateral heads)

Soleus m.

Tibialis anterior m.

L 4
(Dermatome: green)

L 5
(Dermatome: green; gluteus medius m. not shown)

S 1
(Dermatome: yellow; gluteus maximus not shown)

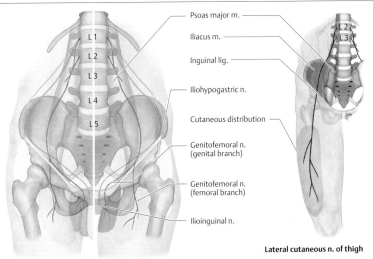

Psoas major m.

Iliacus m.

Inguinal lig.

Iliohypogastric n.

Cutaneous distribution

Genitofemoral n.
(genital branch)

Genitofemoral n.
(femoral branch)

Ilioinguinal n.

L 1
L 2
L 3
L 4
L 5

L 2
L 3

Lateral cutaneous n. of thigh

Cutaneous innervation of the groin
(left, in men; right, in women)

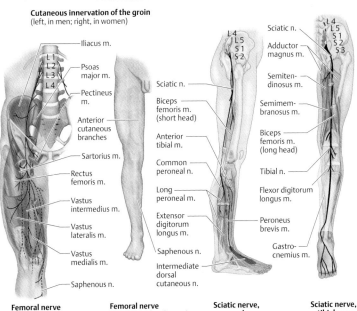

Iliacus m.

Psoas
major m.

Pectineus
m.

Anterior
cutaneous
branches

Sartorius m.

Rectus
femoris m.

Vastus
intermedius m.

Vastus
lateralis m.

Vastus
medialis m.

Saphenous n.

L 1
L 2
L 3
L 4

Sciatic n.

Biceps
femoris m.
(short head)

Anterior
tibial m.

Common
peroneal n.

Long
peroneal m.

Extensor
digitorum
longus m.

Saphenous n.

Intermediate
dorsal
cutaneous n.

L 4
L 5
S 1
S 2

Sciatic n.

Adductor
magnus m.

Semiten-
dinosus m.

Semimem-
branosus m.

Biceps
femoris m.
(long head)

Tibial n.

Flexor digitorum
longus m.

Peroneus
brevis m.

Gastro-
cnemius m.

L 4
L 5
S 1
S 2
S 3

Femoral nerve

Femoral nerve
(cutaneous distribution)

**Sciatic nerve,
peroneal nerve**
(purple: cutaneous
distribution)

**Sciatic nerve,
tibial nerve**
(purple: cutaneous
distribution)

Peripheral Nervous System

37

Normal and Abnormal Function of the Nervous System

2

- Neural Pathways

- Pathophysiology

- Major Syndromes

Reflexes are involuntary and relatively stereo-typed responses to specific stimuli. Afferent nerve fibers conduct the impulses generated by activated receptors to neurons in the central nervous system, which fire impulses that are then transmitted through efferent nerve fibers to the cells, muscles, or organs that carry out the *reflex response*. The pathway as a whole is known as the *reflex arc*. Receptors are found at the origin of all sensory pathways—in the skin, mucous membranes, muscles, tendons, and periosteum, as well as in the retina, inner ear, olfactory mucosa, and taste buds. A reflex response may involve the somatic musculature or the internal organs. Most reflexes are relatively independent of the state of consciousness. An interruption of the reflex arc at any point weakens or abolishes the reflex. *Intrinsic reflexes* are those whose receptors and effectors are located in the same organ (e. g., the quadriceps reflex), while the receptors and effectors of *extrinsic reflexes* are in different organs (e. g., the oculovestibular reflex). Reflexes are important for normal function (e. g., for postural control and goal-directed movement), and an impaired reflex is an important objective finding in clinical neurological examination.

Intrinsic Muscle Reflexes (Phasic Stretch Reflexes, Tendon Reflexes)

Intrinsic muscle reflexes are triggered by stretch receptors within the muscle (annulospiral nerve endings of muscle spindles). The impulses generated at the receptors are conveyed via afferent fast-twitch Ia fibers to spinal alpha-motor neurons, whose efferent α_1 processes excite the agonistic muscle of an opposing muscle pair. The antagonistic muscle is simultaneously inhibited by spinal interneurons. The resulting muscle contraction relaxes the muscle spindles, thereby stopping impulse generation at the stretch receptors. The spinal reflex arc is also under the influence of higher motor centers.

Abnormal reflex responses imply an abnormality of the musculature, the reflex arc, or higher motor centers. The most important reflexes in clinical diagnosis are the biceps (C5–C6), brachioradialis (C5–C6), triceps (C7–C8), adductor (L2–L4), quadriceps (L2/3–L4), posterior tibial (L5), and Achilles (S1–S2) reflexes.

Extrinsic Reflexes

Intrinsic muscle reflexes, discussed above, are monosynaptic, but extrinsic reflexes are polysynaptic: between their afferent and efferent arms lies a chain of spinal interneurons. They may be activated by stimuli of various types, e. g., muscle stretch, touch on the skin (abdominal reflex) or cornea (corneal reflex), mucosal irritation (sneezing), light (eye closure in response to a bright flash), or sound (acoustic reflex). The intensity of the response diminishes if the stimulus is repeated (habituation). Because they are polysynaptic, extrinsic reflexes have a longer latency (stimulus-to-response interval) than intrinsic reflexes. Some important extrinsic reflexes for normal function are the postural and righting reflexes, feeding reflexes (sucking, swallowing, licking), and autonomic reflexes (p. 110).

The *flexor reflex* is triggered by noxious stimulation, e. g., from stepping on a tack. Excitatory interneurons activate spinal cord alpha-motor neurons, which, in turn, excite ipsilateral flexor muscles and simultaneously inhibit ipsilateral extensor muscles via inhibitory interneurons. Meanwhile, the contralateral extensors contract, and the contralateral flexors relax. The response does not depend on pain, which is felt only when sensory areas in the brain have been activated, by which time the motor response has already occurred. This spinal reflex arc, like that of the intrinsic muscle reflexes, is under the influence of higher motor centers.

Abnormalities of the extrinsic reflexes imply an interruption of the reflex arc or of the corticospinal tracts (which convey impulses from higher motor centers). Some clinically important extrinsic reflexes are the abdominal (T6–T12), cremasteric (L1–L2), bulbocavernosus (S3–S4), and anal wink (S3–S5) reflexes.

Reflexes that can be elicited only in the diseased state are called *pathological reflexes*. Pathological reflexes indicating dysfunction of the pyramidal (corticospinal) tract include the Babinski sign (tonic dorsiflexion of the great toe on stimulation of the lateral sole of the foot), the Gordon reflex (same response to squeezing of the calf muscles), and the Oppenheim reflex (same response to a downward stroke of the examiner's thumb on the patient's shin).

Reflex response	Symbol
Absent, cannot be elicited by maneuvers	0
Can only be elicited by maneuvers (e.g., Jendrassik maneuver)	+ −
Diminished	1
Normal intensity	2
Heightened	3
Persistent clonus	4

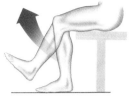

Reflex response
(Proprioceptive muscle reflex)

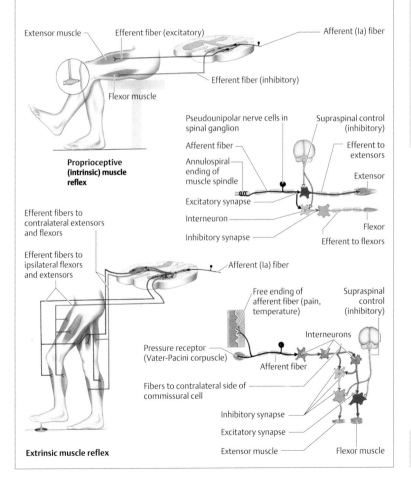

Extensor muscle — Efferent fiber (excitatory) — Afferent (Ia) fiber

Efferent fiber (inhibitory)

Flexor muscle

Proprioceptive (intrinsic) muscle reflex

Pseudounipolar nerve cells in spinal ganglion — Supraspinal control (inhibitory)

Afferent fiber — Efferent to extensors

Annulospiral ending of muscle spindle — Extensor

Excitatory synapse

Interneuron — Flexor

Inhibitory synapse — Efferent to flexors

Efferent fibers to contralateral extensors and flexors

Efferent fibers to ipsilateral flexors and extensors

Afferent (Ia) fiber

Free ending of afferent fiber (pain, temperature) — Supraspinal control (inhibitory)

Interneurons

Pressure receptor (Vater-Pacini corpuscle)

Afferent fiber

Fibers to contralateral side of commissural cell

Inhibitory synapse

Excitatory synapse

Extensor muscle — Flexor muscle

Extrinsic muscle reflex

Motor Function

41

The motor system controls the timing, direction, amplitude, and force of movement through the coordinated opposing actions of agonist and antagonist muscles. It also keeps the body in a stable position through postural and righting reflexes. *Reflex movements* are involuntary, stereotyped responses to stimuli. *Rhythmic movements* have both reflex and voluntary components. *Voluntary movements* are performed at will.

Reflex Movements

Withdrawing a foot from a noxious stimulus or spreading the arms when falling are examples of reflex movements. *Intrinsic muscle reflexes* regulate muscle tone and elasticity and are important for postural control and coordination of muscle groups. Specific functions such as joint stabilization or adjustment of contraction strength are achieved with the aid of inhibitory spinal interneurons. *Extrinsic reflexes* include protective reflexes (flexor response to noxious stimulus, corneal reflex) and postural reflexes (extensor reflex, neck reflex).

Rhythmic Movements

Walking, breathing, and riding a bicycle are rhythmic movements. They are subserved both by spinal reflex arcs and by supraspinal influence from the brain stem, cerebellum, basal ganglia, and motor cortex.

Voluntary Movements

Voluntary movements depend on a sequence of contractions of numerous different muscles that is planned to achieve a desired result (motor program). Hence different parts of the body are able to carry out similar movements *(motor equivalence)* more or less skillfully, e. g., simultaneous rotation of the big toe, foot, lower leg, leg, pelvis and trunk. Voluntary movements incorporate elements of the basic reflex and rhythmic movement patterns; their smooth execution depends on afferent feedback from the visual, vestibular, and proprioceptive systems to motor centers in the spinal cord, brain stem, and cerebral cortex. Further modulation of voluntary movements is provided by the cerebellum and basal ganglia, whose neural output reaches the cortex through thalamic relay nuclei. Fine motor control thus depends on the continuous interaction of multiple centers responsible for the planning (efferent copy) and execution of movement.

Motor cortex (p. 25). Voluntary movements are planned in the motor areas of the cerebral cortex. The *primary motor area* (area 4) regulates the force of muscle contraction and the goal-oriented direction of movement; it mainly controls distal muscle groups. The *supplementary motor area* (medial area 6) plays an important role in complex motor planning. The *premotor area* (lateral area 6) receives nerve impulses from the posterior parietal cortex and is concerned with the visual and somatosensory control of movement; it mainly controls trunk and proximal limb movement.

Cerebellum (p. 54). The cerebellum coordinates limb and eye movements and plays an important role in the maintenance of balance and the regulation of muscle tone.

Basal ganglia (p. 210). The basal ganglia have a close anatomic and functional connection to the motor cortex and participate in the coordination of limb and eye movement.

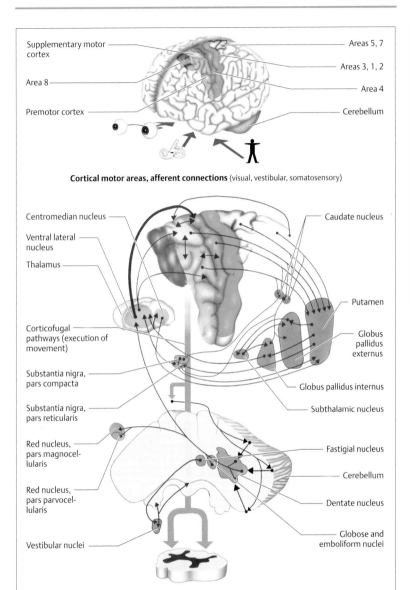

Cortical motor areas, afferent connections (visual, vestibular, somatosensory)

Supplementary motor cortex

Area 8

Premotor cortex

Areas 5, 7

Areas 3, 1, 2

Area 4

Cerebellum

Centromedian nucleus

Ventral lateral nucleus

Thalamus

Corticofugal pathways (execution of movement)

Substantia nigra, pars compacta

Substantia nigra, pars reticularis

Red nucleus, pars magnocellularis

Red nucleus, pars parvocellularis

Vestibular nuclei

Caudate nucleus

Putamen

Globus pallidus externus

Globus pallidus internus

Subthalamic nucleus

Fastigial nucleus

Cerebellum

Dentate nucleus

Globose and emboliform nuclei

Motor pathways
(cortex, basal ganglia, thalamus, brain stem, cerebellum, spinal cord)

Motor Function

43

Pyramidal Tract

Each fiber of the pyramidal tract originates in the *first* or *upper motor neuron*, whose cell body is located in the primary motor area (area 4), primary sensory areas (areas 1–3), the supplementary motor area, or the premotor area (area 6). The fibers descend through the posterior portion of the internal capsule through the cerebral peduncle, pons, and medulla, forming a small bulge (pyramid) on the anterior surface of the medulla. Most of the fibers cross the midline in the decussation of the pyramids and then descend through the spinal cord in the *lateral corticospinal tract*. Among the minority of fibers that do not cross in the pyramidal decussation, most continue in the ipsilateral *anterior corticospinal tract*, crossing the midline in the anterior spinal commissure only once they reach the level of their target motor neurons. The pyramidal tract mainly innervates distal muscle groups in the limbs. In the brain stem, the pyramidal tract gives off fibers to the motor nuclei of the cranial nerves (*corticopontine and corticobulbar tracts*). Fibers from the frontal eye fields (area 8) reach the nuclei subserving eye movement (cranial nerves III, IV, VI) through the pyramidal tract. The motor nuclei of cranial nerves III, IV, VI, and VII (lower two-thirds of the face) are innervated only by the contralateral cerebral cortex; thus, unilateral interruption of the pyramidal tract causes contralateral paralysis of the corresponding muscles. In contrast, the motor nuclei of cranial nerves V (portio minor), VII (frontal branch only), IX, X, XI, and XII receive bilateral cortical innervation, so that unilateral interruption of the pyramidal tract causes no paralysis of the corresponding muscles.

Nonpyramidal Motor Tracts

Other motor tracts lead from the cerebral cortex via the pons to the cerebellum, and from the cerebral cortex to the striatum (caudate nucleus and putamen), thalamus, substantia nigra, red nucleus, and brain stem reticular formation. These fiber pathways are adjacent to the pyramidal tract. Fibers arising from the premotor and supplementary motor areas (p. 43) project ipsilaterally and contralaterally to innervate the muscles of the trunk and proximal portions of the limbs that maintain the erect body posture. Because of the bilateral innervation, paresis due to interruption of these pathways recovers more readily than distal paresis due to a pyramidal lesion. Lesions of the pyramidal tract usually involve the adjacent nonpyramidal tracts as well and cause spastic paralysis; the rare isolated pyramidal lesions cause flaccid paralysis (p. 46).

Corticopontine fibers. Corticopontine fibers originate in the frontal, temporal, parietal, and occipital cortex and descend in the internal capsule near the pyramidal tract. The pontine nuclei project to the cerebellum (p. 54).

Other functionally important tracts. The *rubrospinal tract* originates in the red nucleus, decussates immediately, forms synapses with interneurons in the brain stem, and descends in the spinal cord to terminate in the anterior horn. Rubrospinal impulses activate flexors and inhibit extensors, as do impulses conducted in the medullary portion of the *reticulospinal tract*. On the other hand, impulses conducted in the pontine portion of the *reticulospinal tract* and in the *vestibulospinal tract* activate extensors and inhibit flexors.

Motor Unit

A motor unit is the functional unit consisting of a motor neuron and the muscle fibers innervated by it. The motor neurons are located in the brain stem (motor nuclei of cranial nerves) and spinal cord (anterior horn). The *innervation ratio* is the mean number of muscle fibers innervated by a single motor neuron. The action potentials arising from the cell body of a motor neuron are relayed along its axon to the neuromuscular synapses (motor end plates) of the muscle fibers. The force of muscle contraction depends on the number of motor units activated and on the frequency of action potentials. Innervation ratios vary from 3 for the extraocular muscles and 100 for the small muscles of the hand to 2000 for the gastrocnemius. The smaller the innervation ratio, the finer the gradation of force. The muscle fibers of a motor unit do not lie side by side but are distributed over a region of muscle with a cross-sectional diameter of 5–11 mm.

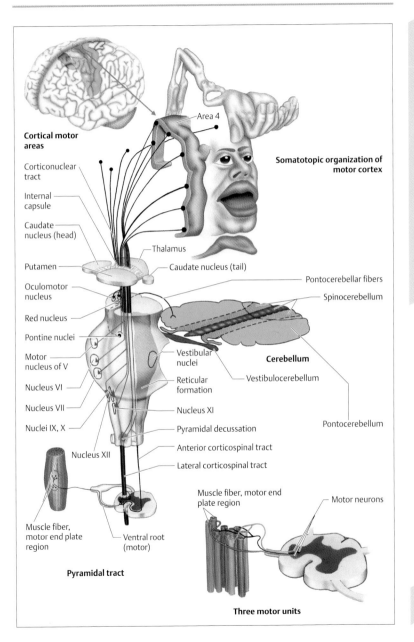

Cortical motor areas

Corticonuclear tract

Internal capsule

Caudate nucleus (head)

Putamen

Oculomotor nucleus

Red nucleus

Pontine nuclei

Motor nucleus of V

Nucleus VI

Nucleus VII

Nuclei IX, X

Nucleus XII

Muscle fiber, motor end plate region

Area 4

Somatotopic organization of motor cortex

Thalamus

Caudate nucleus (tail)

Pontocerebellar fibers

Spinocerebellum

Vestibular nuclei

Cerebellum

Vestibulocerebellum

Reticular formation

Nucleus XI

Pontocerebellum

Pyramidal decussation

Anterior corticospinal tract

Lateral corticospinal tract

Muscle fiber, motor end plate region

Motor neurons

Ventral root (motor)

Pyramidal tract

Three motor units

Motor Function

Paralysis Due to Upper Motor Neuron (UMN) Lesions

The clinical features of paralysis due to lesions of the pyramidal tract (upper motor neuron = UMN) depends on the anatomic site(s) of involvement of other efferent or afferent tracts and nuclei.

Impairment of fine motor function. Voluntary movement of paretic limbs requires greater effort than normal and causes greater muscular fatigue. Moreover, rapid alternating movements are slowed by hypertonia in the opposing agonist and antagonist muscles of paretic limbs. There may be *synkinesia* (involuntary movement of paretic limbs associated with other movements, e. g., yawning), undifferentiated accessory movements (*mass movements*), or *spinal automatisms* (involuntary movements triggered by somatosensory stimuli).

Paralysis. Paralysis of UMN type affects multiple (but not all) muscle groups on one side of the body. Bilaterally innervated movements (e. g., of eyes, jaw, pharynx, neck; see p. 44) may be only mildly paretic, or not at all. Paralysis that is initially total usually improves with time, but recovery may be accompanied by other motor disturbances such as tremor, hemiataxia, hemichorea, and hemiballism. Fine motor control is usually more severely impaired than strength. Neurogenic muscular atrophy does not occur in paralysis of UMN type.

Spasticity. The defining feature of spasticity is a velocity-dependent increase of muscle tone in response to passive stretch. Spasticity is usually, but not always, accompanied by hypertonia. The "clasp-knife phenomenon" (sudden slackening of muscle tone on rapid passive extension) is rare. Spasticity mainly affects the antigravity muscles (arm flexors and leg extensors).

Reflex abnormalities. The intrinsic muscle reflexes are enhanced (enlargement of reflex zones, clonus) and the extrinsic reflexes are diminished or absent. Pathological reflexes such as the Babinski reflex can be elicited.

■ Cerebral lesions

Monoparesis. Isolated lesions of the primary motor cortex (area 4) cause flaccid weakness of the contralateral face, hand, or leg. Lesions affecting adjacent precentral or postcentral areas, or areas deep to the cortex, cause spasticity and possibly an associated sensory deficit. It may be difficult to determine by examination alone whether monoparesis is of upper or lower motor neuron type (p. 50). Accessory movements of antagonistic muscles are present only in paralysis of UMN type.

Contralateral hemiparesis. Lesions of the internal capsule cause spastic hemiparesis. Involvement of corticopontine fibers causes (central) facial paresis, and impairment of corticobulbar fibers causes dysphonia and dysphagia. Sensory disturbances are also usually present. Unilateral lesions in the rostral brain stem cause contralateral spastic hemiparesis and ipsilateral nuclear oculomotor nerve palsy (*crossed paralysis*). For other syndromes caused by brain stem lesions, see p. 70 ff. A rare isolated lesion of the *medullary pyramid* (p. 74) can cause contralateral flaccid hemiplegia without facial paralysis, or (at mid-decussational level) contralateral arm paresis and ipsilateral leg paresis (*Hemiplegia alternans*).

Ipsilateral paresis. Lesions of the lower medulla below the pyramidal decussation (p. 74) cause ipsilateral paralysis and spasticity (as do lesions of the lateral corticospinal tract; see p. 45).

Quadriparesis. *Decortication syndrome* (p. 118) is caused by extensive bilateral lesions involving both the cerebral cortex and the underlying white matter, possibly extending into the diencephalon; midbrain involvement produces the *decerebration syndrome*. Involvement of the pons or medulla causes an initial quadriplegia; in the later course of illness, spinal automatisms may be seen in response to noxious stimuli.

Paraparesis. In rare cases, UMN-type paralysis of both lower limbs accompanied by bladder dysfunction is caused by bilateral, paramedian, precentral cortical lesions (*parasagittal cortical syndrome*). Focal seizures may occur.

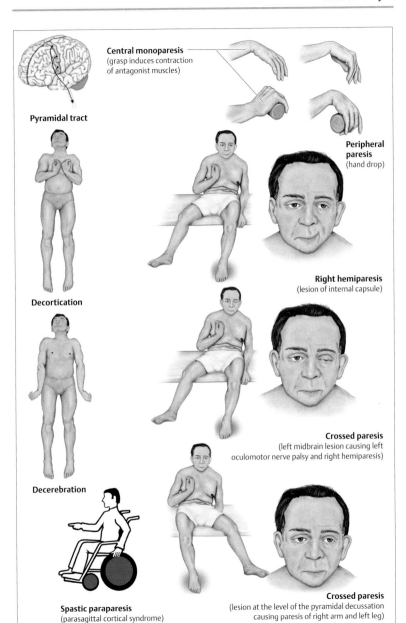

Central monoparesis
(grasp induces contraction
of antagonist muscles)

Pyramidal tract

Peripheral
paresis
(hand drop)

Decortication

Right hemiparesis
(lesion of internal capsule)

Crossed paresis
(left midbrain lesion causing left
oculomotor nerve palsy and right hemiparesis)

Decerebration

Spastic paraparesis
(parasagittal cortical syndrome)

Crossed paresis
(lesion at the level of the pyramidal decussation
causing paresis of right arm and left leg)

Motor Function

47

■ **Spinal Cord Lesions**

The site and extent of a spinal cord lesion can often be determined by clinical examination (p. 32 ff).

Paralysis. Paralysis may be of mixed upper and lower motor neuron type if the lesion affects not only the long fiber tracts but also the anterior horn cells of the spinal cord or their distal processes (root entry zone, spinal nerve roots). Reflex abnormalities are found below the level of the lesion. Central cord lesions cause both paralysis and a dissociated sensory deficit (p. 106).

Posterior cord syndrome. Lesions of the posterior columns of the spinal cord impair vibration and position sense (p. 104 ff). Neck flexion may induce a shocklike paresthesia shooting down the back (*Lhermitte's sign*). There may be hypersensitivity to touch and noxious stimuli in areas of sensory denervation.

Autonomic dysfunction. Spinal cord transection causes acute *spinal shock*, a complete loss of autonomic function below the level of the lesion (bladder, bowel, and sexual function; vasomotor regulation; sweating). Injuries at C4 and above additionally cause respiratory paralysis. The spinal autonomic reflexes (p. 146 ff) may later recover to a variable extent, depending on the site of the lesion. Slowly progressive lesions of the caudal portion of the spinal cord (e. g., intrinsic tumor) usually come to notice because of urinary or sexual dysfunction.

Complete transection. Transection causes immediate flaccid paraplegia or quadriplegia, anesthesia and areflexia below the level of transection, bilateral Babinski signs, and spinal shock (see above). The motor and sensory impairment may begin to improve within 6 weeks if the spinal cord is incompletely transected, ultimately leading to a stable *chronic myelopathy* manifested by spastic paraparesis or quadriparesis and sensory and autonomic dysfunction.

Incomplete transection. Lesions affecting only a portion of the cross-sectional area of the spinal cord cause specific clinical syndromes according to their site (pp. 32, 44, 104), of which the best known are the posterior column syndrome, the anterior horn syndrome (p. 50), the posterior horn syndrome (p. 106), the central cord syndrome (p. 106), the anterior spinal artery syndrome (p. 282), and Brown–Séquard syndrome. In the last-named syndrome, hemisection of the spinal cord causes *ipsilateral* spastic paresis, vasomotor paresis, anhidrosis, and loss of position and vibration sense and somatosensory two-point discrimination, associated with *contralateral* loss of pain and temperature sensations (the so-called dissociated sensory deficit).

Cervical cord lesions. *Upper cervical cord lesions* at the level of the foramen magnum (p. 74) cause neck pain radiating down the arms; shoulder and arm weakness that usually begins on one side, then progresses to include the legs and finally the opposite arm and shoulder; atrophy of the intrinsic muscles of the hand; Lhermitte's sign; cranial nerve deficits (CN X, XI, XII); nystagmus; sensory disturbances on the face; and Horner syndrome. Progressive spinal cord involvement may ultimately impair respiratory function. Lesions at C1 or below do not cause cranial nerve deficits. (C1 root innervates the meninges without dermatome representation.) *Lower cervical cord lesions* (C5–C8) produce the signs and symptoms of complete and incomplete transection discussed above, including segmental sensory and motor deficits. If the lesion involves the spinal sympathetic pathway, Horner syndrome results.

Thoracic cord lesions. Transverse cord lesions at T1 can produce Horner syndrome and atrophy of the intrinsic muscles of the hand. Lesions at T2 and below do not affect the upper limbs. Radicular lesions produce segmental pain radiating in a band from back to front on one or both sides. Localized back pain due to spinal cord lesions is often incorrectly attributed to spinal degenerative disease until weakness and bladder dysfunction appear. Lesions of the upper thoracic cord (T1–T5) impair breathing through involvement of the intercostal muscles.

Lumbar and sacral cord injuries. Lesions at L1 to L3 cause flaccid paraplegia and bladder dysfunction (automatic bladder, p. 156). Iliopsoas weakness may make it difficult or impossible for the patient to sit. Lesions at L4 to S2 impair hip extension and flexion, knee flexion, and foot and toe movement. Lesions at S3 and below produce the *conus medullaris syndrome*: atonic bladder, rectal paralysis, and "saddle" anesthesia of the perianal region and inner thighs. For *cauda equina syndrome*, see pages 318 and 319.

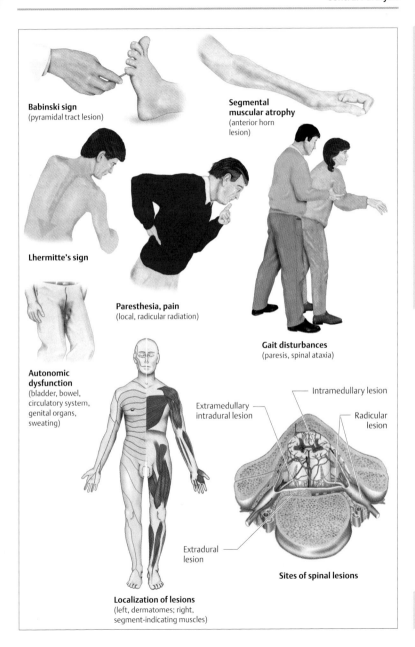

Babinski sign
(pyramidal tract lesion)

Segmental muscular atrophy
(anterior horn lesion)

Lhermitte's sign

Paresthesia, pain
(local, radicular radiation)

Gait disturbances
(paresis, spinal ataxia)

Autonomic dysfunction
(bladder, bowel, circulatory system, genital organs, sweating)

Extramedullary intradural lesion

Intramedullary lesion

Radicular lesion

Extradural lesion

Sites of spinal lesions

Localization of lesions
(left, dermatomes; right, segment-indicating muscles)

Motor Function

49

Signs

Paralysis of peripheral origin can be caused by lesions of the anterior horn (lower motor neuron, LMN), nerve root, peripheral nerve, or motor end plate and must be distinguished from weakness due to disease of the muscle itself (myopathy). Apparent weakness can also be produced by tendon rupture or injury to bones and joints.

Paralysis. Paralysis is accompanied by diminution of muscle tone (flaccidity). The extent of weakness depends on the type, severity, and distribution of LMN or myopathic involvement.

Reflex abnormalities. The intrinsic muscle reflexes are diminished or absent to a degree that may be disproportionate to the degree of weakness: in LMN-type paralysis, loss of reflexes is independent from the loss of strength; in myopathy, it parallels the weakness. Extrinsic reflexes are unaffected unless the effector muscle is atrophic. Pathological reflexes are absent.

Muscle atrophy. Muscle atrophy due to an LMN lesion may be disproportionate to the degree of weakness (either greater or less). Progressive atrophy of paralyzed muscles begins ca. 3 weeks after a peripheral nerve injury. The distribution and severity of muscle atrophy in myopathy depends on the etiology.

Spontaneous movements. Spontaneous movements are seen in affected muscles. *Fasciculations* are involuntary, nonrhythmic contractions of motor units in a relaxed muscle. They are not exclusively caused by anterior horn lesions. *Myokymia* is rhythmic contraction of muscle fibers; if the affected muscle is superficial (e. g., the orbicularis oculi), waves of muscle contraction are visible under the skin.

Lower Motor Neuron (LMN) Lesions

Anterior horn. Loss of motor neurons in the spinal cord paralyzes the motor units to which they belong. The flaccid segmental weakness may begin asymmetrically and is accompanied by severe muscle atrophy. There is no sensory deficit. The intrinsic reflexes of the affected muscles are lost at an early stage. The weakness may be mainly proximal (tongue, pharynx, trunk muscles) or distal (hands, calf muscles) depending on the etiology of anterior horn disease.

Radicular syndrome. A lesion of a single ventral nerve root (caused, for example, by a herniated intervertebral disk) produces weakness in the associated myotome. Muscles supplied by multiple nerve roots are only slightly weakened, if at all, but those supplied by a single root may be frankly paralyzed and atrophic (segment-indicating muscles, cf. Table 2, p. 357). Involvement of the dorsal root produces pain and paresthesia in the associated dermatome, which may be triggered by straining (sneezing, coughing), movement (walking), or local percussion. Autonomic deficits are rare.

Peripheral nerve. Paralysis may be caused by plexus lesions (plexopathy) or by lesions of one or more peripheral nerves (mononeuropathy, polyneuropathy). Depending on the particular segment(s) of nerve(s) affected, the deficit may be purely motor, purely sensory, or mixed, with a variable degree of autonomic dysfunction.

Motor end plate. Disorders of neuromuscular transmission are typified by exercise-induced muscle fatigue and weakness. The degree of involvement of specific muscle groups (eyes, pharyngeal muscles, trunk muscles) depends on the type and severity of the underlying disease. There is no associated sensory deficit. Hyporeflexia characteristically occurs in Lambert–Eaton syndrome and is found in myasthenia gravis to an extent that parallels weakness. Autonomic dysfunction occurs in Lambert–Eaton syndrome and botulism.

Myopathy (see p. 52) **and musculoskeletal lesions** of the tendons, ligaments, joints, and bones may cause real or apparent weakness and thus enter into the differential diagnosis of LMN lesions. They cause no sensory deficit. Musculoskeletal lesions may restrict movement, particularly when they cause pain, sometimes to the extent that the muscle becomes atrophic from disuse. Severe autonomic dysfunction may also occur (p. 110).

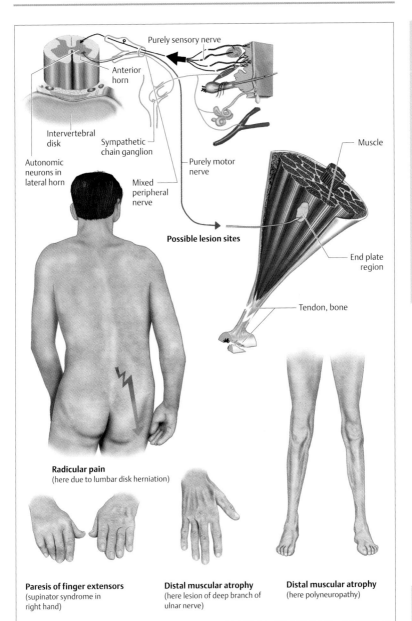

Purely sensory nerve

Anterior horn

Intervertebral disk

Autonomic neurons in lateral horn

Sympathetic chain ganglion

Mixed peripheral nerve

Purely motor nerve

Possible lesion sites

Muscle

End plate region

Tendon, bone

Radicular pain
(here due to lumbar disk herniation)

Paresis of finger extensors
(supinator syndrome in right hand)

Distal muscular atrophy
(here lesion of deep branch of ulnar nerve)

Distal muscular atrophy
(here polyneuropathy)

Motor Function

51

Myopathy

Problems such as muscle weakness, fatigue, stiffness, cramps, tension, atrophy, pain, and involuntary movement do not necessarily signify disease of the muscle itself. Myopathy must be distinguished from neurogenic weakness of UMN or LMN type. Weakness may accompany systemic disease because of a generalized catabolic state or through a specific disease-related impairment of muscle function. Myopathy may be either primary or secondary, i.e., the product of another underlying disease. Different types of myopathy affect different muscle groups: some are generalized (congenital myopathy), while others are mainly either proximal (Duchenne type muscular dystrophy, polymyositis) or distal (myotonic dystrophy, inclusion body myositis), or mainly affect the head and face (mitochondrial myopathy). Myasthenia gravis, strictly speaking a disorder of neuromuscular transmission rather than a form of myopathy, most prominently affects the orbicularis oculi muscle; weakness increases with exercise. Muscle power is commonly graded according to the scale proposed by the British Medical Research Council (MRC) (1976):

0	No muscle contraction
1	Visible or palpable contraction, but no movement
2	Movement occurs, but not against gravity
3	Movement against gravity
4	Movement against gravity and additional resistance
5	Normal muscle power

■ Muscle Atrophy

Myopathy produces atrophy through the impaired development, the destruction, and the impaired regeneration of muscle fibers.

Primary (genetic) myopathies include the progressive muscular dystrophies, myotonic muscular dystrophies, congenital myopathies (e. g., central core disease, nemaline myopathy), and metabolic myopathies (Pompe disease/glycogen storage disease type II, Kearns–Sayre syndrome, carnitine deficiency).

Secondary myopathies include myositis, myopathy due to endocrine disorders (hyperthyroidism and hypothyroidism, hyperparathyroid-

ism), and chronic toxic myopathies (alcohol, corticosteroids, chloroquine).

■ Disorders of Muscle Function

In these disorders, weakness is due to impaired function of the muscle fibers. Persistent weakness can lead to muscle atrophy. The episodic occurrence or worsening of muscle weakness is typical.

Primary myopathies. Hypokalemia- and hyperkalemia-related forms of paralysis belong to this group.

Myasthenic syndromes. Myasthenia gravis and Lambert–Eaton syndrome are characterized by abnormal fatigability of the muscles.

Postviral fatigue syndrome. Mildly increased fatigability of the muscles may persist for weeks after recovery from a viral illness.

■ Muscle Pain and Stiffness

Muscle pain and stiffness restrict movement, causing weakness as a secondary consequence.

Muscle pain. Muscle pain (myalgia, p. 346) at rest and on exertion accompanies muscle trauma (muscle rupture, strain, soreness, compartment syndromes), viral myositis (influenza, Coxsackie virus, herpes simplex virus), fibromyalgia, polymyalgia rheumatica, and muscle cramps and spasms of various causes (malignant hyperthermia, carnitine palmitoyltransferase deficiency, phosphorylase deficiency/glycogen storage disease type V).

Muscle stiffness. Stiffness is prominent in congenital myotonia, neuromyotonia, and cold-induced paramyotonia.

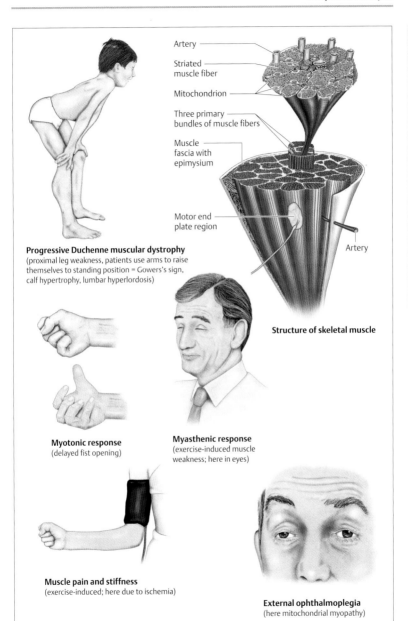

Progressive Duchenne muscular dystrophy
(proximal leg weakness, patients use arms to raise
themselves to standing position = Gowers's sign,
calf hypertrophy, lumbar hyperlordosis)

Artery

Striated
muscle fiber

Mitochondrion

Three primary
bundles of muscle fibers

Muscle
fascia with
epimysium

Motor end
plate region

Artery

Structure of skeletal muscle

Myotonic response
(delayed fist opening)

Myasthenic response
(exercise-induced muscle
weakness; here in eyes)

Muscle pain and stiffness
(exercise-induced; here due to ischemia)

External ophthalmoplegia
(here mitochondrial myopathy)

Motor Function

53

The functions of the cerebellum include the control of balance, posture, gait, and goal-directed movement, and the regulation of muscle tone.

Neural Pathways

Afferent connections. The three large white-matter tracts (peduncles) of the cerebellum convey afferent input to the cerebellar cortex from the cerebral cortex (especially visual areas), pontine nuclei, the brain stem nuclei of the trigeminal, vestibular, and cochlear nerves, and the spinal cord. The *superior cerebellar peduncle* conveys ipsilateral proprioceptive input (p. 104) from the anterior spinocerebellar tract of the spinal cord. The *middle cerebellar peduncle* carries fibers of pontine origin (p. 45). The *inferior cerebellar peduncle* carries fibers from the vestibular nerve and nucleus to the flocculonodular lobe and fastigial nucleus, and from the contralateral inferior olive to the cerebellar hemispheres (olivocerebellar tract), as well as proprioceptive input from the posterior spinocerebellar tract (derived from muscle spindles and destined for the anterior and posterior portions of the paramedian cerebellar cortex) and fibers from the brain stem reticular formation.

Efferent connections. The cerebellar nuclei (fastigial, globose, emboliform, and dentate; p. 43) project via the (contralateral) *superior cerebellar peduncle* to the red nucleus, thalamus, and reticular formation. The thalamus projects in turn to the premotor and primary motor cortex, whose output travels down to the pons, which projects back to the cerebellum, forming a neuroanatomical circuit. Cerebellar output influences (ipsilateral) spinal motor neurons by way of the red nucleus and rubrospinal tract. The *inferior cerebellar peduncle* projects to the vestibular nuclei and brain stem reticular formation (completing the vestibulocerebellar feedback loop) and influences spinal motor neurons by way of the vestibulospinal and reticulospinal tracts.

Functional Systems

The cerebellum can be thought of as containing three separate functional components.

Vestibulocerebellum (archeocerebellum). *Structures:* Flocculonodular lobe and lingula. *Afferent connections:* From the semicircular canals and maculae (p. 56), vestibular nucleus, visual system (lateral geniculate body), superior colliculus, and striate area to the vermis. *Efferent connections:* From the fastigial nucleus to the vestibular nucleus and reticular formation. *Functions:* Control of balance, axial and proximal muscle groups, respiratory movements, and head and eye movements (stabilization of gaze). *Effects of lesions:* Loss of balance (truncal ataxia, postural ataxia > gait ataxia), nystagmus on lateral gaze, and absence of visual fixation suppression (p. 26) resulting in oscillopsia (stationary objects seem to move).

Spinocerebellum (paleocerebellum). *Structures:* Parts of the superior vermis (culmen, central lobule) and inferior vermis (uvula, pyramis), parts of the cerebellar hemispheres (wing of central lobule, quadrangular lobule, paraflocculus). *Afferent connections:* The pars intermedia receives the spinocerebellar tracts, projections from the primary motor and somatosensory cortex, and projections conveying auditory, visual, and vestibular information. *Efferent connections:* From the nucleus interpositus to the reticular formation, red nucleus, and ventrolateral nucleus of the thalamus, which projects in turn to area 4 of the cortex. *Functions:* Coordination of distal muscles, muscle tone (postural control), balance, and velocity and amplitude of saccades. *Effects of lesions:* Gait ataxia > postural ataxia, muscular hypotonia, dysmetria.

Pontocerebellum (neocerebellum). *Structures:* Most of the cerebellar hemispheres, including the declive, folium, and tuber of the vermis. *Afferent connections:* From sensory and motor cortical areas, premotor cortex, and parietal lobes via pontine nuclei and the inferior olive. *Efferent connections:* From the dentate nucleus to the red nucleus and the ventrolateral nucleus of the thalamus, and from these structures onward to motor and premotor cortex. *Functions:* Coordination, speed, and precision of body movement and speech. *Effects of lesions:* Delayed initiation and termination of movement, mistiming of agonist and antagonist contraction in movement sequences, intention tremor, limb ataxia.

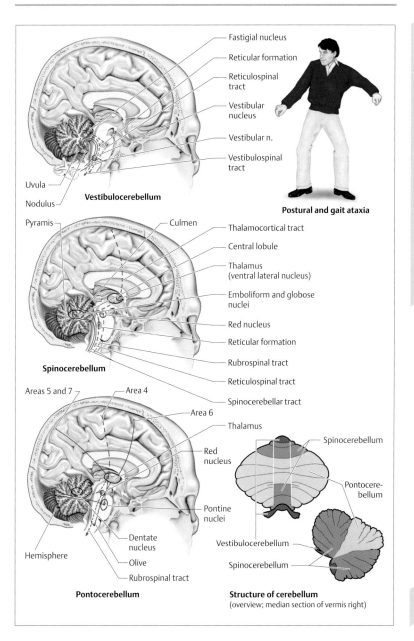

Fastigial nucleus

Reticular formation

Reticulospinal tract

Vestibular nucleus

Vestibular n.

Vestibulospinal tract

Uvula

Nodulus

Vestibulocerebellum

Postural and gait ataxia

Pyramis

Culmen

Thalamocortical tract

Central lobule

Thalamus (ventral lateral nucleus)

Emboliform and globose nuclei

Red nucleus

Reticular formation

Rubrospinal tract

Reticulospinal tract

Spinocerebellar tract

Spinocerebellum

Areas 5 and 7

Area 4

Area 6

Thalamus

Red nucleus

Pontine nuclei

Dentate nucleus

Olive

Hemisphere

Rubrospinal tract

Pontocerebellum

Spinocerebellum

Pontocerebellum

Vestibulocerebellum

Spinocerebellum

Structure of cerebellum
(overview; median section of vermis right)

Motor Function

55

Labyrinth

The vestibular apparatus (labyrinth) consists of the *saccule*, the *utricle*, and three *semicircular canals*, each in a plane approximately at right angles to the others. The labyrinth is filled with fluid (endolymph) and has five receptor organs: the *ampullary crests*, which lie in a dilatation (ampulla) in front of the utricle at the end of each semicircular canal; the *saccular macula* (macula sacculi), a vertically oriented sensory field on the medial wall of the saccule; and the *utricular macula* (macula utriculi), a horizontally oriented sensory field on the floor of the utricle.

Semicircular canals. *Angular acceleration* is sensed by the hair cells of the ampullary crests and the gelatinous bodies (*cupulae*) suspended in the endolymph above them. Rotation about the axis of one of the semicircular canals causes its cupula to deflect in the opposite direction, because it is held back by the more slowly moving endolymph. With persistent rotation at a constant angular velocity (i.e., zero angular acceleration), the cupula returns to its neutral position; but if the rotation should suddenly stop, the cupula is deflected once again, this time in the direction of the original rotation, because it is carried along by the still moving endolymph. The subject feels as if he were rotating counter to the original direction of rotation and also tends to fall in the original direction of rotation.

Maculae. The otolithic membrane of the saccular and utricular maculae is denser than the surrounding endolymph because of the calcite crystals (otoliths) embedded in it. *Linear acceleration* of the head thus causes relative motion of the otolithic membrane and endolymph, resulting in activation of the macular receptor cells (hair cells). The resultant forces lead to activation of the sensory receptors of the maculae.

Neural Pathways

Afferent connections. The *semicircular organs* project mainly to the superior and medial vestibular nuclei, the *macular organs* to the inferior vestibular nuclei. The vestibulocerebellum maintains both afferent and efferent connections with the vestibular nuclei; in particular, the lateral vestibular nucleus receives its major input from the paramedian region of the cerebellar cortex. Fibers reach the vestibular nucleus from the *spinal cord* ipsilaterally, and also bilaterally by way of the fastigial nucleus. The oculomotor nuclei project to the ipsilateral vestibular nuclei through the medial longitudinal fasciculus. The vestibular nuclei are interconnected by internuclear and commissural fibers.

Efferent connections. The vestibulocerebellum projects to the ipsilateral nodulus, uvula, and anterior lobe of the vermis, and to the flocculi bilaterally. The lateral vestibulospinal tract projects ipsilaterally to the motor neurons of the spinal cord and also gives off fibers to cranial nerves X and XI. Fibers to the motor neurons of the contralateral cervical spinal cord decussate in the medial vestibulospinal tract. The *medial longitudinal fasciculus* (p. 86) gives off caudal fibers to the motor neurons of the cervical cord, and rostral fibers bilaterally to the nuclei subserving eye movement. Other fibers cross the midline to the contralateral thalamus, which projects in turn to cortical areas 2 and 3 (primary somatosensory area).

Functional Systems

The vestibular system provides vestibulocochlear input to the cerebellum, spinal cord, and oculomotor apparatus to enable the coordination of head, body, and eye movements. It influences extensor muscle tone and reflexes via the lateral vestibulospinal tract (postural motor system). The medial longitudinal fasciculus permits simultaneous, integrated control of neck muscle tone and eye movements. The oculomotor system (p. 86) communicates with the vestibular nuclei, the cerebellum, and the spinal cord via the medial longitudinal fasciculus and pontine projection fibers; thus the control of eye movements is coordinated with that of body movements. Proprioceptive input concerning joint position and muscle tone reaches the vestibular system from the cerebellum (p. 54). Thalamocortical connections permit spatial orientation. Phenomena such as nausea, vomiting, and sweating arise through interaction with the hypothalamus, the medullary "vomiting center," and the vagus nerve, while the emotional component of vestibular sensation (pleasure and discomfort) arises through interaction with the limbic system.

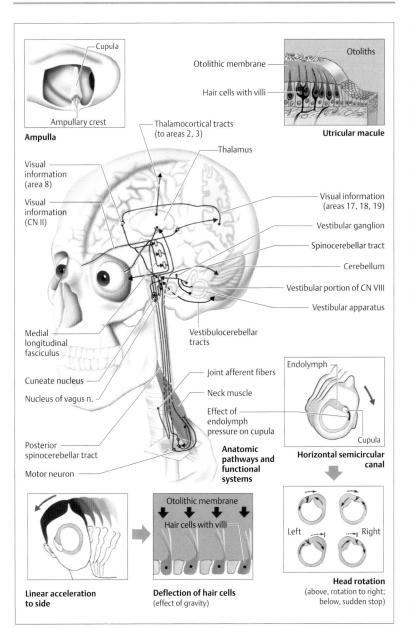

Cupula
Ampullary crest
Ampulla

Otolithic membrane
Hair cells with villi
Otoliths
Utricular macule

Thalamocortical tracts (to areas 2, 3)
Thalamus

Visual information (area 8)
Visual information (CN II)

Visual information (areas 17, 18, 19)
Vestibular ganglion
Spinocerebellar tract
Cerebellum
Vestibular portion of CN VIII
Vestibular apparatus

Medial longitudinal fasciculus

Vestibulocerebellar tracts

Cuneate nucleus
Nucleus of vagus n.

Joint afferent fibers
Neck muscle
Effect of endolymph pressure on cupula

Posterior spinocerebellar tract
Motor neuron

Anatomic pathways and functional systems

Endolymph
Cupula
Horizontal semicircular canal

Left   Right

Head rotation
(above, rotation to right; below, sudden stop)

Otolithic membrane
Hair cells with villi

Linear acceleration to side

Deflection of hair cells
(effect of gravity)

Motor Function

57

Patients often use the word "dizziness" non-specifically to mean lightheadedness, unsteadiness, reeling, staggering, or a feeling of rotation. Dizziness in this broad sense has many possible causes. *Vertigo,* or dizziness in the narrow sense, is the unpleasant illusion that one is moving or that the external world is moving (so-called subjective and objective vertigo, respectively).

Pathogenesis. Vertigo arises from a mismatch between expected and received sensory input (vestibular, visual, and somatosensory) regarding spatial orientation and movement.

Cause. Vertigo occurs as a normal response to certain stimuli (physiological vertigo) or as the result of diseases (pathological vertigo) affecting the labyrinth (peripheral vestibular vertigo), central vestibular system (central vestibular vertigo), or other functional systems (nonvestibular vertigo).

Symptoms and signs. The manifestations of vertigo are the same regardless of etiology. They fall into the following categories: *autonomic* (drowsiness, yawning, pallor, sialorrhea, increased sensitivity to smell, nausea, vomiting), *mental* (decreased drive, lack of concentration, apathy, sense of impending doom), *visual* (oscillopsia = illusory movement of stationary objects), and *motor* (tendency to fall, staggering and swaying gait).

Physiological Vertigo

Healthy persons may experience vertigo when traveling by car, boat, or spaceship (*kinetosis = motion sickness*) or on looking down from a mountain or tall building (*height vertigo*).

Peripheral Vestibular (Labyrinthine) Vertigo (p. 88)

There is usually an acute, severe *rotatory vertigo* directed *away* from side of the labyrinthine lesion, with a tendency to fall *toward* the side of the lesion, horizontal nystagmus *away* from the side of lesion, nausea, and vomiting. Peripheral vestibular vertigo may depend on position, being triggered, for example, when the patient turns over in bed or stands up (*positional vertigo*), or it may be independent of position (*persistent vertigo*). It may also occur in attacks as *episodic vertigo*.

Positional vertigo. Benign, paroxysmal positional vertigo (BPPV) of peripheral origin is usually due to detached otoliths of the utricular macula floating in the posterior semicircular canal (*canalolithiasis*). With every bodily movement, the freely floating otoliths move within the canal, under the effect of gravity. An abnormal cupular deflection results, starting 1–5 seconds after movement and lasting up to 30 seconds. The Dix–Hallpike maneuver is a provocative test for BPPV: the patient is rapidly taken from a sitting to a supine position while the head is kept turned 45° to one side. If nystagmus and vertigo ensue, they are due to canalolithiasis on the side of the ear nearer the ground. The canalith repositioning procedure (CRP), by which particles can be removed from the semicircular canal, involves repeatedly turning the patient's head to the opposite side, then back upright.

Episodic and persistent vertigo may be due to viral infection of the vestibular apparatus (vestibular neuritis, labyrinthitis) or to *Ménière disease,* which is characterized by attacks of rotatory vertigo, tinnitus, hearing loss, and ear pressure. Other causes include labyrinthine fistula and vestibular paroxysm.

Central Vestibular Vertigo (pp. 70 ff and 88)

This type of vertigo is caused by a lesion of the vestibular nuclei, vestibulocerebellum, thalamus, or vestibular cortex, or their interconnecting fibers. Depending on the etiology (e. g., hemorrhage, ischemia, tumor, malformation, infection, multiple sclerosis, "vestibular" epilepsy, basilar migraine), vertigo may be transient or persistent, acute, episodic, or slowly progressive. It may be associated with other neurological deficits depending on the location and extent of the responsible lesion.

Nonvestibular Vertigo

Episodic or persistent nonvestibular vertigo often manifests itself as staggering, unsteady gait, and loss of balance. The possible causes include disturbances of the oculomotor apparatus, cerebellum, or spinal cord; peripheral neuropathy; intoxication; anxiety (phobic attacks of vertigo); hyperventilation; metabolic disorders; and cardiovascular disease.

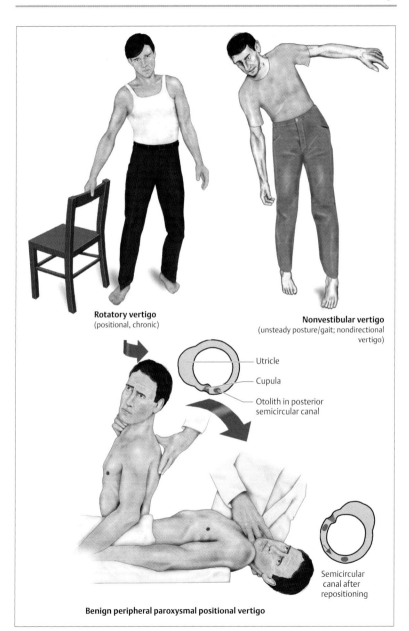

Rotatory vertigo
(positional, chronic)

Nonvestibular vertigo
(unsteady posture/gait; nondirectional vertigo)

Utricle

Cupula

Otolith in posterior semicircular canal

Semicircular canal after repositioning

Benign peripheral paroxysmal positional vertigo

Motor Function

Normal Gait

Posture. The assumption of an *upright posture* and the *maintenance of balance* (postural reflexes) are essential for walking upright. Locomotion requires the unimpaired function of the motor, visual, vestibular, and somatosensory systems. The elderly cannot stand up as quickly and tend to walk somewhat unsteadily, with stooped posture and broader steps, leading to an elevated risk of falling.

Locomotion. Normally, walking can be initiated without hesitation. The *gait cycle* (time between two successive contacts of the heel of one foot with the ground = 2 steps) is characterized by the *gait rhythm* (number of steps per unit time), the *step length* (actually the length of an entire cycle, i.e. 2 steps), and the *step width* (distance

between the lines of movement of the two heels, roughly 5–10 cm). Touchdown is with the heel of the foot. Each leg alternately functions as the supporting leg (*stance phase*, roughly 65 % of the gait cycle), and the advancing leg (*swing phase*, roughly 35 % of the gait cycle). During the *shifting phase*, both feet are briefly in contact with the ground (*double-stance phase*, roughly 25 % of the stance phase). Because the body's center of gravity shifts slightly to the side with each step, the upper body makes small compensatory movements to maintain balance. The arms swing alternately and opposite to the direction of leg movement. Normally, the speed of gait can be changed instantaneously. In old age, the gait sequence is less energetic and more hesitant, and turns tend to be carried out en bloc.

Gait Disturbances

Description	Related Terms	Site of Lesion	Possible Cause
Antalgic gait	Limping gait, leg difference, limp	Foot, leg, pelvis, spinal column	Lumbar root lesion, bone disease, peripheral nerve compression
Steppage gait	Foot-drop gait	Sciatic or peroneal nerve, spinal root L4/5, motor neuron	Polyneuropathy, peroneal paresis; lesions of motor neuron, sciatic nerve, or L4/5 root
Waddling gait	Duchenne gait, Trendelenburg gait, gluteal gait	Paresis of pelvic girdle muscles (Duchenne) or of gluteal abductors (Trendelenburg)	Myopathy, osteomalacia; lesions of the hip joint or superior gluteal nerve; L5 lesion
Toe-walking		Talipes equinus, spasticity	Foot deformity, cerebral palsy, Duchenne muscular dystrophy, habit
Spastic gait	Paraspastic gait, leg circumduction, spastic-ataxic gait, Wernicke–Mann gait	Pyramidal tract, extrapyramidal motor system (supratentorial, infratentorial, spinal)	Unilateral or bilateral central paralysis with spasticity, stiff-man syndrome
Ataxia of gait	Gait ataxia, staggering gait, unsteady gait, tabetic gait, reeling gait	Peripheral nerves, posterior column of spinal cord, spinocerebellar tracts, cerebellum, thalamus, postcentral cortex	Polyneuropathy, disease affecting posterior columns, tabes dorsalis, cerebellar lesion, intoxication, progressive supranuclear palsy
Dystonic gait	Choreiform gait	Basal ganglia	Torsion dystonia, dopa-responsive dystonia, kinesiogenic paroxysmal dystonia, Huntington disease
Start delay	Hypokinetic rigid gait, gait apraxia, festinating gait	Frontal lobe, basal ganglia, extensive white matter lesions	Parkinson disease, frontal lobe lesion, normal-pressure hydrocephalus, Binswanger disease
Psychogenic gait disturbance	Functional gait disturbance		Mental illness, malingering

60

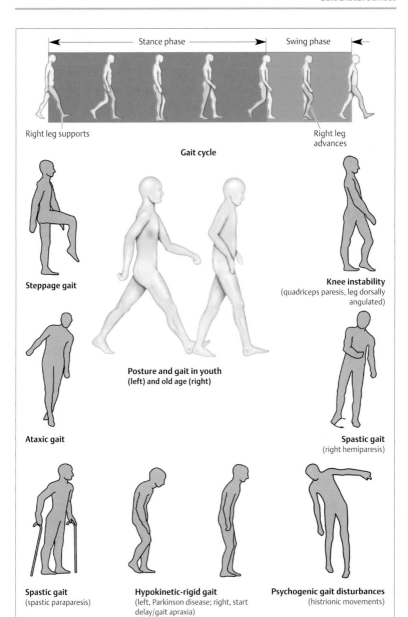

Stance phase → Swing phase ←

Right leg supports

Right leg advances

Gait cycle

Steppage gait

Ataxic gait

Posture and gait in youth (left) and old age (right)

Knee instability
(quadriceps paresis, leg dorsally angulated)

Spastic gait
(right hemiparesis)

Spastic gait
(spastic paraparesis)

Hypokinetic-rigid gait
(left, Parkinson disease; right, start delay/gait apraxia)

Psychogenic gait disturbances
(histrionic movements)

Tremor, the most common movement distur-bance, is an involuntary, rhythmic, oscillating movement of nearly constant amplitude. It can occur wherever movement is subserved by an-tagonistic muscle pairs. Different types of tremor may be classified by the circumstances in which they are activated or inhibited and by their loca-tion, frequency, and amplitude (Table 3, p. 357). Tremor amplitude is the most important deter-minant of disability. Parkinsonian tremor and es-sential tremor are the most common types.

Rest tremor occurs in the absence of voluntary movement and is aggravated by emotional stress (excitement, time pressure) and mental activity (e. g., conversing, reading a newspaper). The tremor subsides when the limbs are moved, but begins again when they return to the resting position. Rest tremor is a typical feature of parkinsonism.

Action tremors occur during voluntary move-ment. *Postural tremor* occurs during main-tenance of a posture, especially when the arms are held outstretched, and disappears when the limbs are relaxed and supported. Essential tremor is a type of postural tremor. *Kinetic tremor* occurs during active voluntary move-ment; it may be worst at the beginning (initial tremor), in the middle (transitory tremor), or at the end of movement (terminal tremor). *Inten-tion tremor*, the type that is worst as the move-ment nears its goal, is characteristic of cerebellar and brain stem lesions. Writing tremor and vocal tremor are examples of *task-specific tremors.* Dystonia-related tremors (e. g., in spasmodic torticollis or writer's cramp) can be suppressed by a firm grip (antagonistic maneuvers).

Frequency. The frequency of tremor in each in-dividual case is relatively invariant and may be measured with a stopwatch or by electromyo-graphy. Different types of tremor have charac-teristic frequencies, listed in the table below, but there is a good deal of overlap, so that differen-tial diagnosis cannot be based on frequency alone.

2.5–5 Hz	Cerebellar tremor, Holmes tremor
3–6 Hz	Parkinsonian tremor
7–9 Hz	Essential tremor, postural tremor in parkinsonism
7–12 Hz	Physiological tremor, exaggerated physiological tremor
12–18 Hz	Orthostatic tremor

Tremor genesis. The tremor of Parkinson disease is due to rhythmic neuronal discharges in the basal ganglia (internal segment of globus pal-lidus, subthalamic nucleus) and thalamus (ven-trolateral nucleus), which are the ultimate result of degeneration of the dopaminergic cells of the substantia nigra that project to the striatum (p. 210). Essential tremor is thought to be due to excessive oscillation in olivocerebellar circuits, which then reaches the motor cortex by way of a thalamic relay. Intention tremor is caused by le-sions of the cerebellar nuclei (dentate, globose, and emboliform nuclei) or their projection fibers to the contralateral thalamus (ven-trolateral nucleus, p. 54). In any variety of tremor, the abnormal oscillations are relayed from the motor cortex through the corticospinal tracts (p. 44) to the spinal anterior horn cells to produce the characteristic pattern of alternating contraction of agonist and antagonist muscles.

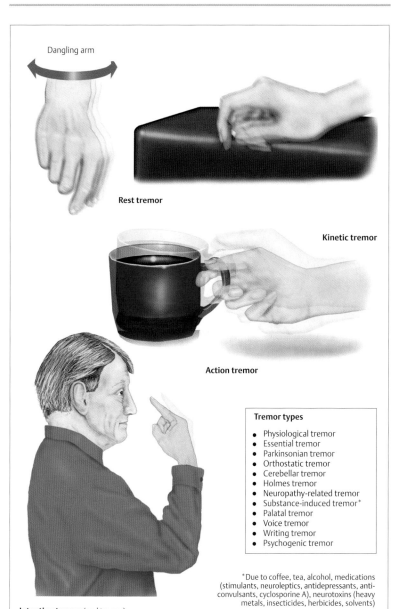

Dangling arm

Rest tremor

Kinetic tremor

Action tremor

Intention tremor (end tremor)

Tremor types

- Physiological tremor
- Essential tremor
- Parkinsonian tremor
- Orthostatic tremor
- Cerebellar tremor
- Holmes tremor
- Neuropathy-related tremor
- Substance-induced tremor*
- Palatal tremor
- Voice tremor
- Writing tremor
- Psychogenic tremor

*Due to coffee, tea, alcohol, medications (stimulants, neuroleptics, antidepressants, anticonvulsants, cyclosporine A), neurotoxins (heavy metals, insecticides, herbicides, solvents)

Motor Function

"Dystonia" is a general term for involuntary movement disorders involving sustained muscle contraction according to a stereotypic pattern, usually resulting in spasmodic or torsional movement and abnormal posture. Dystonic movements are usually exacerbated by voluntary activity. They may arise only during skilled activities such as writing or playing a musical instrument (*action dystonia*). Incomplete relief can be obtained by the avoidance of triggering activities and by the use of antagonistic maneuvers (e. g., placing the fingers on the chin, forehead or neck, or yawning, to counteract cervical dystonia). Dystonia may be classified by its distribution as *focal* (affects only one region of the body), *segmental* (two adjacent regions), *multifocal* (two or more nonadjacent regions), *generalized*, or *lateralized* (hemidystonia), and by its etiology as either *primary* (idiopathic) or *secondary* (symptomatic). Secondary dystonia is usually caused by a disorder of copper, lipid, or amino acid metabolism, or by a mitochondrial disorder (p. 306 ff).

Craniocervical Dystonia

Blepharospasm. Spasmodic contraction of the orbicularis oculi muscle causes excessive blinking and involuntary eye closure. It can often be accompanied by ocular foreign-body sensation and be ameliorated by distracting maneuvers, and is worse at rest or in bright light. There may be involuntary clonic eye closure, tonic narrowing of the palpebral fissure, or difficulty opening the eyes (eye-opening apraxia, p. 128). Blepharospasm may be so severe as to leave the patient no useful vision.

Oromandibular dystonia affects the perioral muscles and the muscles of mastication. In a condition named *Meige syndrome* blepharospasm is accompanied by dystonia of the tongue, larynx, pharynx, and neck.

Cervical dystonia may involve head rotation (*torticollis*), head tilt to one side (*laterocollis*), or flexion or extension of the neck (*anterocollis*, *retrocollis*), often accompanied by tonic shoulder elevation or head tremor. It may be difficult to distinguish nondystonic from dystonic head tremor; only the latter can be improved by antagonistic maneuvers. Dystonia often causes pain, usually in the neck and shoulder.

Arm and Leg Dystonia

These are most often produced by specific, usually complex, activities (*task-specific dystonia*). *Writer's cramp* (graphospasm) and musician's dystonia (for example, while playing the piano, violin, or wind instruments) are well-known examples. Toe or foot dystonia ("striatal foot") is seen in patients with Parkinson disease and dopa-responsive dystonia.

Other Types of Dystonia (see also p. 204)

In *idiopathic torsion dystonia*, focal dystonia of an arm or leg appears in childhood and slowly becomes generalized to include a truncal dystonia causing abnormal posture (scoliosis, kyphosis, opisthotonus). In *spastic dysphonia*, the voice usually sounds strained and forced, and is interrupted by constant pauses (adductor type); less commonly, it becomes breathy or whispered (abductor type). *Dopa-responsive dystonia* (Segawa syndrome) arises in childhood and mainly impairs gait (p. 60), to a degree that varies over the course of the day. *Paroxysmal, autosomal dominant inherited forms of dystonia* are characterized by recurrent dystonic attacks of variable length (seconds to hours). The attacks may be either kinesiogenic (provoked by rapid movements), in which case they usually involve choreoathetosis, or nonkinesiogenic (provoked by caffeine, alcohol, or fatigue).

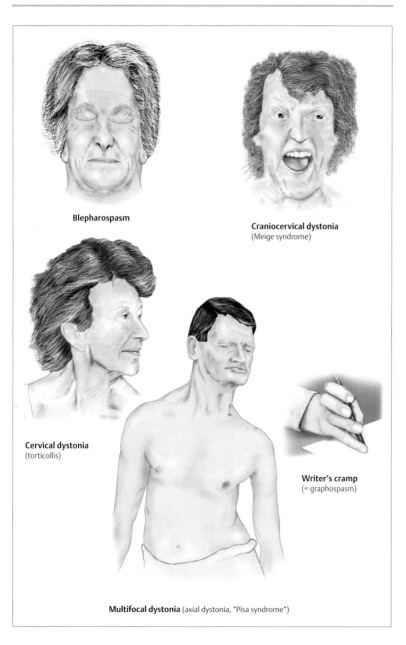

Blepharospasm

Craniocervical dystonia
(Meige syndrome)

Cervical dystonia
(torticollis)

Writer's cramp
(= graphospasm)

Multifocal dystonia (axial dystonia, "Pisa syndrome")

Chorea

Choreiform movements are irregular, abrupt, and seemingly randomly occurring, and usually affect the distal parts of the limbs. In mild chorea, the hyperkinetic movements may be integrated in voluntary movements, such as stroking the hair. More severe cases may involve rapidly changing, bizarre body and limb postures. A combination of choreiform and (distal) dystonic movements is termed *choreoathetosis*. *Huntington disease*, an autosomal dominant disorder, is the best-known cause of chorea (p. 300, 383). Others include hereditary diseases (e. g., neuroacanthocytosis, benign hereditary chorea) and neurodegenerative diseases (e. g., Alzheimer disease, multisystem atrophy). *Secondary chorea* may be caused by infections (e. g., *Sydenham's chorea* due to streptococcal infection; herpes encephalitis, toxoplasmosis), vascular disease (e. g., lupus erythematosus, stroke), brain tumor, drug therapy (e. g., estrogen, neuroleptic drugs), or old age (senile chorea).

Hemiballism (Ballism)

Ballism consists of violent flinging movements of the limbs due to involuntary contraction of the proximal limb muscles, and usually affects only one side of the body (hemiballism). It may be continuous or occur in attacks lasting several minutes. The most common cause is an infarction or other destructive lesion of the subthalamic nucleus (STN). Diminished neural outflow from the STN leads to increased activity in the thalamocortical motor projection (p. 210).

Drug-induced Dyskinesias

Involuntary movements of various kinds may be induced by numerous drugs, most prominently L-*dopa* and *neuroleptic drugs* including phenothiazines, butyrophenones, thioxanthenes, benzamides, and metoclopramide, all of which affect dopaminergic transmission (p. 210).

Acute dystonic reactions (p. 204) involve painful craniocervical or generalized dystonia (opisthotonus, tonic lateral bending and torsion of the trunk = "Pisa syndrome") and are treated with anticholinergic agents (e. g., biperidene).

Tardive (i.e., late) **dyskinesia** is a complication of long-term administration of the so-called classical neuroleptic agents. It is characterized by abnormal, stereotyped movements of the mouth, jaw, and tongue (*orofacial dyskinesia*), sometimes accompanied by respiratory disturbances, grunting, and thrusting movements of the trunk and pelvis. The same drugs may induce tardive *akathisia*, i.e., motor restlessness with a feeling of inner tension and abnormal sensations in the legs; this syndrome must be distinguished from restless legs syndrome (p. 114) and tics (p. 68). These agents also rarely induce tardive craniocervical dystonia, myoclonus, and tremor.

Myoclonus

Myoclonus consists of involuntary, brief, sudden, shocklike muscle contractions producing visible movement. It has a variety of causes and may be focal, segmental, multifocal, or generalized. Its cortical, subcortical, or spinal origin can be determined by neurophysiological testing. Attacks of myoclonus may be spontaneous or may be evoked by visual, auditory, or somatosensory stimuli (reflex myoclonus) or by voluntary movement (postural myoclonus, action myoclonus).

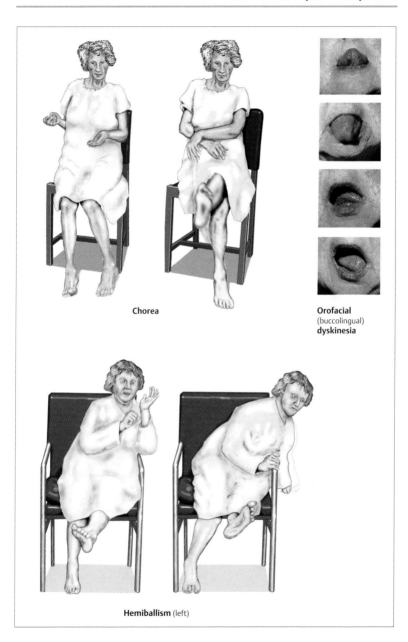

Chorea

Orofacial
(buccolingual)
dyskinesia

Hemiballism (left)

Motor Function

67

Physiological myoclonus. Myoclonus of variable intensity may occur normally as a person falls asleep (*sleep myoclonus*). *Hiccups* (singultus) are myoclonic movements of the diaphragm and normally cease spontaneously. (Severe, intractable hiccups, however, may be produced by lesions of the brain stem.) Normal myoclonic *startle reflexes* are to be distinguished from the rare *startle disorders* such as hyperekplexia, stiff-man syndrome, and startle epilepsy. The myoclonus that occurs in the waking phase after syncope is sometimes mistaken for an epileptic seizure.

Essential myoclonus is a rare hereditary disease characterized by persistent, very brief, multifocal myoclonic movements, accompanied by dystonia. The abnormal movements are improved by small quantities of alcohol.

Myoclonic encephalopathies. Multifocal or generalized action myoclonus is found in association with dementia and tonic-clonic seizures in various types of *progressive myoclonic encephalopathy* (PME), including Lafora disease, myoclonus epilepsy with ragged red fibers (MERRF syndrome), neuronal lipofuscinosis (Kufs disease) and sialidosis type I/II. Epilepsy without dementia is found in progressive myoclonus epilepsy (Unverricht–Lundborg syndrome) and progressive myoclonic ataxia.

Symptomatic myoclonus is associated with many different diseases including Alzheimer disease, corticobasal degeneration, Huntington disease, metabolic disorders (liver disease, lung disease, hypoglycemia, dialysis), encephalitis (Creutzfeldt–Jakob disease, subacute sclerosing panencephalitis), and paraneoplastic syndromes (opsoclonus-myoclonus syndrome). It can also be the result of hypoxic/ischemic brain damage (posthypoxic action myoclonus = Lance–Adams syndrome).

Asterixis consists of brief, irregular flapping movements of the outstretched arms or hands due to sudden pauses in the train of afferent impulses to muscles ("negative" myoclonus). It is not specific for any particular disease. In toxic or metabolic encephalitis, it almost always occurs together with myoclonus.

Tics

Tics are rapid, irregular, involuntary movements (motor tics) or utterances (vocal tics) that interrupt normal voluntary motor activity. They are triggered by stress, anxiety, and fatigue but may also occur at rest; they can be suppressed by a voluntary effort, but tend to re-emerge with greater intensity once the effort is relaxed. Tics are often preceded by a feeling of inner tension. They may be transient or chronic.

Simple tics. Simple motor tics involve isolated movements, e. g., blinking, twitching of abdominal muscles, or shrugging of the shoulders. Simple vocal tics may involve moaning, grunting, hissing, clicking, shouting, throat clearing, sniffing, or coughing.

Complex tics. Complex motor tics consist of stereotyped movements that may resemble voluntary movements, e. g., handshaking, scratching, kicking, touching, or mimicking another person's movements (echopraxia). Complex vocal tics may involve obscene language (coprolalia) or the repetition of another person's words or sentences (echolalia).

Gilles de la Tourette syndrome (often abbreviated to Tourette syndrome) is a chronic disease in which multiple motor and vocal tics begin in adolescence and progress over time. Other features of the disease are personality disturbances, obsessive-compulsive phenomena, and an attention deficit.

Site of possible generators
- Cortical
- Subcortical
- Spinal

Pattern of distribution
- Focal
- Segmental
- Multifocal
- Generalized

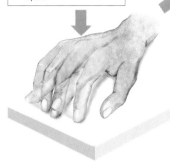

Myoclonus

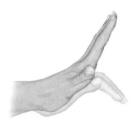

Asterixis
(negative myoclonus)

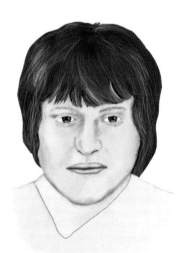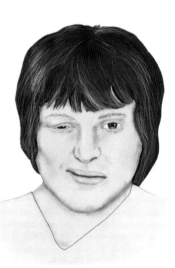

Simple motor tic
(blinking of right eye, left eye normal)

Motor Function

Clinical localization of brain stem lesions depends on knowledge of the tiered arrangement of cranial nerve nuclei, the intramedullary course of cranial nerve fibers, and their spatial relationship to tracts passing up and down the brain stem (see also p. 26). Lesions can be localized to the midbrain, pons, or medulla, and further classified in terms of their location in a cross-sectional plane as anterior, posterior, medial, or lateral. The "classic" brain stem syndromes are rarely seen in actual experience, as the patterns of damage tend to overlap rather than occupy discrete areas of tissue. Brain stem lesions that affect decussating neural pathways proximal to their decussation produce *crossed deficits* (p. 46); thus, some lesions produce ipsilateral cranial nerve palsies and contralateral hemiparesis of the limbs and trunk.

Midbrain Syndromes (Table 4, p. 358)

Lesions of the mid brain may involve its *anterior* portion (cerebral peduncle, Weber syndrome); its *medial* portion (mid brain tegmentum, Benedict syndrome), or its *dorsal* portion (midbrain tectum, Parinaud syndrome). Occlusion of the basilar artery at midbrain level causes *"top of the basilar syndrome"*.

Pontine Syndromes
(p. 72 and Table 5, p. 359)

The syndromes produced by *anterior* and *posterior* pontine lesions are summarized in Table 5.

■ **Paramedian Lesions**

Cause. Multiple lacunar infarcts are the most common cause.

Symptoms and signs. *Unilateral lesions* (mediolateral or mediocentral) cause contralateral paralysis, especially in the distal limb muscles; dysarthria; and unilateral or bilateral ataxia; and, sometimes, contralateral facial and abducens palsies. *Bilateral lesions* cause pseudobulbar palsy and bilateral sensorimotor deficits.

■ **Lateral Pontomedullary Syndrome**

Cause. Infarction or hemorrhage in the territory of the posterior inferior cerebellar artery or aberrant branch of the vertebral artery.

Lesion. As in Wallenberg syndrome (p. 361) with additional involvement of the facial nerve nucleus, vestibular nerve nucleus, and inferior cerebellar peduncle.

Symptoms and signs. As in Wallenberg syndrome with additional ipsilateral findings: facial palsy (nuclear), rotatory vertigo, tinnitus, hearing loss, nystagmus, cerebellar ataxia.

Medullary Syndromes
(p. 73 and Table 6, p. 361)

Lesions usually involve the medial or the lateral portion of the medulla; the lateral medullary syndrome is called Wallenberg syndrome and may be associated with various oculomotor and visual disturbances (p. 86 ff).

Ocular deviation. Vertical deviation (*skew deviation*) in which the ipsilateral eye is lower. Skew deviation may be accompanied by the *ocular tilt reaction*: ipsilateral head tilt, marked extorsion of the ipsilateral eye, and mild intorsion of the contralateral eye.

Nystagmus. *Positional nystagmus* may be horizontal, torsional, or mixed. *See-saw nystagmus* is characterized by intorsion and elevation of one eye and extorsion and depression of the other.

Conjugate deviation to the side of the lesion.

Abnormal saccades. Ocular dysmetria with overreaching (*hypermetria*) when looking to the side of lesion and underreaching (*hypometria*) when looking to the opposite side. Attempted vertical eye movements are executed with diagonal motion.

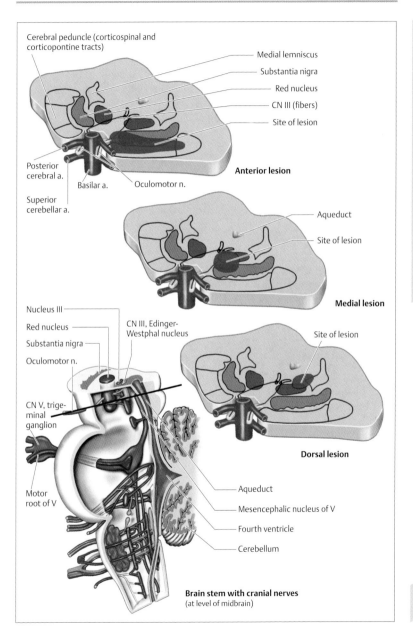

Cerebral peduncle (corticospinal and corticopontine tracts)

Medial lemniscus

Substantia nigra

Red nucleus

CN III (fibers)

Site of lesion

Posterior cerebral a.

Superior cerebellar a.

Basilar a.

Oculomotor n.

Anterior lesion

Aqueduct

Site of lesion

Medial lesion

Nucleus III

Red nucleus

Substantia nigra

Oculomotor n.

CN III, Edinger-Westphal nucleus

Site of lesion

CN V, trigeminal ganglion

Motor root of V

Aqueduct

Mesencephalic nucleus of V

Fourth ventricle

Cerebellum

Dorsal lesion

Brain stem with cranial nerves
(at level of midbrain)

71

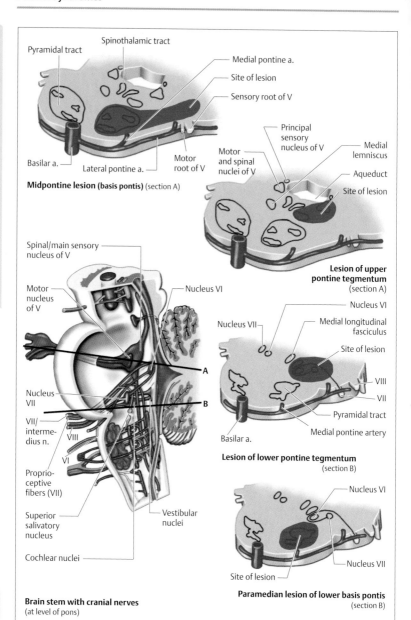

Midpontine lesion (basis pontis) (section A)

Pyramidal tract
Spinothalamic tract
Medial pontine a.
Site of lesion
Sensory root of V
Basilar a.
Lateral pontine a.
Motor root of V
Motor and spinal nuclei of V
Principal sensory nucleus of V
Medial lemniscus
Aqueduct
Site of lesion

Lesion of upper pontine tegmentum (section A)

Spinal/main sensory nucleus of V
Motor nucleus of V
Nucleus VI
Nucleus VII
Nucleus VII
Medial longitudinal fasciculus
Site of lesion
VIII
VII
Pyramidal tract
Medial pontine artery
Nucleus VII
VII/intermedius n.
VIII
VI
Proprioceptive fibers (VII)
Superior salivatory nucleus
Cochlear nuclei
Vestibular nuclei
Basilar a.

Lesion of lower pontine tegmentum (section B)

Nucleus VI
Nucleus VII
Site of lesion

Paramedian lesion of lower basis pontis (section B)

Brain stem with cranial nerves (at level of pons)

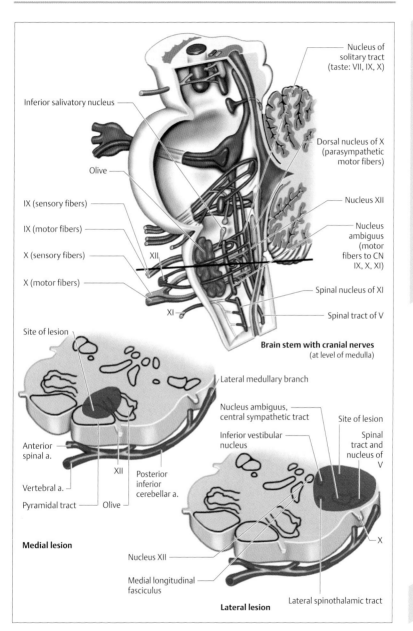

Nucleus of solitary tract (taste: VII, IX, X)

Inferior salivatory nucleus

Dorsal nucleus of X (parasympathetic motor fibers)

Olive

Nucleus XII

IX (sensory fibers)

IX (motor fibers)

Nucleus ambiguus (motor fibers to CN IX, X, XI)

X (sensory fibers)

X (motor fibers)

XII

Spinal nucleus of XI

XI

Spinal tract of V

Brain stem with cranial nerves
(at level of medulla)

Site of lesion

Lateral medullary branch

Nucleus ambiguus, central sympathetic tract

Site of lesion

Inferior vestibular nucleus

Spinal tract and nucleus of V

Anterior spinal a.

XII

Posterior inferior cerebellar a.

Vertebral a.

Pyramidal tract

Olive

X

Medial lesion

Nucleus XII

Medial longitudinal fasciculus

Lateral spinothalamic tract

Lateral lesion

Brain Stem Syndromes

The site of a lesion at the base of the skull can often be deduced from the pattern of cranial nerve involvement.

Site of Lesion	Symptoms	CN[1]	Cause[2]
Olfactory nerve, bulb, and tract	Anosmia, behavioral changes; may progress to Foster Kennedy[3] syndrome	I	Trauma, mass in anterior cranial fossa (meningioma, glioma, osteoma, abscess)
Medial sphenoid wing[4]	Ipsilateral anosmia and optic nerve atrophy, contralateral papilledema	I, II	Medial sphenoid wing meningioma, mass in anterior cranial fossa
Medial/lateral sphenoid wing[4]	Pain in ipsilateral eye, forehead, temple; exophthalmos, diplopia	V/1, III, IV	Medial (eye pain) or lateral (temporal pain) sphenoid wing meningioma
Orbital apex, superior orbital fissure[5]	Ipsilateral: incomplete or complete external ophthalmoplegia, sensory deficit on forehead; papilledema, visual disturbances, optic atrophy	II, III, IV, V/1, VI	Tumor (pituitary adenoma, meningioma, metastasis, nasopharyngeal tumor, lymphoma), granuloma (TB, fungal infection, Tolosa–Hunt syndrome, arteritis), trauma, infraclinoid ICA aneurysm
Cavernous sinus[6]	Ipsilateral symptoms and signs appear earlier than in orbital apex syndrome; exophthalmos[7], Horner syndrome	III, IV, V/1, VI	Same as in orbital apex syndrome + cavernous sinus thrombosis, carotid-cavernous fistula
Optic chiasm[8]	Visual field defects	II	See p. 80
Petrous apex[9]	Ipsilateral facial pain (usually retro-orbital), hearing loss, sometimes also facial palsy	VI, V/1 (to V/3), VIII, (VII)	Inner ear infection, tumor, trauma
Edge of clivus[10]	Ipsilateral mydriasis, may progress to complete oculomotor palsy	III	Intracranial hypertension (p. 158)
Cerebellopontine angle	Ipsilateral hearing loss, tinnitus, deviation nystagmus, facial sensory disturbance, peripheral facial palsy/spasm, abducens palsy, ataxia, headache	VIII, V/1+2, VII, VI	Acoustic neuroma, meningioma, metastasis
Jugular foramen[11]	Ipsilateral: pain in region of tonsils, root of tongue, middle ear; coughing, dysphagia, hoarseness, sternocleidomastoid and trapezius paresis, absence of gag reflex; sensory deficit in root of tongue, soft palate, pharynx, larynx	IX, X, XI	Metastasis, glomus tumor, trauma, jugular vein thrombosis, abscess
Foramen magnum[12]	Same as above + ipsilateral glossoplegia, neck pain, and local spinal symptoms (p. 48)	IX, X, XI, XII	Basilar impression, Klippel–Feil syndrome, local tumor/metastasis

1 CN = cranial nerve (unilateral CN deficits). 2 Only the most common causes are listed; other causes are possible. 3 (Foster) Kennedy syndrome (Foster is the first name). 4 Sphenoid wing syndrome. 5 Orbital apex syndrome, superior orbital fissure syndrome. 6 Cavernous sinus syndrome. 7 Patients with carotid-cavernous fistulae have pulsatile exophthalmos, conjunctival injection, and a systolic bruit that can be heard by auscultation over the eye and temple. 8 Optic chiasm syndrome. 9 Gradenigo syndrome. 10 Clivus syndrome. 11 Jugular foramen syndrome, Vernet syndrome. 12 Collet–Sicard syndrome; may be accompanied by varying degrees of dysfunction of CN IX through XII.

Cranial Nerves

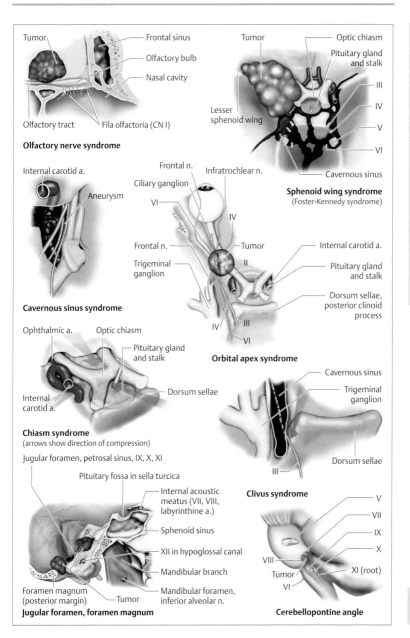

Tumor — Frontal sinus
— Olfactory bulb
— Nasal cavity
Olfactory tract — Fila olfactoria (CN I)

Olfactory nerve syndrome

Tumor — Optic chiasm
— Pituitary gland and stalk
— III
— IV
Lesser sphenoid wing — V
— VI
— Cavernous sinus

Sphenoid wing syndrome
(Foster-Kennedy syndrome)

Internal carotid a.
— Aneurysm

Cavernous sinus syndrome

Frontal n. — Infratrochlear n.
Ciliary ganglion
VI —
IV
Frontal n. — Tumor — Internal carotid a.
Trigeminal ganglion — II — Pituitary gland and stalk
— Dorsum sellae, posterior clinoid process
IV
III
VI

Orbital apex syndrome

Ophthalmic a. — Optic chiasm
— Pituitary gland and stalk
Internal carotid a. — Dorsum sellae

Chiasm syndrome
(arrows show direction of compression)

— Cavernous sinus
— Trigeminal ganglion
— Dorsum sellae
III

Clivus syndrome

Jugular foramen, petrosal sinus, IX, X, XI
Pituitary fossa in sella turcica
— Internal acoustic meatus (VII, VIII, labyrinthine a.)
— Sphenoid sinus
— XII in hypoglossal canal
— Mandibular branch
Foramen magnum (posterior margin) — Mandibular foramen, inferior alveolar n.
— Tumor
Jugular foramen, foramen magnum

— V
— VII
— IX
VIII — X
Tumor — XI (root)
VI

Cerebellopontine angle

Olfactory epithelium. The olfactory mucosa on either side of the nasal cavity occupies an area of approximately 2.5 cm^2 on the roof of the superior nasal concha, extending to the nasal septum. The mucus covering the olfactory epithelium is necessary for olfactory function, because molecules interact with olfactory receptors only when they are dissolved in the mucus. *Olfactory cells* are bipolar sensory cells with a mean lifespan of about 4 weeks. Fine bundles of cilia project from one end of each olfactory cell into the mucus. *Olfactory receptors* located on the cilia are composed of specific receptor proteins that bind particular odorant molecules. Each olfactory cell produces only one type of receptor protein; the cells are thus *chemotopic*, i.e., each responds to only one type of olfactory stimulus. Olfactory cells are uniformly distributed throughout the olfactory mucosa of the nasal conchae.

Olfactory pathway. The unmyelinated axons of all olfactory cells converge in bundles of up to 20 *fila olfactoria* on each side of the nose (these bundles are the true olfactory nerves), which pass through the cribriform plate to the olfactory bulb. Hundreds of olfactory cell axons converge on the dendrites of the mitral cells of the olfactory bulb, forming the *olfactory glomeruli*. Other types of neurons that modulate the olfactory input (e. g., granular cells) are found among the mitral cells. Neural impulses are relayed through the projection fibers of the olfactory tract to other areas of the brain including the prepiriform cortex, limbic system, thalamus (medial nucleus), hypothalamus, and brain stem reticular formation. This complex interconnected network is responsible for the important role of smell in eating behavior, affective behavior, sexual behavior, and reflexes such as salivation. The *trigeminal nerve* supplies the mucous membranes of the nasal, oral, and pharyngeal cavities. Trigeminal receptor cells are also stimulated by odorant molecules, but at a higher threshold than the olfactory receptor cells.

Olfactory Disturbances (Dysosmia)

Olfactory disturbances can be classified as either *quantitative* (anosmia, hyposmia, hyperosmia) or *qualitative* (parosmia, cacosmia). Congenital olfactory disturbances manifest themselves as *partial anosmia* ("olfactory blindness"). The perceived intensity of a persistent odor decreases or disappears with time (*olfactory adaptation*). External factors such as an arid environment, cold, or cigarette smoke impair the ability to smell; diseases affecting the nasopharyngeal cavity impair both smell and taste. Odors and emotions are closely linked and can influence each other. The perception of smell may be qualitatively changed (*parosmia*) because of autonomic (hunger, stress) and hormonal changes (pregnancy) or disturbances such as ozena, depression, traumatic lesions, or nasopharyngeal empyema. *Olfactory hallucinations* can be caused by mediobasal and temporal tumors (focal epilepsy), drug or alcohol withdrawal, and psychiatric illnesses such as schizophrenia or depression.

Tests of smell. One nostril is held closed, and a bottle containing a test substance is held in front of the other. The patient is then asked to inhale and report any odor perceived. In this subjective test, odor perception per se is more important than odor recognition. Odor perception indicates that the peripheral part of the olfactory tract is intact; odor recognition indicates that the cortical portion of the olfactory pathway is also intact. More sophisticated tests may be required in some cases. Because there is bilateral innervation, unilateral lesions proximal to the anterior commissure and cortical lesions may not cause anosmia.

Anosmia/hyposmia. Unilateral anosmia may be caused by a tumor (meningioma). *Korsakoff syndrome* can render the patient unable to identify odors. Viral infections (influenza), heavy smoking, and toxic substances can damage the olfactory epithelium; trauma (disruption of olfactory nerves, frontal hemorrhage), tumors, meningitis, or radiotherapy may damage the olfactory pathway. Parkinson disease, multiple sclerosis, Kallmann syndrome (congenital anosmia with hypogonadism), meningoencephalocele, albinism, hepatic cirrhosis, and renal failure can also cause olfactory disturbances.

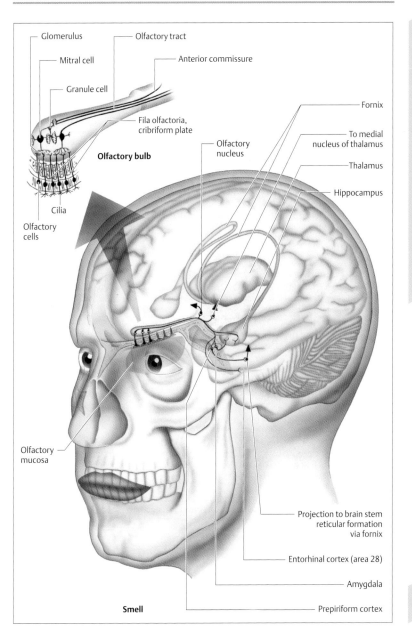

Glomerulus

Mitral cell

Granule cell

Olfactory tract

Anterior commissure

Fila olfactoria, cribriform plate

Olfactory bulb

Cilia

Olfactory cells

Olfactory mucosa

Olfactory nucleus

Fornix

To medial nucleus of thalamus

Thalamus

Hippocampus

Projection to brain stem reticular formation via fornix

Entorhinal cortex (area 28)

Amygdala

Prepiriform cortex

Smell

Taste buds. Each taste bud contains 50–150 gustatory cells. Taste buds are found on the margins and furrows of the different types of gustatory papillae (fungiform, foliate, and vallate) and are specific for one of the four primary tastes, *sweet*, *sour*, *salty*, and *bitter*. The lifespan of each gustatory cell is approximately one week. Filaments called *microvilli* projecting from the cells' upper poles are coated with gustatory receptor molecules. Stimulation of the gustatory cell at its receptors by the specific taste initiates a molecular transduction process, resulting in depolarization of the cell. Each taste bud responds to multiple qualities of taste, but at different sensitivity thresholds, resulting in a characteristic taste profile. For example, one papilla may be more sensitive to "sweet," another to "sour." The higher the concentration of the tasted substance, the greater the number of gustatory cells that fire action potentials. Complex tastes are encoded in the different patterns of receptor stimulation that they evoke.

Gustatory pathway. Sensory impulses from the tongue are conveyed to the brain by three pathways: from the anterior two-thirds of the tongue via the lingual nerve (V/3) to the chorda tympani, which arises from the facial nerve (nervus intermedius); from the posterior third of the tongue via the glossopharyngeal nerve; and from the epiglottis via the vagus nerve (fibers arising from the inferior ganglion). Sensory impulses from the soft palate travel via the palatinate nerves to the pterygopalatine ganglion and onward through the greater petrosal nerve and nervus intermedius. All gustatory information arrives at the nucleus of the solitary tract, which projects, through a thalamic relay, to the postcentral gyrus. The gustatory pathway is interconnected with the olfactory pathway through the hypothalamus and amygdala. It has important interactions with the autonomic nervous system (facial sweating and flushing; salivation) and with affective centers (accounting for like and dislike of particular tastes).

Gustatory Disturbances (Dysgeusia)

When smell is impaired, the patient loses the capacity for fine differentiation of tastes but is able to distinguish the primary tastes (sweet, sour, salty, bitter). For example, chocolate pudding can be identified as "sweet" but not as "chocolate." Diminished taste (hypogeusia) is more common than complete loss of taste (ageusia).

Tests of taste. Taste thresholds on each side of the tongue are tested with the tongue outstretched. A test solution is applied to the tongue with a cotton swab for 20 to 30 seconds. The patient is then asked to point to the corresponding region of a map divided into "sweet", "sour", "salty" and "bitter" zones. The test solutions contain glucose (sweet), sodium chloride (salty), citric acid (sour), or quinine (bitter). The mouth is rinsed with water between test solutions. The taste zones are not organized in a strict topographic pattern. *Electrogustometry* can be used for precise determination of the taste thresholds but it is time-consuming and requires a high level of concentration on the part of the patient.

Ageusia/hypogeusia. Dry mouth (Sjögren syndrome), excessive alcohol consumption, smoking, spicy food, chemical burns, medications (e.g., lithium, L-dopa, aspirin, cholestyramine, amitryptiline, vincristine, carbamazepine), radiotherapy, infectious diseases (influenza), and stomatitis (thrush) can damage the taste buds. *Lesions of the chorda tympani* producing unilateral gustatory disturbances are seen in patients with peripheral facial palsy, chronic otitis media, and cholesteatoma. Lesions of cranial nerves V, IX, or X lead to taste distortion (especially of bitter, sour, and salty) in the posterior third of the tongue, in combination with paresthesia (sensation of burning or numbness). Gustatory disturbances may also be caused by damage to the central gustatory pathway, e.g., by trauma, brain tumors, carbon monoxide poisoning, or multiple sclerosis. The sense of taste can also change because of aging (especially sweet and sour), pregnancy, diabetes mellitus, hypothyroidism, and vitamin deficiencies (A, B_2).

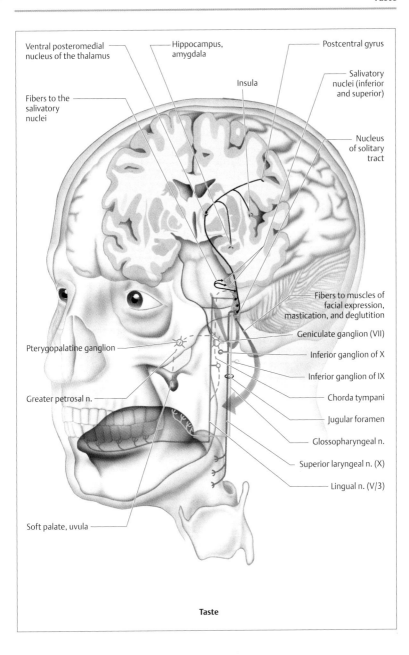

Ventral posteromedial nucleus of the thalamus

Hippocampus, amygdala

Postcentral gyrus

Insula

Salivatory nuclei (inferior and superior)

Fibers to the salivatory nuclei

Nucleus of solitary tract

Fibers to muscles of facial expression, mastication, and deglutition

Geniculate ganglion (VII)

Pterygopalatine ganglion

Inferior ganglion of X

Inferior ganglion of IX

Greater petrosal n.

Chorda tympani

Jugular foramen

Glossopharyngeal n.

Superior laryngeal n. (X)

Lingual n. (V/3)

Soft palate, uvula

Taste

Retina. Visible light is electromagnetic radiation at wavelengths of 400–750 nanometers. The *dioptric system* (cornea, aqueous humor of the anterior and posterior ocular chambers, pupil, lens, vitreous body) produces a miniature, upside-down mirror image of the visual field on the retina. The fovea, located in the center of the macula at the posterior pole of the eyeball, is the area of sharpest vision in daylight. Blood is supplied to the eye by the ophthalmic artery via the ciliary arteries (supplies the choroid) and the central retinal artery (supplies the retina). The optic disk, the central retinal artery that branches from it, and the central retinal vein can be examined by *ophthalmoscopy*.

Visual pathway. The visual pathway begins in the retina (first three neurons) and continues through the optic nerve to the optic chiasm, from which it continues as the optic tract to the lateral geniculate body. The *optic radiation* arises at the lateral geniculate body and terminates in the *primary* (area 17) and *secondary visual areas* (areas 18, 19) of the occipital lobe. The fibers of the retinal neuronal network converge at the *optic disk* before continuing via the optic nerve to the *optic chiasm*, in which the medial (nasal) fibers cross to the opposite side. The right optic tract thus contains fibers from the temporal half of the right retina and the nasal half of the left retina. The *lateral geniculate body* is the site of the fourth neuron of the optic pathway. Its efferent fibers form the optic radiation, which terminates in the visual cortex (striate cortex) of the occipital lobe. The central foveal area has the largest cortical representation. The visual pathway is interconnected with midbrain nuclei (medial, lateral, and dorsal terminal nuclei of the pretectal region; superior colliculus), nonvisual cortical areas (somatosensory, premotor, and auditory), the cerebellum, and the pulvinar (posterior part of thalamus).

Visual field. The *monocular visual field* is the portion of the external world seen with one eye, and the *binocular visual field* is that seen by both eyes. The visual fields of the two eyes overlap; the overall visual field therefore consists of a central zone of clear binocular vision produced by the left and right central foveae, a peripheral binocular zone, and a monocular zone. Partial decussation at the optic chiasm brings visual information from the right (left) side of the world to the left (right) side of the brain. The visual field is topographically represented at all levels of the visual pathway from retina to cortex; lesions at any level of the pathway cause visual field defects of characteristic types. If the images on the two retinas are displaced by more than a certain threshold distance, double vision (diplopia) results. This is most commonly due to disturbances of the extraocular muscles, e. g., paralysis of one or more of these muscles (p. 86).

Stereoscopic vision. Three-dimensional visual perception (stereoscopic vision) is produced by comparison of the slightly different images in the two eyes. Stereoscopic vision is very important for depth perception, though depth can be judged to some extent, through other cues, with monocular vision alone.

Color vision. Testing of color vision requires standard definition of the colors red, blue, and green. The visual threshold for various colors, each defined as a specific mixture of the three primary colors, is determined with a standardized color perception chart. *Disturbances of color vision* may be due to disturbances of the dioptric system, the retina, or the visual pathway. Cortical lesions cause various kinds of visual agnosia. Lesions of area 18 may make it impossible for patients to recognize colors despite intact color vision (color agnosia), or to recognize familiar objects (object agnosia) or faces (prosopagnosia). Patients with lesions of area 19 have intact vision but cannot recognize or describe the objects that they see. Spatial orientation may be impaired (visuospatial agnosia), as may the inability to draw pictures. Persons with visual agnosia may need to touch objects to identify them.

Limbic system. Connections with the limbic system (hippocampus, amygdala, parahippocampal gyrus; p. 144) account for the ability of visual input to evoke an emotional response.

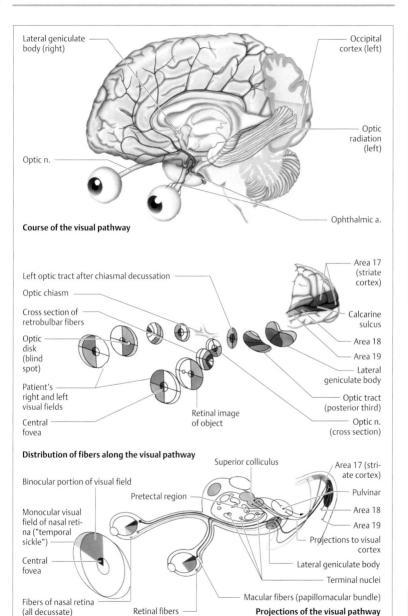

Course of the visual pathway

Lateral geniculate body (right)

Occipital cortex (left)

Optic radiation (left)

Optic n.

Ophthalmic a.

Distribution of fibers along the visual pathway

Left optic tract after chiasmal decussation

Optic chiasm

Cross section of retrobulbar fibers

Optic disk (blind spot)

Patient's right and left visual fields

Central fovea

Retinal image of object

Area 17 (striate cortex)

Calcarine sulcus

Area 18

Area 19

Lateral geniculate body

Optic tract (posterior third)

Optic n. (cross section)

Projections of the visual pathway

Binocular portion of visual field

Pretectal region

Superior colliculus

Monocular visual field of nasal retina ("temporal sickle")

Central fovea

Fibers of nasal retina (all decussate)

Retinal fibers

Area 17 (striate cortex)

Pulvinar

Area 18

Area 19

Projections to visual cortex

Lateral geniculate body

Terminal nuclei

Macular fibers (papillomacular bundle)

Cranial Nerves

Examination. The visual fields of both eyes should always be jointly assessed. The *confrontation test*, in which the examiner "confronts" the patient's visual field with his or her own, intact, contralateral visual field, is used to check for visual field defects. For the test to be performed correctly, the patient and the examiner must first fixate along the same line. The examiner then slowly moves a white or red object (at least 1 cm in diameter) from the periphery of the visual field toward the center in a number of different directions, and determines where the patient can and cannot see it. Alternatively, the examiner may raise one or more fingers and ask the patient to count them (a useful test for small children, and for persons whose vision is so poor that it cannot be tested by the first method). The perceived *brightness* (unequal in patients with hemianopsia) of the hand in the nasal and temporal portions of the visual field is also determined. The *red vision test* enables the detection of a central scotoma as an area in which the red color is perceived as less intense. More detailed information can be obtained by further ophthalmological testing (Goldmann perimetry, automatic perimetry).

Visual field defect (scotoma). The thin myelinated fibers in the center of the optic nerve, which are derived from the papillomacular bundle, are usually the first to be affected by optic neuropathy (*central scotoma*). From the optic chiasm onward, the right and left visual fields are segregated into the left and right sides of the brain. Unilateral lesions of the retina and optic nerve cause monocular deficits, while retrochiasmatic lesions cause homonymous defects (quadrantanopsia, hemianopsia) that do not cross the vertical meridian, i.e., affect one side of the visual field only. Anterior retrochiasmatic lesions cause incongruent visual field defects, while posterior retrochiasmatic lesions lead to congruent visual field defects. Temporal lobe lesions cause mildly incongruent, contralateral, superior homonymous quadrantanopsia. Bitemporal visual field defects (heteronymous hemianopsia) have their origin in the chiasm. Unilateral retrochiasmatic lesions cause visual field defects but do not impair visual acuity. Organic visual field defects widen progressively with the distance of test objects from the eye, whereas psychogenic ones are constant ("tubular fields").
Prechiasmatic lesions may affect the retina, papilla (= optic disk), or optic nerve. Transient episodes of monocular blindness (amaurosis fugax) see p. 372 (table 22 a). Acute or subacute unilateral blindness may be caused by optic or retrobulbar neuritis, papilledema (intracranial mass, pseudotumor cerebri), cranial arteritis, toxic and metabolic disorders, local tumors, central retinal artery occlusion, or central retinal vein occlusion.

Chiasmatic lesions. Lesions of the optic chiasm usually produce bitemporal visual field defects. Yet, because the medial portion of the chiasm contains decussating fibers while its lateral portions contain uncrossed fibers, the type of visual field defect produced varies depending on the exact location of the lesion. As a rule, anterior chiasmatic lesions that also involve the optic nerve cause a central scotoma in the eye on the side of the lesion and a superior temporal visual field defect (junction scotoma) in the contralateral eye. Lateral chiasmatic lesions produce nasal hemianopsia of the ipsilateral eye; those that impinge on the chiasm from both sides produce binasal defects. Dorsal chiasmatic lesions produce bitemporal hemianopic paracentral scotomata. Double vision may be the chief complaint of patients with bitemporal scotomata.

Retrochiasmatic lesions. Depending on their location, retrochiasmatic lesions produce different types of *homonymous unilateral scotoma*: the defect may be congruent or incongruent, quadrantanopsia or hemianopsia. As a rule, temporal lesions cause contralateral superior quadrantanopsia, while parietal lesions cause contralateral inferior quadrantanopsia. Complete hemianopsia may be caused by a relatively small lesion of the optic tract or lateral geniculate body, or by a more extensive lesion more distally along the visual pathway. Sparing of the temporal sickle (p. 80) indicates that the lesion is located in the occipital interhemispheric fissure. *Bilateral homonymous scotoma* is caused by bilateral optic tract damage. The patient suffers from "tunnel vision" but the central visual field remains intact (sparing of macular fibers). Cortical blindness refers to subnormal visual acuity due to bilateral retrogeniculate lesions. Bilateral *altitudinal* homonymous hemianopsia (i.e., exclusively above or exclusively below the visual equator) is due to extensive bilateral damage to the temporal lobe (superior scotoma) or parietal lobe (inferior scotoma).

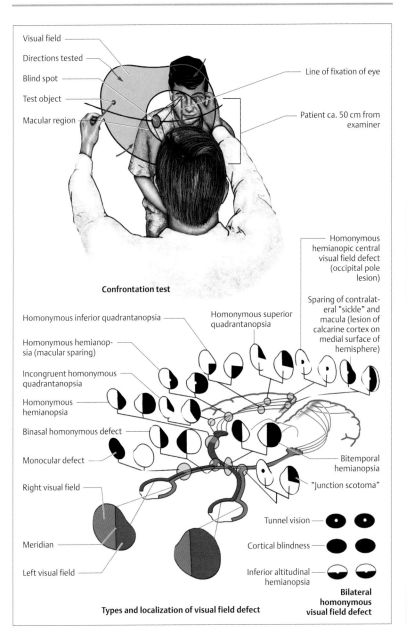

Visual field

Directions tested

Blind spot

Test object

Macular region

Line of fixation of eye

Patient ca. 50 cm from examiner

Confrontation test

Homonymous hemianopic central visual field defect (occipital pole lesion)

Sparing of contralateral "sickle" and macula (lesion of calcarine cortex on medial surface of hemisphere)

Homonymous inferior quadrantanopsia

Homonymous superior quadrantanopsia

Homonymous hemianopsia (macular sparing)

Incongruent homonymous quadrantanopsia

Homonymous hemianopsia

Binasal homonymous defect

Monocular defect

Bitemporal hemianopsia

"Junction scotoma"

Right visual field

Meridian

Tunnel vision

Cortical blindness

Left visual field

Inferior altitudinal hemianopsia

Bilateral homonymous visual field defect

Types and localization of visual field defect

The visual axes of the eyes are directed straight ahead on primary gaze (i.e., 23° inward from the more lateral axes of the orbits). Movements of the eyes are mediated by six extraocular muscles on each side. The lateral and medial rectus muscles are responsible for horizontal eye movements. Vertical eye movements are subserved by the superior and inferior rectus as well as superior and inferior oblique muscles. The rectus muscles elevate and depress the eye when it is abducted, the oblique muscles when it is adducted. The two muscles of each synergistic pair (e. g., the left lateral rectus and right medial rectus muscles) receive equal degrees of innervation (Hering's law).

Vestibulo-ocular reflex (VOR). Impulses arising in the semicircular canals in response to rapid movement of the head induce reflex movement of the eyes in such a way as to stabilize the visual image (p. 26). For example stimulation of the horizontal semicircular canal activates the ipsilateral medial rectus and contralateral lateral rectus muscles, while inhibiting the ipsilateral lateral rectus and contralateral medial rectus muscles. The VOR makes the eyes move in the direction opposite to the head movements, at the same angular velocity.

Optokinetic reflex. Optokinetic nystagmus (OKN) is triggered by large-scale, moving visual stimuli and serves to stabilize the visual image during slow head movement. OKN is characterized by slow, gliding conjugate movement of the eyes in the direction of an object moving horizontally or vertically across the visual field, in alternation with rapid return movements in the opposite direction (saccades). OKN is intact in psychogenic (pseudo) blindness.

Fixation. Fixation is active adjustment of the gaze (with or without the aid of eye movement) to keep a visualized object in focus.

Saccades. Saccades are rapid, jerky conjugate movements of the eyes that serve to adjust or set the point of fixation of an object on the fovea. Saccades may be spontaneous, reflexive (in response to acoustic, visual, or tactile stimuli), or voluntary; the rapid phase of nystagmus is a saccade. The speed, direction, and amplitude of a saccadic movement are determined before it is carried out and cannot be influenced voluntarily during its execution. Shifts of visual fixation by more than 10° are accompanied by head movements.

Slow ocular pursuit. Voluntary ocular pursuit can occur only when triggered by a moving visual stimulus (e. g., a passing car). Conversely, fixation of the gaze on a resting object while the head is moving leads to gliding eye movements. Fixation-independent ocular pursuit also occurs during somnolence and the early stages of sleep ("floating" eye movements).

Vergence movements (convergence and divergence) are mirror-image movements of the two eyes toward or away from the midline, evoked by movement of an object toward or away from the head in the sagittal plane. They serve to center the visual image on both foveae and are accompanied by an adjustment of the curvature of the lens (accommodation) to keep the object in focus.

Neural pathways. The *medial longitudinal fasciculus* (MLF) interconnects the nuclei of cranial nerves III, IV, and VI. The MLF also connects with fibers conveying information to and from the cervical musculature, vestibular nuclei, cerebellum, and cerebral cortex and thus mediates the coordination of eye movements with movements of the body and head. Saccades are produced by two parallel systems: *Voluntary eye movements* are subserved by the frontal system, which consists of the frontal eye fields (areas 4, 6, 8, 9), the supplementary eye field (area 6), the dorsolateral prefrontal cortex (area 46), and a portion of the parietal cortex (area 7). It projects to the contralateral paramedian pontine reticular formation (PPRF), which coordinates vertical and horizontal saccades. Vertical and torsional eye movements are controlled by the rostral interstitial nucleus of the MLF and by the interstitial nucleus of Cajal. *Reflex eye movements* are initiated in the visual cortex (area 17) and temporal lobe (areas 19, 37, 39) and modulated in the superior colliculus (collicular system). *Vergence and accommodation* are mediated by the pretectal area in the vicinity of the oculomotor nucleus.

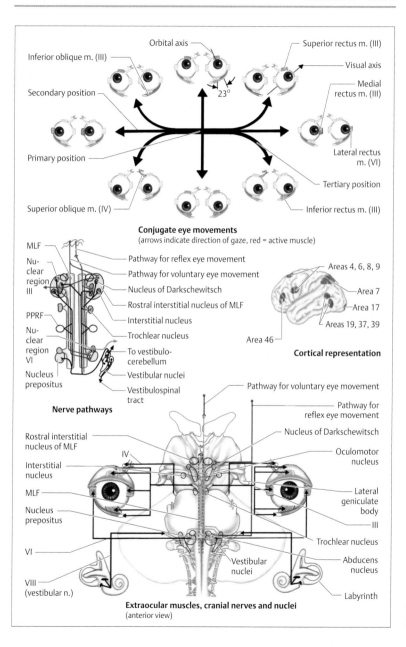

Conjugate eye movements
(arrows indicate direction of gaze, red = active muscle)

Nerve pathways

Cortical representation

Extraocular muscles, cranial nerves and nuclei
(anterior view)

Cranial Nerves

85

Peripheral Oculomotor Disturbances

Weakness of an extraocular muscle results in diplopia, which is most pronounced in the direction of action of the affected muscle (p. 85). The cause may be a lesion in the muscle itself, in the cranial nerve that supplies it, or in the cranial nerve nucleus.

Examination. The more peripheral of the two images seen by the patient is always derived from the affected eye. The impaired eye movement may be seen directly by observation of conjugate eye movements in the nine cardinal directions of gaze (p. 85). Next, the examiner has the patient look in the direction of greatest image displacement, covers first one eye and then the other, and asks the patient each time which of the two images has disappeared. The more peripheral image disappears when the affected eye is covered. Alternatively, the patient can be asked to look at a point of light while a red glass is held in front of one eye; if the more peripheral image is red, then the eye with the glass is the affected eye. Another test is to rapidly cover and uncover one eye and then the other while the patient looks in the cardinal directions of gaze. The greatest ocular deviation and the greatest adjustment of the unaffected eye (secondary angle of deviation) occur when the patient looks in the direction of the paretic muscle. As a rule, these tests are helpful when a single muscle is acutely weak; more sophisticated ophthalmological tests are needed if the weakness is chronic or affects more than one muscle.

Oculomotor nerve palsy. When a compressive lesion causes *complete oculomotor nerve palsy*, the patient complains of diplopia (with double image displacement) only when the ptotic eyelid is passively elevated. The affected eye is turned downward (action of the intact superior oblique muscle) and outward (intact lateral rectus muscle) on primary gaze, and the pupil is fixed, dilated, and irregularly shaped. The involved eye can still be abducted (intact CN VI), and looking down causes intorsion (intact CN IV). *Incomplete oculomotor nerve palsy* because of nuclear or myopathic lesions may differentially affect the intraocular and extraocular muscles supplied by CN III and cause different types of diplopia and pupillary disorders (p. 90).

Trochlear nerve palsy. The affected eye points upward and toward the nose on primary gaze. Diplopia is worst when the affected eye looks toward the nose and downward.

Abducens nerve palsy. The affected eye deviates toward the nose on primary gaze. Horizontal diplopia is worst on looking toward the side of the affected eye.

Supranuclear and Internuclear Oculomotor Disturbances

Internuclear ophthalmoplegia (INO) is characterized by inability to adduct one eye, combined with nystagmus of the other, abducted eye (dissociated nystagmus), on attempted lateral gaze. It is due to a lesion of the medial longitudinal fasciculus (MLF) on the side of the nonadducting eye and at a level between the nuclei of CN III and CN VI. Bilateral MLF lesions cause bilateral INO. Both eyes can adduct normally during convergence. More rostral lesions lead to convergence paresis without nystagmus; more caudal lesions lead to paresis of the lateral rectus muscle. Multiple sclerosis and vascular disorders are the most common causes of INO.

Unilateral pontine lesions cause ipsilateral gaze palsy (the gaze points away from the side of the lesion) but leave vertical eye movement largely intact. Co-involvement of the MLF leads to *one-and-a-half syndrome* (ipsilateral pontine gaze palsy + INO), e. g., paresis of conjugate gaze to the left and impaired adduction of the left eye on looking to the right.

Supratentorial lesions. Extensive cortical or subcortical hemispheric lesions produce *contralateral gaze palsy* (patient gazes toward the side of the lesion). Slow reflex movements of the eyes in all directions are still possible because the optokinetic reflex is not affected. In occipital lesions, the optokinetic reflex is absent; voluntary eye movements are preserved, but the eyes can no longer follow slowly moving objects. Abnormal, diffuse elevation of activity within a hemisphere (e. g., because of an epileptic seizure) causes *contralateral gaze deviation*.

For further information on horizontal and vertical gaze palsy, see page 70.

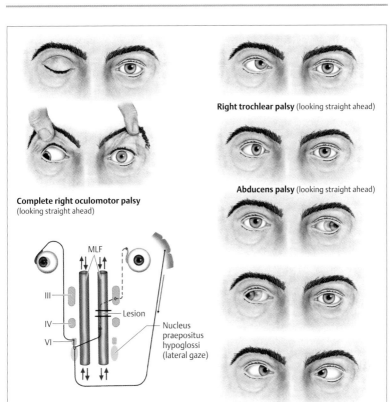

Complete right oculomotor palsy
(looking straight ahead)

**Neuroanatomy of internuclear ophthalmoplegia
(INO)** (shown: left INO on rightward gaze)

Right trochlear palsy (looking straight ahead)

Abducens palsy (looking straight ahead)

Bilateral INO
(leftward, rightward, and downward gaze)

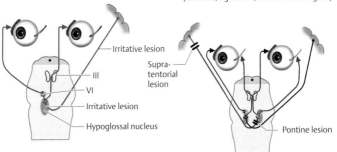

Rightward gaze deviation
(irritative lesion: left, supratentorial; right, pontine)

Conjugate supranuclear paresis of leftward gaze
(right supratentorial lesion or left pontine destructive lesion)

Cranial Nerves

87

Nystagmus is involuntary rhythmic movement of the eyes consisting of slow movement in one direction and rapid return movement in the other. The slow component is caused by disturbances of the motor and stabilizing systems of the eye (p. 84) or because of ocular muscle paresis; the fast component represents the rapid return movement of pontine generators. Although the slow component is the actual pathological component of nystagmus, the direction of nystagmus is conventionally said to be that of its fast component, which is easier to detect. The intensity of nystagmus increases when the patient gazes in the direction of the fast component. Nystagmus can be further classified according to the type of movement as *pendular, circular, or torsional (rotatory)*.

Examination. The examiner first observes the eyes on primary gaze, then during horizontal and vertical pursuit (fixation of gaze on a slowly moving object) and vergence. Nystagmus of labyrinthine origin is observed best with Frenzel spectacles (preventing visual fixation and giving the examiner a magnified view of the eyes). The following features of nystagmus are assessed: *positional-dependence, coordination* (conjugate, dissociated), *direction* (horizontal, vertical, rotatory, retracting, pendular), *amplitude* (fine, medium, coarse), and *frequency* (slow, moderate, fast).

Physiological Nystagmus

Physiological nystagmus serves to stabilize the visual image while the head and body are moving or when the individual looks at a moving object. The different types include *congenital nystagmus* (often X-linked recessive; fixation nystagmus is most pronounced when gazing fixedly on an object; the direction of nystagmus is usually horizontal), *spasmus nutans* (pendular nystagmus beginning in the first year of life; often accompanied by nodding of the head and torticollis; disappears spontaneously), *end-position nystagmus* (occurs during rapid movement; extreme lateral gaze; usually only a few beats), and *optokinetic nystagmus* (its absence is pathological; see p. 84).

Pathological Nystagmus

Gaze-evoked nystagmus occurs only in certain direction(s) of gaze. The main causes are drug intoxication and brain stem or cerebellar disturbances. A slower and coarser *gaze-paretic nystagmus* may be seen in association with supranuclear or peripheral *gaze palsy*, beating in the direction of the paretic gaze. Peripheral palsy of an eye muscle may cause unilateral nystagmus of the affected eye.

Spontaneous nystagmus is that which occurs when the eyes are in the primary position; it is usually caused by vestibular dysfunction and is rarely congenital.

Peripheral vestibular nystagmus (cf. p. 58) can be seen in patients with benign paroxysmal positional vertigo, vestibular neuritis, Ménière disease, vascular compression of the vestibular nerve, and labyrinthine fistula. Nystagmus decreases on fixation and increases when fixation is blocked (lid closure, Frenzel spectacles). Most patients exhibit rotatory nystagmus that either beats continually toward the nonaffected ear, or else begins a short time after a change of position (*positional nystagmus* toward the lower ear, see p. 58).

Central vestibular nystagmus (p. 58) is caused by lesions of the brain stem (vestibular nuclei, vestibulocerebellum) or of the thalamocortical projections. It is usually accompanied by other brain stem or cerebellar signs, does not decrease on fixation, depends on the direction of gaze, and usually persists. Central *positional nystagmus* does not exhibit latency, is not affected by the rate of positional change, occurs with changes of position to either side, beats toward the higher ear, and is not exhaustible, stopping only when the patient is returned to the neutral position. Because positional information from vestibular, visual, and somatosensory systems is integrated in the vestibulo-ocular reflex (VOR; see pp. 26, 84), the phenomena associated with nystagmus can be explained as functional disturbances in one of the major three spatial planes of action of the VOR. Lesions cause an imbalance between the neural inputs to the VOR concerning the two sides of the affected plane. Depending on which plane is affected, the resulting nystagmus may be *horizontal* (horizontal plane; lesion of the vestibular nuclei), *vertical* (sagittal plane; pontomesencephalic, pontomedullary, or floccular lesion), or *torsional* (coronal plane; pontomesencephalic or pontomedullary lesion). Vertical nystagmus (upbeat or downbeat) is always due to a central lesion.

Direction of nystagmus

Primary gaze

Gaze-evoked nystagmus
(no nystagmus on primary gaze)

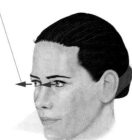

Horizontal plane = yaw
(tendency to fall to ipsilateral side; diminished
response to caloric testing in ipsilateral ear)

Spontaneous nystagmus

Retraction nystagmus
(bilateral dorsal midbrain
lesion)

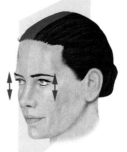

Sagittal plane = pitch
(tendency to fall forward/backwards;
"elevator" sensation)

Primary gaze

Peripheral vestibular nystagmus (no nystagmus on primary gaze)

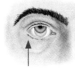
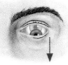

Skew deviation (vertical disconjugate gaze)
Vertical up- and downbeat nystagmus (brain stem lesion)

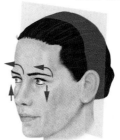

Frontal plane = roll
(tendency to fall sideways, lateropulsion)

**Central vestibular nystagmus,
spatial planes**

The colored part of the eye, or *iris* (Greek "rainbow"), is the posterior wall of the anterior ocular chamber. Its inner edge forms the margin of the pupil. The sphincter pupillae muscle contracts the pupil, and the dilator pupillae muscle dilates it. The upper eyelid contains two muscles: the superior tarsal muscle receives sympathetic innervation, and the levator palpebrae superioris muscle is innervated by the oculomotor nerve.

Nerve Pathways

Parasympathetic fibers. The preganglionic fibers arise in the accessory oculomotor nucleus (*Edinger–Westphal nucleus*), travel in the oculomotor nerve along its outer edge, and enter the ciliary ganglion. The postganglionic fibers travel to the ciliary and sphincter pupillae muscles in the short ciliary nerves (of which there are up to 20). The parasympathetic fibers and all others on the outer aspect of CN III receive their blood supply from the pial vessels, while fibers in the interior of the nerve are supplied by the vasa nervorum.

Sympathetic fibers. The central sympathetic fibers exit from the posterolateral portion of the hypothalamus (first preganglionic neurons), then pass ipsilaterally through the tegmentum of the mid brain and pons and through the lateral medulla to form a synapse onto the second preganglionic neurons in the intermediolateral cell column of the spinal cord (ciliospinal center), at levels C8–T2. Most of the fibers exit the spinal cord with the ventral root of T1 and join with the sympathetic trunk, which lies adjacent to the pleural dome at this level. They travel with the ansa subclavia around the subclavian artery and pass through the inferior (stellate) and middle cervical ganglia to the superior cervical ganglion, where they form a (third) synapse onto the postganglionic neurons. Postganglionic fibers to the pupil travel along the course of the internal carotid artery (carotid plexus) and the ophthalmic artery, then in the nasociliary nerve (a branch of CN V) and, finally, the long ciliary nerves, which innervate the dilator pupillae muscle. Other postganglionic fibers of the sympathetic system pass to the sweat glands, the orbital muscles (bridging the inferior orbital fissure), the superior and inferior tarsal muscles, and the conjunctival vessels. Fibers to the sweat glands arise at the T3–T4 level and form a synapse with the third neuron in the stellate ganglion; thus, nerve root lesions at C8–T2 do not impair sweating.

Light Reflex

The light reflex regulates the diameter of the pupils according to the amount of light falling on the eye. Each pupil constricts in response to light and dilates in the dark. The afferent arm of the reflex arc consists of fibers of the optic nerve that decussate in the optic chiasm, then pass around the lateral geniculate body and terminate in the mid brain pretectal area, both ipsilaterally and contralaterally. The parasympathetic fibers are the efferent arm. The Edinger–Westphal nuclei of the two sides are connected to each other by interneurons; thus, impulses from each optic nerve arrive at both Edinger–Westphal nuclei, and light falling on one eye leads to contraction of both the ipsilateral pupil (direct light reflex) and the contralateral pupil (consensual light reflex). The pupillary diameter in moderate ambient light is normally 3–4 mm. Excessive pupillary constriction (<2 mm) is referred to as *miosis*, and excessive dilatation (>5 mm) as *mydriasis*. *Anisocoria* (inequality of the diameters of the pupils) often indicates a diseased state (see below); it may be physiological but, if so, is usually mild.

The Near Response: Convergence, Pupilloconstriction, Accommodation

When a subject watches an approaching object, three things happen: the eyes converge through the action of the medial rectus muscles; the pupils constrict; and the curvature of the lens increases through the action of the ciliary muscle (accommodation). The near response may be initiated voluntarily (by squinting) but is most often the result of a reflex, whose afferent arm consists of the visual pathway to the visual cortex. The efferent arm for convergence consists of descending fibers to the pretectal convergence center (*Perlia's nucleus*) and onward to the oculomotor nucleus (nuclear area for the medial rectus muscles); the efferent arm for pupilloconstriction and accommodation is the parasympathetic projection of the Edinger–Westphal nucleus through the oculomotor nerve to the sphincter pupillae and ciliary muscles.

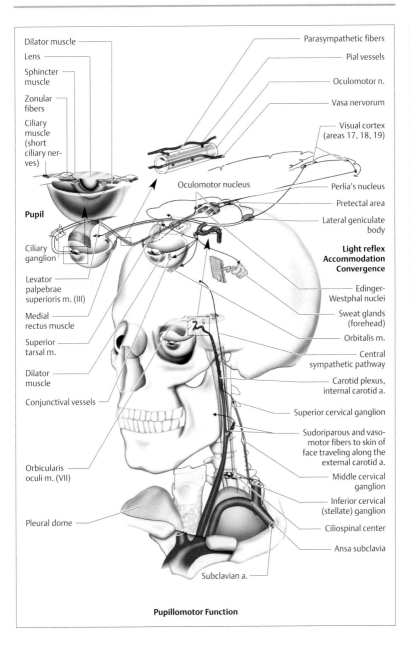

Dilator muscle

Lens

Sphincter muscle

Zonular fibers

Ciliary muscle (short ciliary nerves)

Pupil

Ciliary ganglion

Levator palpebrae superioris m. (III)

Medial rectus muscle

Superior tarsal m.

Dilator muscle

Conjunctival vessels

Orbicularis oculi m. (VII)

Pleural dome

Oculomotor nucleus

Subclavian a.

Parasympathetic fibers

Pial vessels

Oculomotor n.

Vasa nervorum

Visual cortex (areas 17, 18, 19)

Perlia's nucleus

Pretectal area

Lateral geniculate body

Light reflex Accommodation Convergence

Edinger-Westphal nuclei

Sweat glands (forehead)

Orbitalis m.

Central sympathetic pathway

Carotid plexus, internal carotid a.

Superior cervical ganglion

Sudoriparous and vaso-motor fibers to skin of face traveling along the external carotid a.

Middle cervical ganglion

Inferior cervical (stellate) ganglion

Ciliospinal center

Ansa subclavia

Cranial Nerves

Cranial Nerves

Examination. The size and shape of the pupils are first assessed in diffuse light with the patient looking at a distant object to prevent the near response. The room is then darkened and the direct light reflex of each pupil is tested at varying light intensities (by varying the distance of the lamp from the eye). If both pupils constrict when illuminated, there is no *efferent* pupillary defect. Next, in the *swinging flashlight test*, the examiner indirectly illuminates one eye with a bright light for ca. 2 seconds, then quickly switches the light to the other eye, and back again, some 5–7 times. The normal finding is that the two pupils are always of equal diameter; an abnormal finding indicates asymmetry of the *afferent* arm of the light reflex on the two sides, e. g., because of an optic nerve lesion (Marcus Gunn pupillary escape phenomenon). If either of these tests is abnormal, or if the pupils are significantly unequal, the near response should be tested and the direct and consensual light reflexes should be tested separately in each eye. It is easier to identify which pupil is abnormal by observing *both* phases of the light response (constriction and dilatation): both are slower in the abnormal pupil. In *light–near dissociation*, the pupils constrict as part of the near response, but not in response to light. Pharmacological pupil testing may be necessary in some cases.

Parasympathetic Denervation (Unilateral Mydriasis)

Oculomotor palsy (p. 86) is accompanied by mydriasis only when the parasympathetic fibers on the margin of the oculomotor nerve are affected. This is usually *not* the case in ischemic neuropathy of CN III (e. g., in diabetes mellitus), because the marginal fibers receive their blood supply from pial vessels (p. 90). A *tonic pupil* is a mydriatic pupil with light–near dissociation. This condition may be due to local causes (infection, temporal arteritis) or to systemic diseases such as Adie syndrome (+ reduction/absence of tendon reflexes in the legs) and Ross syndrome (+ hyporeflexia + segmental hypohidrosis). The use of anticholinergic agents (atropine eyedrops, scopolamine patch) causes iatrogenic mydriasis.

Sympathetic Denervation (Unilateral Miosis)

Horner syndrome is produced by a lesion at any site along the sympathetic pathway to the eye and is characterized by unilateral miosis (with sluggish dilatation) and ptosis; anhidrosis (absence of sweating) and enophthalmos are part of the syndrome but are of no practical diagnostic value. The affected pupil will fail to dilate in response to the instillation of 5% cocaine eyedrops. *Preganglionic* lesions (i.e., those proximal to the superior cervical ganglion) can be distinguished from *postganglionic* lesions by the instillation of 5% pholedrine eyedrops (at least three days after the cocaine test); the miotic pupil dilates *more* than the normal pupil if the lesion is preganglionic, symmetrically if it is postganglionic. Central Horner syndrome (*first preganglionic neuron*) may be due to lesions of hypothalamus, brain stem, or cervicothoracic spinal cord; the *second preganglionic neuron* may be affected by lesions of the brachial plexus, apical thorax, mediastinum, or neck; the *postganglionic neuron* may be affected by carotid dissection or lesions of the skull base.

Supranuclear Lesions

Lesions above the oculomotor nucleus tend to cause bilateral pupillary dysfunction; the most common cause is dorsal compression of the midbrain (Parinaud syndrome; p. 358). Neurosyphilis produces *Argyll–Robertson pupils*—unequal, irregularly miotic pupils with a variable degree of iris atrophy, and light–near dissociation.

Coma (see also p. 118)

The cause of coma may be structural, metabolic, or toxic. *Pupilloconstriction* is produced by opiates, alcohol, and barbiturates, *pupillary dilation* by atropine poisoning (mushrooms, belladonna), tricyclic antidepressants, botulinum toxin, cocaine, and other drugs. Focal lesions (clivus, midbrain) may cause unilateral or bilateral pupillary areflexia and mydriasis. Unilateral miosis is seen in central Horner syndrome, and bilateral miosis (pinpoint pupils) in acute pontine dysfunction.

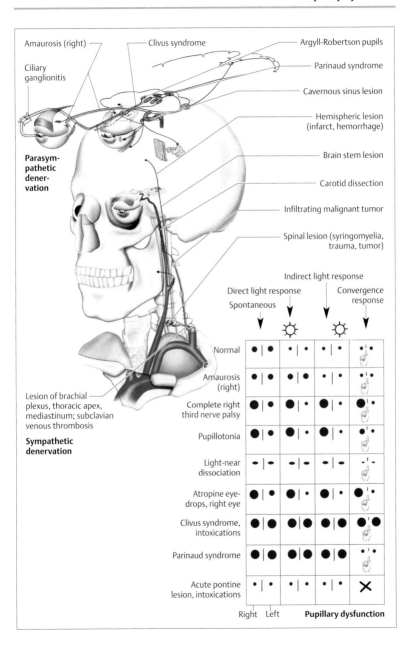

Amaurosis (right)

Clivus syndrome

Argyll-Robertson pupils

Ciliary ganglionitis

Parinaud syndrome

Cavernous sinus lesion

Hemispheric lesion (infarct, hemorrhage)

Parasym-pathetic dener-vation

Brain stem lesion

Carotid dissection

Infiltrating malignant tumor

Spinal lesion (syringomyelia, trauma, tumor)

Lesion of brachial plexus, thoracic apex, mediastinum; subclavian venous thrombosis

Sympathetic denervation

Indirect light response

Direct light response

Convergence response

Spontaneous

	Spontaneous	Direct light response	Indirect light response	Convergence response
Normal				
Amaurosis (right)				
Complete right third nerve palsy				
Pupillotonia				
Light-near dissociation				
Atropine eye-drops, right eye				
Clivus syndrome, intoxications				
Parinaud syndrome				
Acute pontine lesion, intoxications				

Right   Left   **Pupillary dysfunction**

Cranial Nerves

93

Peripheral Connections of the Trigeminal Ganglion

Ophthalmic nerve (V/1). V/1 gives off a recurrent branch to the tentorium cerebelli and falx cerebri (*tentorial branch*) and the lacrimal, frontal, and nasociliary nerves, which enter the orbit through the superior orbital fissure. The *lacrimal nerve* supplies the lacrimal gland, conjunctiva, and lateral aspect of the upper eyelid. The *frontal nerve* divides into the supratrochlear nerve, which supplies the inner canthus, and the supraorbital nerve, which supplies the conjunctiva, upper eyelid, skin of the forehead, and frontal sinus. Finally, the *nasociliary nerve* gives off branches to the skin of the medial canthus, bridge and tip of the nose, the mucous membranes of the nasal sinus (anterior ethmoid nerve) and sphenoid sinus, and the ethmoid cells (posterior ethmoid nerve).

Maxillary nerve (V/2). Before entering the foramen rotundum, V/2 gives off a *middle meningeal branch* that innervates the dura mater of the medial cranial fossa and the middle meningeal artery. Other branches innervate the skin of the zygomatic region and temple (*zygomatic nerve*), and of the cheek (*infraorbital nerve*). The infraorbital nerve enters the orbit through the inferior orbital fissure, then exits from it again through the infraorbital canal; it innervates the cheek and the maxillary teeth (superior alveolar nerve).

Mandibular nerve (V/3). V/3 gives off a meningeal branch (nervus spinosus) just distal from its exit from the foramen ovale that reenters the cranial cavity through the foramen spinosum to supply the dura mater, part of the sphenoid sinus, and the mastoid air cells. In its further course, V/3 gives off the *auriculotemporal nerve* (supplies the temporomandibular joint, skin of the temple in front of the ear, external auditory canal, eardrum, parotid gland, and anterior surface of the auricle), the *lingual nerve* (tonsils, mucous membranes of the floor of the mouth, gums of the lower front teeth, and mucosa of the anterior two-thirds of the tongue), the *inferior alveolar nerve* (teeth of the lower jaw and lateral gums), the *mental nerve* (lower lip, skin of the chin, and gums of front teeth), and the *buccal nerve* (buccal mucosa).

The motor root of CN V contains motor fibers from the trigeminal motor nucleus in the pons and joins the mandibular nerve to innervate the muscles of mastication (temporalis, masseter, and medial and lateral pterygoid muscles), hyoid muscles (anterior belly of the digastric muscle, mylohyoid muscle), muscles of the soft palate (tensor veli palatini muscle), and tensor tympani muscle.

Central Connections of the Trigeminal Ganglion

Sensory fibers mediating epicritic sensation terminate in the *principal sensory nucleus* of the trigeminal nerve, which is located in the pons. Fibers terminating in this nucleus also form the afferent arm of the corneal reflex, whose efferent arm is the facial nerve. Fibers mediating protopathic sensation terminate in the *spinal nucleus* of the trigeminal nerve, a column of cells that extends down the medulla to the upper cervical spinal cord. The spinal nucleus is somatotopically organized: its uppermost portion is responsible for perioral sensation, while lower portions serve progressively more peripheral areas of the face in an "onion-skin" arrangement. The caudal portion of the spinal nucleus of the trigeminal nerve also receives fibers from cranial nerves VII, IX, and X carrying nociceptive impulses from the ear, posterior third of the tongue, pharynx, and larynx.

Mesencephalic nucleus of trigeminal nerve. This midbrain nucleus, too, contains pseudounipolar neurons, whose long dendrites pass through the trigeminal ganglion without forming a synapse and carry afferent impulses from masticatory muscle spindles and pressure receptors (for regulation of the force of chewing).

Trigeminocortical tracts. Output fibers of the spinal nucleus of the trigeminal nerve decussate in the brain stem and ascend, by way of the *trigeminal lemniscus* (adjacent to the spinothalamic tract) and the medial lemniscus, to the ventral posteromedial (VPM) and posterior nuclei of the thalamus, where the third neuron of the sensory pathway is located. These thalamic nuclei project via the internal capsule to the postcentral gyrus. The supranuclear innervation of the *motor nucleus* of the trigeminal nerve is from the caudal portions of the precentral gyrus (bilaterally), by way of the corticonuclear tract.

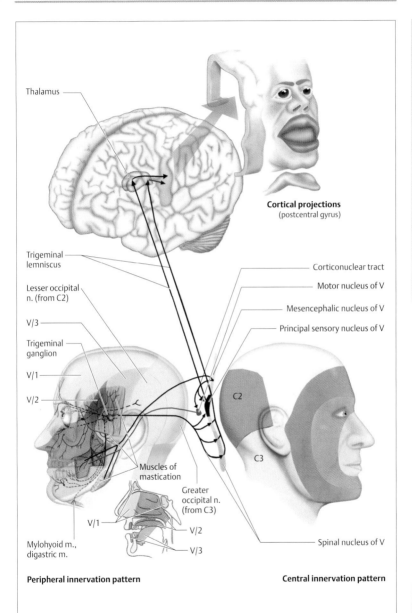

Thalamus

Cortical projections
(postcentral gyrus)

Trigeminal lemniscus

Corticonuclear tract

Lesser occipital n. (from C2)

Motor nucleus of V

Mesencephalic nucleus of V

V/3

Principal sensory nucleus of V

Trigeminal ganglion

V/1

V/2

C2

Muscles of mastication

C3

Greater occipital n. (from C3)

V/1

V/2

V/3

Mylohyoid m., digastric m.

Spinal nucleus of V

Peripheral innervation pattern

Central innervation pattern

Nerve Pathways

Central motor pathway. The corticonuclear tract originates in the precentral cortex (area 8), passes in front of the pyramidal tract in the genu of the internal capsule, then travels in the medial portion of the ipsilateral cerebral peduncle to reach the facial nucleus in the lower pons. The supranuclear fibers serving the upper facial muscles (frontalis and corrugator supercilii muscles, upper part of orbicularis oculi muscle, superior auricular muscle) decussate incompletely in the pons, so that these muscles have bilateral supranuclear innervation; fibers serving the remaining muscles decussate completely, so that they have contralateral innervation only. The precentral cortex is responsible for the voluntary component of facial expression, while *nonpyramidal motor connections* subserve the automatic and emotive components of facial expression. These anatomical facts explain the *dissociated functional deficits* that set supranuclear facial palsies apart from nuclear or subnuclear palsies, and enable their further differentiation into cortical and subcortical types (see below).

Peripheral motor pathway. The facial nucleus and its efferent fibers are somatotopically organized. The emerging fibers first run dorsomedially, then turn anterolaterally to pass around the abducens nucleus (inner genu of facial nerve), and exit the brain stem as the facial nerve in the cerebellopontine angle, near CN VI and VIII. The facial nerve enters the internal acoustic meatus together with the nervus intermedius and CN VIII, then leaves the meatus to enter the facial canal; it passes between the cochlea and labyrinth, then turns back again (outer genu of facial nerve). After leaving the skull at the stylomastoid foramen, it continues inside the parotid gland and gives off motor branches to all muscles of facial expression as well as the platysma, ear muscles, stapedius, digastric (posterior belly), and stylohyoid muscles.

Sensory and parasympathetic fibers (nervus intermedius). Sensory fibers from the geniculate ganglion travel to the superior salivatory nucleus, nucleus of the tractus solitarius (p. 78), and spinal nucleus of the trigeminal nerve (p. 94). *Taste fibers* from the anterior two-thirds of the tongue (lingual nerve) and the soft palate (greater petrosal nerve) join the chorda tympani. Preganglionic parasympathetic fibers travel in the greater petrosal nerve to the pterygopalatine ganglion, from which postganglionic fibers pass to the lacrimal, nasal, and palatine glands; other preganglionic fibers travel in the chorda tympani to the submandibular ganglion, from which postganglionic fibers pass to the sublingual and submandibular glands. Connections via the contralateral medial lemniscus to the thalamus and postcentral gyrus, and to the hypothalamus, subserve reflex salivation in response to the smell and taste of food. The facial nerve carries *sensory fibers* from the external auditory canal, eardrum, external ear, and mastoid region (posterior auricular nerve), as well as *proprioceptive fibers* from the muscles it innervates.

Functional Systems

The voluntary component of facial expression is mediated by the precentral cortex, in which the face is somatotopically represented. Only the upper facial muscles have bilateral supranuclear innervation; thus, a central supranuclear facial palsy does not affect eye closure or the ability to knit one's brow. Yet facial palsy that spares the upper face is not necessarily of supranuclear origin: because the facial nucleus and nerve are also somatotopically organized, incomplete lesions of these structures may also produce a similar appearance. An important and sometimes helpful distinguishing feature is that a supranuclear palsy may affect facial expression in the lower face in a dissociated fashion. Supranuclear facial palsy due to a *cortical* lesion impairs voluntary facial expression, but tends to spare emotional expression (laughing, crying); that due to a *subcortical* lesion (e. g., in Parkinson disease or hereditary dystonia) does just the opposite.

The following reflexes are of clinical significance (A = afferent arm, E = efferent arm): *orbicularis oculi reflex* (blink reflex; A: V/1; E: VII); *corneal reflex* (A: V/1; E: VII); *sucking reflex* (A: V/2, V/3, XI; E: V, VII, IX, X, XII), *palmomental reflex* (A: thenar skin/muscles; E: VII), *acoustic blink reflex* (A: VIII; E: VII), *visual blink reflex* (A: II; E: VII), *orbicularis oris reflex* (snout reflex; A: V/2; E: VII).

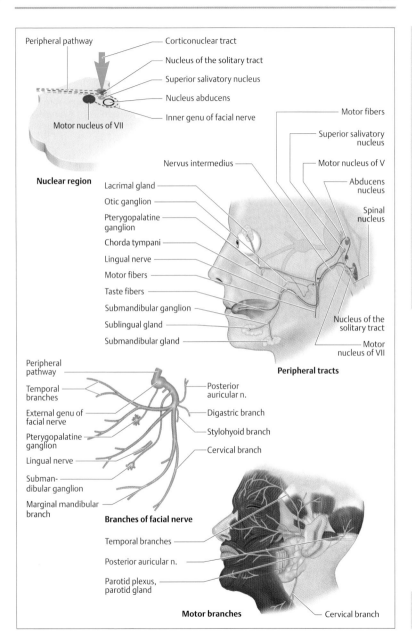

Peripheral pathway

Corticonuclear tract

Nucleus of the solitary tract

Superior salivatory nucleus

Nucleus abducens

Inner genu of facial nerve

Motor nucleus of VII

Motor fibers

Superior salivatory nucleus

Motor nucleus of V

Abducens nucleus

Spinal nucleus

Nervus intermedius

Nuclear region

Lacrimal gland

Otic ganglion

Pterygopalatine ganglion

Chorda tympani

Lingual nerve

Motor fibers

Taste fibers

Submandibular ganglion

Sublingual gland

Submandibular gland

Nucleus of the solitary tract

Motor nucleus of VII

Peripheral tracts

Peripheral pathway

Temporal branches

External genu of facial nerve

Pterygopalatine ganglion

Lingual nerve

Submandibular ganglion

Marginal mandibular branch

Posterior auricular n.

Digastric branch

Stylohoid branch

Cervical branch

Branches of facial nerve

Temporal branches

Posterior auricular n.

Parotid plexus, parotid gland

Motor branches

Cervical branch

Cranial Nerves

97

Examination. Motor function is assessed at rest (asymmetry of face/skin folds, atrophy, spontaneous movements, blink rate) and during voluntary movement (forehead, eyelids and brows, cheeks, mouth region, platysma). Trigeminal nerve dysfunction (V/1) causes unilateral or bilateral *absence* of the *blink reflex*; facial palsy may impair or abolish the blink response, but lagophthalmos persists, because the extraocular muscles are unimpaired. Similar logic applies to other facial nerve reflexes (p. 96). If the patient complains of loss of taste, it is tested accordingly (p. 78). *Lacrimation* can be tested with the Schirmer test, which, however, is positive only if tear flow is minimal or absent. The *salivation test* is used to measure the flow of saliva from the submandibular and sublingual glands. The *stapedius reflex* is tested by measuring the contraction of the stapedius muscle in response to an acoustic stimulus.

Facial Nerve Lesions

Site of Lesion	Clinical Features
Cortex or internal capsule	Contralateral central facial palsy (+ pyramidal tract lesion, p. 46). Emotional component of facial expression is unimpaired
Brainstem, facial nucleus	Pontine syndrome (p. 70, 72, 359), myokymia
Cerebellopontine angle	Ipsilateral peripheral facial palsy (+V/1–2, VI, VIII; p. 74). Hemifacial spasm ipsilateral.
Base of skull, internal acoustic meatus	Peripheral facial palsy (+ other cranial nerve palsies; p. 74)
Geniculate ganglion	Peripheral facial palsy, dysgeusia, hyposalivation, diminished lacrimation, ear ache, hyperacusis (due to absence of stapedius reflex)
Facial canal distal to geniculate ganglion	Peripheral facial palsy, dysgeusia, hyposalivation (but normal lacrimation), hyperacusis
Proximal to stylomastoid foramen	Peripheral facial palsy, dysgeusia, hyposalivation, intact stapedius reflex
Stylomastoid foramen	Purely motor peripheral facial palsy
Parotid gland, facial region	More or less complete, purely motor facial palsy; palsy due to lesions of individual branches of the facial nerve

For signs and symptoms of facial nerve lesions, see Table 7 on p. 362.

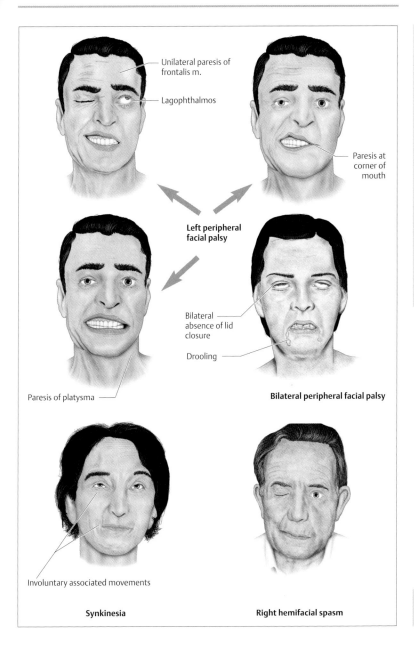

Unilateral paresis of frontalis m.

Lagophthalmos

Paresis at corner of mouth

Left peripheral facial palsy

Bilateral absence of lid closure

Drooling

Paresis of platysma

Bilateral peripheral facial palsy

Involuntary associated movements

Synkinesia

Right hemifacial spasm

Cranial Nerves

Perception of Sound

Sound waves enter the ear through the external acoustic meatus and travel through the ear canal to the tympanic membrane (eardrum), setting it into vibration. Vibrations in the 20–16 000 Hz range (most sensitive range, 2000–5000 Hz) are transmitted to the auditory ossicles (malleus, incus, stapes). The base of the stapes vibrates against the oval window, creating waves in the perilymph in the vestibular canal (*scala vestibuli*) of the cochlea; these waves are then transmitted through the connecting passage at the cochlear apex (*helicotrema*) to the perilymph of the tympanic canal (*scala tympani*). (Oscillations of the round window compensate for volume changes caused by oscillations of the oval window. Sound waves can also reach the cochlea by direct conduction through the skull bone.) *Migrating waves* are set in motion along the basilar membrane of the cochlear duct; they travel from the stapes to the helicotrema at decreasing speed, partly because the basilar membrane is less tense as it nears the cochlear apex. These waves have their amplitude maxima at different sites along the basilar membrane, depending on frequency (*tonotopicity*): there results a frequency-specific excitation of the receptor cells for hearing—the hair cells of the organ of Corti, which is adjacent to the basilar membrane as it winds through the cochlea.

Cochlear Nerve

The tonotopicity of the basilar membrane causes each hair cell to be tuned to a specific sound frequency (*spectral analysis*). Each hair cell is connected to an afferent fiber of the cochlear nerve inside the organ of Corti. The cochlear nerve is formed by the central processes of the bipolar neurons of the cochlear ganglion (the first neurons of the auditory pathway); it exits from the petrous bone at the internal acoustic meatus, travels a short distance in the subarachnoid space, and enters the brain stem in the cerebellopontine angle. Central auditory processing involves interpretation of the pattern and temporal sequence of the action potentials carried in the cochlear nerve.

Auditory Pathway

As it ascends from the cochlea to the auditory cortex, the auditory pathway gives off collateral projections to the cerebellum, the oculomotor and facial nuclei, cervical motor neurons, and the reticular activating system, which form the afferent arm of the acoustically mediated reflexes.

Axons of the cochlear nerve originating in the cochlear apex and base terminate in the anterior and posterior cochlear nuclei, respectively. These nuclei contain the second neurons of the auditory pathway. Fibers from the *posterior cochlear nucleus* decussate in the floor of the fourth ventricle, then ascend to enter the lateral lemniscus and synapse in the inferior colliculus (third neuron). The inferior colliculus projects to the medial geniculate body (fourth neuron), which, in turn, projects via the acoustic radiation to the auditory cortex. The acoustic radiation passes below the thalamus and runs in the posterior limb of the internal capsule. Fibers from the *anterior cochlear nucleus* also decussate, mainly in the trapezoid body, and synapse onto the next (third) neuron in the olivary nucleus or the nucleus of the lateral lemniscus. This branch of the auditory pathway then continues through the lateral lemniscus to the inferior colliculus and onward through the acoustic radiation to the auditory cortex.

The *primary auditory cortex* (area 41: Heschl's gyrus, transverse temporal gyri) is located in the temporal operculum (i.e., the portion of the temporal lobe overlying the insula and separated from it by the sylvian cistern). Areas 42 and 22 make up the *secondary auditory cortex*, in which auditory signals are further processed, recognized, and compared with auditory memories. The auditory cortex of each side of the brain receives information from both ears (contralateral more than ipsilateral); unilateral lesions of the central auditory pathway or auditory cortex do not cause clinically relevant hearing loss.

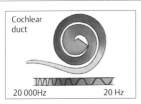

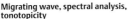

20 000Hz   20 Hz

Migrating wave, spectral analysis, tonotopicity

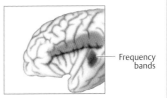

Frequency bands

Auditory cortex

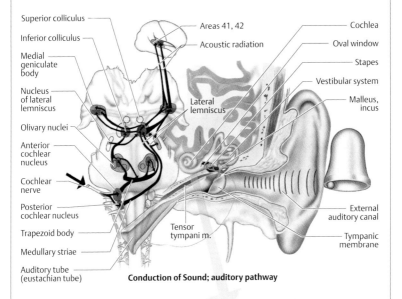

Superior colliculus

Inferior colliculus

Medial geniculate body

Nucleus of lateral lemniscus

Olivary nuclei

Anterior cochlear nucleus

Cochlear nerve

Posterior cochlear nucleus

Trapezoid body

Medullary striae

Auditory tube (eustachian tube)

Areas 41, 42

Acoustic radiation

Lateral lemniscus

Tensor tympani m.

Cochlea

Oval window

Stapes

Vestibular system

Malleus, incus

External auditory canal

Tympanic membrane

Conduction of Sound; auditory pathway

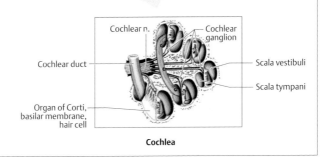

Cochlear n.

Cochlear ganglion

Cochlear duct

Organ of Corti, basilar membrane, hair cell

Scala vestibuli

Scala tympani

Cochlea

Cranial Nerves

Impairment of swallowing (deglutition) is called *dysphagia*; pain on swallowing is called *odynophagia*. Dysphagia or vomiting due to neurological disease often causes *aspiration* (entrance of solid or liquid food into the airway below the vocal cords). *Globus hystericus* is a foreign-body sensation in the swallowing pathway independent of the act of swallowing. Despite its name, it is not always psychogenic; organic causes include Zenker diverticulum and gastroesophageal reflux.

Deglutition

Mechanism. The food is ground by the teeth and moistened with saliva to form *chyme*, which is molded by the tongue into an easily swallowed bolus (oral preparatory phase). The tongue pushes the bolus into the oropharynx (oral phase) to initiate the reflex act of swallowing (pharyngeal phase). The lips and jaw close, the soft palate rises to seal off the nasopharynx, and the bolus bends the epiglottis backward. The bolus is pushed further back by the tongue, respiration briefly ceases, and the raised larynx occludes the airway. The upper esophageal sphincter slackens (cricopharyngeus, inferior pharyngeal constrictor, smooth muscle of upper portion of esophagus). Pressure from the tongue and pharyngeal peristalsis push the bolus past the epiglottis and into the esophagus (esophageal phase). The larynx is lowered, respiration is reinstated, and esophageal peristalsis propels the bolus into the stomach.

Nerve pathways. Fibers of CN V/2, VII, IX, and X to the nucleus ambiguus and the nucleus of the tractus solitarius (p. 78) make up the afferent arm of the swallowing reflex. The motor swallowing center (one on each side) lies adjacent to these nuclei and is associated with the upper medullary reticular formation; it coordinates the actions of the numerous muscles involved in swallowing. Efferent signals reach these muscles through CN V/3, VII, IX, X, and XII. Crossed and uncrossed supranuclear innervation is derived from the cerebral cortex (precentral and postcentral gyri, frontoparietal operculum, premotor cortex, and anterior insular region). Spinal motor neurons also participate (C1–C4).

Neurological Disturbances of Deglutition
(See Table 8 on p. 362)

The disturbance usually manifests itself at the beginning of the act of swallowing (e. g., a feeling of food stuck in the throat, the escape of liquid or solid food through the nose, choking, coughing). Associated inflammation of the swallowing pathway may cause odynophagia. Chronic dysphagia causes inadequate nutrition and weight loss. Neurogenic dysphagia usually impairs the swallowing of liquids more than solids; soft, chilled foods (like pudding or yogurt) are often easier to swallow. Sensory disturbances in the larynx and trachea, a diminished cough reflex, and muscle weakness may cause aspiration, sometimes unremarked by the patient (silent aspiration). The diagnostic evaluation of dysphagia may require special tests such as radiocinematography, video endoscopy, manometry, and pH measurement.

Cranial Nerves

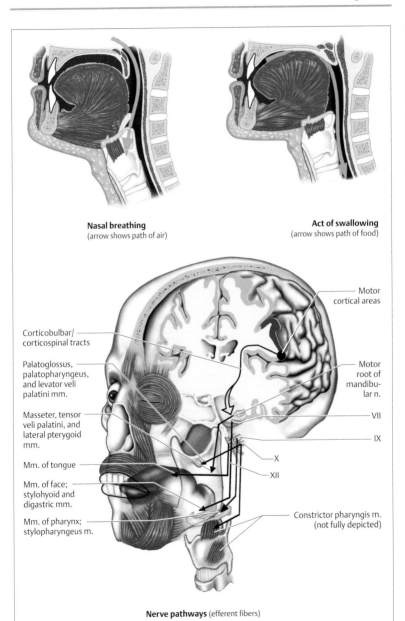

Nasal breathing
(arrow shows path of air)

Act of swallowing
(arrow shows path of food)

Motor
cortical areas

Corticobulbar/
corticospinal tracts

Palatoglossus,
palatopharyngeus,
and levator veli
palatini mm.

Motor
root of
mandibu-
lar n.

Masseter, tensor
veli palatini, and
lateral pterygoid
mm.

VII

IX

Mm. of tongue

X

Mm. of face;
stylohyoid and
digastric mm.

XII

Mm. of pharynx;
stylopharyngeus m.

Constrictor pharyngis m.
(not fully depicted)

Nerve pathways (efferent fibers)

There are two functionally and anatomically distinct types of somatic sensation and pain. The spatially and temporally precise perception of light tactile, noxious, and temperature stimuli is called *epicritic sensation*, and the more diffuse perception of stronger tactile, noxious, and temperature stimuli is called *protopathic sensation*. Sensation in the deep tissues (muscles, viscera) is predominantly protopathic.

Receptors

Sensory stimuli affect the nervous system by physically interacting with *receptors*. *Exteroceptors* respond to external stimuli (mechanical, thermal, optic, acoustic, olfactory, gustatory); *interoceptors* respond to internal stimuli (stretch, pressure, chemical irritation of internal organs). A stimulus activates a receptor only if it is sufficiently intense (above threshold). Receptors are classified according to their activating stimuli: *mechanoreceptors* (pressure, touch; proprioceptive sensations such as joint postion, muscle contraction, muscle stretch; hearing, sense of balance), *thermoreceptors* (heat, cold), *chemoreceptors* (pain, smell, itch, taste), and *photoreceptors* (light). *Cutaneous receptors* include both "free" nerve endings and specially adapted receptors (e. g., corpuscles of Meissner and Vater-Pacini). The former type mainly subserve pain and temperature sense, the latter tactile sensation (touch, pressure, vibration). In hair-covered skin there are tactile receptors around the hair roots.

Nerve Pathways

From the receptor, information is transmitted to the afferent fibers of the pseudounipolar spinal ganglion cells, whose efferent fibers reach the spinal cord by way of the dorsal root. A synapse onto a second neuron in the sensory pathway is made either immediately, in the posterior horn of the spinal cord (protopathic system), or more rostrally, in the brain stem (epicritic/lemniscal system). The highest level of the somatosensory pathway is the contralateral primary somatosensory cortex. The somatotopic organization of the somatosensory pathway is preserved at all levels.

Posterior column (epicritic/lemniscal system).
Fibers mediating sensation in the legs are in the fasciculus gracilis (medial), while those for the arms are in the fasciculus cuneatus (lateral). These fibers synapse onto the second sensory neuron in the corresponding somatosensory nuclei of the lower medulla (nucleus gracilis, nucleus cuneatus), which emit fibers that decussate and ascend in the contralateral medial lemniscus to the thalamus (ventral posterolateral nucleus, VPL). VPL projects to the postcentral gyrus by way of the internal capsule.

Anterolateral column (protopathic system).
Fibers of the protopathic pathway for *somatic sensation* (strong pressure, coarse touch) enter the spinal cord through the dorsal root and then ascend two or more segments before making a synapse in the ipsilateral posterior horn. Fibers originating in the posterior horn decussate in the anterior commissure of the spinal cord and enter the *anterior spinothalamic tract*, which is somatotopically arranged: fibers for the legs are anterolateral, fibers for the arms are posteromedial. The anterior spinothalamic tract traverses the brain stem adjacent to the medial lemniscus and terminates in VPL, which, in turn, projects to the postcentral gyrus. The protopathic pathway for *pain* (as well as tickle, itch, and temperature sensation) is organized in similar fashion: Central fibers of the first sensory neuron ascend 1 or 2 segments before making a synapse in the substantia gelatinosa of the posterior horn. Fibers from the posterior horn decussate and enter the lateral spinothalamic tract, which, like the anterior spinothalamic tract, projects to VPL; VPL projects in turn to the postcentral gyrus.

Spinocerebellar tracts (spinocerebellar system).
These tracts mediate proprioception. Fibers originating from muscles spindles and tendon organs make synapses onto the neurons of *Clarke's column* within the posterior horn at levels T1–L2, whose axons form the posterior spinocerebellar tract (ipsilateral) and the anterior spinocerebellar tract (both ipsilateral and contralateral). These tracts terminate in the spinocerebellum (p. 54).

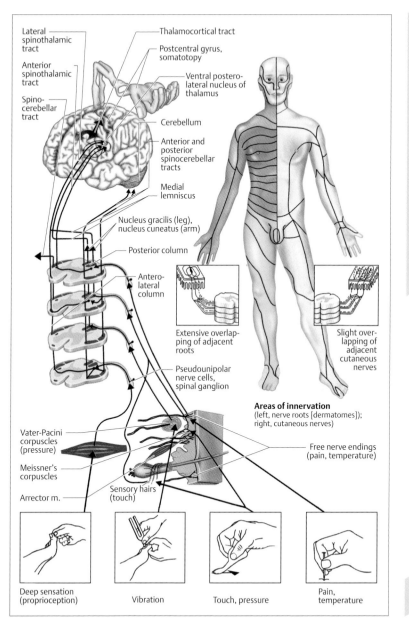

Lateral spinothalamic tract

Thalamocortical tract

Postcentral gyrus, somatotopy

Anterior spinothalamic tract

Ventral postero-lateral nucleus of thalamus

Spino-cerebellar tract

Cerebellum

Anterior and posterior spinocerebellar tracts

Medial lemniscus

Nucleus gracilis (leg), nucleus cuneatus (arm)

Posterior column

Antero-lateral column

Extensive overlapping of adjacent roots

Slight overlapping of adjacent cutaneous nerves

Pseudounipolar nerve cells, spinal ganglion

Areas of innervation
(left, nerve roots [dermatomes]); right, cutaneous nerves)

Vater-Pacini corpuscles (pressure)

Free nerve endings (pain, temperature)

Meissner's corpuscles

Arrector m.

Sensory hairs (touch)

Deep sensation (proprioception)

Vibration

Touch, pressure

Pain, temperature

Sensation

Sensory Disturbances

Examination. Somatic sensation is tested with the patient's eyes closed. The examiner tests each primary modality of *superficial sensation* (touch, pain, temperature), the patient's ability to distinguish different qualities of each modality (sharp/blunt, hot/cold, different intensities, two-point discrimination), and more complex sensory modalities (stereognosis, graphesthesia). Next, sensation to pressure and vibration stimuli are tested, as is acrognosis (posture sense), to evaluate *proprioception*. Sensory disturbances commonly cause disturbances of posture (tests: Romberg test, standing on one leg) or gait (p. 60).

Interpretation of findings. There is a wide range of normal findings. Apparent abnormalities should be interpreted in conjunction with findings of other types, such as abnormal reflexes or paresis. Sensory dysfunction may involve not only a diminution or absence of sensation (*hypesthesia, anesthesia*), but also sensations of abnormal type (*paresthesia*, such as prickling or formication) or spontaneous pain (*dysesthesia*, often of burning type). Patients often use the colloquial term "numbness" to mean hypesthesia, anesthesia, or paresthesia; the physician should ask specific questions to determine what is meant.

Localization of Sensory Disturbances

Clinical Features	Site of Lesion	Possible Causes[1]
Localized sensory disturbance (not in a dermatomal or peripheral nerve distribution)[2]	Cutaneous nerves/ receptors	Skin lesions, scars, lepromatous leprosy (dissociated sensory deficit[3] distally in the limbs, tip of nose, external ear)
Often pain and paresthesia at first, then sensory deficit, in a distribution depending on the site of the lesion	Distal peripheral nerve	Mononeuropathy (compression, tumor), mononeuritis multiplex (involvement of multiple peripheral nerves by vasculitis, diabetes mellitus, etc.)
Distal symmetrical sensory disturbances	Distal peripheral nerves	Polyneuropathy (diabetes mellitus, alcohol, drug/toxic, Guillain–Barré syndrome)
Bilateral symmetrical or asymmetrical thigh pain	Peripheral nerves, lumbar plexus	Diabetes mellitus
Multiple sensory and motor deficits in a single limb	Plexus	Trauma, compression, infection, ischemia, tumor, metabolic disturbance
Unilateral or bilateral, monoradicular or polyradicular deficits	Nerve root	Herniated disk, herpes zoster, Guillain–Barré syndrome, tumor, carcinomatous meningitis, paraneoplastic syndrome
Spinal ataxia, incomplete or complete cord transection syndrome (p. 48)	Spinal cord	Vascular, tumor, inflammatory/multiple sclerosis, hereditary, metabolic disease, trauma, malformation
Loss of position and vibration sense in the upper limbs and trunk, Lhermitte's sign	Craniocervical junction	Tumor, basilar impression
Contralateral dissociated or crossed sensory deficit (p. 70 ff)	Brainstem	Vascular, tumor, multiple sclerosis
Contralateral paresthesia and sensory deficits, pain, loss of vibration sense	Thalamus	Vascular (p. 170), tumor, multiple sclerosis
Paresthesia, contralateral sensory deficits (astereognosis, loss of position sense and two-point discrimination, inability to localize a stimulus, agraphesthesia)	Postcentral cortex	Vascular, tumor, trauma

1 The listing of possible causes is necessarily incomplete. **2** May be factitious or psychogenic.
3 Impairment or loss of pain and temperature sensation with preserved touch sensation.

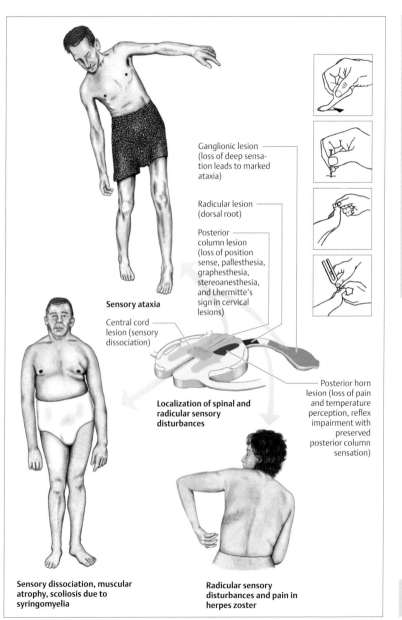

Ganglionic lesion (loss of deep sensation leads to marked ataxia)

Radicular lesion (dorsal root)

Posterior column lesion (loss of position sense, pallesthesia, graphesthesia, stereoanesthesia, and Lhermitte's sign in cervical lesions)

Sensory ataxia

Central cord lesion (sensory dissociation)

Localization of spinal and radicular sensory disturbances

Posterior horn lesion (loss of pain and temperature perception, reflex impairment with preserved posterior column sensation)

Sensory dissociation, muscular atrophy, scoliosis due to syringomyelia

Radicular sensory disturbances and pain in herpes zoster

Sensation

107

Pain is an unpleasant sensory and emotional experience associated with actual or potential tissue damage, or described in terms of such damage (International Association for the Study of Pain).

Pathogenesis

Pain results from the interaction of a noxious (i.e., pain-producing) stimulus with a receptor, and the subsequent transmission and processing of pain-related signals in the PNS and CNS; the entire process is called *nociception*. Pain evokes a behavioral response involving nocifensor activity as well as motor and autonomic reflexes.

Pain reception. Nociceptors for mechanical, thermal, and chemical stimuli are found in all body organs except the brain and spinal cord. By releasing neuropeptides, the nociceptors can produce a neurogenic sterile inflammatory response that enhances nociception (*peripheral sensitization*).

Pain transmission. Nociceptive impulses travel in peripheral nerves to the posterior horn of the spinal cord. Here, the incoming information is processed by both pain-specific and nonspecific (wide dynamic range) neurons. *Central sensitization* processes arising at this level may lower the nociceptor threshold and promote the development of chronic pain (such as phantom limb pain after amputation). Ascending impulses reach the brain through the spinothalamic and spinoreticular tracts as well as other pathways to a number of different brain regions involved in nociception.

Pain processing. The *reticular formation* regulates arousal reactions, autonomic reflexes, and emotional responses to pain. The *thalamus* relays and differentiates nociceptive stimuli. The *hypothalamus* mediates autonomic and neuroendocrine responses. The *limbic system* (p. 144) mediates emotional and motivation-related aspects of nociception. The *somatosensory cortex* is mainly responsible for pain differentiation and localization. *Descending pathways* that originate in these CNS areas also modulate nociception.

Neurotransmitters and neuropeptides are involved in nociception on different levels. Various neurotransmitters and neuropeptide systems play a role in the mechanism of action of one or more currently used analgesic agents (effective drugs in parantheses): glutamate (memantine); substance P (capsaicin); histamine (antihistamines); serotonin/norepinephrine (antidepressants); GABA (baclofen, diazepam); prostaglandins (nonsteroidal anti-inflammatory drugs); enkephalin, endorphin, dynorphin (opiates, opioids).

Types of Pain (See Table 9, p. 363)

Nociceptive pain, the "normal" type of pain, is that which arises from actual or potential tissue damage and results from the activation of nociceptors and subsequent processing in an intact nervous system. *Somatic pain* is the variety of nociceptive pain mediated by somatosensory afferent fibers; it is usually easily localizable and of sharp, aching, or throbbing quality. Postoperative, traumatic, and local inflammatory pain are often of this variety. *Visceral pain* is harder to localize (e.g., headache in meningitis, biliary colic, gastritis, mesenteric infarction) and may be dull, cramplike, piercing, or waxing and waning. It is mediated peripherally by C fibers and centrally by spinal cord pathways terminating mainly in the limbic system. This may explain the unpleasant and emotionally distressing nature of visceral pain. Visceral pain may be felt in its site of origin or may be *referred* to another site (e.g., from the diaphragm to the shoulder).

Neuropathic pain is that which is caused by damage to nerve tissue. It is always *referred* to the sensory distribution of the affected neural structure: e.g., calf pain in S1 radiculopathy, frontal headache in tentorial meningioma, unilateral bandlike abdominal pain in schwannoma of a thoracic spinal nerve root. (Note that neuropathic pain is not necessarily due to neuropathy. The less misleading synonym "neurogenic pain" is not as widely used.)

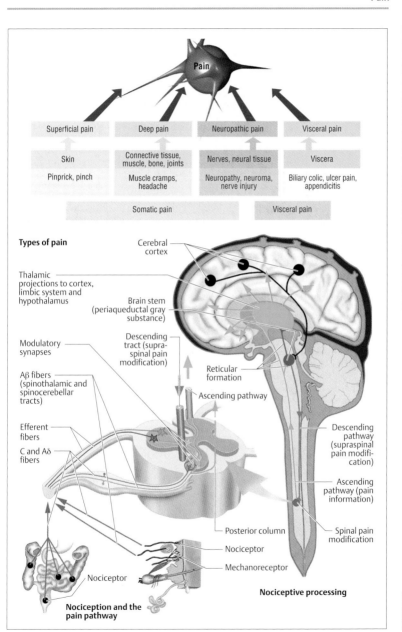

Types of pain

Nociception and the pain pathway

Nociceptive processing

Head's Zones

Visceral pain is not felt in the internal organ where it originates, but is rather referred to a cutaneous zone (of Head) specific to that organ. This phenomenon is explained by the arrival of sensory impulses from both the internal organ and its related zone of Head at the posterior horn at the same level of the spinal cord; the brain thus (mis)interprets the visceral pain as originating in the related cutaneous zone. The pain may be described as burning, pulling, pressure, or soreness, and there may be cutaneous hyperesthesia to light touch. Certain etiologies (e. g., angina pectoris, cholecystitis, gastric ulcer, intestinal disease) can produce ipsilateral mydriasis. In addition to the zones of Head, referred pain may also be felt in muscles and connective tissue (pressure points, as in Blumberg's sign or McBurney's point). Physicians should beware of mistaking referred for local pain.

Spinal Autonomic Reflexes

The afferent arm of these reflexes originates in the internal organs and terminates on the sympathetic preganglionic neurons in the intermediolateral and intermediomedial cell columns of the spinal cord at levels T1 through L2 (p. 140). Typical examples are the *viscerovisceral reflex* (causing meteorism in colic and anuria in myocardial infarction), the *viscerocutaneous reflex* (a visceral stimulus leads to sweating and hyperemia in the corresponding zone of Head), the *cutivisceral reflex* (reduction of colic, myogelosis, etc., by warm compresses or massage), the *visceromotor reflex* (defensive muscle contraction in response to visceral stimulus), and the *vasodilatory axon reflex* (dermographism). Any abnormality of these reflexes may be an important sign of impaired autonomic function (cardiovascular, gastrointestinal, thermoregulatory, or urogenital), particularly in patients with spinal cord disorders.

Complex Regional Pain Syndrome (CRPS)

The International Association for the Study of Pain (IASP) recommends the term CRPS for a set of painful disorders of apparently related pathophysiology, which are further classified into CRPS type I (*reflex sympathetic dystrophy*; without peripheral nerve injury) and CRPS type II (*causalgia*; with peripheral nerve injury). CRPS usually results from a traumatic or other injury to a limb, often in conjunction with prolonged disuse. The pain is persistent and diffuse, and of burning, stabbing, or throbbing quality, often in association with allodynia (pain evoked by a normally nonpainful stimulus) and hyperpathia (abnormally intense pain evoked by a normally painful stimulus). It is generally not in a radicular or peripheral nerve distribution. It may be accompanied by motor disturbances (paresis, disuse of limb), autonomic disturbances (sweat secretion or circulatory disturbances), trophic changes (edema, muscle atrophy, joint swelling, bone destruction), and reactive mental changes (depression, anxiety). The diagnosis of CRPS is based on criteria defined by the IASP and requires the exclusion of other disease processes such as fracture, vasculitis, thrombosis, radicular lesion, rheumatoid arthritis, etc. Its pathogenetic mechanism is unknown.

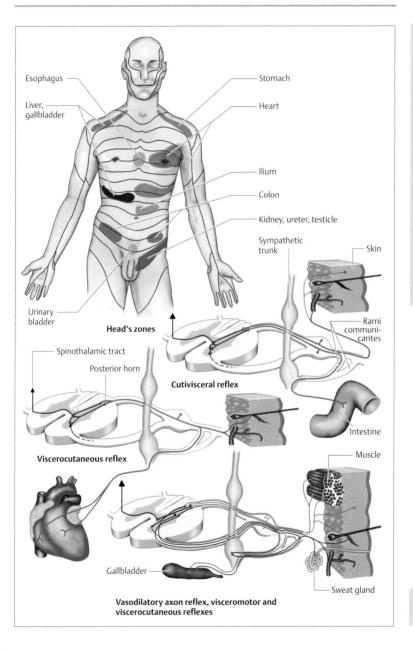

Esophagus

Liver, gallbladder

Stomach

Heart

Ilium

Colon

Kidney, ureter, testicle

Sympathetic trunk

Skin

Urinary bladder

Head's zones

Rami communicantes

Spinothalamic tract

Posterior horn

Cutivisceral reflex

Intestine

Viscerocutaneous reflex

Muscle

Gallbladder

Sweat gland

Vasodilatory axon reflex, visceromotor and viscerocutaneous reflexes

Pain

Circadian Rhythm

The human sleep–wake cycle has a period of approximately 24 hours, as the term *circadian* (Latin *circa* + *dies*) implies. If all external time indicators are removed, the circadian rhythm persists but the times of waking and going to sleep become later each day. The circadian rhythm is thought to be regulated by the suprachiasmatic nucleus of the hypothalamus (p. 142). Retinohypothalamic connections tie the circadian rhythm to environmental light conditions. There is also a retinal projection to the pineal gland; the melatonin produced there has a rhythm-shifting effect.

Not only sleeping and waking but also many other bodily functions, including cardiovascular and respiratory function, hormone secretion, mitosis rate, intracranial pressure, and attentiveness, follow a circadian pattern (*chronobiology*). Circadian variation in performance is important in the workplace and elsewhere. Some diseases are associated with certain times of the day (*chronopathology*)—certain types of epileptic seizures, asthma, cluster headache, gastroesophageal reflux disease, myocardial infarction, vertricular tachycardia.

Sleep

Sleep is divided into REM sleep, in which rapid eye movements occur, and non-REM (NREM) sleep. *Polygraphic recordings* (EEG, EOG, EMG) can distinguish these two types of sleep and are used to subdivide NREM sleep into four stages, the last two of which constitute deep sleep (see Table 10, p. 363).

Normal sleep occurs in cycles lasting 90–120 minutes, of which there are thus four or five during a normal night's sleep of ca. 8 hours' duration. Sleep cycles are regulated by activating and deactivating systems (cholinergic REM-on neurons, noradrenergic REM-off neurons) located mainly in the brain stem. The exact physiological significance of sleep is not known. Sleep appears to play a role in regenerative metabolic processes, cognitive functions, and memory.

Sleep Profile

The sleep–wake rhythm changes with age. Neonates sleep 16–18 hours a day at irregular intervals. By age 1 year, the sleep pattern stabilizes to roughly 12 hours of sleep alternating with 12 hours of waking. Adults sleep for 4–10 hours nightly, with the median value ca. 8 hours. As adults age, they tend to take longer and more frequent naps, sleep less deeply, and lie in bed longer in the morning. The *sleep architecture* changes with age: neonates have 50% REM sleep, but adults only 18%. After age 50, stages 3 and 4 account for only about 5% of sleep. Persons differ in their sleep–wake patterns (*somnotypes*): there are morning types ("larks") and night types ("night owls"); bedtimes vary by two or more hours among these individuals.

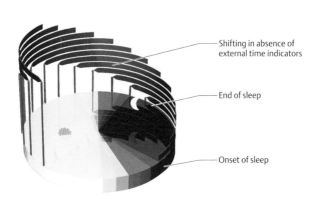

Shifting in absence of
external time indicators

End of sleep

Onset of sleep

Circadian rhythm

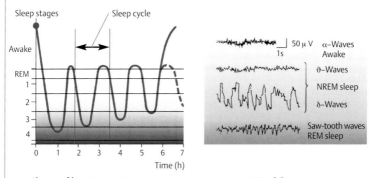

Sleep stages | Sleep cycle

Awake

REM
1
2
3
4

0 1 2 3 4 5 6 7
Time (h)

Sleep profile (4 sleep cycles)

50 μV   α–Waves
1s   Awake

ϑ–Waves

NREM sleep

δ–Waves

Saw-tooth waves
REM sleep

EEG of sleep stages

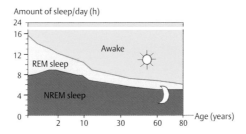

Amount of sleep/day (h)
24
16
12
8
4
0

Awake

REM sleep

NREM sleep

2 10 30 60 80
Age (years)

Changes in sleep structure with age

Sleep

113

Sleep Disorders

More than 100 sleep disorders have been described to date. Sleep disorders may involve insufficient, interrupted, or absent sleep (*insomnia*), or an excessive need for sleep, including during the day (*hypersomnia*). They may involve respiratory disturbances during sleep (snoring, sleep apnea, asthma), involuntary movement disorders, parasomnias, pharmacologically active substances (medications, illegal drugs, alcohol, coffee, smoking), or systemic disease.

The prerequisite to treatment is an adequate diagnostic assessment, which begins with the determination whether the sleep disorder is primary or secondary (i.e., the result of another disease or condition).

Primary Sleep Disorders (Dyssomnias)

Intrinsic sleep disorders. *Psychogenic insomnia* is characterized by increased mental tension (inability to relax, anxiety, brooding) and excessive concern about sleep itself (constant complaining about an inability to fall asleep or stay asleep, or about waking up too early). Sleep often improves in a new environment (e.g., on vacation).

Pseudoinsomnia is a subjective feeling of disturbed sleep in the absence of objective evidence (i.e., normal polysomnography).

Restless legs syndrome (RLS) is characterized by ascending abnormal sensations in the legs when they are at rest (e.g., when the patient watches television, or before falling asleep) accompanied by an urge to move the legs. It is sometimes present as a genetic disorder with autosomal dominant inheritance. *Periodic leg movements* during sleep are repeated, abrupt twitching movements of the legs that may persist for minutes to hours. These two movement disorders may appear together or in isolation; both may be either primary or secondary (due to, e.g., uremia, tricyclic antidepressant use, or iron deficiency).

Narcolepsy is characterized by daytime somnolence and frequent, sudden, uncontrollable episodes of sleep (imperative sleep), which tend to occur in restful situations (e.g., reading, hearing a lecture, watching TV, long automobile rides). It may be associated with cataplexy (sudden, episodic loss of muscle tone without unconsciousness), sleep paralysis (inability to move or speak when awaking from sleep), and hypnagogic hallucinations (visual or acoustic hallucinations while falling asleep). Polysomnography reveals a short sleep latency and an early onset of REM sleep. The presence of HLA antigens (DR2, DQw1, DQB1*0602) is nonspecific, as is the absence of hypocretin-1 (orexin A) in the cerebrospinal fluid.

Obstructive sleep apnea is characterized by daytime somnolence with frequent dozing, nocturnal respiratory pauses, and loud snoring. Impaired concentration, decreased performance, and headaches are also common.

Extrinsic sleep disorders. Sleep may be disturbed by external factors such as noise, light, mental stress, and medication use.

Disturbance of the circadian rhythm. Sleep may be disturbed by shift work at night or by intercontinental travel (*jet lag*).

Parasomnias. These disorders include confusion on awakening (sleep drunkenness), sleepwalking (somnambulism), nightmares, sleep myoclonus, bedwetting (enuresis), and nocturnal grinding of the teeth (bruxism).

Secondary Sleep Disorders

Psychogenic sleep disorders. Depression (of various types) can impair sleep, though paradoxically sleep deprivation can ameliorate depression. Depressed persons typically complain of early morning awakening, nocturnal restlessness, and difficulty in starting the day. Sleep disturbances are also common in patients suffering from psychosis, mania, anxiety disorders, alcoholism, and drug abuse.

Neurogenic sleep disorders. Sleep can be impaired by dementia, Parkinson disease, dystonia, respiratory disturbances secondary to neuromuscular disease (muscular dystrophy, amyotrophic lateral sclerosis), epilepsy (nocturnal attacks), and headache syndromes (cluster headaches, migraine). *Fatal familial insomnia* is a genetic disorder of autosomal dominant inheritance (p. 252).

Sleep disorders due to systemic disease. Sleep can be impaired by pulmonary diseases (asthma, COPD), angina pectoris, nocturia, fibromyalgia, and chronic fatigue syndrome.

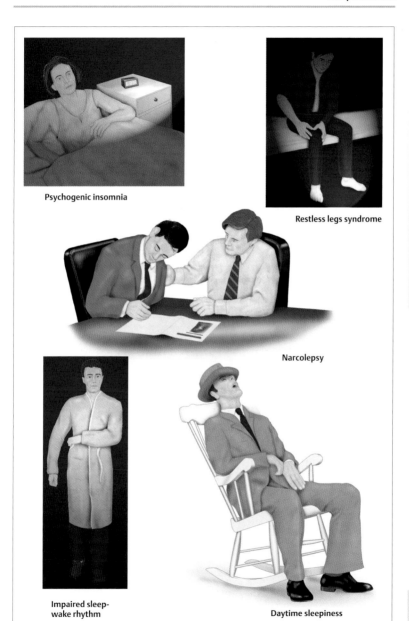

Psychogenic insomnia

Restless legs syndrome

Narcolepsy

Impaired sleep-
wake rhythm

Daytime sleepiness

Sleep

115

Consciousness is an active process with multiple individual components, including wakefulness, arousal, perception of oneself and the environment, attention, memory, motivation, speech, mood, abstract/logical thinking, and goal-directed action. Psychologists and philosophers have long sought to understand the nature of consciousness.

Clinical assessment of consciousness tests the patients' perception of themselves and their environment, behavior, and responses to external stimuli. Findings are expressed in terms of three categories: *level of consciousness* (state/clarity of consciousness, quantitative level of consciousness, vigilance, alertness, arousability); *content of consciousness* (quality of consciousness, awareness); and *wakefulness*. Changes in any of these categories tend to affect the others as well. Morphologically, the level of consciousness is associated with the *reticular activating system* (RAS). This network is found along the entire length of the brain stem reticular formation (p. 26), from the medulla to the intralaminar nuclei of the thalamus. The RAS has extensive bilateral projections to the cerebral cortex; the cortex also projects back to the RAS. Neurotransmission in these systems is predominantly with acetylcholine, monoamines (norepinephrine, dopamine, serotonin), GABA (inhibitory), and glutamate (excitatory).

In the *normal state of consciousness*, the individual is fully conscious, oriented, and awake. All of these categories undergo circadian variation (depending on the time of day, a person may be fully awake or drowsy, more or less concentrated, with organized or disorganized thinking), but normal consciousness with full wakefulness can always be restored by a vigorous stimulus.

Acute Disturbances of Consciousness

Confusion affects the content of consciousness—attention, concentration, thought, memory, spatiotemporal orientation, and perception (lack of recognition). It may also be associated with changes in the level of consciousness (fluctuation between agitation and somnolence) and in wakefulness (impaired sleep–wake cycle with nocturnal agitation and daytime somnolence). *Delirium* is characterized by visual hallucinations, restlessness, suggestibility, and autonomic disturbances (tachycardia, blood pressure fluctuations, hyperhidrosis).

Somnolence is a mild reduction of the *level of consciousness* (drowsiness, reduced spontaneous movement, psychomotor sluggishness, and delayed response to verbal stimuli) while the patient *remains arousable*: he or she is easily awakened by a stimulus, but falls back asleep once it is removed. The patient responds to noxious stimuli with direct and goal-directed defensive behavior. Orientation and attention are mildly impaired but improve on stimulation.

Stupor is a significant reduction of the *level of consciousness*. These patients require vigorous and repeated stimulation before they open their eyes and look at the examiner. They answer questions slowly and inadequately, or not at all. They may lie motionless or display restless or stereotyped movements. Confusion reflects concomitant impairment of the content of consciousness.

Disorders of arousal. Wakefulness normally follows a circadian rhythm (p. 112). Sleep apnea syndrome, narcolepsy, and parasomnia are disorders of arousal (dyssomnias, p. 114). *Hypersomnia* is caused by bilateral paramedian thalamic infarcts, tumors in the third ventricular region, and lesions of the midbrain tegmentum (p. 70 ff). The level and content of consciousness may also be affected. In patients with bilateral paramedian thalamic infarction, for example, there may be a sudden onset of confusion, followed by somnolence and coma. After recovery from the acute phase, these patients are apathetic and their memory is impaired ("thalamic dementia").

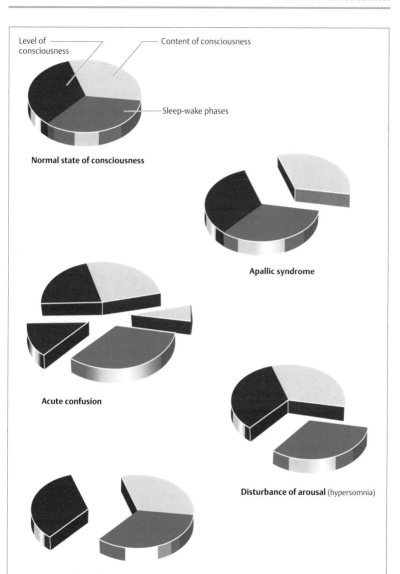

Level of consciousness

Content of consciousness

Sleep-wake phases

Normal state of consciousness

Apallic syndrome

Acute confusion

Disturbance of arousal (hypersomnia)

Somnolence, stupor

Coma

Coma (from the Greek for "deep sleep") is a state of unconsciousness in which the individual lies motionless, with eyes closed, and cannot be aroused even by vigorous stimulation. Coma reflects a loss of the structural or functional integrity of the RAS (p. 116) or the areas to which it projects. Coma may be produced by an extensive brain stem lesion or by extensive bihemispheric cerebral lesions, as well as by metabolic, hypoxic/ischemic, toxic, or endocrine disturbances. In the syndrome of *transtentorial herniation* (see p. 162), a large unihemispheric lesion can cause coma by compressing the midbrain and the diencephalic RAS. Even without herniation, however, large unihemispheric lesions can transiently impair consciousness.

Coma Staging

The degree of impairment of consciousness is correlated with the extent of the causative lesion. The severity and prognosis of coma are judged from the patient's response to stimuli. There is no universally accepted grading system for coma. Proper documentation involves an exact description of the stimuli given and the responses elicited, rather than isolated items of information such as "somnolent" or "GCS 10." Coma scales (e. g., the Glasgow Coma Scale) are useful for the standardization of data for statistical purposes but do not replace a detailed documentation of the state of consciousness.

Spontaneous movement. Assessment of motor function yields clues to the site of the lesion (p. 44 ff) and the etiology of coma. The examiner should note the pattern of breathing, any utterances, yawning, swallowing, coughing, and movements of the limbs (twitching of the face or hands may indicate epileptic activity; there may be myoclonus or flexion/extension movements).

Stimuli. Lesions of the mid brain or lower diencephalon produce the *decerebration syndrome* (arm/leg extension with adduction and internal rotation of the arms, pronation and flexion of the hands), while extensive bilateral lesions at higher levels produce the *decortication syndrome* (arm/hand flexion, arm supination, leg extension) (p. 47). These pathological flexion and extension movements occur spontaneously or in response to external stimuli (verbal stimu-

lation, tickling around the nose, pressure on the knuckles or other bones) whether the cause of coma is structural or metabolic. Withdrawal of the limb from the stimulus usually means that the pyramidal pathway for the affected limb is intact. Stereotyped flexion or extension movements are usually seen in patients with severe damage to the pyramidal tract.

Brain stem reflexes (p. 26). Structural lesions of the brain stem usually impair the function of the internal and external eye muscles (p. 70 ff), while supratentorial lesions generally do not, unless they secondarily affect the brain stem. Coma in a patient with intact brain stem reflexes is likely to be due to severe bihemispheric dysfunction (if no further objective deficit is found, coma may be psychogenic or factitious; see p. 120). Physicians should be aware that coma due to intoxication or drug overdose (p. 92) may be difficult to distinguish from that due to structural damage by clinical examination alone. Preservation of the vestibulo-ocular reflex (VOR) and of the doll's eyes reflex is compatible with either a bihemispheric lesion or a toxic or metabolic disorder. The VOR induces conjugate eye movement only if its brain stem pathway is intact (from the cervical spinal cord to the oculomotor nucleus). Nonetheless, the VOR may be absent in some cases of toxic coma (due to, e. g., alcohol, barbiturates, phenytoin, pancuronium, or tricyclic antidepressants).

Abnormalities of the respiratory pattern (p. 151) are of limited localizing value. *Cheyne–Stokes respiration* is characterized by regular waxing and waning of the tidal volume, punctuated by apneic pauses. It has a number of causes, including bihemispheric lesions and metabolic disorders. Slow, shallow respiration usually reflects a metabolic or toxic disorder. Rapid, deep respiration (*Kussmaul's respiration*) usually reflects a pontine or mid brain lesion, or metabolic acidosis. Medullary lesions and extensive supratentorial damage produce ataxic, cluster, or gasping respiration.

Spontaneous movements						
Motor response (defensive response) to sensory stimulus	Specifically localized	Directed	Decortication	Decerebration	Flexion/ extension	Absent
Pupillary diameter						
Pupillary light reflex (direct and indirect)	Immediate	Delayed	Sluggish	Sluggish or absent	Absent	Absent
Vestibulo-ocular reflex (doll's-eyes reflex)						
Vestibulo-ocular reflex (cold water in either ear; test in left ear shown)						
	Normal		Stages of coma	Diminishing responses and reflexes		

Disturbances of Consciousness

Disturbances of Consciousness

Comalike Syndromes

Locked-in syndrome (p. 359) is a "de-efferented state" in which the patient is fully conscious but can make no spontaneous movements except lid and vertical eye movements. There may be reflex extension of the arms and legs in response to mild stimuli such as repositioning in bed or tracheal suction. Physicians and nurses must remember that these patients can perceive themselves and their surroundings fully even though they may be unable to communicate. Possible causes include basilar artery occlusion, head trauma, pontine hemorrhage, central pontine myelinolysis, and brain stem encephalitis; a similar clinical picture may be produced by myasthenia gravis, Guillain–Barré syndrome, or periodic paralysis (see pp. 326, 338).

Persistent vegetative state (apallic syndrome) is caused by extensive injury to the cerebral cortex, subcortical white matter, or thalamus. The patients are awake but unconscious (loss of cortical function). Periods in which the eyes are open and move spontaneously, in conjugate fashion, seemingly with fixation, alternate with a state resembling sleep (eyes closed, regular breathing). The patient may blink in response to visual stimuli (rapid hand movements, light), perhaps creating the impression of conscious perception, but does not obey verbal commands. The limbs may be held in a decorticate or decerebrate posture (p. 46). There may be nondirected movements of the arms, legs, head, and jaw, as well as utterances, sucking movements, and lip-licking. The patient may also yawn spontaneously or in response to perioral stimuli. Autonomic disturbances include profuse sweating, tachycardia, urinary and fecal incontinence, and hyperventilation. Optokinetic nystagmus is absent, but the vestibulo-ocular reflex can often be elicited. Spontaneous respiration is preserved. Swallowing is usually possible, but food is kept in the mouth so long than no effective oral nutrition is possible. The persistent vegetative state confers a high mortality. When it lasts for more than a year, improvement is unlikely.

Akinetic mutism. In this syndrome, the patient is awake but the drive to voluntary movement is severely impaired and the patient does not speak (mutism). External stimuli evoke no more than brief ocular fixation without head movement. Possible causes include bifrontal lesions, hydrocephalus, and lesions of the cingulate gyrus or in the third ventricular region. One should keep in mind that other diseases, among them Guillain–Barré syndrome, amyotrophic lateral sclerosis, periodic paralysis, and myasthenia gravis, can present with akinetic mutism or with a similar but less severe syndrome called *abulia* (reduced drive, sluggish voluntary movements, reduced verbal response).

Psychogenic disturbances of consciousness are relatively rare and difficult to diagnose. The lack of arousability can be either an expression of a psychiatric disease (conversion or acute stress reaction, severe depression, catatonic stupor) or a deliberate fabrication. Clues are sometimes found in the case history or on neurological examination (e. g., presence of aversive reflexes, active eye closing, preserved optokinetic and vestibulo-ocular nystagmus, catalepsy, stereotyped posture).

Death

Death is medically and legally defined as the total and irreversible cessation of all brain function (hence the synonymous term, "brain death"). Spontaneous respiration (a function of the brain stem) is absent, though the heart may continue beating and other organs may still function if supportive measures are maintained (ventilation, pressor medications). All organ systems cease to function when these are discontinued.

The clinical determination of death is based on the following criteria: coma; lack of spontaneous respiration (apnea test); lack of response to noxious stimuli (with the possible exception of spinal reflexes); absence of brain stem reflexes (pupillary, corneal, cough, gag, and oculovestibular reflexes). The diagnosis of death requires the exclusion of possibly similar-appearing states such as toxic, metabolic, and endocrine disorders, pharmacological relaxation and sedation, and hypothermia. Major structural damage of the brain is present in all cases (though not necessarily demonstrable on all imaging studies). Ancillary diagnostic testing (EEG, Doppler sonography, evoked potentials, perfusion scintigraphy, cerebral angiography, MRI) may support the diagnosis but is generally not legally required (Table 11, p. 364).

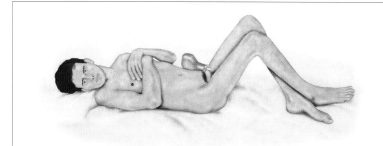

Apallic syndrome
(persistent vegetative state)

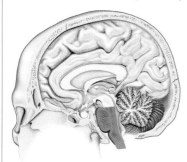

Lesion causing locked-in syndrome

Lesion causing apallic syndrome

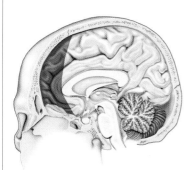

Bifrontal lesion
(causing akinetic mutism)

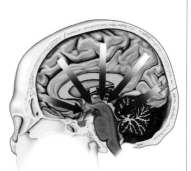

Lesion causing death (total
absence of brain function)

Disturbances of Consciousness

Personality is the set of physical and psychological traits that distinguish one individual from another. It evolves over time under the influence of changes in brain function, as well as other internal and external factors. These include neurobiological factors (heredity, structure and function of the nervous system), physiological factors (endocrine, metabolic), socialization (formation of language, thought, emotion, and action according to societal norms and value systems), individualization (consciousness of one's own individuality), sexuality, temperament, intelligence, life experiences, education, economic status, and individual will. Changes in personality cause gradual or abrupt changes in behavior. Some neurological diseases produce behavioral changes; the clinical picture depends mainly on the location of the disturbance.

Frontal Lobe Lesions

The frontal lobe includes the motor cortex (areas 4, 6, 8, 44), the prefrontal cortex (areas 9–12 and 45–47), and the cingulate gyrus (p. 144). It is responsible for the planning, monitoring, and performance of motor, cognitive, and emotional functions (*executive functions*). Frontal lobe syndromes may be due to either cortical or subcortical damage and thus cannot be reliably localized without neuroimaging. The typical syndromes listed here are useful for classification but do not imply a specific diagnosis or exact localization of the underlying lesion.

Lateralized syndromes. *Left frontal lobe lesions*, depending on their location and extent, can produce right hemiparesis or hemiplegia, transcortical motor aphasia and diminished verbal output (p. 126), buccofacial apraxia (p. 128), and/or depression or anxiety. *Right frontal lobe lesions* can produce left hemiparesis or hemiplegia, left hemineglect (p. 132), mania, and/or increased psychomotor activity.

Nonlateralized syndromes. *Fronto-orbital lesions* produce increased drive, memory impairment with confabulation, and disorientation. Disinhibition and impaired insight into one's own behavior may produce abnormal facetiousness (German *Witzelsucht*), abnormal social behavior (loss of distance, sexual impulsiveness), indifference, or carelessness.

Lesions of the *cingulate gyrus* and *premotor cortex* produce syndromes ranging from abulia (loss of drive) to akinetic mutism (p. 120) and generally characterized by apathy, loss of interest, inertia, loss of initiative, decreased sexual activity, loss of emotion, and loss of planning ability. Urinary and fecal incontinence occur because of the loss of (cortical) perception of the urge to urinate and defecate. Altered voiding frequency or sudden voiding is the result.

These patients are usually impaired in their capacity for *divided attention* (the processing of new information and adaptation to altered requirements, i.e., flexibility) and for *directed attention* (selective attention to a particular thing or task). Their attention span is short, they are easily distracted, they have difficulty in the execution of motor sequences, and they tend to perseverate (to persist in a particular activity or thought). Increased distractibility and prolonged reaction times impair performance in the workplace and in everyday activities such as driving.

Lesions of pathways. Lesions in pathways connecting the frontal lobe to other cortical and subcortical areas (p. 24) can produce frontal lobe-type syndromes, as can other diseases including multisystem atrophy, Parkinson disease, Alzheimer disease, normal-pressure hydrocephalus, and progressive supranuclear palsy.

Lesions of the corpus callosum. See p. 24.

Behavioral Manifestations of Neurological Disease

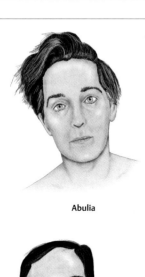

Abulia

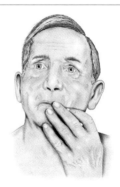

Concentration and attention
deficits

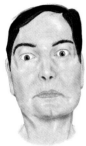

Anxiety, misperceptions

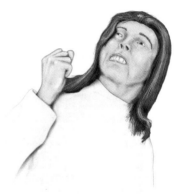

Defensiveness, irritability,
psychomotor agitation

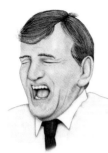

Pathological crying and laughing

Language is a means of transmitting and processing information, organizing sensory perceptions, and expressing thoughts, feelings, and intentions. The content of language encompasses the past, present, and future. The development of language does not necessarily require speech and audition: deaf-mutes learn to communicate with sign language. Language is most easily acquired in childhood. Linguistic messages are transmitted and received through speaking and hearing, writing and reading, or (in the case of sign language) the production and interpretation of gestures. The cerebral language areas are located in the left hemisphere in over 90% of right-handers and in 60% of left-handers; the remaining individuals have bihemispheric or (in 1–2%) exclusively right-hemispheric dominance for language. The left (dominant) hemisphere is responsible for the cognitive processing of language, while the right (nondominant) hemisphere produces and recognizes the emotional components of language (*prosody* = emphasis, rhythm, melody). Language is subserved by subcortical nuclei as well (left thalamus, left caudate nucleus, associated fiber pathways). Language function depends on the well-coordinated activity of an extensive neural network in the left hemisphere. It is simplistic to suppose that language is understood and produced by means of a unidirectional flow of information through a chain of independently operating brain areas linked together in series. Rather, it has been shown that any particular linguistic function (such as reading, hearing, or speaking) relies on the simultaneous activation of multiple, disparate cortical areas. Yet the simplified model of language outlined below (proposed by Wernicke and further elaborated by Geschwind) usually suffices for the purposes of clinical diagnosis.

Hearing and speaking. Acoustic signals are transduced in the inner ear into neural impulses in the cochlear nerve, which ascend through the auditory pathway and its relay stations to the primary and secondary auditory cortex (p. 100). From here, the information is sent to *Wernicke's area* (the "posterior language area"), consisting of Wernicke's area proper, in the superior temporal gyrus (Brodmann area 22), as well as the angular and supramarginal gyri (areas 39, 40). The *angular gyrus* processes auditory, visual,

and tactile information, while Wernicke's area proper is the center for the understanding of language. It is from here that the arcuate fasciculus arises, the fiber tract that conveys linguistic information onward to *Broca's area* (areas 44 and 45; the "anterior language area"). Grammatical structures and articulation programs are represented in Broca's area, which sends its output to the motor cortex (speech, p. 130). Spoken language is regulated by an auditory feedback circuit in which the utterer hears his or her own words and the cortical language areas modulate the speech output accordingly.

Reading and writing. The visual pathway conveys visual information to the primary and secondary visual cortex (p. 80), which, in turn, project to the angular gyrus and Wernicke's area, in which visually acquired words are understood, perhaps after a prior "conversion" to phonetic form. Wernicke's area then projects via the arcuate fasciculus to Broca's area, as discussed above; Broca's area sends its output to the motor cortex (for speech or, perhaps, to the motor hand area for writing). This pathway enables the recognition and comprehension of written language, as well as reading out loud.

Examination. The clinical examination of language includes spontaneous speech, naming of objects, speech comprehension, speech repetition, reading, and writing. The detailed assessment of aphasia requires the use of test instruments such as the Aachen aphasia test, perhaps in collaboration with neuropsychologists and speech therapists. Disturbances of speech may be classified as *fluent* or *nonfluent*. Examples of the former are paragrammatism (faulty sentence structure), meaningless phrases, circumlocution, semantic paraphasia (contextual substitution, e.g., "leg" for "arm"), phonemic paraphasia (substitution of one letter for another, e.g., "tan" for "can"), neologisms (nonexistent words), and fluent gibberish (jargon). Examples of the latter are agrammatism (word chains without grammatical structure), echolalia (repetition of heard words), and automatism (repeating the same word many times). *Prosody* and *dysarthria* (if present; p. 130) are evaluated during spontaneous speech. *Anomia* is the inability to name objects. Patients with *aphemia* can read, write, and understand spoken language but cannot speak.

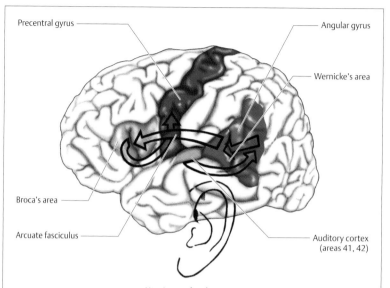

Precentral gyrus

Angular gyrus

Wernicke's area

Broca's area

Arcuate fasciculus

Auditory cortex
(areas 41, 42)

Hearing spoken language

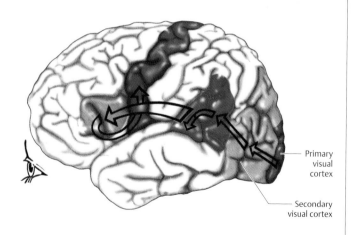

Primary
visual
cortex

Secondary
visual cortex

Reading written language

Behavioral Manifestations of Neurological Disease

Aphasia is an acquired disturbance of language. Lesions at various sites produce different types of aphasia; focal lesions do not cause total loss of all language functions simultaneously. The side of cerebral dominance for language can be determined by the Wada test (intracarotid amobarbital procedure, IAP), in which amobarbital is injected first into one internal carotid artery and then into the other, under angiographic control, to selectively anesthetize each hemisphere (this is done, for example, before cortical resections for epilepsy). *Crossed aphasia*, i.e., aphasia due to a right hemispheric lesion in a right-handed patient, is rare. Aphasia usually improves markedly within a few weeks of onset and may continue to improve gradually over the first year, even if the symptoms temporarily appear to have stabilized. Improvement beyond one year is rare and usually minor.

Aphasia in bilingual and multilingual persons (usually) affects all of the languages spoken. The severity of involvement of each language depends on the age at which it was acquired, premorbid language ability, and whether the languages were learned simultaneously or sequentiallly. Aphasia is most commonly due to stroke or head trauma and may be accompanied by apraxia.

Global aphasia involves all aspects of language and severely impairs spoken communication. The patient cannot speak spontaneously or can only do so with great effort, producing no more than fragments of words. Speech comprehension is usually absent; at best, patients may recognize a few words, including their own name. Perseveration (persistent repetition of a single word/subject) and neologisms are prominent, and the ability to repeat heard words is markedly impaired. Patients have great difficulty naming objects, reading, writing, and copying letters or words. Their ability to name objects, read, and write, except for the ability to copy letters of the alphabet or isolated words, is greatly impaired. Language automatism (repetition of gibberish) is a characteristic feature. *Site of lesion:* Entire distribution of the middle cerebral artery, including both Broca's and Wernicke's areas.

Broca's aphasia (also called anterior, motor, or expressive aphasia) is characterized by the absence or severe impairment of spontaneous speech, while comprehension is only mildly impaired. The patient can speak only with great effort, producing only faltering, nonfluent, garbled words. Phonemic paraphasic errors are made, and sentences are of simple construction, often with isolated words that are not grammatically linked (agrammatism, "telegraphic" speech). Naming, repetition, reading out loud, and writing are also impaired. *Site of lesion:* Broca area; may be due to infarction in the distribution of the pre-rolandic artery (artery of the precentral sulcus).

Wernicke's aphasia (also called posterior, sensory, or receptive aphasia) is characterized by severe impairment of comprehension. Spontaneous speech remains fluent and normally paced, but paragrammatism, paraphasia, and neologisms make the patient's speech partially or totally incomprehensible (word salad, jargon aphasia). Naming, repetition of heard words, reading, and writing are also markedly impaired. *Site of lesion:* Wernicke's area (area 22). May be due to infarction in the distribution of the posterior temporal artery.

Transcortical aphasia. Heard words can be repeated, but other linguistic functions are impaired: spontaneous speech in transcortical *motor* aphasia (syndrome similar to Broca's aphasia), language comprehension in transcortical *sensory* aphasia (syndrome similar to Wernicke's aphasia). *Site of lesion:* Motor type, left frontal lobe bordering on Broca's area; sensory type, left temporo-occipital junction dorsal to Wernicke's area. Watershed infarction is the most common cause (p. 172).

Amnestic (anomic) aphasia. This type of aphasia is characterized by impaired naming and word-finding. Spontaneous speech is fluent but permeated with word-finding difficulty and paraphrasing. The ability to repeat, comprehend, and write words is essentially normal. *Site of lesion:* Temporoparietal cortex or subcortical white matter.

Conduction aphasia. Repetition is severely impaired; fluent, spontaneous speech is interrupted by pauses to search for words and by phonemic paraphasia. Language comprehension is only mildly impaired. *Site of lesion:* Arcuate fasciculus or insular region.

Subcortical aphasia. Types of aphasia similar to those described may be produced by subcortical lesions at various sites (thalamus, internal capsule, anterior striatum).

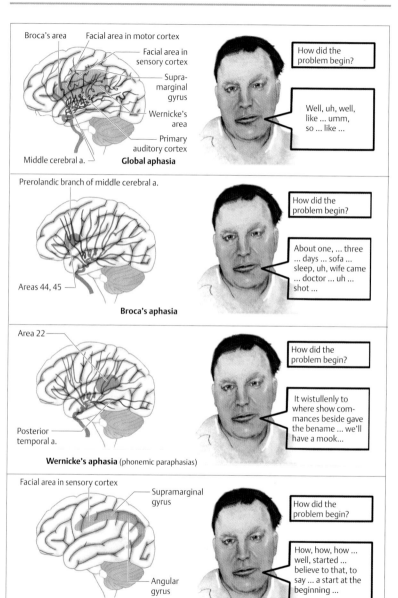

Global aphasia

Broca's area — Facial area in motor cortex — Facial area in sensory cortex — Supra-marginal gyrus — Wernicke's area — Primary auditory cortex — Middle cerebral a.

How did the problem begin?

Well, uh, well, like ... umm, so ... like ...

Broca's aphasia

Prerolandic branch of middle cerebral a. — Areas 44, 45

How did the problem begin?

About one, ... three ... days ... sofa ... sleep, uh, wife came ... doctor ... uh ... shot ...

Wernicke's aphasia (phonemic paraphasias)

Area 22 — Posterior temporal a.

How did the problem begin?

It wistullenly to where show com-mances beside gave the bename ... we'll have a mook...

Transcortical (sensory) aphasia

Facial area in sensory cortex — Supramarginal gyrus — Angular gyrus

How did the problem begin?

How, how, how ... well, started ... believe to that, to say ... a start at the beginning ...

Agraphia. Agraphia is the acquired inability to write. Agraphia may be *isolated* (due to a lesion located in area 6, the superior parietal lobule, or elsewhere) or accompanied by other disturbances: *aphasic agraphia* is fluent or nonfluent, depending on the accompanying aphasia; *apraxic agraphia* is due to a lesion of the dominant parietal lobe; *spatial agraphia*, in which the patient has difficulty writing on a line and only writes on the right side of the paper, is due to a lesion of the nondominant parietal lobe; *alexia with agraphia* may be seen in the absence of aphasia. *Micrographia* (abnormally small handwriting) is found in *Parkinson disease* (p. 206) and is not pathogenetically related to agraphia. Various forms of agraphia are common in Alzheimer disease. *Examination:* The patient is asked to write sentences, long words, or series of numbers to dictation, to spell words, and to copy written words.

Alexia. Alexia is the acquired inability to read. In *isolated alexia* (alexia without agraphia), the patient cannot recognize entire words or read them quickly, but can decipher them letter by letter, and can understand verbally spelled words. The ability to write is unaffected. The responsible lesion is typically in the left temporo-occipital region with involvement of the visual pathway and of callosal fibers. *Anterior alexia* (difficulty and errors in reading aloud; impaired ability to write, spell, and copy words) is usually associated with Broca's aphasia. *Central alexia* (combination of alexia and agraphia) is usually accompanied by right-left disorientation, finger agnosia, agraphia, and acalculia (Gerstmann syndrome; lesions of the angular and supramarginal gyri), or by Wernicke's aphasia. Other features include the inability to understand written language or to spell, write, or copy words. *Examination:* The patient is asked to read aloud and to read individual words, letters, and numbers; the understanding of spelled words and instructions is tested.

Acalculia. Acalculia is an acquired inability to use numbers or perform simple arithmetical calculations. Patients have difficulty counting change, using a thermometer, or filling out a check. Lesions of various types may cause acalculia. *Examination:* The patient is asked to perform simple arithmetical calculations and to read numbers.

Apraxia. There are several kinds of apraxia; in general, the term refers to the inability to carry out learned motor tasks or purposeful movements. Apraxia is often accompanied by aphasia.

Ideomotor apraxia involves the faulty execution (parapraxia) of acquired voluntary and complex movement sequences; it can be demonstrated most clearly by asking the patient to perform pantomimic gestures. It can involve the face (*buccofacial apraxia*) or the limbs (*limb apraxia*). It is due to a lesion in the association fiber pathways connecting the language, visual, and motor areas to each other and to the two hemispheres (disconnection syndrome). *Examination* (pantomimic gestures on command): face (open eyes, stick out tongue, lick lips, blow out a match, pucker, suck on a straw); arms (turn a screw, cut paper, throw ball, comb hair, brush teeth, snap fingers); legs (kick ball, stamp out cigarette, climb stairs). The patient may perform the movement in incorrect sequence, or may carry out a movement of the wrong type (e. g., puffing instead of sucking).

Ideational apraxia is impairment of the ability to carry out complex, learned, goal-directed activities in proper logical sequence. A temporal or parietal lesion may be responsible. *Examination:* The patient is asked to carry out pantomimic gestures such as opening a letter, making a sandwich, or preparing a cup of tea.

Apraxia-like syndromes. The following disturbances are termed "apraxia" even though actual parapraxia is absent: *Lid-opening apraxia* (p. 64) is difficulty opening the eyes on command. *Gait apraxia* is characterized by difficulty initiating gait and by short steps (p. 160). *Dressing apraxia* is often seen in patients with nondominant parietal lobe lesions. They cannot dress themselves and do not know how to position a shirt, shoes, trousers, or other items of clothing to put them on correctly. An underlying impairment of spatial orientation is responsible.

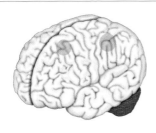

Sites of lesions causing agraphia

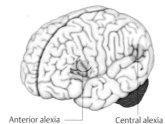

Anterior alexia — Central alexia

Topography of lesions in alexia

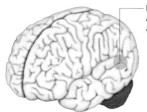

Numerical alexia/agraphia, anarithmia

Sites of lesions causing acalculia

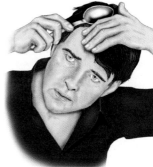

Ideomotor apraxia

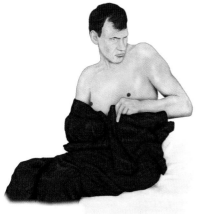

Dressing apraxia

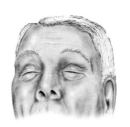

Lid-opening apraxia

Speech

The neural basis of speech. Speech-related movement programs generated in the premotor cortex (area 6) are modulated by information from the cerebellum and basal ganglia and are relayed to the motor cortex (inferior portion of the precentral gyrus, area 4) for implementation. The motor cortex projects by way of the corticopontine and corticobulbar tracts to the *motor cranial nerve nuclei* in the brain stem. CN V (mandibular nerve) controls the muscles that open and close the jaw (masseter, temporalis, medial and lateral pterygoid muscles). CN VII controls facial expression and labial articulation; CN X and, to a lesser extent, IX control motility of the soft palate, pharynx, and larynx; CN XII controls tongue movement. Speech-related impulses to the respiratory muscles travel (among other pathways) from the motor cortex to the spinal anterior horn cells. Connections to the basal ganglia and cerebellum are important for the coordination of speech. *Sensory impulses* from the skin, mucous membranes, and muscles return to the brain through CN V (maxillary and mandibular nerves), IX, and X. These impulses are processed by a neural network (reticular formation, thalamus, precentral cortex) mediating feedback control of speech. The central innervation of the speech pathway is predominantly bilateral; thus, dysarthria due to unilateral lesions is usually transient.

Voice production (phonation). Voice production by the larynx (phonation) through the vibrating vocal folds (cords) yields sound at a fundamental frequency with a varying admixture of higher-frequency components, which lend the voice its *timbre* (musical quality); timbre depends on the resonant cavities above the vocal folds (pharynx, oral cavity, nasal cavity). The *volume* of the voice is regulated by stretching and relaxation of the vocal folds and by adjustment of air pressure in the larynx. The air flow necessary for phonation is produced in the respiratory tract (diaphragm, lungs, chest, and trachea). The individual structural characteristics of the larynx, particularly the length of the vocal folds, determine the pitch of a person's voice. A *whisper* is produced when the vocal folds are closely apposed and do not vibrate.

Creation of the sounds of speech (articulation). The sounds of speech are created by changing the configuration of the physiological resonance spaces and articulation zones. The resonance spaces can be altered by movement of the velum (which separates the oral and pharyngeal cavities) and tongue (which divides the oral cavity). Each vowel (a, e, i, o, u) is associated with a specific partitioning of the oral cavity by the tongue. The palate, teeth, and lips are the articulation zones with which consonants are produced (g, s, b, etc.).

Dysarthria, Dysphonia

Dysarthria (impaired articulation) and dysphonia (impaired phonation and resonance) result from a disturbance of the neural control mechanism for speech (sensory portion, motor portion, or both). Diagnostic assessment requires both analysis of the patient's vocal output (breathing, phonation, resonance, articulation; speed, coordination, and prosody of speech) and the determination of any associated neurological findings (e.g. dysphagia, hyperkinesia, cranial nerve deficits). For responsible lesions and syndromes, see Table 12 (p. 365).

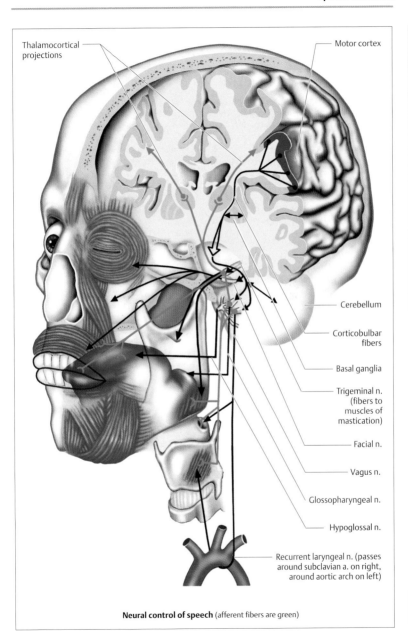

Thalamocortical projections

Motor cortex

Cerebellum

Corticobulbar fibers

Basal ganglia

Trigeminal n. (fibers to muscles of mastication)

Facial n.

Vagus n.

Glossopharyngeal n.

Hypoglossal n.

Recurrent laryngeal n. (passes around subclavian a. on right, around aortic arch on left)

Neural control of speech (afferent fibers are green)

Agnosia is defined as a disturbance of recognition in which perception, attention, and general intelligence are (largely) unimpaired.

Disturbances of Body Image Perception

Autotopagnosia (body-image agnosia) is the inability to correctly orient or perceive different body parts; patients cannot obey commands to point to parts of their own or the examiner's body (e. g., foot, hand, nose). The responsible lesion is usually, though not always, in the temporoparietal region (angular and supramarginal gyri). An aphasic patient may appear to have autotopagnosia because he cannot understand verbal instructions; but aphasia may also coexist with true autotopagnosia. *Finger agnosia* is the inability to identify, name, or point to fingers. These patients cannot mimic the examiner's finger movements or copy finger movements of their own contralateral hidden hand with the affected hand. *Right–left disorientation* is the inability to distinguish the right and left sides of one's own or another's body; these patients cannot obey a command to raise their left hand or touch it to their right ear. This type of disorientation can cause *dressing apraxia* (p. 128) and similar problems.

Anosognosia is the unawareness or denial of a neurological deficit, such as hemiplegia. Patients may claim that they only want to give the paralyzed side a rest, or attempt to demonstrate that their condition has improved without realizing that they are moving the limb on the unaffected side. Most such patients have extensive lesions of the nondominant hemisphere. Anosognosia may also accompany visual field defects due to unilateral or bilateral lesions of the visual cortex (homonymous hemianopsia, cortical blindness). The most striking example of this is *Anton syndrome*, in which cortically blind patients act as if they could see, and will even "describe" details of their surroundings (incorrectly) without hesitation.

Disturbances of Spatial Orientation

A number of different types of agnosia impair the awareness of one's position relative to the surroundings, i.e., *spatial orientation*. Parieto-occipital lesions are commonly responsible.

Constructional apraxia is characterized by the inability to represent spatial relationships in drawings, or with building blocks. Affected patients cannot copy a picture of a bicycle or clock. Everyday activities are impaired by the inability to draw diagrams, read (analog) clocks, assemble pieces of equipment or tools, or write words in the correct order (*spatial agraphia*).

Hemineglect is the inability to consciously perceive, react to, or classify stimuli on one side in the absence of a sensorimotor deficit or exceeding what one would expect from the severity of the sensorimotor deficit present. Hemineglect may involve unawareness of one side of the body (one-sided tooth brushing, shaving, etc.) or of one side of an object (food may be eaten from only one side of the plate, eyeglasses may be looked for on only one side of the room). When addressed, the patient always turns to the healthy side. Neurological examination reveals that double simultaneous stimulation (touch, finger movement) of homologous body parts (same site, e. g., face or arm) is not felt on the affected side (*extinction phenomenon*). In addition, perception of stimuli on the affected side is quantitatively lower than on the healthy side, there is limb akinesia despite normal strength on the side of the lesion, and spatial orientation is impaired (e. g., the patient copies only half of a clock-face).

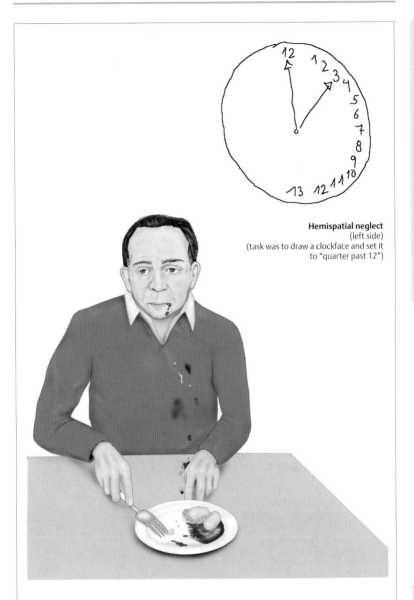

Hemispatial neglect
(left side)
(task was to draw a clockface and set it
to "quarter past 12")

Hemispatial neglect (left side)

Memory

Memory involves the acquisition, storage, recall, and reproduction of information. Memory depends on intact functioning of the limbic system (p. 144) and areas of the brain that are connected to it.

Declarative or *explicit memory* (i.e., memory for facts and events) can be consciously accessed and depends on intact functioning of the mediobasal portion of the temporal lobe. The duration of information storage may be relatively short (short-term, immediate, and working memory) or long (long-term memory). Verbal (telephone number) or visuospatial information (how to find a street) can be directly recalled from *short-term memory*. The entorhinal cortex plays a key role in these memory functions: all information from cortical regions (frontal, temporal, parietal) travels first to the entorhinal cortex and then, by way of the parahippocampal and perirhinal cortex, to the hippocampus. There is also a reciprocal projection from the hippocampus back to the entorhinal cortex. *Long-term memory* stores events of personal history that occurred at particular times (*episodic memory* for a conversation, one's wedding day, last year's holiday; orbitofrontal cortex) as well as conceptual, non–time-related knowledge (*semantic memory* for the capital of Spain, the number of centimeters in a meter, the meaning of the word "stethoscope"; subserved by different cortical regions).

Nondeclarative (procedural, implicit) memory, on the other hand, cannot be consciously accessed. Learned motor programs (riding a bicycle, swimming, playing the piano), problem-solving (rules), recognition of information acquired earlier (priming), and conditioned learning (avoiding a hot burner on the stove, sitting still in school) belong to this category. Nondeclarative memory is mediated by the basal ganglia (motor function), neocortex (priming), cerebellum (conditioning), striatum (agility), amygdala (emotional responses), and reflex pathways.

Examination. Only disturbances of declarative memory (*amnesia*) can be studied by clinical examination. *Short-term memory:* the acquisition of new information is tested by having the patient repeat a series of numbers or groups of words and asking for this information again

5–10 minutes later. The patient's *orientation* (name, place of residence/address, time/date) and *long-term memory* (place of birth, education, place of employment, family, general knowledge) are also tested by directed questioning.

Memory Disorders (Amnesia)

Forgetfulness. Verbal memory does not decline until approximately age 60, and even then only gradually, if at all. Aging is, however, often accompanied by an evident decline in information processing ability and attention span (*benign senescent forgetfulness*). These changes occur normally, yet to a degree that varies highly among individuals, and they are often barely measurable. They are far less severe than full-blown dementia, but they may be difficult to distinguish from incipient dementia.

Amnesia. *Anterograde amnesia* is the inability to acquire (declarative) information, for later recall, from a particular moment onward; *retrograde amnesia* is the inability to remember (declarative) information acquired before a particular moment (p. 269). Amnestic patients commonly *confabulate* (i.e., fill in gaps in memory with fabricated, often implausible information); they may be disoriented and lack awareness of their own memory disorder. For individual symptoms and their causes, see Table 13 (p. 365).

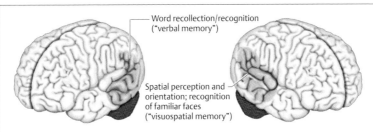

Word recollection/recognition
("verbal memory")

Spatial perception and
orientation; recognition
of familiar faces
("visuospatial memory")

Temporal cortical representation

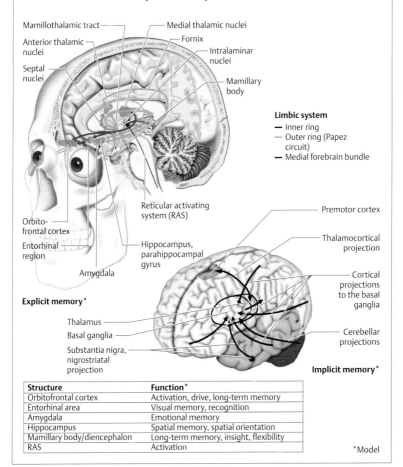

Mamillothalamic tract

Anterior thalamic
nuclei

Septal
nuclei

Medial thalamic nuclei

Fornix

Intralaminar
nuclei

Mamillary
body

Limbic system
— Inner ring
— Outer ring (Papez
circuit)
— Medial forebrain bundle

Orbito-
frontal cortex

Entorhinal
region

Amygdala

Reticular activating
system (RAS)

Hippocampus,
parahippocampal
gyrus

Explicit memory*

Premotor cortex

Thalamocortical
projection

Cortical
projections
to the basal
ganglia

Cerebellar
projections

Thalamus

Basal ganglia

Substantia nigra,
nigrostriatal
projection

Implicit memory*

Structure	Function*
Orbitofrontal cortex	Activation, drive, long-term memory
Entorhinal area	Visual memory, recognition
Amygdala	Emotional memory
Hippocampus	Spatial memory, spatial orientation
Mamillary body/diencephalon	Long-term memory, insight, flexibility
RAS	Activation

*Model

135

Dementia is a newly occurring, persistent, and progressive loss of cognitive function. Both short-term and long-term memory are impaired, in conjunction with at least one of the following disorders: aphasia, apraxia, agnosia, or impairment of abstract thinking, decision-making ability, visuospatial performance, planned action, or personality. Professional, social and interpersonal relationships deteriorate, and the sufferer finds it increasingly difficult to cope with everyday life without help. The diagnosis of dementia requires the exclusion of disturbances of consciousness (e. g., delirium) and of psychiatric disease (e. g., depression, schizophrenia). The differential diagnosis also includes benign senescent forgetfulness ("normal aging," in which daily functioning is unimpaired) and amnestic disorders. Approximately 90 % of all cases of dementia are caused by Alzheimer disease (p. 297) or cerebrovascular disorders; diverse etiologies account for the rest. The physician confronted with a case of incipient dementia must distinguish primary dementia from that secondary to another disease (Table 14, p. 366). The objective is early determination of the etiology of dementia, especially when these are treatable or reversible.

Examination. The patient or another informant should be asked for an account of the duration, type, and extent of problems that arise in everyday life. The clinical examination is used to ascertain the type and severity of cognitive deficits and any potential underlying disease. Standardized examining instruments are useful for precise documentation and differentiation of the cognitive deficits. Rapid tests for dementia, such as the Mini-Mental Status Examination, mini-syndrome test, and clock/numbers test, are useful for screening. Function-specific neurophysiological tests permit diagnostic assessment of individual aspects of cognition including orientation, attention, concentration, memory, speech, and visual constructive performance. Laboratory tests (ESR[1], differential blood count, electrolytes, liver function tests, BUN[2], creatinine, glucose, vitamin B_{12}, folic acid, TPHA[3], TSH[4], and HIV[5]), EEG, and diagnostic imaging techniques (CT[6], MRI[7], SPECT[8], and PET[9]) provide further useful information for classification and determination of the cause of dementia. None of these diagnostic techniques alone can pinpoint the etiology of dementia; definitive diagnosis practically always requires multiple tests and examinations. Diagnostic imaging is of particular importance in patients with the subacute onset of cognitive impairment or amnesia (< 1 month), fluctuation or acute worsening of symptoms, papilledema, visual field defects, headaches, a recent head injury, known malignancies, epilepsy, a history of stroke, urinary incontinence, or an abnormal gait.

---

[1]ESR   Erythrocyte sedimentation rate
[2]BUN   Blood urea nitrogen
[3]TPHA   Treponema pallidum hemagglutination test
[4]TSH   Thyroid-stimulating hormone
[5]HIV   Human immunodeficiency virus
[6]CT   Computerized tomography
[7]MRI   Magnetic resonance imaging
[8]SPECT   Single photon emission computerized tomography
[9]PET   Positron emission tomography

Additional diagnostic tests to be performed as needed: Coagulation profile, serum protein electrophoresis, serum ammonia, parathyroid hormone, cortisol, rheumatoid factor, antinuclear antibodies, blood alcohol, serum/urine drug levels, copper/ceruloplasmin, lactate/pyruvate, hexosaminidase, CSF tests, molecular genetic analysis.

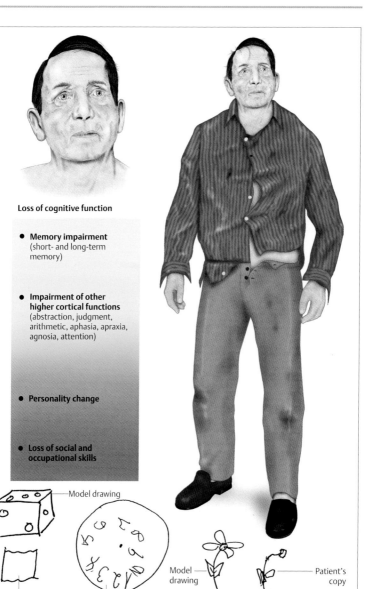

Loss of cognitive function

- **Memory impairment**
  (short- and long-term memory)

- **Impairment of other higher cortical functions**
  (abstraction, judgment, arithmetic, aphasia, apraxia, agnosia, attention)

- **Personality change**

- **Loss of social and occupational skills**

Model drawing

Patient's copy

Clock face (patient's drawing)

Model drawing

Patient's copy

Personality change, cognitive impairment

Patients with symptoms and signs that are unusual, difficult to classify, or resistant to treatment are often referred to a neurologist for a determination whether the patient's problem is "organic" or "psychogenic." Many such patients make a diagnostic and therapeutic odyssey from one medical or paramedical office to another, and have a long list of positive findings to show for it. In other patients, symptoms and signs may arise acutely or subacutely, perhaps in repeated episodes, creating the impression of a serious illness. The physician's primary objectives must be (1) to identify the possible physical or psychosocial causes of the problem, and at the same time (2) to avoid unnecessary or dangerous diagnostic tests. A correct diagnosis requires time, solid knowledge of the relevant anatomy and physiology, and the ability to recognize the psychosocial dynamics that may have given rise to the patient's complaints.

If detailed neurological examination reveals no abnormality and the symptoms cannot be attributed to any neurological disease, the physician should consider potential psychosocial causes. These may be *unconscious* (e. g., an inner conflict of which the patient is unaware) or *conscious* (e. g., a deliberate attempt to acquire the financial benefits and increased attention associated with illness). The underlying cause may be an unresolved social conflict (familial, professional, financial) or some other mental disorder (depression, anxiety, obsessive-compulsive disorder, personality disorder). Organic dysfunction and objective signs of illness are disproportionately mild in relation to the patient's complaints, unrelated to them, or entirely absent.

Conversion disorders (previously termed "conversion hysteria") often present with a single (pseudoneurological) symptom, such as psychogenic amnesia, stupor, mutism, seizures, paralysis, blindness, or sensory loss. It has been theorized that such symptoms serve to resolve unconscious inner conflicts. The diagnosis may be particularly difficult to make in patients who simultaneously suffer from organic neurological or psychiatric disease (e. g., hyperventilation in epilepsy, headaches in depression, paralysis in multiple sclerosis).

Somatoform disorders, according to current psychiatric terminology, are mental disorders characterized by "repeated presentation of physical symptoms, together with persistent requests for medical investigations, in spite of repeated negative findings and reassurances by doctors that the symptoms have no physical basis" (ICD-10, WHO, 1992). In *somatization disorder*, the patient asks for treatment of multiple, recurrent, and frequently changing symptoms, which often affect multiple organ systems (e. g. headaches + bladder dysfunction + leg pains + breathing disorder). In *hypochondriacal disorder* (previously termed "hypochondriasis"), the patient is less concerned about the symptoms themselves, and more preoccupied with the supposed presence of a serious disease. The fears persist despite repeated, thorough examination, normal test results, and medical reassurance. Any mild abnormalities that may happen to be found, e. g. of heartbeat, respiration, or intestinal function, or skin changes, only amplify the patient's anxiety. *Persistent somatoform pain disorder* involves complaints of "persistent, severe, and distressing pain, which cannot be explained fully by a physiological process or a physical disorder" (ICD-10), though an organic cause of pain is often present as well. The physical impairment that the patient attributes to pain may actually be due to a lack of fulfillment in familial, professional, or social relationships. For these patients, dealing with the pain may become the major "purpose in life."

Malingering is not a mental disorder, but rather the deliberate, premeditated feigning of illness to achieve a goal (e. g., feigning of headaches to obtain opiates).

Simulated or intentionally induced (factitious) symptoms may serve no clear purpose (neither the resolution of an unconscious conflict, nor any obvious kind of gain); they may be present in the simulator (*Münchhausen syndrome*) or in a child or other person under their care (*Münchhausen-by-proxy*). The *peregrinating patient (hospital hopper)* demands diagnostic tests from one physician after another, but negative results can never put the patient's fears to rest. Patients with *Ganser syndrome* give approximate or fatuous answers to simple questions, possibly creating the impression of dementia.

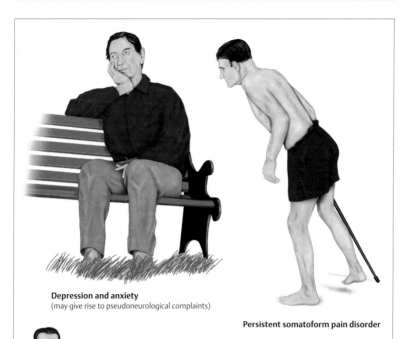

Depression and anxiety
(may give rise to pseudoneurological complaints)

Persistent somatoform pain disorder

Factitious gait disturbance

Hypochondriacal disorder

The autonomic nervous system (ANS) is so called because its functions are normally not subject to direct voluntary control. It regulates hormonal and immunological processes as well as the functioning of major organ systems (cardiovascular, respiratory, gastrointestinal, urinary, and reproductive systems).

ANS, Central Portion

Central components of the ANS are found in the cerebral cortex (insular, entorhinal, orbitofrontal, and frontotemporal areas), the hypothalamus, the limbic system, the mid brain (periaqueductal gray substance), the medulla (nucleus of the solitary tract, ventrolateral and ventromedial areas of the medulla), and the spinal cord (various tracts and nuclei, discussed in further detail below).

Afferent connections. Afferent impulses enter the ANS from spinal tracts (anterolateral fasciculus = spinothalamic + spinocerebellar + spinoreticular tracts), brain stem tracts (arising in the reticular formation), and corticothalamic tracts, and from the *circumventricular organs.* The latter are small clusters of specialized neurons, lying on the surface of the ventricular system, that sense changes in the chemical composition of the blood and the cerebrospinal fluid (i.e., on both sides of the blood–CSF barrier). These organs include the organum vasculosum of the lamina terminalis (in the roof of the third ventricle behind the optic chiasm ⇨ cytokines/ fever), the subfornical organ (under the fornices between the foramina of Monro ⇨ angiotensin II/blood pressure and fluid balance), and the area postrema (rostral to the obex on each side of the fourth ventricle ⇨ cholecystokinin/ gastrointestinal function, food intake).

Efferent connections. Projections from the hypothalamus and brain stem, particularly from the brain stem reticular formation, travel to the lateral horn of the thoracolumbar spinal cord, where they form synapses onto the *sympathetic* neurons of the spinal cord. The latter, in turn, project preganglionic fibers to the sympathetic ganglia (p. 147). The *parasympathetic* neurons receive input from higher centers in similar fashion and project in turn to parasympathetic ganglia that are generally located near the end organs they serve. The hypothalamus regulates *hormonal* function through its regulator hormones as well as efferent neural impulses.

Neurotransmitters. The main excitatory neurotransmitter is *glutamate*, and the main inhibitory neurotransmitter is γ-*aminobutyric acid* (GABA). Modulating neurotransmitters include acetylcholine, amines, neuropeptides, purines, and nitric oxide (NO).

ANS, Peripheral Portion (p. 146)

The sympathetic and parasympathetic components are both structurally and functionally segregated.

Spinal nuclei. *Sympathetic* spinal neurons lie in the lateral horn (intermediolateral and intermediomedial cell columns) of the thoracolumbar spinal cord (T1–L2) and are collectively termed the *thoracolumbar system. Parasympathetic* spinal neurons lie in the brain stem (with projections along CN III, VII, IX, X) and the sacral spinal cord (S2–S4), and are collectively termed the *craniosacral system.* The intestine has its own autonomic ganglia, which are located in the myenteric and submucous plexuses (p. 154).

Afferent connections. Afferent impulses to the ANS enter the spinal cord via the dorsal roots, and the brain stem via CN III, VII, IX and X.

Efferent connections. The projecting fibers of the spinal autonomic neurons (preganglionic fibers) exit the spinal cord in the ventral roots and travel to the paravertebral and prevertebral ganglia, where they synapse onto the next neuron of the pathway. The *sympathetic* preganglionic fibers (unmyelinated; white ramus communicans) travel a short distance to the paravertebral sympathetic chain, and the postganglionic fibers (unmyelinated; gray ramus communicans) travel a relatively long distance to the effector organs. An exception to this rule is the *adrenal medulla*: playing, as it were, the role of a sympathetic chain ganglion, it receives *long* preganglionic fibers and then, instead of giving off postganglionic fibers, secretes epinephrine into the bloodstream. The *parasympathetic* preganglionic fibers are long; they project to ganglia near the effector organs, which, in turn, give off short postganglionic processes.

Neurotransmitters. *Acetylcholine* is the neurotransmitter in the sympathetic and parasympathetic ganglia. The neurotransmitters of the postganglionic fibers are *norepinephrine* (sympathetic) and *acetylcholine* (parasympathetic). *Neuromodulators* include neuropeptides (substance P, somatostatin, vasoactive intestinal

Autonomic Nervous System

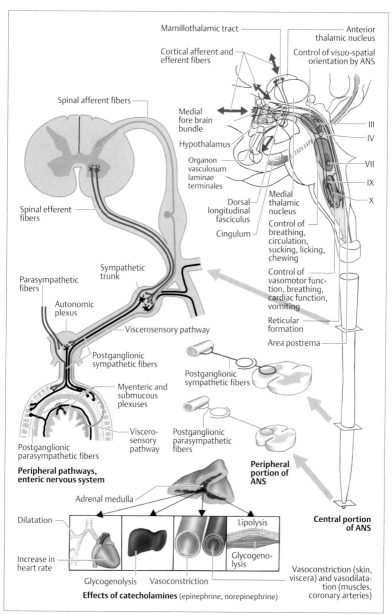

Mamillothalamic tract

Anterior thalamic nucleus

Cortical afferent and efferent fibers

Control of visuo-spatial orientation by ANS

Spinal afferent fibers

Medial fore brain bundle

Hypothalamus

III

IV

VII

IX

X

Organon vasculosum laminae terminales

Spinal efferent fibers

Dorsal longitudinal fasciculus

Cingulum

Medial thalamic nucleus

Control of breathing, circulation, sucking, licking, chewing

Control of vasomotor function, breathing, cardiac function, vomiting

Reticular formation

Area postrema

Sympathetic trunk

Parasympathetic fibers

Autonomic plexus

Viscerosensory pathway

Postganglionic sympathetic fibers

Postganglionic sympathetic fibers

Myenteric and submucous plexuses

Postganglionic parasympathetic fibers

Viscerosensory pathway

Postganglionic parasympathetic fibers

Peripheral portion of ANS

Peripheral pathways, enteric nervous system

Adrenal medulla

Dilatation

Lipolysis

Glycogenolysis

Increase in heart rate

Glycogenolysis

Vasoconstriction

Central portion of ANS

Vasoconstriction (skin, viscera) and vasodilatation (muscles, coronary arteries)

Effects of catecholamines (epinephrine, norepinephrine)

141

polypeptides, thyrotropin-releasing hormone, cholecystokinin, bombesin, calcitonin-gene-related peptide, neuropeptide Y, galanin, oxytocin, enkephalins) and nitric oxide.

The hypothalamus lies in the anterior portion of the diencephalon, below the thalamus and above the pituitary gland. It forms part of the wall and floor of the third ventricle. Among its anatomical components are the preoptic area, infundibulum, tuber cinereum, and mamillary bodies. It is responsible for the control and integration of endocrine function, thermoregulation (p. 152), food intake (p. 154), thirst, cardiovascular function (p. 148), respiration (p. 150), sexual function (p. 156), behavior and memory (p. 122 ff), and the sleep–wake rhythm (p. 112). Under the influence of changes in the external and internal environment, and the emotional state of the individual, the hypothalamus controls the activity of the ANS through its neural and humoral outflow.

Neuroendocrine Control
(Table 15, p. 367)

The neuroendocrine control circuits of the hypothalamic-pituitary axis regulate the plasma concentration of numerous hormones.

Adenohypophysis (anterior lobe of pituitary gland). Various regulatory hormones (releasing and inhibiting hormones) are secreted by hypothalamic neurons into a local vascular network, through which they reach the adenohypophysis to regulate the secretion of pituitary hormones into the systemic circulation. Among the pituitary hormones, the *glandotropic* hormones (TSH, ACTH, FSH, LH) induce the release of further hormones (effector hormones) from the endocrine glands, which, in turn, affect the function of the end organs, while the *aglandotropic* pituitary hormones (growth hormone, prolactin) themselves exert a direct effect on the end organs. Finally, the plasma concentration of the corresponding effector hormones and aglandotropic pituitary hormones affects the hypothalamic secretion of regulatory hormones in a negative feedback circuit (closed regulatory loop).

Neurohypophysis (posterior lobe of pituitary gland). A subset of hypothalamic neurons projects axons to the neurohypophysis. The bulb-like endings of these axons store oxytocin and antidiuretic hormone and secrete them directly into the bloodstream (neurosecretion). These hormones act directly on their effector organs. The ensuing effects are sensed by the hypothalamus, thus closing the regulatory loop.

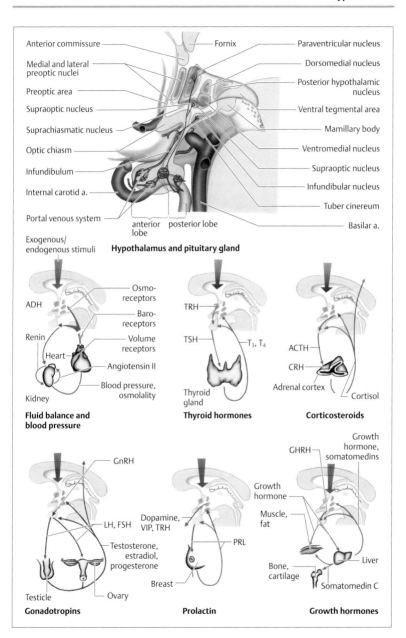

Anterior commissure — Fornix — Paraventricular nucleus

Medial and lateral preoptic nuclei — Dorsomedial nucleus

Preoptic area — Posterior hypothalamic nucleus

Supraoptic nucleus — Ventral tegmental area

Suprachiasmatic nucleus — Mamillary body

Optic chiasm — Ventromedial nucleus

Infundibulum — Supraoptic nucleus

Internal carotid a. — Infundibular nucleus

Portal venous system — Tuber cinereum

anterior lobe / posterior lobe — Basilar a.

Hypothalamus and pituitary gland

Exogenous/endogenous stimuli

ADH

Osmo-receptors

Baro-receptors

Renin

Volume receptors

Heart — Angiotensin II

Kidney — Blood pressure, osmolality

Fluid balance and blood pressure

TRH

TSH — T_3, T_4

Thyroid gland

Thyroid hormones

ACTH

CRH

Adrenal cortex — Cortisol

Corticosteroids

GnRH

LH, FSH

Testosterone, estradiol, progesterone

Testicle — Ovary

Gonadotropins

Dopamine, VIP, TRH

PRL

Breast

Prolactin

GHRH — Growth hormone, somatomedins

Growth hormone

Muscle, fat

Bone, cartilage

Liver

Somatomedin C

Growth hormones

Limbic System

The limbic system consists of a number of separate structures with complex interconnections. Its function is only partly understood, but it is clear that it plays an important role in memory, emotion, and behavior.

■ Structure

The limbic system consists of inner and outer portions, both of which resemble a ring (Latin *limbus*). The outer portion extends from rostral structures (the septal and preoptic areas) in a craniocaudal arch (cingulate gyrus) to the temporal lobe, all the way to the temporal pole (hippocampus, entorhinal cortex). The inner portion extends from the hypothalamus and mamillary body via the fornix to the dentate gyrus, hippocampus, and amygdala.

■ Nerve pathways

The neuroanatomical loop, hippocampus ⇨ fornix ⇨ mammillary body ⇨ mammillothalamic tract ⇨ anterior thalamic nucleus ⇨ cingulate gyrus ⇨ cingulum ⇨ hippocampus, is called the *Papez circuit*. Numerous fiber tracts, many of them bilateral, connect the limbic system to the thalamus, cortex, olfactory bulb (p. 76), and brain stem. The *medial forebrain bundle* links the septal and preoptic areas with the hypothalamus and midbrain. Fibers from the amygdala pass in the stria terminalis, which occupies the groove between the caudate nucleus and the thalamus, to the septal area and hypothalamus. Short fibers from the amygdala also project to the hippocampus. The *anterior commissure* connects the two amygdalae, and the commissure of the fornix connects the two hippocampi.

■ Functions of the limbic system
(Table 16, p. 368)

The limbic system controls emotional processes, such as those involved in anger, motivation, joy, sexuality, sleep, hunger, thirst, fear, aggression, and happiness. These processes are closely linked with cognition and memory (p. 134). The amygdala plays a key role in these events (emotional memory), integrating new, incoming information with the stored contents of memory. This integration determines the neural output of the limbic system, which affects the individual's physical state and behavioral responses.

ANS, Peripheral Portion (p. 146 ff)

The peripheral portion of the ANS (p. 140) subserves a number of autonomic reflexes (p. 110). Nociceptive, mechanical, and chemical stimuli interact with their respective receptors to induce the generation of afferent impulses, which then travel to the spinal autonomic neurons, whose efferent output, as described in previous sections, controls the function of the heart, smooth muscles, and glands. The activity of the spinal sympathetic neurons is subject to supraspinal regulation by the autonomic centers of the brain. Most organs of the body receive both sympathetic and parasympathetic innervation. This double innervation enables synergistic coordination of multiple organ systems (e. g., acceleration of breathing and blood flow during physical exercise).

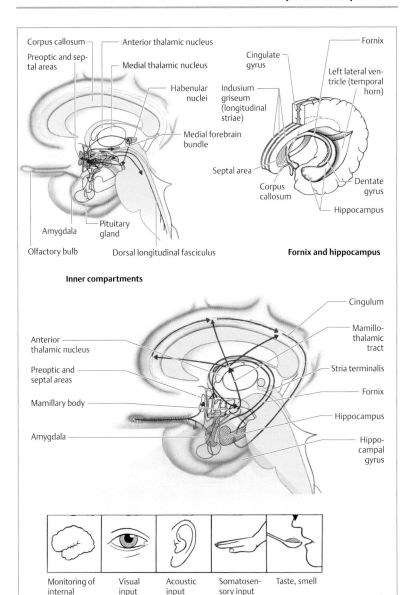

Corpus callosum

Preoptic and septal areas

Anterior thalamic nucleus

Medial thalamic nucleus

Habenular nuclei

Medial forebrain bundle

Amygdala

Pituitary gland

Olfactory bulb

Dorsal longitudinal fasciculus

Cingulate gyrus

Indusium griseum (longitudinal striae)

Septal area

Corpus callosum

Fornix

Left lateral ventricle (temporal horn)

Dentate gyrus

Hippocampus

Fornix and hippocampus

Inner compartments

Anterior thalamic nucleus

Preoptic and septal areas

Mamillary body

Amygdala

Cingulum

Mamillo-thalamic tract

Stria terminalis

Fornix

Hippocampus

Hippo-campal gyrus

Monitoring of internal environment

Visual input

Acoustic input

Somatosensory input

Taste, smell

Outer compartments

Sympathetic End Effect[1] (Receptor Type[2])	Effector Organ	Parasympathetic End Effect[1]
	Eye	
Contraction ⇨ mydriasis (α_1)	Dilator pupillae m.	—
Contraction ⇨ lid elevation	Tarsal m.	—
—	Sphincter pupillae m.	Constriction ⇨ miosis (light response)
—	Ciliary m.	Contraction ⇨ accommodation (near response)
—	Lacrimal gland	Secretion
Light mucous secretion (α_1)	*Salivary glands*	Heavy serous secretion
	Thoracic organs	
Relaxation (β_2)	Bronchial smooth muscle	Constriction
Secretion: ⇩ (α_1), ⇧ (β_2)	Bronchial glands	⇧Secretion
⇧Heart rate (β_1)	Sinoatrial node	⇩ Heart rate
⇧Contractility (β_1)	Myocardium	Slightly ⇩ contractility
	Abdominal organs	
Glycogenolysis, gluconeogenesis (α_1, β_2)	Liver	—
Dilatation (β_2)	Gallbladder, biliary tract	Contraction
⇩ Motility (α_2, β_2)	Intestine	⇧Motility
Contraction (α_1)	Sphincters	Relaxation
⇩ Insulin secretion (α_2)	Pancreas	—
⇧ Renin secretion (β_1)	Kidney	—
⇧ Secretion[3]	Adrenal medulla	—
Contraction (α_1)	Urinary sphincter	Relaxation
Relaxation (β_2)	Urinary detrusor	Contraction
Contraction (pregnancy, α_1)	Uterus	Varies (cycle-dependent)
Ejaculation (α_1)	Male genitalia	Erection
	Skin	
Secretion: ⇧generalized (cholinergic), localized[4]	Sweat glands	—
Contraction (α_1)	Arrector muscles of hair	—
	Blood vessels	
Vasoconstriction (α_1, α_2)	Cutaneous arteries	Vasodilatation
Vasoconstriction (α_1), vasodilatation (β_2)	Arteries of skeletal muscle	Vasodilatation
Vasoconstriction (α_1)	Cerebral arteries	Vasodilatation
Vasoconstriction (α_1, α_2), Vasodilatation (β_2)	Coronary arteries	Slight vasoconstriction
Vasoconstriction (α_1)	Abdominal arteries	—
Vasoconstriction (α_1, α_2)	Veins	—

1 The action of the respective organ is listed in this column. 2 These are mainly membrane receptors for epinephrine and norepinephrine (adrenoceptors). Norepinephrine mainly acts on α and β_1 receptors; epinephrine acts on all types of adrenoceptors. *Sympathomimetic* ⇨ increases sympathetic nervous activity (adrenoceptor agonist); *sympatholytic* ⇨ reduces sympathetic nervous activity (adrenoceptor antagonist, receptor blocker); *parasympathomimetic* ⇨ muscarinic receptor agonist; *indirect parasympathomimetic* ⇨ blocks acetylcholinesterase; *parasympatholytic (anticholinergic)* ⇨ muscarinic receptor antagonist; *antiparasympathotonic* ⇨ botulinum toxin. 3 Preganglionic sympathetic fibers; transmitter acetylcholine. 4Palms of hands (adrenergic sweating).

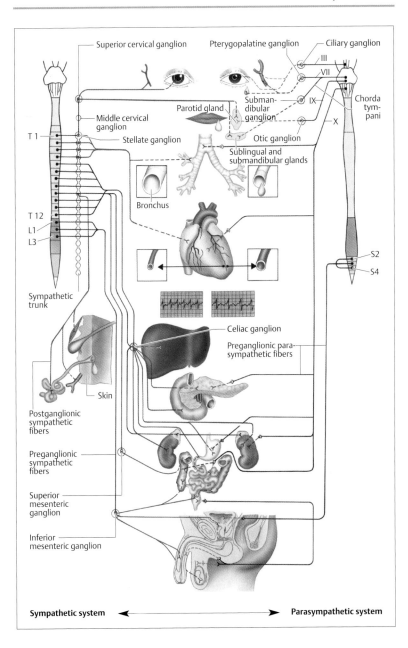

Superior cervical ganglion

Pterygopalatine ganglion

Ciliary ganglion

III

VII

Chorda tympani

Parotid gland

Submandibular ganglion

Middle cervical ganglion

IX

Stellate ganglion

X

T 1

Otic ganglion

Sublingual and submandibular glands

Bronchus

T 12

L1

L3

S2

S4

Sympathetic trunk

Celiac ganglion

Preganglionic parasympathetic fibers

Skin

Postganglionic sympathetic fibers

Preganglionic sympathetic fibers

Superior mesenteric ganglion

Inferior mesenteric ganglion

Sympathetic system ←————————→ **Parasympathetic system**

Autonomic Nervous System

Sympathetic efferent impulses cause arterial and venous vasoconstriction, acceleration of the heart rate, activation of the renin–angiotensin–aldosterone system, and secretion of epinephrine/norepinephrine from the adrenal medulla. Blood pressure and blood volume rise, and blood is redistributed away from the vascular beds of skin (pallor), intestinal organs, and kidneys in favor of the heart and brain. Conversely, parasympathetic efferent impulses cause vasodilation and a decrease in heart rate. The normal arterial blood pressure is no higher than 140 mmHg systolic and 90 mmHg diastolic. **Afferent connections.** *Baroreceptors* (pressure sensors) are located between the media and adventitia of the arterial wall in the carotid sinus (innervated by CN IX), the aortic arch (X), and the brachiocephalic trunk (X). The impulses they generate are conveyed to the *nucleus of the solitary tract* (NST) in the dorsolateral medulla; the polysynaptic relay proceeds via interneurons to the anterolateral portion of the *caudal medulla* (CM), which in turn projects to inhibitory neurons in the anterolateral portion of the *rostral medulla* (RM). Other fibers from the NST project to the *nucleus ambiguus* (NA). Other baroreceptors, found in the atria and venae cavae near their entrance to the heart, sense the volume status of the vascular system and generate impulses that travel by way of CN X to the NST and hypothalamus. *Cerebral ischemia* ($\uparrow CO_2$ in extracellular fluid and CSF; p. 162) leads to increased sympathetic activity. Mechanical, nociceptive, metabolic, and respiratory influences also affect the medullary and hypothalamic centers that regulate the circulatory system.

Efferent connections. Sympathetic impulses travel from the (inhibitory) RM to the interomediolateral cell column of the spinal cord, which projects to the adrenal medulla and, through a relay in the sympathetic ganglia, to the heart, blood vessels, and kidney. The parasympathetic outflow of the NST is relayed in the nucleus ambiguus, by way of CN X, to the heart and blood vessels.

Central nervous regulation. The sympathetic and parasympathetic innervation of the circulatory system act synergistically. Both are ultimately controlled by the hypothalamus, which projects not only to the intermediolateral cell column (sympathetic), but also to the NST and nucleus ambiguus (parasympathetic). Afferent impulses from the skeletal muscles, baroreceptors, and vestibular organs reach the fastigial nucleus of the cerebellum, which has an excitatory projection to the NST and an inhibitory projection to the RM. Cortical projections to circulatory control centers enable the cardiovascular system to function as needed in the course of voluntary, planned movements.

Syndromes (Table 17, p. 369)

Neurogenic arrhythmias may be of supraventricular or ventricular origin and are commonly associated with subarachnoid and intracerebral hemorrhage, head trauma, ischemic stroke, multiple sclerosis, epileptic seizures, brain tumors, carotid sinus syndrome (cardioinhibitory type), glossopharyngeal neuralgia and hereditary QT syndrome. They also sometimes occur in the immediate postoperative period after major neurosurgical procedures.

Neurogenic ECG abnormalities (ST depression or elevation, T-wave inversion) can occur in the setting of cerebral hemorrhage or infarction but are often difficult to distinguish from changes due to myocardial ischemia.

Hemodynamic abnormalities. *Hypertension:* Cerebral hemorrhage, Cushing reflex (accompanied by bradycardia) in response to elevated ICP, porphyria, Wernicke encephalopathy (accompanied by arrhythmia), and posterior fossa tumors. *Hypotension:* Head injuries, spinal lesions (syringomyelia, trauma, myelitis, funicular myelosis), multisystem atrophy, progressive supranuclear palsy, Parkinson disease, peripheral neuropathies (e. g., in diabetes mellitus, amyloidosis, Guillain–Barré syndrome, or renal failure). *Neurocardiogenic syncope* (vasovagal syncope) is due to pooling of venous blood in the arms and legs. Underfilling of the left ventricle activates baroreceptors, which, in turn, project via CN X to the NST. The ensuing increase of parasympathetic outflow, if large enough, sets off a "neurocardiogenic cascade" that leads to presyncope and syncope (p. 200). The characteristic features include decreased sympathetic activity, increased epinephrine secretion from the adrenal medulla, and decreased norepinephrine secretion, resulting in vasodilatation. Hyperexcitability of the vagus nerve (bradycardia) is also seen.

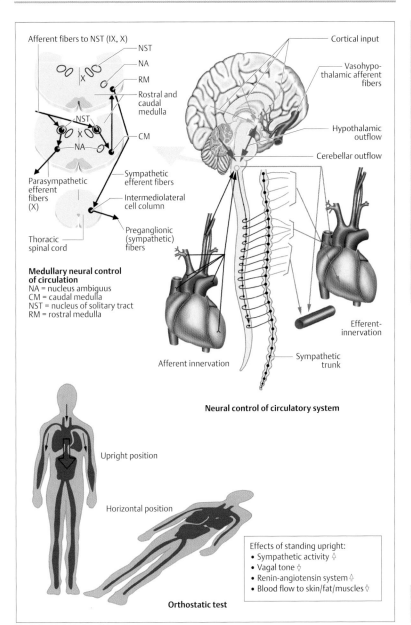

Afferent fibers to NST (IX, X)
NST
NA
RM
Rostral and caudal medulla
CM

Parasympathetic efferent fibers (X)

Sympathetic efferent fibers
Intermediolateral cell column

Thoracic spinal cord

Preganglionic (sympathetic) fibers

Medullary neural control of circulation
NA = nucleus ambiguus
CM = caudal medulla
NST = nucleus of solitary tract
RM = rostral medulla

Cortical input
Vasohypo-thalamic afferent fibers
Hypothalamic outflow
Cerebellar outflow

Efferent-innervation
Sympathetic trunk
Afferent innervation

Neural control of circulatory system

Upright position

Horizontal position

Effects of standing upright:
• Sympathetic activity ⇧
• Vagal tone ⇩
• Renin-angiotensin system ⇧
• Blood flow to skin/fat/muscles ⇩

Orthostatic test

Autonomic Nervous System

Respiration ensures an adequate oxygen supply for the body's tissues and maintains acid–base hemostasis.

Respiratory movements. Inspiration can be achieved by contraction of the diaphragm (*diaphragmatic respiration*) or of the intercostal muscles (*costal respiration*). The *auxiliary respiratory muscles* of the shoulder girdle further enlarge the chest cavity, if required, for deep breathing. Expiration is largely passive. The muscles of the abdominal wall and the latissimus dorsi muscle serve as *auxiliary expiratory muscles*. Other muscles (genioglossus, pharyngeal constrictor, and laryngeal muscles) keep the upper airway open during respiration.

Afferent connections. Chemoreceptors responding to arterial pH and O_2 and CO_2 concentration are found in the carotid glomus (innervated by CN IX), aortic arch (X), and para-aortic bodies (X). Impulses arising in these chemoreceptors, and in *mechanoreceptors* in the respiratory muscles (sensory afferent connections ⇨ phrenic nerve, intercostal nerves 2–12, CN IX) and in the lungs (bronchodilatation ⇨ pulmonary plexus, sympathetic nerve T1–T4), travel to the *dorsal respiratory group* of nuclei (DRG) anterior to the nucleus of the solitary tract, from which they are relayed, via interneurons, to the *ventral respiratory group* (VRG) in the medulla. The DRG also receives afferent input from the cardiovascular system, which is thus able to influence respiratory function. Changes in the pH and CO_2 concentration of the extracellular fluid (ECF) and cerebrospinal fluid (CSF) are also directly sensed by medullary chemoreceptors. Respiration is further influenced by a wide variety of other phenomena, e. g., cold, heat, hormones, reflexes (sneezing, coughing, yawning, swallowing), sleep, mental state (anxiety, fear), speaking, singing, laughing, muscle activity (physical work, sports), sexual activity, and body temperature.

Efferent connections. The laryngopharyngeal muscles and bronchoconstrictors are innervated by CN X. The phrenic nerve (diaphragm, C3–C5) and motor branches of the spinal nerves (intercostal nerves 2–9/T2–T11 ⇨ intercostal muscles; intercostal nerves 6–12/T6–T12 ⇨ abdominal wall muscles) supply the auxiliary respiratory muscles.

Respiratory rhythm. Rhythmic breathing is achieved by oscillating, alternately inhibitory

and excitatory *neural control circuits* within the VRG. As inspiration progresses, the inspiratory neuron groups of the VRG are progressively inhibited (Hering–Breuer reflex), while the expiratory neuron groups are excited. The respiratory rhythm is influenced by afferent input from chemoreceptors reflecting changes in the composition of the blood (decreases in pH and O_2 concentration, rise in CO_2 concentration ⇨ deeper respiration, ⇧ respiratory rate) or of the ECF and CSF (decrease in pH, rise in CO_2 concentration ⇨ deeper respiration, ⇧ respiratory rate). The VRG is influenced by pontine nuclei.

Syndromes (Table 18, p. 370)

Pathological breathing patterns may be due to metabolic, toxic, or mechanical factors (obstructive sleep apnea) or to a lesion of the nervous system (p. 118). Morning headaches, fatigue, daytime somnolence, and impaired concentration may reflect a (nocturnal) breathing disorder. Neurogenic or myogenic breathing disorders often come to medical attention because of coughing attacks or food "going down the wrong pipe." Neurological diseases are often complicated by respiratory dysfunction. The respiratory parameters (respiratory drive, coughing force, blood gases, vital capacity) should be carefully monitored over time so that intubation and/or tracheostomy for artificial ventilation can be performed as necessary.

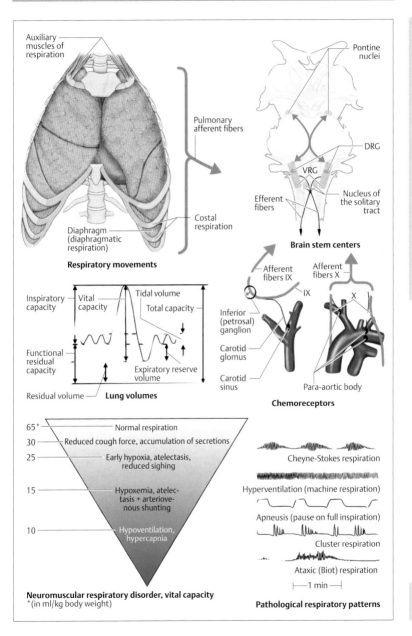

Auxiliary muscles of respiration

Pontine nuclei

Pulmonary afferent fibers

DRG

VRG

Efferent fibers

Nucleus of the solitary tract

Costal respiration

Diaphragm (diaphragmatic respiration)

Respiratory movements

Brain stem centers

Afferent fibers IX

Afferent fibers X

IX

X

Inferior (petrosal) ganglion

Carotid glomus

Carotid sinus

Para-aortic body

Chemoreceptors

Inspiratory capacity

Vital capacity

Tidal volume

Total capacity

Functional residual capacity

Expiratory reserve volume

Residual volume — **Lung volumes**

65* — Normal respiration

30 — Reduced cough force, accumulation of secretions

25 — Early hypoxia, atelectasis, reduced sighing

15 — Hypoxemia, atelectasis + arteriovenous shunting

10 — Hypoventilation, hypercapnia

Neuromuscular respiratory disorder, vital capacity
*(in ml/kg body weight)

Cheyne-Stokes respiration

Hyperventilation (machine respiration)

Apneusis (pause on full inspiration)

Cluster respiration

Ataxic (Biot) respiration

⊢—1 min—⊣

Pathological respiratory patterns

Thermoregulation

The temperature of the body is a function of heat absorption, heat production, and heat elimination. Core body temperature normally fluctuates from approximately 36 °C in the morning to 37.5 °C in the late afternoon. It can be influenced by the menstrual cycle, pregnancy, and other hormonal factors, as well as by eating behavior and digestion, and it varies with age.

Neural control. The thermoregulatory center lies in the preoptic and anterior region of the hypothalamus (p. 142). Heat is *eliminated* through the skin (heat radiation, convection, sweating ⇨ cooling by evaporation), respiration (evaporation), and blood circulation (heat transport from the interior to the surface, cutaneous blood flow). Heat is *produced* by metabolic processes (under the influence of thyroid hormones) and by muscle contraction (shivering, voluntary movement). *Thermoreceptors* in the skin, spinal cord, medulla, and midbrain generate afferent impulses that travel to the hypothalamic control center; the cutaneous receptors project to the hypothalamus by way of the spinothalamic tract. Thermoreceptors are also present in the hypothalamus itself. The hypothalamus makes extensive connections with other regions of the brain. Its major *efferent pathways* relating to thermoregulation (vasomotor and sudoriparous pathways) pass by way of the ipsilateral lateral funiculus of the spinal cord to the spinal sympathetic nuclei (thoracolumbar system). These then give rise to fibers that travel by way of the ventral roots to the sympathetic chain ganglia; postganglionic fibers travel with the peripheral nerves to the skin. *Sudoriparous fibers* are found only in the ventral roots of T2/3 to L2/3, yet they innervate the skin of the entire body; thus, their distribution is not the same as the dermatomal distribution of sensation. Sudoriparous fibers to the head travel along the internal and external carotid arteries and then join branches of the trigeminal nerve to arrive at the skin. The neurotransmitter for the sympathetic innervation of the sweat glands is acetylcholine.

Disturbances of body temperature. *Central hyperthermia* is an elevation of body temperature due to impaired thermoregulation by the central nervous system. Its mechanism may involve either excessive heat production, excessive heat absorption (e. g., in a hot environment), or inadequate heat elimination. *Fever* may be defined as an oral temperature greater than 37.2 °C in the morning or 37.7 °C in the afternoon (rectal temperature 0.6 °C higher). Its cause is generally not an impairment of thermoregulation, but rather a change in the set point for temperature established by the hypothalamic thermoregulatory center. Such a change can be brought about by circulating pyrogenic cytokines (e. g., interleukin-1, tumor necrosis factor, interferon-α) that exert an effect on hypothalamic function by interacting with the circumventricular organs (p. 140). *Hypothermia* is defined as a core temperature below 35 °C.

Syndromes

Disturbances of thermoregulatory sweating. *Examination:* Useful tests include palpation of the skin to appreciate its moisture and temperature, the quantitative sudomotor axon reflex test (QSART), the sympathetic skin response (SSR), iodine–starch test (Minor test), and the ninhydrin test.

Generalized anhidrosis (which confers a risk of hyperthermia) may be idiopathic or may be due to lesions in the hypothalamus or in the spinal cord above T3/4 . Monoradicular lesions or cervical or lumbosacral polyradicular lesions do not impair sweating. Lesions of the sympathetic trunk cause segmental anhidrosis. *Plexus lesions* and *isolated or combined neuropathies* produce anhidrosis in the area of a sensory deficit. Lesions from the level of the stellate ganglion upward cause anhidrosis as a component of Horner syndrome. Sweating of the palms and soles is not influenced by thermoregulatory mechanisms but rather by the emotional state (fear, nervousness).

Central hyperthermia may be due to hypothalamic lesions (infarction, hemorrhage, tumor, encephalitis, neurosarcoidosis, trauma), intoxications (anticholinergic agents, salicylates, amphetamines, cocaine), acute spinal cord transection above T3/4, delirium, catatonia, malignant neuroleptic syndrome, malignant hyperthermia, dehydration, heat stroke, and generalized tetanus.

Fever. The symptoms include malaise, shivering, feeling cold, chills, nausea, vomiting, and somnolence. The heart rate and blood pressure rise, thermoregulatory sweating diminishes, and the peripheral blood volume is redistributed to the core of the body. Simple febrile convulsions in children under 5 years of age generally do not lead to epilepsy or other neurological complications.

Autonomic Nervous System

152

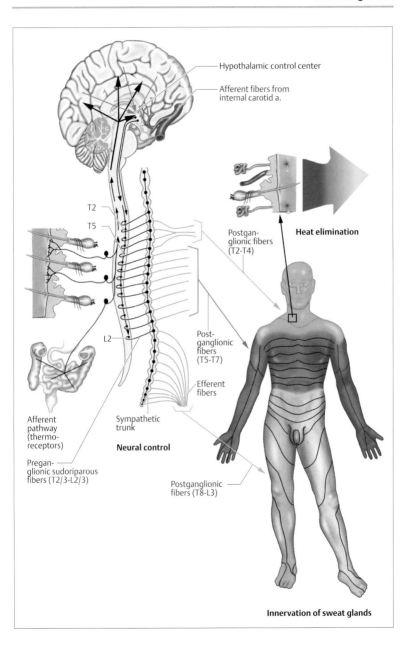

Hypothalamic control center

Afferent fibers from
internal carotid a.

T2

T5

Postgan-
glionic fibers
(T2–T4)

Heat elimination

Post-
ganglionic
fibers
(T5–T7)

Efferent
fibers

L2

Afferent
pathway
(thermo-
receptors)

Sympathetic
trunk

Neural control

Pregan-
glionic sudoriparous
fibers (T2/3–L2/3)

Postganglionic
fibers (T8–L3)

Innervation of sweat glands

Autonomic Nervous System

153

The uptake, transport, storage, and digestion of food, the absorption of nutrients, and the elimination of waste matter are under the influence of both the extrinsic autonomic nervous system and the intrinsic autonomic nervous system of the intestine.

The **extrinsic system** modulates the function of the intrinsic enteric system in coordination with the function of other organs of the body. Brain stem nuclei subserve the gastrointestinal and enterocolic reflexes, while cortical, limbic (hypothalamus, amygdala) and cerebellar centers (fastigial nucleus) mediate the perception of satiety, the enteral response to hunger and odors, and emotional influences on alimentary function. The *parasympathetic innervation* (neurotransmitter: acetylcholine) of the esophagus, stomach, small intestine, and proximal portion of the large intestine is through the vagus nerve, while that of the distal portion of the large intestine and anal sphincter is derived from segments S2–S4. Parasympathetic activity stimulates intestinal motility (peristalsis) and glandular secretion. *Sympathetic innervation* (transmitter: norepinephrine) is from the superior cervical ganglion to the upper esophagus, from the celiac ganglion to the lower esophagus and stomach, and from the superior and inferior mesenteric ganglia to the colon. Sympathetic activity inhibits peristalsis, lowers intestinal blood flow, and constricts the sphincters of the gastrointestinal tract (lower esophageal sphincter, pylorus, inner anal sphincter).

The **intrinsic system (enteric system)** consists of the myenteric and submucous ganglionic plexuses (p. 141), which are independent neural networks of sensory and motor neurons and interneurons. The enteric autonomic nervous system receives chemical, nociceptive, and mechanical stimuli, processes this neural input, and produces efferent impulses affecting gastrointestinal glandular secretion and smooth-muscle contraction.

Syndromes (Table 19, p. 370)

Neurological diseases most commonly affect gastrointestinal function by impairing motility, less commonly by impairing resorptive and secretory processes. The differential diagnosis must include gastrointestinal dysfunction of nonneurological (often obstructive) origin. Specialized diagnostic testing is usually indicated.

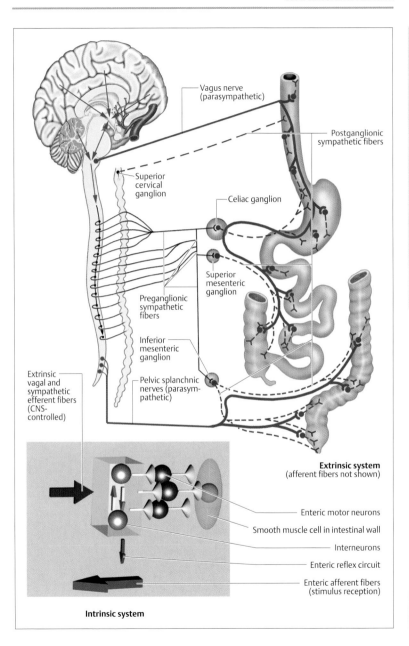

Vagus nerve (parasympathetic)

Postganglionic sympathetic fibers

Superior cervical ganglion

Celiac ganglion

Preganglionic sympathetic fibers

Superior mesenteric ganglion

Inferior mesenteric ganglion

Extrinsic vagal and sympathetic efferent fibers (CNS-controlled)

Pelvic splanchnic nerves (parasympathetic)

Extrinsic system
(afferent fibers not shown)

Enteric motor neurons

Smooth muscle cell in intestinal wall

Interneurons

Enteric reflex circuit

Enteric afferent fibers (stimulus reception)

Intrinsic system

Autonomic Nervous System

155

Bladder Function

The urinary bladder stores (continence) and voids (micturition) the urine produced by the kidneys. *Parasympathetic fibers* arising in segments S2–S4 (sacral micturition center, detrusor nucleus) and traveling through the pelvic plexus activate the detrusor muscle of the bladder. *Sympathetic fibers* arising from segments T10–L2 and traveling through the hypogastric plexus inhibit the detrusor (β-adrenergic receptors) and stimulate the vesical neck (trigone, internal sphincter; α-adrenergic receptors). *Somatic motor impulses* arising from segments S2–S4 (Onuf's nucleus) travel through the pudendal nerve to the external sphincter and the pelvic floor muscles. *Somatosensory fibers* from the bladder travel along the hypogastric and pelvic nerves to spinal levels T10–L2 and S2–S4, conveying information about the state of bladder stretch (overdistention is painful). The *central nervous system* (frontal lobes, basal ganglia) subserves the voluntary inhibition of detrusor contraction. The pontine micturition center, which triggers the act of micturition, is under the influence of afferent impulses relating to the state of bladder stretch; its output passes to somatic motor neurons in the spinal cord that synergistically innervate the detrusor and external sphincter muscles.

Continence. An intact bladder closure mechanism is essential for normal filling (up to 500 ml). Closure involves contraction of the vesical neck and external sphincter urethrae and pelvic floor muscles, and relaxation of the detrusor muscle (dome of the bladder).

Micturition. Once a urine volume of 150–250 ml has accumulated, stretch receptors generate impulses that pass to the pontine micturition center and also produce the sensation of bladder distention. Micturition begins when the dome of the bladder is stimulated to contract while the vesical neck and pelvic floor muscles relax. Contraction of the muscles of the abdominal wall increases the intravesical pressure and facilitates micturition.

Neurogenic bladder dysfunction (Table 20, p. 371). Additional diagnostic tests are performed in collaboration with a urologist or gynecologist as deemed necessary on the basis of the case history and neurological findings.

Useful diagnostic aids include laboratory testing (urinalysis and renal function), ultrasound examination (kidney, bladder, pelvis), urodynamic testing, micturition cystourethrography, and neurophysiological studies (evoked potentials, urethroanal/bulbocavernosus reflex).

Sexual Function

The genital organs receive sympathetic (T11–L2), parasympathetic (S2–S4), somatic motor (Onuf's nucleus), and somatosensory innervation (S2–S4) and are under supraspinal control, mostly through hypothalamic projections to the spinal cord. Hormonal factors also play an important role (p. 142). Neurological disease often causes sexual dysfunction (erectile dysfunction, ejaculatory dysfunction) in combination with bladder dysfunction. Isolated sexual dysfunction is more often due to psychological factors (depression, anxiety), diabetes mellitus, endocrine disorders, and atherosclerosis.

Autonomic Nervous System

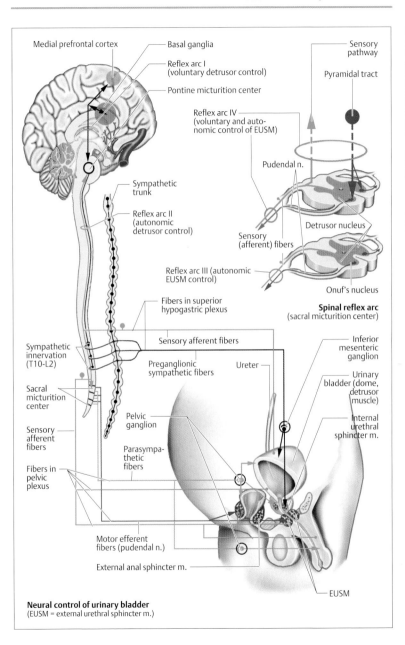

Medial prefrontal cortex

Basal ganglia

Reflex arc I
(voluntary detrusor control)

Pontine micturition center

Sensory
pathway

Pyramidal tract

Reflex arc IV
(voluntary and auto-
nomic control of EUSM)

Pudendal n.

Sympathetic
trunk

Reflex arc II
(autonomic
detrusor control)

Sensory
(afferent) fibers

Detrusor nucleus

Reflex arc III (autonomic
EUSM control)

Onuf's nucleus

Fibers in superior
hypogastric plexus

Spinal reflex arc
(sacral micturition center)

Sympathetic
innervation
(T10–L2)

Sensory afferent fibers

Preganglionic
sympathetic fibers

Ureter

Inferior
mesenteric
ganglion

Urinary
bladder (dome,
detrusor
muscle)

Sacral
micturition
center

Pelvic
ganglion

Internal
urethral
sphincter m.

Sensory
afferent
fibers

Parasympa-
thetic
fibers

Fibers in
pelvic
plexus

Motor efferent
fibers (pudendal n.)

External anal sphincter m.

EUSM

Neural control of urinary bladder
(EUSM = external urethral sphincter m.)

Autonomic Nervous System

The intracranial pressure (ICP) corresponds to the pressure that the contents of the skull exert on the dura mater.

Intracranial Hypertension

The normal intracranial pressure (ICP) is 60–120 mmH$_2$O, which corresponds to 5–15 mmHg. An ICP greater than 30 mmHg impairs cerebral blood flow; an ICP greater than 50 mmHg for more than 30 minutes is fatal; an ICP greater than 80 mmHg for any length of time can cause brain damage. Intracranial hypertension may be either acute (developing in hours to days) or chronic (lasting for weeks or months). Its manifestations are progressively more severe as the ICP rises, but are not specific; thus, the diagnosis cannot be made from the signs of intracranial hypertension alone but requires either the demonstration of a causative lesion (e. g., subdural hematoma, encephalitis, brain tumor, hydrocephalus) or direct measurement of the intracranial pressure. Treatment is indicated when the ICP persistently exceeds 20 mmHg, when plateau waves are found, or when the pulse amplitude rises. Individual cases may manifest a variety of different signs of intracranial hypertension, either in slow or rapid alternation, or all at the same time. Compression of the brain stem by a space-occupying lesion (p. 118) has similar clinical manifestations; the diagnostic differentiation of brain stem compression from intracranial hypertension is critical. Lumbar puncture is contraindicated in cases of suspected or documented intracranial hypertension, as the resulting increase in the already high craniospinal pressure gradient may lead to brain herniation.

■ **Clinical Features** (Table 21, p. 371)

Headache due to intracranial hypertension ranges in intensity from mild to unbearable. Patients typically report a pressing, bifrontal headache that is most severe upon awakening in the morning or after naps in the daytime. It is exacerbated by lying flat, coughing, abdominal straining, or bending over, and ameliorated by sitting or standing. It may wake the patient from sleep. Often, both mild daytime headaches and more severe nighttime headaches are present.

Nausea due to intracranial hypertension is often independent of movement of the head or of other abdominal complaints, and its intensity is not correlated with that of headache. It may be mild or severe.

Projectile vomiting may occur without warning or after a brief sensation of nausea upon sitting up or moving the head. Initially, vomiting mainly occurs suddenly, in the morning (on an empty stomach).

Eye movements and vision. Compression of CN III or VI causes paresis of extraocular muscles or pupillary dilatation (p. 92). *Papilledema* often affects the eye on the side of the causative lesion first, and then gradually the other eye as well. The older the patient, the less likely that papilledema will occur as a sign of intracranial hypertension; its absence thus cannot be taken as ruling out intracranial hypertension. Early papilledema is characterized by hyperemia, blurred papillary margins, dilated veins, loss of venous pulsations (may be absent normally), and small hemorrhages around the papilla. Full-blown papilledema is characterized by disk elevation, engorged veins, tortuous vessels around the papilla, and streaky hemorrhages. If intracranial hypertension persists, *chronic papilledema* will develop in weeks or months, characterized by grayish-white optic nerve atrophy and small vessel caliber. Acute papilledema generally does not affect the visual fields or visual acuity (unlike papillitis, which should be considered in the differential diagnosis); but physical exertion or head movement may cause transient amblyopic attacks lasting several seconds (foggy or blurred vision, or blindness). Chronic papilledema, on the other hand, can cause an impairment visual acuity, concentric visual field defects, and even blindness.

Gait disturbances. An unsteady, slow, hesitant, gait with small steps and swaying from sided to side is sometimes seen.

Behavioral changes. Impairment of memory, attention, concentration, and planning ability, confusion, slowed reactions, and changes in personal habits are often observed by relatives and friends.

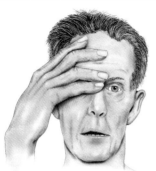

Headache

Streaky hemorrhage

Mild disk elevation (0.5 diopters), ill-defined margins

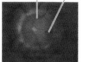

Early papilledema

Elevated (3–5 diopters) and enlarged disk with irregular margins

Infarcts (cotton-wool spots)

Dilated vein

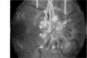

Papilledema
(fully developed)

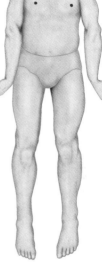

Herniation
(decerebration syndrome)

Nausea

Disk elevation (5 diopters)

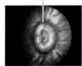

Chronic papilledema

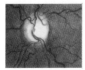

Optic nerve atrophy

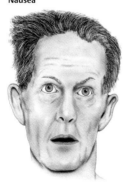

Behavioral change

Herniation syndromes (p. 162). *Transtentorial herniation* causes an ipsilateral oculomotor nerve palsy (ptosis, mydriasis, and secondary ophthalmoplegia), contralateral hemiplegia, and decerebration syndrome (p. 46). Downward herniation of the contents of the posterior fossa into the foramen magnum causes neck pain and stiffness, a head tilt, and shoulder paresthesiae. If medullary compression is also present, respiratory and circulatory disorders, cerebellar fits, and obstructive hydrocephalus may develop. Upward herniation of the contents of the posterior fossa across the tentorial notch causes a decerebration syndrome in which the ipsilateral pupil is initially constricted and later dilated.

Pseudotumor cerebri causes headache (holocephalic, bilateral frontal/occipital), visual disturbances of varying severity (enlarged blind spot, blurred vision, loss of vision, or diplopia due to abducens palsy), and bilateral papilledema. CT and MRI scans reveal the absence of an intracranial mass (normal ventricular size, thickening of optic nerve, "empty sella" = intrasellar expansion of the suprasellar cisterns, with or without sellar dilatation). CSF tests are normal except for an elevated opening pressure (>250 mmH$_2$O). The etiology of pseudotumor cerebri is multifactorial; it occurs most commonly in obese young women. Its differential diagnosis includes intracranial venous or venous sinus thrombosis, drug toxicity (high doses of vitamin A, tetracycline, NSAIDs), elevated CSF protein level (spinal tumor, Guillain–Barré syndrome), or endocrine changes (pregnancy, Addison disease, Cushing syndrome, hypothyroidism).

Intracranial Hypotension

Spontaneous drainage of cerebrospinal fluid by means of lumbar puncture is no longer possible when the CSF pressure is below 20 mmH$_2$O (patient is lying flat); when it is below 0 mmH$_2$O, air is sucked through the LP needle into the subarachnoid space and travels upward to the head, where air bubbles can be seen on a CT scan. For causes of low intracranial pressure see Table 22 (p. 372).

▪ Symptoms

Severe headache (nuchal, occipital, or frontal) is provoked by sitting, standing, or walking, and subsides when the patient lies flat. It is exacerbated by abdominal straining, coughing, and the Valsalva maneuver. Other symptoms include nausea, vomiting, and dizziness. Unilateral or bilateral abducens palsy, tinnitus, ear pressure, or neck stiffness may also occur. Subdural fluid collections (hematoma due to rupture of the bridging veins, hygroma arising from local CSF collection due to rupture of the arachnoid membrane) are rare. Intracranial hypotension may be caused by a CSF leak; patients may report occasional loss of watery fluid from the nose or ear (traces visible on pillows).

Normal-pressure hydrocephalus (NPH) is a chronic form of communicating hydrocephalus that reflects an impairment of CSF circulation and resorption, sometimes in the aftermath of subarachnoid hemorrhage, head trauma, or chronic meningitis, but often without discernible cause. Symptoms develop over several weeks or months. *Gait disturbances* (gait apraxia, hydrocephalic astasia-abasia) begin as unsteadiness, difficulty climbing stairs, leg fatigue, a small-stepped gait, and frequent stumbling and falling, and then typically progress to an inability to stand, sit, or turn over in bed. The associated *behavioral changes* (p. 132 ff) are variable and may include impaired spatial orientation, reduced psychomotor drive (abulia), mild memory disturbances, or even dementia. *Bladder dysfunction* such as urge incontinence and polyuria develop as the condition progresses. Patients ultimately lose the perception of bladder distension and thus void uncontrollably.

Pathogenesis

ICP depends on the volume of nervous tissue, CSF, and blood inside the nondistensible cavity formed by the skull and vertebral canal. An increase in the volume of one of these three components must be offset by a compensatory mechanism (Monro–Kellie doctrine) such as an adjustment of the CSF or (venous) blood volume, expansion or the lumbosacral dural sheath, or deformation of the brain. When the capacity of such mechanisms is exhausted, the ICP decompensates. *Compliance* is defined as the first derivative of volume as a function of ICP, i.e., the ratio of a small, incremental change in

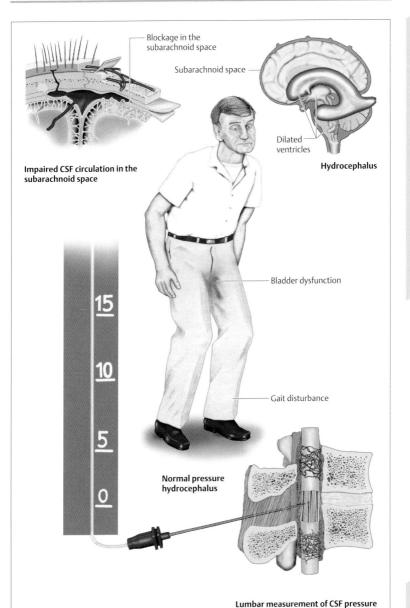

Blockage in the subarachnoid space

Subarachnoid space

Impaired CSF circulation in the subarachnoid space

Dilated ventricles

Hydrocephalus

Bladder dysfunction

Gait disturbance

Normal pressure hydrocephalus

Lumbar measurement of CSF pressure

volume to the change in ICP that it produces. Compliance is thus an index of the ability to compensate for changes in volume. Decreased compliance leads to ICP decompensation. *Elastance* is the reciprocal of compliance, hence indicating the inability to compensate for changes in volume.

CSF volume. *Hydrocephalus* is defined as abnormal dilatation of the ventricular system. It occurs because of disturbances of CSF circulation and/or resorption. Hydrocephalus due to a blockage of the CSF pathway at some point within the ventricular system is called *noncommunicating* or *obstructive hydrocephalus*. Hydrocephalus due to impaired CSF resorption at the arachnoid villi is called *communicating* or *malresorptive hydrocephalus*. *Acute hydrocephalus* is characterized by ventricular dilatation with acute intracranial hypertension. Hydrocephalus with normal ICP and without progression of ventricular dilatation is called arrested, compensated or *chronic hydrocephalus*. So-called *normal-pressure hydrocephalus* occupies an intermediate position between these two conditions. *External hydrocephalus* is a dilatation of the subarachnoid space with no more than mild enlargement of the ventricles.

Cerebral Blood Flow

Cerebral blood flow (CBF) is a function of the cerebral perfusion pressure (CPP), which normally ranges from 70 to 100 mmHg, and the cerebral vascular resistance (CVR): CBF = CPP/CVR. CBF is maintained at a constant value of approximately 50 ml/100 g/min as long as the mean arterial pressure (MAP)[1] remains in the relatively wide range from 50 to 150 mmHg (cerebral autoregulation). When the patient is lying flat, CPP = MAP – ICP. A rapid rise in the systemic arterial pressure is followed by a slow, delayed rise in ICP; chronic arterial hypertension usually does not affect the ICP. On the other hand, any elevation of the *venous pressure* (normal central venous pressure: 40–120 mmH$_2$O) due to Valsalva maneuvers, hypervolemia, right heart failure, changes in body position, or obstruction of jugular venous drainage elevates the ICP by a comparable amount. *Acidosis* (defined as pH < 7.40), which may be due to hypoxia, ischemia, or hypoventilation, causes cerebral vasodilatation and increased cerebral blood volume, thereby elevating the ICP. Chronic obstructive pulmonary disease can elevate the ICP by this mechanism. On the other hand, *alkalosis* (e. g., due to hyperventilation) reduces the cerebral blood volume and thus also the ICP. CBF and ICP are elevated in fever and low in hyperthermia.

Intracranial Space-occupying Lesions

Extra-axial or intra-axial compression of brain tissue elevates the ICP, calling compensatory mechanisms into play; once these have been exhausted, mass displacement of brain tissue occurs, possibly resulting in herniation. The distribution of pressure within the cranial cavity is a function of the structure of the brain and the partitioning of the cavity by dural folds (p. 6). Different herniation syndromes occur depending on the site and extent of the causative lesion: subfalcine herniation involves movement of the cingulate gyrus under the falx cerebri; transtentorial herniation involves movement of the medial portion of the temporal lobe across the tentorial notch; upward posterior fossa herniation involves movement of the brain stem and cerebellum across the tentorial notch; and downward posterior fossa herniation involves movement of the cerebellar tonsils across the foramen magnum.

In *cerebral edema*, accumulation of water and electrolytes in brain tissue causes an increase in brain volume. *Vasogenic cerebral edema* is due to increased capillary permeability and mainly affects white matter; it is caused by brain tumor, abscess, infarction, trauma, hemorrhage, and bacterial meningitis. *Cytotoxic cerebral edema* affects both white and gray matter and is due to fluid accumulation in all cells of the brain (neurons, glia, endothelium) because of hypoxia/ischemia or acute hypotonic hyperhydration (water intoxication, dysequilibrium syndrome, inadequate ADH syndrome). *Hydrocephalic* (interstitial) brain edema is found in the walls of the cerebral ventricles and results from movement of fluid from the ventricles into the adjacent tissue in the setting of acute hydrocephalus.

[1]The MAP can be estimated with the following formulas: MAP = [(systolic BP) + (2 × diastolic BP)] × 1/3 or, equivalently, MAP = diastolic BP + [(BP amplitude) × 1/3]

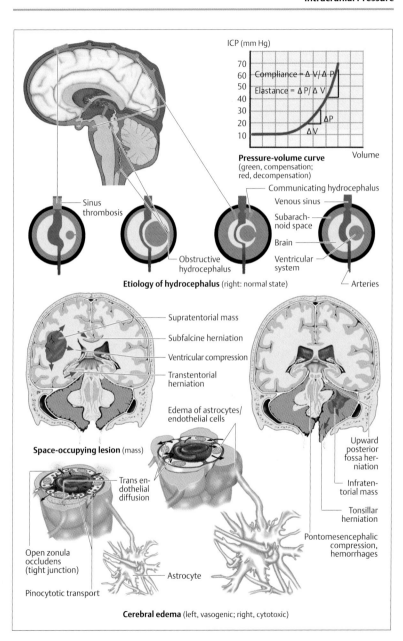

ICP (mm Hg)

Compliance = Δ V/ Δ P
Elastance = Δ P/ Δ V

ΔP
ΔV

Volume

Pressure-volume curve
(green, compensation;
red, decompensation)

Communicating hydrocephalus

Venous sinus

Subarach-
noid space

Brain

Sinus
thrombosis

Obstructive
hydrocephalus

Ventricular
system

Arteries

Etiology of hydrocephalus (right: normal state)

Supratentorial mass

Subfalcine herniation

Ventricular compression

Transtentorial
herniation

Edema of astrocytes/
endothelial cells

Upward
posterior
fossa her-
niation

Infraten-
torial mass

Tonsillar
herniation

Pontomesencephalic
compression,
hemorrhages

Space-occupying lesion (mass)

Trans en-
dothelial
diffusion

Open zonula
occludens
(tight junction)

Astrocyte

Pinocytotic transport

Cerebral edema (left, vasogenic; right, cytotoxic)

3 Neurological Syndromes

- Brain Disorders

- Spinal Disorders

- Peripheral Neuropathies

- Myopathies

Stroke

A *stroke* is an acute focal or global impairment of brain function resulting from a pathological process (e.g. thrombus, embolus, vessel rupture) of the blood vessels. Its causes, in order of decreasing frequency, are *ischemia* (80%), spontaneous *intracerebral or intraventricular hemorrhage* (15%), and *subarachnoid hemorrhage* (5%). The signs and symptoms of stroke are usually not specific enough to enable identification of its etiology without further diagnostic studies. CT, MRI, cerebrovascular ultrasonography, ECG, and laboratory testing are usually needed.

Symptoms and Signs

The clinical manifestations of stroke persist, by definition, for more than 24 hours, and are often permanent, though partial recovery is common. The duration of symptoms and signs seems not to be correlated with the etiology of stroke.

Ischemia. A *transient ischemic attack* (TIA) differs from a stroke (by definition) in that its symptoms and signs resolve completely within 24 hours. The vast majority of TIAs resolve within one hour, and only 5% last longer than 12 hours. Patients with *crescendo TIAs* (a rapid succession of TIAs) have a high risk of developing a (completed) stroke, which can cause neurological deficits that are either minor (minor stroke) or major (disabling stroke, major stroke). A stuttering, fluctuating, or progressive course of stroke development (*stroke in evolution*) is uncommon.

Hemorrhage. Nontraumatic intracerebral hemorrhages usually cause acute neurological deficits that persist thereafter. If deficits worsen after the initial hemorrhage, the cause is either recurrent hemorrhage or a complication of the initial hemorrhage (cerebral edema, electrolyte imbalance, or heart disorder).

Type of Deficit	Clinical Manifestations
Weakness (pp. 46 ff, 70)	Acute hemi-, mono-, or quadriparesis/quadriplegia (ca. 80–90%); loss of coordination and balance; hyperkinesia (during or after stroke), e. g. hemichorea, hemiballism, or (rarely) dystonia
Sensory loss (pp. 70 ff, 106)	Injury of postcentral cortex or subcortical area ⇨ distal sensory (often also motor) deficit in contralateral limbs. Paresthesiae and loss of stereognosis, graphesthesia, topesthesia, and acrognosis are prominent
Oculomotor and visual disturbances (pp. 70, 82 ff)	Conjugate horizontal eye movements, disjugate gaze, nystagmus, diplopia. Visual field defects (p. 82), transient monocular blindness (= amaurosis fugax)
Headache (p. 182)	May be caused by subarachnoid hemorrhage, temporal arteritis, venous sinus thrombosis, arterial dissection, cerebellar hemorrhage, massive intracerebral hemorrhage (rare)
Impairment of consciousness (pp. 116, 204)	TIA and stroke generally do not impair consciousness (exception: brainstem stroke, massive supratentorial stroke with bilateral cortical dysfunction)
Behavioral changes (p. 122 ff)	Aphasia, confusion (must be distinguished from aphasia), impairment of memory, neglect, impaired affect control (compulsive crying and/or laughing), apraxia. Mental changes, especially depression and anxiety disorders, are common after stroke
Dysarthria and dysphagia (pp. 102, 130)	Severe dysarthria is often accompanied by coughing, difficulty chewing, and dysphasia. *Pseudobulbar palsy* ⇨ loss of voluntary motor control (e. g., swallowing, speaking, tongue movement) with preservation of involuntary movements (e. g., yawning, coughing, laughing)
Dizziness (p. 58)	Cerebellum, brainstem (vertigo, nausea, nystagmus)
Epileptic seizures (p. 192 ff)	Simple partial, complex partial, or generalized tonic-clonic seizures may occur during or after a stroke
Respiratory disorders (p. 150)	*Hiccups* (singultus) often occur in stroke, particularly in lateral medullary infarction. Central hyperventilation is associated with a poor prognosis. Bihemispheric lesions may cause Cheyne–Stokes respiration (p. 118)

Minor complications of stroke: Mild unilateral arm paresis, moderate sensory loss, mild dysarthria; these patients can care for themselves. *Major complications*: Aphasia, spastic hemiplegia, and hemianopsia; these patients generally need nursing care.

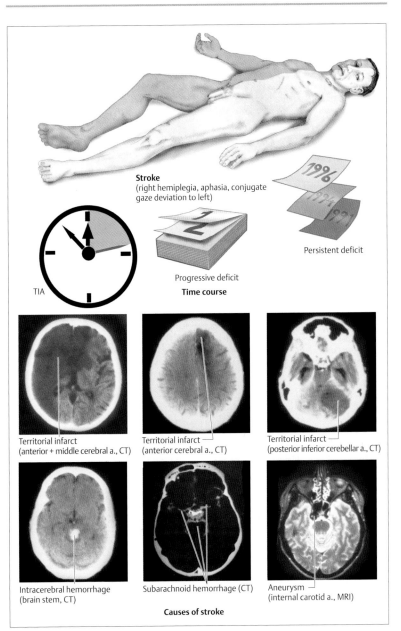

Stroke
(right hemiplegia, aphasia, conjugate gaze deviation to left)

Persistent deficit

Progressive deficit

Time course

TIA

Territorial infarct
(anterior + middle cerebral a., CT)

Territorial infarct
(anterior cerebral a., CT)

Territorial infarct
(posterior inferior cerebellar a., CT)

Intracerebral hemorrhage
(brain stem, CT)

Subarachnoid hemorrhage (CT)

Aneurysm
(internal carotid a., MRI)

Causes of stroke

Stroke Syndromes: Carotid Artery Territory

■ Brachiocephalic Trunk

Brachiocephalic trunk occlusion by emboli from the aortic arch has the same clinical manifestations as internal carotid artery (ICA) occlusion. Patients with adequate collateral flow remain asymptomatic.

■ Common Carotid Artery (CCA)

CCA occlusion is very rare and, even when it occurs, is usually asymptomatic, because of an adequate collateral supply. When symptoms do occur, they are the same as those of ICA occlusion.

■ Internal Carotid Artery (ICA)

Territorial infarcts affect the middle cerebral artery (MCA) more often than the anterior cerebral artery (ACA). If the ICA is occluded and collateral flow via the circle of Willis is inadequate, extensive infarction occurs in the anterior two-thirds of the hemisphere, including the basal ganglia. Symptoms include partial or total blindness in the ipsilateral eye, impairment of consciousness (p. 116), contralateral hemiplegia and hemisensory deficit, homonymous hemianopsia, conjugate gaze deviation to the side of the lesion, and partial Horner syndrome. ICA infarcts in the dominant hemisphere produce global aphasia. The occipital lobe can also be affected if the posterior cerebral artery (PCA) arises directly from the ICA (so-called fetal origin of the PCA). *Border zone infarcts* occur in distal vascular territories with inadequate collateral flow. They affect the "watershed" areas between the zones of distribution of the major cerebral arteries in the high parietal and frontal regions, as well as subcortical areas at the interface of the lenticulostriate and leptomeningeal arterial zones.

Ophthalmic artery. Occlusion leads to sudden blindness ("black curtain" phenomenon or centripetal shrinking of the visual field), which is often only temporary (*amaurosis fugax* = *transient monocular blindness*). Thorough diagnostic evaluation is needed, as the same clinical syndrome can be produced by other ophthalmological diseases (Table 22a, p. 372).

Anterior choroidal artery (AChA). Infarction in the AChA territory, depending on its precise lo-

cation and extent, can produce contralateral motor, sensory, or mixed deficits, hemiataxia, homonymous quadrantanopsia (both upper and lower), memory impairment, aphasia, and hemineglect.

Anterior cerebral artery (ACA). Contralateral hemiparesis is usually more distal than proximal, and more prominent in the lower than in the upper limb (sometimes only in the lower limb). Infarction in the territory of the *central branches* of the ACA (A1 segment, recurrent artery of Heubner) produces brachiofacial hemiparesis, sometimes accompanied by dystonia. Bilateral ACA infarction (when the arteries of both sides share a common origin) and infarctions of the *cortical branches* of the ACA produce abulia (p. 120), Broca aphasia (dominant hemisphere), perseveration, grasp reflex, palmomental reflex, paratonic rigidity (*gegenhalten*), and urinary incontinence. Lesions in the superior and medial frontal gyri or the anterior portion of the cingulate gyrus cause bladder dysfunction. Disconnection syndromes due to lesions of the corpus callosum are characterized by ideomotor apraxia, dysgraphia, and tactile anomia of the left arm.

Middle cerebral artery (MCA). Main trunk (M1) occlusion produces contralateral hemiparesis or hemiplegia with a corresponding hemisensory deficit, homonymous hemianopsia, and global aphasia (dominant side) or contralateral hemineglect with limb apraxia (nondominant side). Occlusion of the *posterior main branch* produces homonymous hemianopsia or quadrantanopsia as well as Wernicke or global aphasia (dominant side) or apraxia and dyscalculia (nondominant side); *central main branch* occlusion produces contralateral brachiofacial weakness and sensory loss; *anterior branch* occlusion on the dominant side additionally produces Broca aphasia. Occlusion of *peripheral branches* produces monoparesis of the face, hand, or arm. Occlusions of the *lenticulostriate arteries*, depending on their precise location, produce (purely motor) hemiparesis/hemiplegia, or hemiparesis with ataxia (*lacunar infarct*, p. 172).

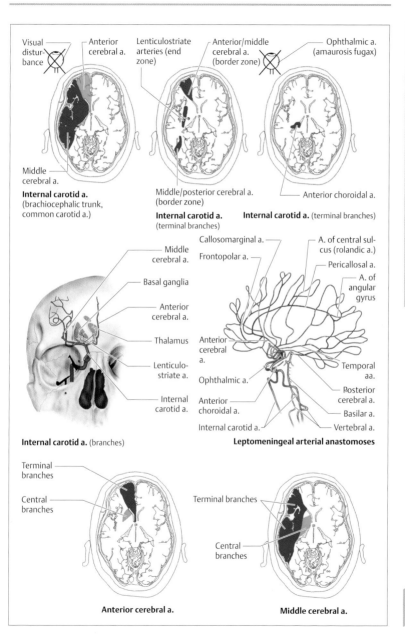

Visual disturbance

Anterior cerebral a.

Lenticulostriate arteries (end zone)

Anterior/middle cerebral a. (border zone)

Ophthalmic a. (amaurosis fugax)

Middle cerebral a.

Internal carotid a.
(brachiocephalic trunk, common carotid a.)

Middle/posterior cerebral a. (border zone)

Internal carotid a.
(terminal branches)

Anterior choroidal a.

Internal carotid a. (terminal branches)

Middle cerebral a.

Basal ganglia

Anterior cerebral a.

Thalamus

Lenticulo-striate a.

Internal carotid a.

Internal carotid a. (branches)

Callosomarginal a.

Frontopolar a.

A. of central sulcus (rolandic a.)

Pericallosal a.

A. of angular gyrus

Anterior cerebral a.

Ophthalmic a.

Anterior choroidal a.

Internal carotid a.

Temporal aa.

Posterior cerebral a.

Basilar a.

Vertebral a.

Leptomeningeal arterial anastomoses

Terminal branches

Central branches

Anterior cerebral a.

Terminal branches

Central branches

Middle cerebral a.

Stroke Syndromes: Vertebrobasilar Territory

■ Subclavian Artery

High-grade subclavian stenosis or occlusion proximal to the origin of the vertebral artery may cause a reversal of blood flow in the vertebral artery, which worsens with exertion of the ipsilateral arm (*subclavian steal*). Rapid arm fatigue and pain often result; less common are vertigo and other brain stem signs. The arterial blood pressure is measurably different in the two arms.

■ Vertebral Artery (VA)

VA occlusion produces variable combinations of symptoms and signs, including homonymous hemianopsia, dysarthria, dysphagia, unilateral or bilateral limb paralysis with or without sensory deficit, ataxia, drop attacks (due to medullary ischemia), and impairment of consciousness. Unilateral VA occlusion (e. g., due to dissection) can lead to infarction in the territory of the posterior inferior cerebellar artery.

■ Cerebellar Arteries

Large cerebellar infarcts can cause brain stem compression and hydrocephalus.

Posterior inferior cerebellar artery (PICA). Dorsolateral medullary infarction produces (usually incomplete) *Wallenberg syndrome* (p. 361). Often, only branches to the cerebellum are affected (⇨ vertigo, headache, ataxia, nystagmus, lateropulsion).

Anterior inferior cerebral artery (AICA). AICA occlusion is rare. It produces ipsilateral hearing loss, Horner syndrome, limb ataxia, and dissociated facial sensory loss, as well as contralateral dissociated sensory loss on the trunk and limbs (mainly the upper limbs) and nystagmus.

Superior cerebellar artery (SCA). SCA occlusion can produce ipsilateral Horner syndrome, limb ataxia, dysdiadochokinesia, and CN VI and VII palsy, as well as contralateral hypesthesia and hypalgesia.

■ Basilar Artery (BA)

Basilar artery occlusion. Thrombotic occlusion of the BA may be heralded several days in advance by nonspecific symptoms (unsteadiness, dysarthria, headache, mental changes). BA occlusion causes impairment of consciousness (ranging from somnolence to coma), mental syndromes (hallucinations, confabulation, psychoses), quadriparesis, and oculomotor disorders (diplopia, vertical or horizontal gaze palsy). Apical BA occlusion (p. 359) is caused by cardiac or arterial emboli. *Pontine infarction* sparing the posterior portion of the pons (tegmentum) produces quadriplegia and mutism with preservation of sensory function and vertical eye movements (*locked-in syndrome*, pp. 120, 359).

Paramedian infarction in the BA territory usually affects the pons (pp. 72, 359 ff).

Dorsolateral infarction affects the cerebellum, with a corresponding clinical picture. Occlusion of the labyrinthine artery (a branch of the AICA) produces rotatory vertigo, nausea, vomiting and nystagmus.

■ Posterior Cerebral Artery (PCA)

PCA occlusion is rare and produces symptoms and signs similar to those of MCA infarction. Unilateral occlusion of a *cortical branch* produces homonymous hemianopsia with sparing of the macula (supplied by the MCA), while bilateral occlusion produces cortical blindness and, occasionally, Anton syndrome (p. 132). *Central branch* occlusion leads to thalamic infarction (p. 106; Dejerine–Roussy syndrome), resulting in transient contralateral hemiparesis, spontaneous pain ("thalamic pain"), sensory deficits, ataxia, abasia, choreoathetosis, "thalamic hand" (flexion of the metacarpophalangeal joints with hyperextension of the interphalangeal joints), and homonymous hemianopsia. If branches to the midbrain are affected, an ipsilateral CN III palsy results, accompanied by variable contralateral deficits including hemiparesis/hemiplegia, (rubral) tremor, ataxia, and nystagmus. Isolated hemihypesthesia is associated with thalamic lacunar infarction.

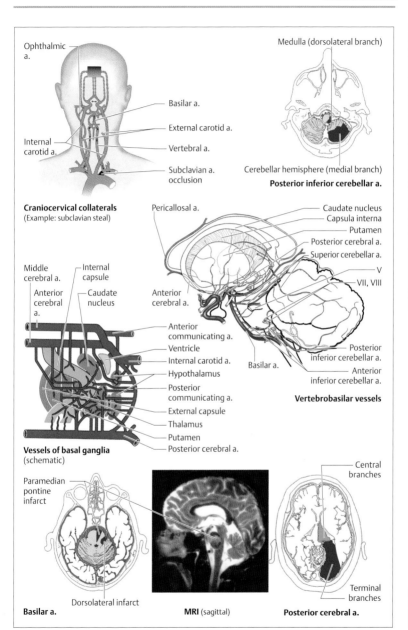

Ophthalmic a.

Basilar a.

External carotid a.

Internal carotid a.

Vertebral a.

Subclavian a. occlusion

Craniocervical collaterals
(Example: subclavian steal)

Medulla (dorsolateral branch)

Cerebellar hemisphere (medial branch)
Posterior inferior cerebellar a.

Pericallosal a.

Caudate nucleus
Capsula interna
Putamen
Posterior cerebral a.
Superior cerebellar a.
V
VII, VIII

Middle cerebral a.

Internal capsule

Anterior cerebral a.

Caudate nucleus

Anterior cerebral a.

Anterior communicating a.

Ventricle

Internal carotid a.

Hypothalamus

Posterior communicating a.

External capsule

Thalamus

Putamen

Posterior cerebral a.

Vessels of basal ganglia
(schematic)

Basilar a.

Posterior inferior cerebellar a.

Anterior inferior cerebellar a.

Vertebrobasilar vessels

Paramedian pontine infarct

Central branches

Terminal branches

Dorsolateral infarct

Basilar a.

MRI (sagittal)

Posterior cerebral a.

Central Nervous System

171

■ Risk Factors

The risk of stroke increases with *age* and is higher in men than in women at any age. Major risk factors include arterial hypertension (>140 mmHg systolic, >90 mmHg diastolic), diabetes mellitus, heart disease, cigarette smoking, hyperlipoproteinemia (total cholesterol >5.0 mmol/l, LDL >3 mmol/l, HDL <0.9–1.2 mmol/l), elevated plasma fibrinogen, and obesity. Symptomatic or asymptomatic carotid artery stenosis, elevated plasma homocysteine levels, erythrocytosis, anti-phospholipid antibodies, alcohol abuse (≥60 g of alcohol ≙ 75 cl of wine per day in men, ≥40 g in women). Drug abuse (amphetamines, heroin, cocaine), a sedentary lifestyle, and low socioeconomic status (unemployment, poverty) also increase the risk of stroke.

■ Causes

Embolism (ca. 70%) is the most common cause of stroke. Emboli arise from local atheromatous lesions (atheromatous thromboembolism) on the walls of large arteries (macroangiopathy) of the brain or heart (cardiac embolism in atrial fibrillation, valvular heart disease, ventricular thrombus, and myxoma).

Thrombosis (ca. 25%). Occlusion of a small end-artery (microangiopathy, small vessel disease) causes lacunar infarction. The cause is hyaline (lipohyalinosis) or proximal sclerosis of penetrating arteries (lenticulostriate, thalamoperforating or pontine arteries, central branches). Causal factors include hypertension, diabetes, and blood–brain barrier disruption leading to deposition of plasma proteins in the arterial wall. Microangiopathy-related hemodynamic changes sometimes cause *hemodynamic infarction*.

Rare causes (ca. 5%) include hematological diseases (e. g., coagulopathy, abnormal blood viscosity, anemia, leukemia) and arterial processes (dissection, vasculitis, migraine, fibromuscular dysplasia, moyamoya, vasospasm, amyloid angiopathy, and CADASIL = cerebral autosomal dominant arteriopathy with subcortical infarcts and leukoencephalopathy).

■ Infarct Types

Lacunar infarcts ("small deep infarcts"). Lacunes are small (≤1.5 cm in diameter), round or oval infarcts in the subcortical periventricular region or brain stem. Classic lacunar syndromes include purely motor hemiparesis (internal capsule, corona radiata, pons), contralateral purely sensory deficit (thalamus, internal capsule), ataxic hemiparesis (internal capsule, corona radiata, pons), and dysarthria with clumsiness of one hand (= clumsy hand–dysarthria syndrome; internal capsule, pons). The presence of multiple supratentorial and infratentorial lacunes is termed the *lacunar state* ("état lacunaire") and is clinically characterized by pseudobulbar palsy (p. 367), small-step gait ("marche à petit pas"), urinary incontinence, and affective disorders (compulsive crying). For leukoaraiosis, see p. 298.

Territorial infarcts are those limited to the distribution of the ACA, MCA, or PCA. With the exception of striatocapsular infarcts (internal capsule, basal ganglia), these infarcts are predominantly cortical. Embolic territorial infarcts often undergo secondary hemorrhage ("hemorrhagic conversion").

End zone infarcts. *Low-flow infarction* in the subcortical white matter is due to extracranial high-grade vessel stenosis and/or inadequate collateral flow.

Border zone infarcts (p. 168) also result from hemodynamic disturbances due to microangiopathy. They are found at the interface ("watershed") between adjacent vascular territories, and can be either anterior (MCA–ACA ⇨ contralateral hemiparesis and hemisensory deficit, mainly in the lower limb and sparing the face, with or without aphasia) or posterior (MCA–PCA ⇨ contralateral hemianopsia and cortical sensory deficit, with or without aphasia).

Global cerebral hypoxia/ischemia. The causes include cardiac arrest with delayed resuscitation, hemorrhagic shock, suffocation, and carbon monoxide poisoning. Global cerebral hypoxia/ischemia causes bilateral necrosis of brain tissue, particularly in the basal ganglia and white matter.

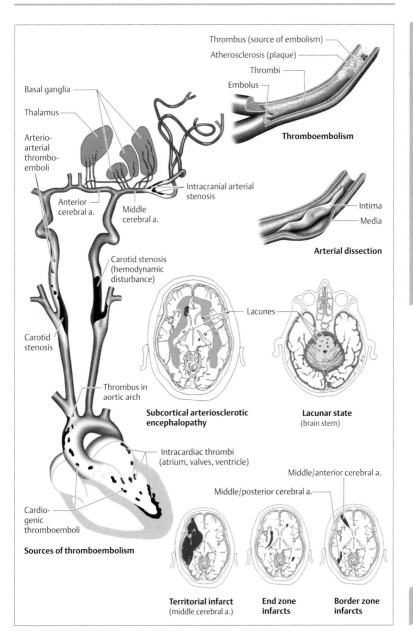

Thrombus (source of embolism)

Atherosclerosis (plaque)

Thrombi

Embolus

Thromboembolism

Basal ganglia

Thalamus

Arterio-arterial thrombo-emboli

Anterior cerebral a.

Middle cerebral a.

Intracranial arterial stenosis

Intima

Media

Arterial dissection

Carotid stenosis (hemodynamic disturbance)

Carotid stenosis

Lacunes

Thrombus in aortic arch

Subcortical arteriosclerotic encephalopathy

Lacunar state (brain stem)

Intracardiac thrombi (atrium, valves, ventricle)

Middle/anterior cerebral a.

Middle/posterior cerebral a.

Cardio-genic thromboemboli

Sources of thromboembolism

Territorial infarct (middle cerebral a.)

End zone infarcts

Border zone infarcts

Stroke Pathophysiology

Hemodynamic insufficiency. Cerebrovascular autoregulation is normally able to maintain a relatively constant cerebral blood flow (CBF) of 50–60 ml/100 g brain tissue/min as long as the mean arterial pressure (MAP) remains within the range of 50–150 mmHg (p. 162). The regional cerebral blood flow (rCBF) is finely adjusted according to local metabolic requirements (coupling of CBF and metabolism). If the MAP falls below 50 mmHg, and in certain pathological states (e. g., ischemia), autoregulation fails and CBF declines. Vascular stenosis or occlusion induces compensatory vasodilatation downstream, which increases the cerebral blood volume and CBF (*vascular reserve*); the extent of local brain injury depends on the availability of collateral flow, the duration of hemodynamic insufficiency, and the vulnerability of the particular brain region affected. Major neurological deficits arise only when CBF falls below the critical *ischemia threshold* (ca. 20 ml/100 g/min).

Hypoperfusion. If adequate CBF is not reestablished, clinically evident neurological dysfunction ensues (breakdown of cerebral metabolism ⇨ EEG and evoked potential change). Prolonged, severe depression of CBF below the *infarction threshold* of ca. 8–10 ml/100 g/min causes progressive and irreversible abolition of all cellular metabolic processes, accompanied by structural breakdown (necrosis). Infarction occurs where hypoperfusion is most severe; the area of tissue surrounding the zone of infarction in which the CBF lies between the thresholds for ischemia and infarction is called the *ischemic penumbra*. Brain tissue in the zone of infarction is irretrievably lost, while that in the ischemic penumbra is at risk, but potentially recoverable. The longer the ischemia lasts, the more likely infarction will occur; thus, *time is brain*. The zones of infarction and ischemia are well demonstrated by recently developed MRI techniques (DWI, PWI).[1,2]

Stroke Treatment

Primary prevention involves the therapeutic modification or elimination of risk factors. Patients with asymptomatic stenosis are given *antiplatelet therapy* (APT) consisting of aspirin, aspirin–dipyridamole combination, or clopidogrel. *Endarterectomy* may be indicated in asymptomatic high-grade stenosis (>80%[4] or >90%[3]). *Anticoagulants* may be indicated in patients with atrial fibrillation without rheumatic valvular heart disease, depending on their individual risk profile (TIAs, age, comorbidities).

Acute treatment is based on the existence of a 3–6-hour interval between the onset of ischemia and the occurrence of maximum irreversible tissue damage (*treatment window*). *General treatment measures* include the assurance of adequate cardiorespiratory status (normal blood oxygenation is essential for the survival of the ischemic penumbra); because autoregulation of CBF in the penumbra is impaired, the systolic BP should be maintained above 160 mmHg. The serum glucose level should not be allowed to exceed 200 mg/100 ml. Balanced fluid replacement should be provided, and fever, if it occurs, should be treated. Physicians should be vigilant in the recognition and treatment of complications such as aspiration (secondary to dysphagia), deep venous thrombosis (secondary to immobility of a plegic limb), cardiac arrhythmia, pneumonia, urinary tract infection, and pressure sores. Rehabilitation measures include physical, occupational, and speech therapy, as well as psychological counseling of the patient and family.

Special treatment measures: APT (after exclusion of hemorrhage); thrombolysis, treatment of cerebral edema, surgical decompression in space-occupying cerebellar or MCA infarcts, and anticonvulsants, as needed.

Secondary prevention. APT (TIA, mild stroke, atherothrombotic stroke); oral anticoagulation (cardiac embolism, arterial dissection); endarterectomy (in symptomatic carotid stenosis >70%[4], or >80%[3], or after mild strokes). The potential utility and indications of carotid angioplasty and stenting in the treatment of carotid stenosis are currently under intensive study.

---

[1]Diffusion-weighted imaging (DWI) demonstrates the zone of infarction; the early CT signs of infarction (blurring of insular cortex, hypodensity of basal ganglia, cortical swelling) are less reliable.

[2]Perfusion-weighted imaging (PWI) demonstrates the ischemic penumbra and zone of oligemia (tissue at risk).

[3]Data from the European Carotid Surgery Trial (ECST).

[4]Data from the North American Symptomatic Carotid Endarterectomy Trial (NASCET).

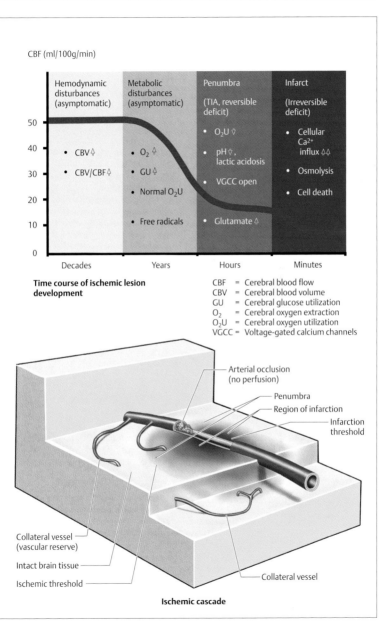

Time course of ischemic lesion development

CBF = Cerebral blood flow
CBV = Cerebral blood volume
GU = Cerebral glucose utilization
O_2 = Cerebral oxygen extraction
O_2U = Cerebral oxygen utilization
VGCC = Voltage-gated calcium channels

Ischemic cascade

Clinical Features

Spontaneous (i.e., nontraumatic) intracranial hemorrhage may be epidural, subdural (p. 267), subarachnoid, intraparenchymal, or intraventricular. Its site and extent are readily seen on CT (somewhat less well on MRI) and determine its clinical manifestations.

■ Subarachnoid Hemorrhage (SAH)

Symptoms and signs. The typical presentation of aneurysmal rupture (by far the most common cause of SAH) is with a very severe headache of abrupt onset ("the worst headache of my life"), often initially accompanied by nausea, vomiting, diaphoresis, and impairment of consciousness. The neck is stiff, and neck flexion is painful. There may also be focal neurological signs, photophobia, and/or backache. Subarachnoid blood can be seen on CT within 24 hours of the hemorrhage in roughly 90% of cases. If SAH is suspected but the CT is negative, a diagnostic lumbar puncture must be performed.

Complications. The initial hemorrhage may extend beyond the subarachnoid space into the brain parenchyma, the subarachnoid space, and/or the ventricular system. A ruptured saccular aneurysm may rebleed at any time until it is definitively treated; the rebleed risk is highest on the day of onset (day 0), and 40% in the ensuing 4 weeks. The greater the amount of blood in the subarachnoid cisterns, the more likely that *vasospasm* and *delayed cerebral ischemia* will occur; the risk is highest between days 4 and 12. Clotted blood blocking the ventricular system or the arachnoid villi can lead to *hydrocephalus*, of obstructive or malresorptive type, respectively (p. 162). Other complications include cerebral edema, hyponatremia, neurogenic pulmonary edema, seizures, and cardiac arrhythmias.

■ Intracerebral Hemorrhage

Intraparenchymal hemorrhages of arterial origin are to be distinguished from secondary hemorrhages into arterial or venous infarcts.

General features. Sudden onset of headache, impairment of consciousness, nausea, vomiting, and focal neurological signs, with acute progression over minutes or hours.

Hemorrhage into the basal ganglia. *Putaminal hemorrhage* produces contralateral hemiparesis/hemiplegia and hemisensory deficit, conjugate horizontal gaze deviation, homonymous hemianopsia, and aphasia (dominant side) or hemineglect (nondominant side). *Thalamic hemorrhage* produces similar manifestations and also vertical gaze palsy, miotic, unreactive pupils, and (sometimes) convergence paresis. The very rare *caudate hemorrhages* are characterized by confusion, disorientation, and contralateral hemiparesis. Hemorrhage into the *basal ganglia and internal capsule* leads to coma, contralateral hemiplegia, homonymous hemianopsia, and aphasia (dominant side).

Lobar hemorrhage usually originates at the gray–white matter junction and extends inward into the white matter, producing variable clinical manifestations. *Frontal lobe:* Frontal headache, abulia, contralateral hemiparesis (arm more than leg). *Temporal lobe:* Pain around the ear, aphasia (dominant side), confusion, upper quadrantanopsia. *Parietal lobe:* Temporal headache, contralateral sensory deficit, aphasia, lower quadrantanopsia. *Occipital lobe:* Ipsilateral periorbital pain, hemianopsia.

Cerebellar hemorrhages are usually restricted to one hemisphere. They produce nausea, vomiting, severe occipital headache, dizziness, and ataxia.

Brain stem hemorrhage. Pontine hemorrhage is the most common type, producing coma, quadriplegia/decerebration, bilateral miosis (pinpoint pupils), "ocular bobbing," and horizontal gaze palsy. Locked-in syndrome may ensue.

General complications. Intraventricular extension of hemorrhage, hydrocephalus, cerebral edema, intracranial hypertension, seizures, and hemodynamic changes (often a dangerous elevation of blood pressure).

■ Intraventricular Hemorrhage

Intraventricular hemorrhage only rarely originates in the ventricle itself (choroid plexus). It is much more commonly the intraventricular extension of an aneurysmal SAH or other brain hemorrhage.

Symptoms and signs. Acute onset of headache, nausea, vomiting, impairment of consciousness or coma.

Complications. Extension of hemorrhage, hydrocephalus, seizures.

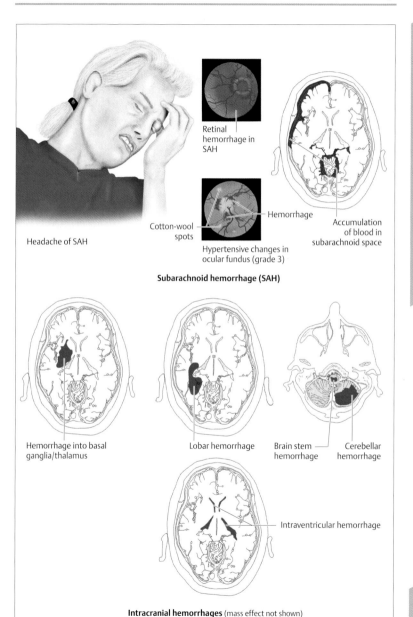

Headache of SAH

Retinal hemorrhage in SAH

Cotton-wool spots

Hemorrhage

Hypertensive changes in ocular fundus (grade 3)

Accumulation of blood in subarachnoid space

Subarachnoid hemorrhage (SAH)

Hemorrhage into basal ganglia/thalamus

Lobar hemorrhage

Brain stem hemorrhage

Cerebellar hemorrhage

Intraventricular hemorrhage

Intracranial hemorrhages (mass effect not shown)

Central Nervous System

177

Central Nervous System

Pathogenesis

Subarachnoid hemorrhage (SAH). Roughly 85% of cases of SAH are caused by rupture of a saccular aneurysm at the base of the skull. Another 10% are caused by nonaneurysmal lesions (whose nature is not, at present, understood), with bleeding mainly in the perimesencephalic cisterns (p. 8). Other, rare, causes include vertebral artery dissection, arteriovenous malformation (AVM), cavernoma, hypertension, anticoagulation, and trauma.

Aneurysm. An aneurysm is not a congenital lesion, but a progressive, localized dilatation of an arterial wall. *Saccular aneurysms* tend to develop at branching sites of the internal carotid artery (ICA), the anterior communicating artery, and the proximal middle cerebral artery (MCA). *Fusiform aneurysms* usually appear as an elongated, twisted, and dilated segment (dolichoectasis) of the basilar artery or supraclinoid ICA. Most are due to atherosclerosis. Spontaneous hemorrhage is rare; ischemia due to arterio-arterial embolism is more common. The rare *septic-embolic aneurysms* (mycotic aneurysms) may be secondary to endocarditis, meningoencephalitis, hemodialysis, or intravenous drug administration. They are located in distal vessel segments, particularly in the MCA, and may cause SAH, massive hemorrhage, or infarction with secondary hemorrhage.

Vascular malformations. *Arteriovenous malformations* (AVMs) are congenital lesions consisting of a tangled web of arteries and veins with pathological arteriovenous shunting. Most are located near the surface of the cerebral hemispheres. AVMs tend to enlarge over time and may become calcified. They may cause subarachnoid or intracerebral hemorrhage at any age. They become clinically manifest either through a hemorrhage or through headache, seizures, or focal neurological signs (aphasia, hemiparesis, hemianopsia).

Cavernomas are compact, often calcified, aggregations of dilated blood vessels and connective tissue in the brain and leptomeninges. They rarely bleed (ca. 0.5%/year). Some cause seizures and focal deficits; others are discovered on MRI scans as an incidental finding.

Intracerebral hemorrhage. Hypertension is the most common cause; other causes include aneurysm, AVM, cerebral amyloid angiography, moyamoya, coagulopathy (leukemia, thrombocytopenia, therapeutic anticoagulation), cerebral vasculitis, cerebral venous thrombosis, drug abuse (cocaine, heroin), alcohol, metastases, and brain tumors. *Massive hypertensive hemorrhage* is thought to be caused by pressure-induced rupture of arterioles and microaneurysms. The high pressure and a kind of chain reaction involving multiple microaneurysms is thought to explain the size of these hemorrhages (despite the small caliber of the ruptured vessels). The recurrent, mainly cortical, bleeding associated with cerebral *amyloid angiopathy* is due to the fragility of leptomeningeal and cortical small vessels in whose walls amyloid deposits have accumulated.

Dural fistula is an abnormal anastomosis between dural arteries and a venous sinus. Hemorrhage is rare; they may cause pulsating tinnitus, headache, papilledema, and visual disturbances.

Treatment

Aneurysmal hemorrhage. Cautious transport, bed rest, analgesia, admission to a neurosurgical unit, and angiography to establish the diagnosis and define the anatomy of the aneurysm(s). The timing of surgical clipping depends on the site and clinical severity of the hemorrhage, the aneurysm's configuration, and the age and general medical condition of the patient. Inoperable cases can be managed with intravascular neuroradiological techniques ("embolization"; filling with Guglielmi detachable coils (GDC) is currently favored).

Hemorrhage from an AVM may be treated with surgery, embolization, and/or stereotactic radiosurgery, depending on its site and extent. **Cavernomas** that bleed are usually excised.

Intracerebral hemorrhage is often treated conservatively, unless it impairs consciousness or causes a progressive neurological deficit. Major cerebellar hemorrhage (rule of thumb: >3 cm) is life-threatening unless treated neurosurgically.

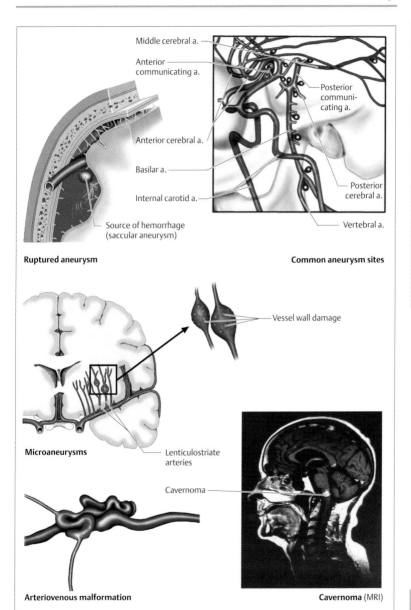

Middle cerebral a.

Anterior communicating a.

Posterior communicating a.

Anterior cerebral a.

Basilar a.

Internal carotid a.

Posterior cerebral a.

Vertebral a.

Source of hemorrhage (saccular aneurysm)

Ruptured aneurysm

Common aneurysm sites

Vessel wall damage

Microaneurysms

Lenticulostriate arteries

Cavernoma

Arteriovenous malformation

Cavernoma (MRI)

Central Nervous System

Sinus Thrombosis

Symptoms and signs. *Aseptic sinus thrombosis* most commonly affects the superior sagittal sinus and produces initial headache, vomiting, and focal epileptic seizures, followed by monoparesis or hemiparesis, papilledema, abulia, and impairment of consciousness. Blockage of venous outflow causes cerebral edema and rupture of the distended cerebral veins upstream from the thrombosis. *Septic sinus thrombosis* is heralded by fever, chills, and malaise. Pain, redness, and swelling of the eye or ear may develop, in addition to focal neurological signs. Transverse and sigmoid sinus thromboses are often secondary to ear and mastoid infections, while cavernous sinus thrombosis is often due to infections about the face (orbit, paranasal sinuses, teeth).

Etiology. Aseptic sinus thrombosis may occur during or after pregnancy, or secondary to the use of oral contraceptives, deficiencies of protein C, protein S, antithrombin III, or factor V, dehydration, polycythemia vera, leukemia, Behçet disease, trauma, surgical procedures, and malignancy. Septic sinus thrombosis often occurs by secondary spread of infections about the head (sinusitis, otitis media, mastoiditis, facial furuncle). *Identification:* CT or MRI angiography generally suffices to demonstrate the occluded sinus; conventional angiography is rarely needed.

Treatment. *Aseptic thrombosis:* anticoagulation. *Septic thrombosis* (pp. 226, 375): antibiotics and surgical management of the source of infection.

Cerebral Vasculitis

Primary vasculitis arises in the cerebral arteries and veins themselves, while *secondary vasculitis* is a sequela of another disease (see *Causes*, below).

Symptoms and signs. Cerebral vasculitis produces variable symptoms and signs, including recurrent ischemia, intracerebral or subarachnoid hemorrhage, persistent headache, focal epilepsy, gradually progressive focal neurological signs, dementia, behavioral abnormalities, cranial nerve palsies, and meningismus. Vasculitis may also affect vessels of the spinal cord (transverse cord syndrome) and those supplying the peripheral nerves (painful mononeuropathy).

Causes. *Isolated cerebral angiitis (idiopathic)* is difficult to diagnose because its findings are nonspecific (elevated CSF protein, EEG and MRI abnormalities). Leptomeningeal biopsy may be needed. *Primary or secondary vasculitides* of various kinds affect the vessels of the central nervous system (CNS), peripheral nervous system (PNS) and/or skeletal muscles to a variable extent (see table).

Treatment. Infectious vasculitis is treated with antiviral or antibacterial agents, as needed, while autoimmune vasculitis is treated with corticosteroids and immune suppressants (cyclophosphamide, azathioprine).

Syndrome	CNS	PNS	Muscle
Churg–Strauss syndrome	++	+++	+
Wegener granulomatosis	++	++	+
Behçet disease	++	+/–	–
Lymphomatoid granulomatosis	++	+/–	–
Syphilis, tuberculosis, herpes zoster, bacterial meningitis, fungal infection	++	+/–	+/–
Temporal arteritis	+	+/–	–
Polyarteritis nodosa	+	+++	+
Takayasu arteritis	+	–	–
Lymphoma	+	+	–

+++ usual, ++ common, + occasional, +/– rare, – absent

(From Moore and Calabrese, 1994)

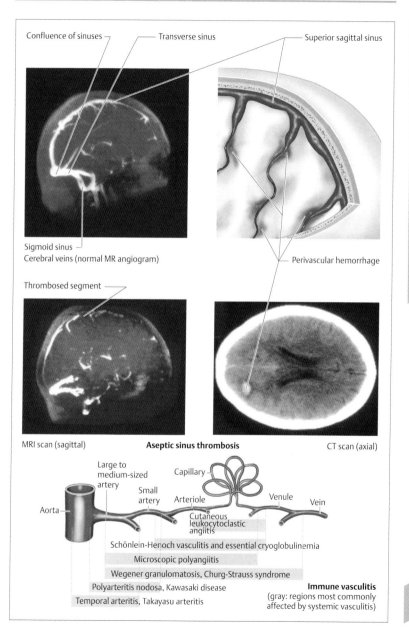

Confluence of sinuses

Transverse sinus

Superior sagittal sinus

Sigmoid sinus
Cerebral veins (normal MR angiogram)

Perivascular hemorrhage

Thrombosed segment

MRI scan (sagittal)

Aseptic sinus thrombosis

CT scan (axial)

Large to medium-sized artery

Small artery

Capillary

Arteriole

Venule

Vein

Aorta

Cutaneous leukocytoclastic angiitis

Schönlein-Henoch vasculitis and essential cryoglobulinemia

Microscopic polyangiitis

Wegener granulomatosis, Churg-Strauss syndrome

Polyarteritis nodosa, Kawasaki disease

Temporal arteritis, Takayasu arteritis

Immune vasculitis
(gray: regions most commonly affected by systemic vasculitis)

Central Nervous System

181

Tension Headache

Tension headache often involves painful cervical muscle spasm, may change with the weather, and is frequently ascribed by patients and others to cervical spinal degenerative disease, visual disturbance, or life stress. It consists of a bilateral, prominent nuchal pressure sensation that progresses over the course of the day. Patients may report feeling as if their head were being squeezed in a vise or by a band being drawn ever more tightly around it, or as if their head were about to explode, though the pain is rarely so severe as to impede performance of the usual daily tasks, e. g., at work. It may be accompanied by malaise, anorexia, lack of concentration, emotional lability, chest pain, and mild hypersensitivity to light and noise. Unlike migraine, it is not aggravated by exertion (e. g., climbing stairs), nor does it produce vomiting or focal neurological deficits. It can be *episodic* (< 15 days/month, pain lasting from 30 minutes to 1 week) or *chronic* (> 15 days/month for at least 6 months). Some patients suffer from pericranial tenderness (posterior cervical, masticatory, and cranial muscles). Isolated attacks of sudden, stabbing pain (*ice-pick headache*) may occur on one side of the head or neck. Tension headache rarely wakes the patient from sleep. Its cause usually cannot be determined, though it may be due to disorders of the temporomandibular joint or psychosomatic troubles such as stress, depression, anxiety, inadequate sleep, or substance abuse. Tension headache combined with migraine is termed *combination headache*.
Pathogenesis. It is theorized that diminished activity of certain neurotransmitters (e. g., endogenous opioids, serotonin) may lead to abnormal nociceptive processing (p. 108) and thus produce a pathological pain state.

Headache Due to Vascular Processes (Other than Migraine)

The nociceptive innervation of the extracranial and intracranial vessels is of such a nature that pain arising from them is often projected to a site in the head that is some distance away from the responsible lesion. Thus, specific diagnostic studies are usually needed to pinpoint the location of the disturbance. The pain may *precede* the actual vascular event (arterial dissection, arteriovenous malformation, vasculitis), may *occur simultaneously* with the event (subarachnoid hemorrhage, intracerebral hemorrhage, epidural hematoma, cerebral venous thrombosis, giant cell arteritis, carotidynia, venous outflow obstruction in goiter or mediastinal processes, pheochromocytoma, preeclampsia, malignant hypertension), or may *follow* the event (subdural hematoma, intracerebral hemorrhage, endarterectomy).

Chronic Daily Headache

Rational treatment is based on the classification of primary daily headache by clinical characteristics (see Table 23, p. 373), and of secondary (symptomatic) headache by etiology.

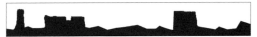

Persistent, variably severe headache

• Depression

• Anxiety

• Stress

• Noise

• Alcohol

• Medications

• Transient stabbing pain

• Episodic

• Chronic

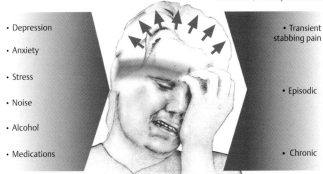

Tension headache

Central Nervous System

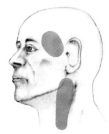

Carotid artery (common, external, internal)

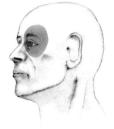

Internal carotid a., cavernous sinus

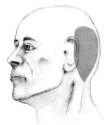

Vertebral, basilar, posterior cerebral arteries; transverse/sigmoid sinus

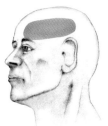

Superior sagittal sinus

Referred pain due to cerebrovascular lesions

Migraine

Migraine is a periodic headache often accompanied by nausea and sensitivity to light and noise (photophobia and phonophobia). A typical attack consists of a *prodromal phase* of warning (premonitory) symptoms, followed by an *aura*, the actual *headache phase*, and a *resolution phase*. Attack characteristics often change over time. Attacks often tend to occur in the morning or evening but may occur at any time. They typically last 4–72 hours.

■ Symptoms and Signs

Prodromal phase. The migraine attack may be preceded by a period of variable prodromal phenomena lasting a few hours to two days. Most patients complain of sensitivity to smells and noise, irritability, restlessness, drowsiness, fatigue, lack of concentration, depression, and polyuria. In children, the chief complaints are abdominal pain and dizziness.

Aura. This is the period preceding the focal cerebral symptoms of the actual migraine headache. Some patients experience attacks without an aura (common migraine), while others have attacks with an aura (classic migraine) that develops over 5–20 minutes and usually lasts less than one hour, but may persist as long as one week (prolonged aura). In some cases, the aura is not followed by a headache ("migraine equivalent"). Auras typically involve visual disturbances, which can range from undulating lines (resembling hot air rising), lightning flashes, circles, sparks or flashing lights (photopsia), or zig-zag lines (fortification figures, teichopsia, scintillating scotoma). The visual images, which may be white or colored, cause gaps in the visual field and usually have scintillating margins. Unilateral paresthesiae (tingling or cold sensations) may occur. Emotional changes (anxiety, restlessness, panic, euphoria, grief, aversion) of variable intensity are relatively common.

Headache phase. Most patients (ca. 60%) complain of pulsating, throbbing, or continuous pain on one side of the head (hemicrania). Others have pain in the entire head, particularly behind the eyes ("as if the eye were being pushed out"), in the nuchal region, or in the temples. Migraine headache worsens on physical exertion and is often accompanied by anorexia, malaise, nausea, and vomiting.

Resolution phase. This phase is characterized by listlessness, lack of concentration, and increased pain sensitivity in the head.

■ Pathogenesis

During the interval between attacks, various disturbances (genetically determined) may be observed, e.g., cerebral hypomagnesemia, elevated concentration of excitatory amino acids (glutamate, aspartate), and increased reactivity of cranial blood vessels. The cumulative effect of these disturbances is a heightened sensitivity to nociceptive stimuli (migraine pain threshold). Impulses from the cortex, thalamus, and hypothalamus activate the so-called *migraine center* responsible for the generation of migraine attacks, putatively located in the brain stem (serotonergic raphe nuclei, locus ceruleus). The migraine center triggers *cortical spreading depression* (suppression of brain activity across the cortex) accompanied by oligemia, resulting in an aura. Trigeminovascular input from meningeal vessels is relayed to the brain stem, via projecting fibers to the thalamus and then, by the parasympathetic efferent pathway, back to the meningeal vessels (*trigeminal autonomic reflex circuit*). Perivascular trigeminal C-fiber endings (*trigeminovascular system*) are stimulated to release vasoactive neuropeptides such as substrate P, neurokinin A, and calcitonin gene-regulated polypeptide (CGRP), causing a (sterile) *neurogenic inflammatory response*. Vasoconstriction and vascular hyperesthesia with subsequent vasodilatation spread via trigeminal axon reflexes. The perception of pain is mediated by the pathway from the trigeminal nerve to the nucleus caudalis, thalamus (p. 94) and cortex. Trigeminal impulses also reach autonomic centers.

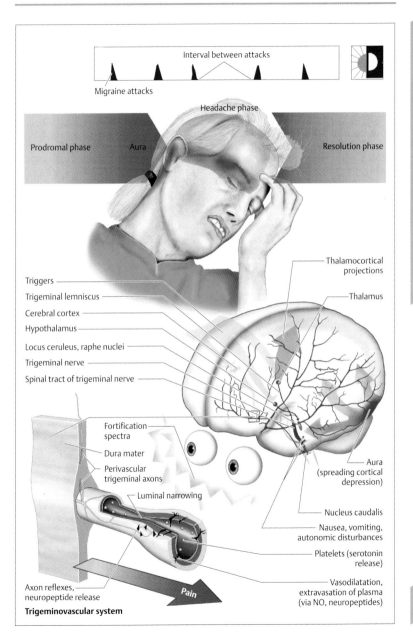

Interval between attacks

Migraine attacks

Headache phase

Prodromal phase Aura Resolution phase

Thalamocortical projections

Triggers
Trigeminal lemniscus
Cerebral cortex
Hypothalamus
Locus ceruleus, raphe nuclei
Trigeminal nerve
Spinal tract of trigeminal nerve

Thalamus

Fortification spectra
Dura mater
Perivascular trigeminal axons
Luminal narrowing

Aura (spreading cortical depression)

Nucleus caudalis
Nausea, vomiting, autonomic disturbances
Platelets (serotonin release)
Vasodilatation, extravasation of plasma (via NO, neuropeptides)

Axon reflexes, neuropeptide release
Pain
Trigeminovascular system

Trigeminal Neuralgia

Trigeminal neuralgia (*tic douloureux*) is characterized by the sudden onset of excruciating, intense stabbing pain (during waking hours). Several brief attacks (<2 minutes each) generally occur in succession. The pain is almost always precipitated by a trigger stimulus or activity (e.g., chewing, speaking, swallowing, touching the face, cold air, tooth brushing, shaving) and is located in the distribution of one or two branches of the trigeminal nerve, usually V/2 and/or V/3. Involvement of V/1, all three branches, or both sides of the face is uncommon. The attacks may persist for weeks to months or may spontaneously remit for weeks, or even years, before another attack occurs. Trigeminal neuralgia in the V/3 distribution is often mistaken for odontogenic pain, sometimes resulting in unnecessary tooth extraction. Typical (idiopathic) trigeminal neuralgia must be distinguished from secondary forms of the syndrome (see below).

Pathogenesis. *Idiopathic trigeminal neuralgia* ⇨ much evidence points to microvascular compression of the trigeminal nerve root (usually by a branch of the superior cerebellar artery) where it enters the brain stem, leading to the development of ephapses or suppression of central inhibitory mechanisms. *Symptomatic trigeminal neuralgia* ⇨ cerebellopontine angle tumors, multiple sclerosis, vascular malformations.

Cluster Headache (CH)

Episodic cluster headache. Attacks of very severe burning, searing, stabbing, burning, needlelike, or throbbing pain develop over a few minutes on one side of the head, behind or around the eye, and may extend to the forehead, temple, ear, mouth, jaw, throat, or nuchal region. If untreated, attacks last ca. 15 minutes to 3 hours. They are predominantly nocturnal, waking the patient from sleep, but can also occur during the day. Attacks come in episodes (clusters) consisting of 1–3 daily bouts of pain for up to 8 weeks. A seasonal pattern of occurrence may be observed. During a cluster, the pain can be triggered by alcoholic drinks, histamines, or nitrates. Temporal pressure or the application of heat to the eye may alleviate the pain. Unlike migraine patients, who seek peace and quiet, these patients characteristically pace restlessly, and may even strike their aching head with a fist. The headache may be accompanied by ipsilateral *ocular* (watery eyes, conjunctival injection, incomplete Horner syndrome, photophobia), *nasal* (nasal congestion, rhinorrhea), and *autonomic* manifestations (facial flushing, tenderness of temporal artery, nausea, diarrhea, polyuria, fluctuating blood pressure, cardiac arrhythmia). Cluster headache is more common in men.

Chronic cluster headache. Attacks do not occur in clusters, but rather persist for more than one year at a time, punctuated by remissions lasting no longer than two weeks. Chronic cluster headache may arise primarily, or else as a confluence of clusters in what began as episodic cluster headache.

Pathogenesis. One hypothesis attributes CH to dilatation of the carotid artery within the carotid canal, causing compression of the periarterial sympathetic plexus. There is also evidence suggesting a role for inflammatory dilatation of the intracavernous venous plexus. The result is abnormal function of the sympathetic and parasympathetic fibers in the region of the cavernous sinus (⇨ autonomic dysfunction, activation of trigeminovascular system).

Chronic Paroxysmal Hemicrania (CPH)

CPH is a very rare condition characterized by the daily onset of pain similar to that of cluster headache. The daily attacks of CPH are much more frequent (10–20 times/day) and shorter (5–30 minutes) than those of cluster headache. The pain of CPH typically responds to indomethacin.

Sinus Headache

The pain of frontal, sphenoid, or ethmoid nasal sinusitis is usually felt in the middle of the forehead and above the eyes. That of maxillary sinusitis radiates to the upper jaw and zygomatic region and worsens when the patient bends forward.

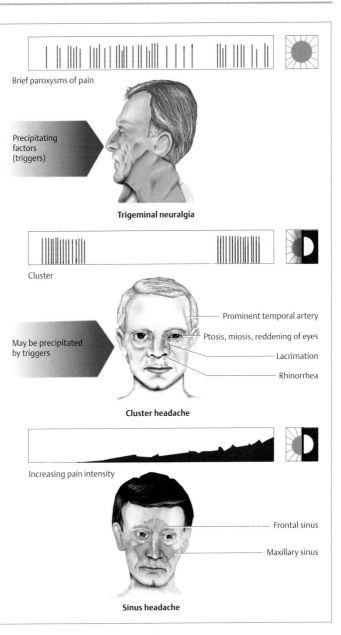

Brief paroxysms of pain

Precipitating factors (triggers)

Trigeminal neuralgia

Cluster

May be precipitated by triggers

Prominent temporal artery

Ptosis, miosis, reddening of eyes

Lacrimation

Rhinorrhea

Cluster headache

Increasing pain intensity

Frontal sinus

Maxillary sinus

Sinus headache

Nociceptive Transmission

The brain tissue itself is insensitive to pain. The major cranial and proximal intracranial vessels and dura mater of the supratentorial compartment derive nociceptive innervation from the ophthalmic nerve (V/1, p. 94), while those of the posterior fossa are innervated by C2 branches. Because nociceptive impulses from the anterior and middle fossae, the venous sinuses, the falx cerebri, and the upper surface of the tentorium travel through V/1, the pain that is experienced is referred to the ocular and frontoparietal regions; similarly, pain arising from the lower surface of the tentorium, the posterior cranial fossa, and the upper 2–3 cervical vertebrae (mediated by C2) is referred to the occipital and nuchal region. Small regions of the dura mater are innervated by CN IX and X; pain arising here is, accordingly, referred to the throat or ear. These neuroanatomical connections also explain the referral of pain from the upper cervical region to the eye (shared trigeminal innervation), and why tension and migraine headache can cause pain in the neck.

Cervical Syndrome (Upper Cervical Syndrome)

Cervical syndrome typically causes pain in the frontal, ocular, and nuchal regions. The pain is usually continuous, without any circadian pattern, but may be more severe during the day or night. It may be worsened by active or passive movement of the head. It is usually due to a lesion affecting the C2 root and is characterized by muscle spasm, tenderness, and restricted neck movement. The diagnosis is based on the typical clinical findings, and cannot be based solely on radiographic evidence of degenerative disease of the cervical spine. For other causes of neck pain, see Table 23 (p. 373). For *cervical distortion* (whiplash), see p. 272. For *Posttraumatic headache*, see p. 270.

Substance-Induced Headache

Acute headache can be induced by a number of vasoactive substances. Triggers include alcohol consumption or withdrawal ("hangover"), caffeine or nicotine withdrawal, sodium glutamate, cocaine, marijuana, nitrates, and dihydropyridines (calcium antagonists). The headache is usually a pressing, piercing, or pulsating pain, and is typically bifrontal or frontotemporal. It may be accompanied by nausea, chest tightness, dizziness, abdominal complaints, lack of concentration, or impairment of consciousness.

Rebound headache. Persons suffering from recurrent or chronic headache are at risk for the excessive or uncontrolled use of medications, singly or in combination (analgesics, benzodiazepines, ergot alkaloids, combined preparations). This may result in daily *rebound headache*, persisting from morning to night and characterized by pressurelike or pulsating, unilateral or bilateral pain, accompanied by malaise, nausea, vomiting, phonophobia, and photophobia. Patients may also complain of lack of concentration, disturbed sleep, blurred or flickering vision, a feeling of cold, and mood swings. These patients change medications frequently and tend to take medication even at the first sign of mild pain, because they fear a recurrence of severe pain. Eventually, drug tolerance develops, resulting in persistent headache. The original migraine or tension headache may be largely masked by the rebound headache. Other drug side effects may include ergotism, gastritis, gastrointestinal ulcers, renal failure, physical dependence, and epileptic seizures (withdrawal seizures).

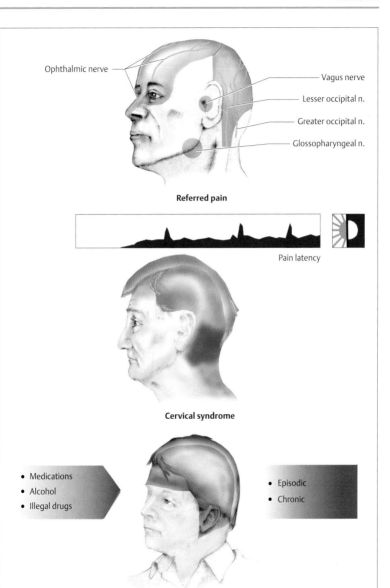

Ophthalmic nerve

Vagus nerve

Lesser occipital n.

Greater occipital n.

Glossopharyngeal n.

Referred pain

Pain latency

Cervical syndrome

- Medications
- Alcohol
- Illegal drugs

- Episodic
- Chronic

Substance-induced headache

Treatment

The proper treatment of headache depends on its cause. Episodic or chronic tension headache and migraine are by far the most common types of headache. Structural lesions are a rare cause of headache ($<5\%$ of all headaches); such headaches typically start suddenly, worsen quickly, and represent a new type of pain that the patient has never had before. If a structural lesion is suspected, neuroimaging studies should be performed.

■ General Treatment Measures

Good patient–physician communication is essential for the diagnosis and treatment of headache. The most important clues to differential diagnosis are derived from the case history. The medication history must be obtained, and psychological factors must also be considered; headache is often associated with anxiety, e. g., fear of a brain tumor, of a mental illness, or of not having one's complaints taken seriously. Patients must be instructed how they themselves can improve their symptoms (behavioral modification) through lifestyle changes (e. g., avoidance of alcohol, dietary changes, physical exercise, adequate sleep) and nonpharmacological measures (relaxation training, biofeedback, stress management, keeping a pain diary).

■ Acute Treatment

Type of Headache	General Measures	Pharmacotherapy
Episodic tension headache	Behavioral therapy, ice packs	Peppermint oil to forehead and temples; aspirin, acetaminophen, ibuprofen, or naproxen
Migraine	Rest, ice packs	Antiemetic (metoclopramide or domperidone) + aspirin or acetaminophen; if ineffective, triptans[1]
Cluster headache	Hot compresses	Oxygen inhalation; if ineffective, triptan s.c. or ergotamine
Chronic paroxysmal hemicrania		Indomethacin
Trigeminal neuralgia	Avoidance of triggers	Carbamazepine, gabapentin, phenytoin, baclofen, or pimozide[2]

1 This group includes sumatriptan, almotriptan, eletriptan, frovatriptan, naratriptan, rizatriptan, and zolmitriptan.
2 Patients with primary or secondary resistance to medical treatment should be treated neurosurgically (percutaneous thermocoagulation or retroganglionic glycerol instillation; microvascular decompression).

■ Prophylaxis

Type of Headache	General Measures	Pharmacotherapy
Episodic or chronic tension headache	Behavioral therapy	Tricyclic antidepressants (e. g., amitryptiline, doxepin, amitryptiline oxide)
Migraine	Behavioral therapy	*1st line*: Beta-blockers (e. g., metoprolol, propranolol); *2nd line*: flunarizine or valproate; *3rd line*: methysergide or pizotifen
Episodic cluster headache	Avoidance of alcohol (during cluster), nitrates, histamines, and nicotine	Prednisone, ergotamine, verapamil, methysergide, or lithium
Chronic cluster headache		Lithium, verapamil, or pizotifen

Central Nervous System

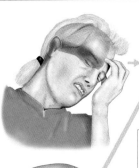

 Neck stiffness

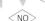 YES → CT[1] →

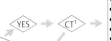
- Hemorrhage[2]
- Abscess
- Hydrocephalus
- Neoplasia
- Pseudotumor cerebri

Normal →

Lumbar puncture ⇨ meningoencephalitis, spinal hemorrhage, leptomeningeal metastases; pseudotumor cerebri

NO

- Migraine
- Tension headache
- Substance-induced headache (nitrates, glutamate, analgesics)
- Sinusitis
- Cervical syndrome
- Temporal arteritis
- After lumbar puncture
- Systemic lupus erythematosus

Doppler, MRI; MR angiotomography, angiography ⇨ arterial dissection, venous sinus thrombosis, cerebral infarction

Diagnostic classification
(acute or subacute headache)

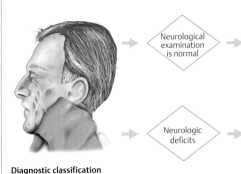

Neurological examination is normal ⇨

- Sinusitis
- Trigeminal neuralgia
- Cluster headache
- Atypical facial pain
- Herpes zoster
- Chronic paroxysmal hemicrania
- Oromandibular dysfunction, odontogenic
- Acute glaucoma
- Optic neuritis
- Temporal arteritis
- Thalamic pain

Neurologic deficits ⇨

- Cluster headache
- Diabetic neuropathy
- Lesion in cavernous sinus
- Supra- or infratentorial mass
- Lesion of brain stem or trigeminal nerve
- Herpes zoster
- Tolosa-Hunt syndrome

Diagnostic classification
(facial pain)

[1] Computed tomography
[2] Subarachnoid hemorrhage (SAH), intracerebral/intraventricular hemorrhage

Central Nervous System

Epilepsy: Seizure Types

An epileptic seizure (convulsion, fit) is a sign of brain dysfunction (p. 198). Seizures generally last no more than 2 minutes; the *postictal period* may be marked by impairment of consciousness or focal neurological signs. The type and extent of motor, sensory, autonomic and/or psychological disturbance during the seizure (seizure semiology) reflects the location and extent (localized/generalized) of brain dysfunction. Seizure classification, including the differentiation of true epileptic from nonepileptic seizures (pseudoseizures or psychogenic seizures, p. 202), is essential for effective treatment.

■ **Partial (Focal) Seizures**

Focal or *partial seizures* reflect paroxysmal discharges restricted to a part of the affected hemisphere. By definition, *simple partial seizures* are those in which consciousness is not impaired, while *complex partial seizures* (psychomotor seizures) are those in which consciousness is impaired. A sensory or behavioral disturbance preceding a focal or generalized seizure with motor manifestations is called a seizure *aura*. Some features of partial seizures are listed in the table below.

The semiology of simple and complex partial seizures depends on their site of origin (focus) and the brain areas to which they spread (see table, p. 194). They may become *secondarily generalized*, evolving into generalized paroxysmal attacks or tonic-clonic seizures. The initial symptoms and signs vary depending on the location of the epileptic focus.

Feature	Simple Partial Seizures	Complex Partial Seizures
Consciousness	Unaffected	Impaired
Duration	Seconds to minutes	Minutes
Symptoms and signs	Depend on site of origin; no postictal confusion	Depend on site of origin; postictal confusion
Age group	Any age	Any age
Ictal EEG	Contralateral epileptiform discharges; in many cases, no interictal abnormalities are detected	Unilateral or bilateral epileptiform discharges, diffuse or focal

(Adapted from Gram, 1990)

Central Nervous System

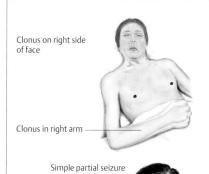

Clonus on right side of face

Ictal EEG: Focal activity on left (frontoprecentral spike waves)

Clonus in right arm

50 μ V |___
        1s

Simple partial seizure

Oral automatisms (licking, chewing, lip smacking)

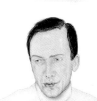

Ictal EEG: Bilateral frontotemporal activity (rhythmic θ waves)

Oral automatisms (snorting, throat clearing, chewing)

50 μ V |___
        1s

Complex partial seizure

Partial seizures (focal epilepsy)

Interictal phase	Prodromal phase	Tonic phase	Clonic phase	Postictal phase	
Normal EEG	Focal or generalized dysrhythmia and slowing	Ictal β and α spike waves	Rhythmic slowing with occasional spikes	Extinction phase	Irregular and high δ and sub-δ wave activity

Generalized seizures (schematic representation of ictal EEG in grand mal seizure)

Site of focus	Seizure type	Symptoms and signs
Frontal lobe	Simple or complex partial seizures with or without secondary generalization (hypermotor frontal lobe seizures)	Adversive head movement and other complex motor phenomena (mainly in legs), e. g., pelvic movements, ambulatory automatisms, swimming movements, fencing posture, staring, laughing, outcries, genital fumbling, autonomic dysfunction, speech arrest. Mood changes may also occur. Seizures occur several times a day with an abrupt onset. The unvarying course of the seizures may suggest hysteria. Brief postictal confusion
Temporal lobe	Complex partial seizures with or without secondary generalization	Ascending epigastric sensations (nausea, heat sensation); olfactory/gustatory hallucinations; compulsive thoughts, feeling of detachment, déjà-vu, jamais-vu; oral and other automatisms (psychomotor attacks); dyspnea, urinary urgency, palpitations; macropsia, micropsia; postictal confusion
Parietal lobe	Simple partial seizures with or without secondary generalization	Sensory and/or motor phenomena (jacksonian seizures); pain (rare)
Occipital lobe	Simple partial seizure with or without secondary generalization	Unformed visual hallucinations (sparks, flashes)

(Adapted from Gram, 1990)

■ **Generalized Seizures**

Generalized epilepsy reflects paroxysmal discharges occurring in both hemispheres. The seizures may be either *convulsive* (e. g., generalized tonic-clonic seizure ⇨ GTCS) or *nonconvulsive* (myoclonic, tonic, or atonic seizures; absence seizures). Generalized seizures are classified by their clinical features.

Feature	Absence Seizure	Myoclonic Seizure	Atonic (Astatic) Seizure	Tonic-clonic Seizure
Consciousness	Impaired	Unaffected	Impaired	Impaired
Duration	A few (≤ 30) seconds	1–5 seconds	A few seconds	1–3 minutes
Symptoms and signs	Brief absence, vacant gaze and blinking followed by immediate return of mental clarity; automatisms (lip smacking, chewing, fiddling, fumbling) may occur	Sudden, bilaterally synchronous jerks in arms and legs; often occur in series	Sudden loss of muscle tone causing severe falls	Initial cry (occasionally); falls (loss of muscle tone); respiratory arrest; cyanosis; tonic, then clonic seizures; muscle relaxation followed by deep sleep. Tongue biting, urinary and fecal incontinence
Age group	Children and adolescents	Children and adolescents	Infants and children	Any age
Ictal EEG	Bilateral regular 3 (2–4) Hz spike waves	Polyspike waves, spike waves, or sharp and slow waves	Polyspike waves, flattening or low-voltage fast activity	Often obscured by muscle artifacts

(Adapted from Gram, 1990)

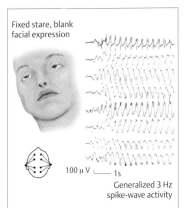

Fixed stare, blank facial expression

100 μV ⊢—— 1 s

Generalized 3 Hz spike-wave activity

Absence

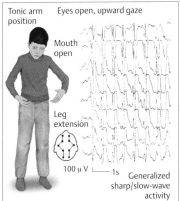

Tonic arm position   Eyes open, upward gaze

Mouth open

Leg extension

100 μV ⊢—— 1 s

Generalized sharp/slow-wave activity

Tonic seizure
(in myoclonic/astatic epilepsy)

Central Nervous System

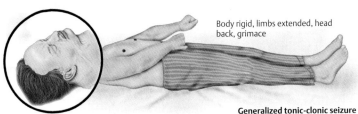

Body rigid, limbs extended, head back, grimace

Generalized tonic-clonic seizure
(Grand mal, tonic phase; transition to clonic phase with forceful, rhythmic convulsions)

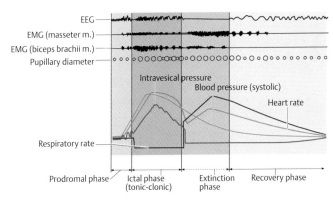

EEG

EMG (masseter m.)

EMG (biceps brachii m.)

Pupillary diameter

Intravesical pressure

Blood pressure (systolic)

Heart rate

Respiratory rate

Prodromal phase   Ictal phase (tonic-clonic)   Extinction phase   Recovery phase

Tonic-clonic grand mal seizure (temporal course)

Epilepsy: Classification

The etiology and prognosis of epilepsy depend on its clinical type. All forms of epilepsy (e. g., absence epilepsy of childhood, juvenile myoclonic epilepsy, temporal lobe epilepsy, frontal lobe epilepsy, reflex epilepsy) are characterized by *recurrent* paroxysmal attacks; thus classification cannot be based on a single seizure. *Epileptic syndromes* vary in seizure pattern, cause, age at onset, precipitating factors, EEG changes, and prognosis (e. g., neonatal convulsions, infantile spasms and salaam seizures = West syndrome, Lennox–Gastaut syndrome, temporal lobe seizures). Seizures triggered by fever, substance abuse, alcohol, eclampsia, trauma, tumor, sleep deprivation, or medications are designated as *isolated nonrecurring seizures* or *acute epileptic reactions*. *Status epilepticus* is a single prolonged seizure or a series of seizures without full recovery in between. Any type of seizure (convulsive or nonconvulsive) may appear under the guise of status epilepticus. In *grand mal status epilepticus*, patients do not regain consciousness between seizures.

Location-related (focal, partial) *epilepsy* can be differentiated from *generalized epilepsies* and *epileptic syndromes* on the basis of the seizure pattern. Seizures that cannot be classified because of inadequate data on focal or generalized seizure development are called *unclassified epilepsy* or *epileptic syndrome*. Other terms used in classification refer to seizure etiology (e. g., idiopathic, cryptogenic, symptomatic).

Type of Epilepsy	Features
Location-related	Partial (focal) seizures
Generalized	Generalized convulsive seizures (GCS)
Idiopathic	No known cause other than genetic predisposition. No manifestations other than epileptic seizures. Characteristic age of onset
Cryptogenic	Assumed to reflect a CNS disorder of unidentified type. (Once the cause is identified, epilepsy is classified as symptomatic.)
Symptomatic	Due to an identified CNS disorder or lesion

Type of Epilepsy	Etiology	Epilepsy/Epileptic Syndrome
Location-related (focal, localized, partial)	Idiopathic (characteristic age of onset)	Benign epilepsy of childhood with centrotemporal spikes; epilepsy of childhood with occipital paroxysms
	Cryptogenic or symptomatic	Variable expression depending on cause and location (e. g., temporal, frontal, parietal, or occipital lobe epilepsy)
Generalized	Idiopathic (characteristic age of onset)	Absence epilepsy of childhood (pyknolepsy); juvenile absence epilepsy; juvenile myoclonic epilepsy (impulsive petit mal); awakening grand mal epilepsy (GTCS); epilepsy with specific triggers (reflex epilepsy)
	Cryptogenic or symptomatic	West syndrome (infantile spasms, salaam seizures); Lennox–Gastaut syndrome; myoclonic-astatic epilepsy; epilepsy with myoclonic absence
	Symptomatic	Early myoclonic encephalopathy (unspecific etiology); seizures secondary to various diseases
Unsure whether focal or generalized	Idiopathic or symptomatic	Neonatal convulsions; acquired epileptic aphasia (Landau–Kleffner syndrome)
Variably focal and generalized	Symptomatic (situation-related seizure)	Febrile convulsions; isolated seizure or isolated status epilepticus; acute metabolic or toxic triggers

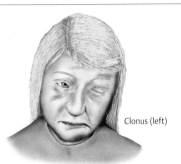

Clonus (left)

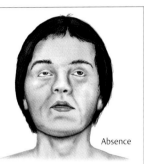

Absence

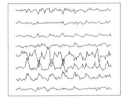

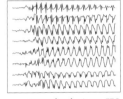

Partial seizure, EEG
(right temporoparietal δ-wave activity)

Generalized seizure, EEG
(generalized 3 Hz spike-wave pattern)

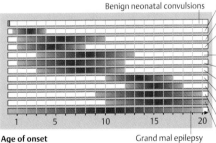

Benign neonatal convulsions

Febrile convulsions
Lennox-Gastaut syndrome
Epilepsy with myoclonic-astatic seizures
Benign focal epilepsy of childhood
Epilepsy with spike waves during sleep
Pyknolepsy
Juvenile absence epilepsy
Impulsive petit mal
Awakening grand mal epilepsy
Benign juvenile focal epilepsy

Age of onset

Grand mal epilepsy

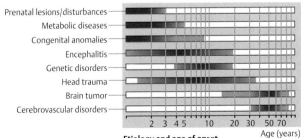

Prenatal lesions/disturbances
Metabolic diseases
Congenital anomalies
Encephalitis
Genetic disorders
Head trauma
Brain tumor
Cerebrovascular disorders

Age (years)

Etiology and age of onset

Causes. Some patients have a *genetic* predisposition to epilepsy, particularly those with generalized epilepsies. Some hereditary diseases are associated with epilepsy (e.g., tuberous sclerosis, Sturge–Weber syndrome, mitochondrial encephalopathies, sphingolipidoses). *Acquired* forms of epilepsy may be focal (possibly with secondary generalization), bilateral, or diffuse (primary generalized epilepsies). The causes include developmental disorders, pyridoxine deficiency, hippocampal sclerosis, brain tumors, head trauma, cerebrovascular disturbances, alcohol, drug abuse, medications, and CNS infections.

Pathophysiology. Seizure activity in the brain is thought to be initiated by a preponderance of excitatory over inhibitory postsynaptic potentials (EPSP, IPSP), resulting in depolarization of nerve cell membranes. Such a depolarization may appear on the EEG as an interictal spike, an initial spike component, or an abrupt depolarization with superimposed high-frequency action potentials (*paroxysmal depolarization shift, PDS*). The synchronous discharges of large numbers of neurons result in an epileptic seizure. Seizure activity is terminated by active processes such as transmembrane ion transport via sodium–potassium pumps, adenosine release, and the liberation of endogenous opiates, whose combined effect is membrane hyperpolarization, manifested as slow-wave activity in the EEG. Factors favoring the development of seizures include changes in the concentration of electrolytes (Na^+, K^+, Ca^{2+}), excitatory amino acids (glutamic acid), and inhibitory amino acids (GABA), irregular interneuron connections, and abnormal afferent connections from subcortical structures ($\Rightarrow$ diencephalon, thalamus, brain stem). In focal epilepsy, the epileptic focus is surrounded by an "inhibitory margin", while the paroxysmal activity of generalized epilepsy is spread throughout the brain.

General treatment measures. *Lifestyle changes* (sleep–wake rhythm, avoidance of seizure triggers); *chronic use of anticonvulsant medication.* Patients with partial seizures preceded by long auras may be able to abort their seizures while still in the aura phase by various concentration techniques (seizure interruption methods).

Antiepileptic drugs (AEDs). AEDs work by a variety of mechanisms, e.g., inhibition of voltage-gated sodium channels (carbamazepine, oxcarbazepine, lamotrigine, phenytoin, valproic acid) or thalamic calcium channels (ethosuximide), or interaction with inhibitory GABA receptors (benzodiazepines, phenobarbital, gabapentin, tiagabine, levetiracetam) or excitatory glutamate receptors (phenobarbital, felbamate, topiramate). Antiepileptic therapy is generally started in patients who have had a single seizure and are thought to be at risk of recurrence, in those with an epileptic syndrome, and in those who have had two or more seizures within 6 months. AEDs used to treat focal, unclassified, and symptomatic tonic-clonic seizures include carbamazepine, gabapentin, lamotrigine, oxcarbazepine, topiramate, levetiracetam, phenytoin, phenobarbital, and primidone; those used to treat generalized seizures include valproic acid, ethosuximide (absences), primidone, phenobarbital (epilepsy associated with myoclonic seizures, tonic-clonic seizures), and lamotrigine. Treatment is always begun with a single drug (monotherapy); if this ineffective, another drug is used instead of or in addition to the first (combination therapy). Antiepileptic therapy can be discontinued in some cases if the risk of seizure recurrence is judged to be low.

Other measures. Surgery (indicated in patients with drug-resistant focal epilepsy and/or resectable lesions, such as brain tumors or unilateral mesial temporal sclerosis). Vagus nerve stimulation by means of an implanted neurocybernetic prosthesis (NCP) is a form of treatment whose efficacy remains controversial.

Prognosis (Table 24, p. 373). Antiepileptic drugs prevent seizure recurrence in roughly 70% of patients, reduce the frequency of seizures in 25%, and are ineffective in 5% (drug resistance), especially those with Lennox–Gastaut syndrome, symptomatic myoclonic epilepsy, and cryptogenic syndromes.

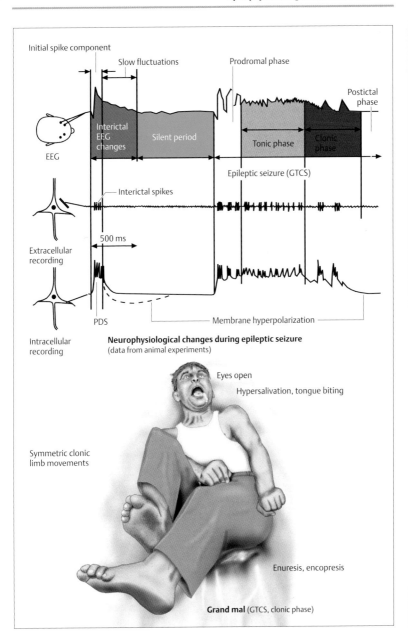

Neurophysiological changes during epileptic seizure
(data from animal experiments)

Grand mal (GTCS, clonic phase)

The differentiation of epileptic from nonepileptic seizures is of major prognostic and therapeutic importance. Nonepileptic seizures may or may not involve loss of consciousness. *Pseudoseizures* resemble epileptic seizures (p. 192 ff), but are of nonepileptic origin. This broad category includes syncope, psychogenic seizures, and simulated seizures. "Pseudoseizure," in the narrower sense, is a synonym for "psychogenic seizure."

Nonepileptic seizures are misdiagnosed as epileptic seizures in nearly 20% of patients, roughly 15% of whom are unnecessarily treated with antiepileptic drugs; conversely, some 10% of all epileptic seizures are misdiagnosed as nonepileptic seizures; 20–30% of patients have both epileptic and nonepileptic seizures. In case of doubt, the patient should be referred to a specialist or specialized epilepsy center.

■ Syncope

Syncope is defined as a brief loss of consciousness, often involving a fall, due to transient cerebral ischemia or hypoxia (see Table 25, p. 374 for potential causes). In 45% of cases, the cause can be determined from the history and physical examination. Important anamnestic clues include triggers such as excitement or anxiety, precipitating situations (blood drawing, prolonged standing, urination, coughing fits, pain), heart disease, mental illness (generalized anxiety disorder, depression, somatization disorders), and medications. The patient should be evaluated for possible blood pressure abnormalities and for cardiac or neurological disorders (p. 148). EEG yields the diagnosis in only about 2% of cases. Only rare cases of syncope are due to TIA (p. 166). Syncope clinically resembles an epileptic seizure in some ways, but differs in others (see table, below).

Clinical Feature	Syncope	Epileptic Seizure
Triggers	Common	No
Time of day	Mostly diurnal; does not awaken patient from sleep	Day or night; awakens patient from sleep
Skin coloration	Pale	Cyanotic or normal
Premonitory symptoms	Tinnitus, visual blurring or blackout, feeling faint, lightheadedness	None or aura
Type of fall	Collapse or fall over stiffly (often backwards)	Fall over stiffly
Duration	Usually < 30 seconds	1–3 minutes or longer
Abnormal movements (myoclonus)	Frequent, arrhythmic, multifocal to generalized, last < 30 seconds	Always generalized, 1–2 minutes
Eyes	Open	Closed
Urinary incontinence	Occasional	Common
Postictal confusion	Brief or absent	Longer-lasting
Tongue-biting	Occasional	Common
Prolactin, creatine kinase	Normal	Elevated
Typical EEG changes	Absent	Common
Focal neurological deficit	Absent	Occasional

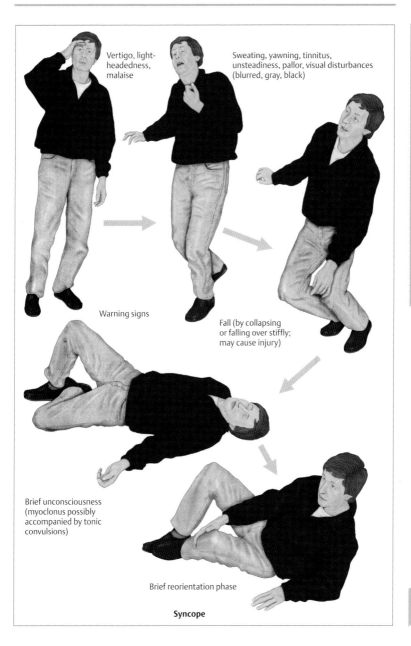

Vertigo, light-headedness, malaise

Sweating, yawning, tinnitus, unsteadiness, pallor, visual disturbances (blurred, gray, black)

Warning signs

Fall (by collapsing or falling over stiffly; may cause injury)

Brief unconsciousness (myoclonus possibly accompanied by tonic convulsions)

Brief reorientation phase

Syncope

Central Nervous System

201

■ Psychogenic Seizures

Nonorganic, nonepileptic seizures arising from psychological factors do not involve loss of consciousness. They are involuntary and unintentional, and thus must be differentiated from *simulated seizures*, which are voluntarily, consciously, and intentionally produced events. Psychogenic seizures may resemble *frontal lobe seizures* (p. 194) and are more common in women than men. About 40% of patients with psychogenic seizures also suffer from true epileptic seizures. The case history often reveals characteristic risk factors, which may be *biographical* (family difficulties, abuse, divorce, sexual assault in childhood), *somatic* (genetic predisposition), *psychiatric* (conflicts, stress, psychosocial gain from illness behavior, mental illness), or *social* (poor living and working conditions). Patients often meet the psychiatric diagnostic criteria for a conversion disorder (F44.5 according to the ICD-10). Epileptic seizures in family members, or in the patients themselves, may serve as the prototype for psychogenic seizures.

Premonitory signs. Psychogenic seizures can be induced or terminated by suggestion. They may be preceded by a restless, anxious, or fearful state. They usually occur in the presence of others (an "audience") and do not occur when the patient is asleep.

Seizure semiology. Psychogenic seizures usually take a dramatic course, with a variable ending. Their semiology is usually of a type more likely to incite sympathy and pity in onlookers than fear or revulsion. Typical features include an abrupt fall or slow collapse, jerking of the limbs, tonic contraction of the body, writhing (*arc de cercle*), calling out, shouting, rapid twisting of the head and body, and forward pelvic thrusting; the sequence of movements is usually variable. The eyes are usually closed, but sometimes wide open and staring; the patient squeezes the eyes shut when passive opening is attempted. Urinary incontinence or injury (self-mutilation) may also occur. Tongue-bite injuries, if present, are usually at the tip of the tongue (those in true epileptic fits are usually lateral). The patient is less responsive than normal to external stimuli, including painful stimuli, but not unconscious (squeezes eyelids shut when the eyes are touched, drops arm to the side when it is held over the patient's face and released). The patient's skin is not pale or cyanotic during the ictus. Patients who hyperventilate during psychogenic seizures may have carpopedal spasms. Psychogenic seizures often last longer than epileptic seizures.

Postictal phase. No focal neurological deficits can be detected, though there may be a psychogenic postictal stupor. The serum prolactin level is not elevated (which, however, does not rule out a true epileptic seizure). The seizure may be terminated abruptly by suggestion, or by departure of the "audience." Some patients recall the seizure to some extent, while others emphatically deny memory of it.

■ Panic Disorder (ICD-10 ⇨ F41.0)

Panic disorder is characterized by sudden, unexpected and apparently unprovoked attacks of intense anxiety, which may range in severity from a general feeling of restlessness to a mortal dread. The attacks usually last 5–30 minutes and may awaken the patient from sleep. Accompanying symptoms include feelings of detachment from the environment, i.e., *depersonalization* (detachment from one's own body, floating state) and *derealization* (sensation of being in a dream or nightmare, feeling of unreality); autonomic and other physical symptoms of variable severity, including *cardiovascular* (tachycardia, palpitations, pallor, chest pain or pressure), *gastrointestinal* (nausea, dry mouth, dysphagia, diarrhea), *respiratory* (hyperventilation, dyspnea, smothering sensation), and other manifestations (tremor, twitching of the limbs, dizziness, paresthesia, mydriasis, urinary urgency, sweating). The differential diagnosis includes epilepsy (aura, simple partial seizures), hyperthyroidism, hyperventilation syndrome, pheochromocytoma, heart disease, and hypoglycemia.

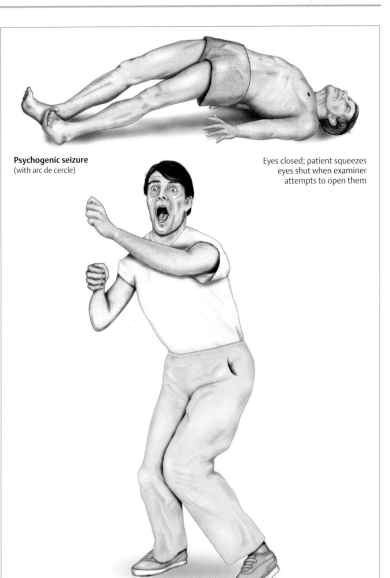

Psychogenic seizure
(with arc de cercle)

Eyes closed; patient squeezes
eyes shut when examiner
attempts to open them

Panic attack (hyperventilation, psychomotor restlessness)

■ Drop Attacks

Sudden, unprovoked, and unheralded falls without loss of consciousness are most common in patients over 65 years of age. Some 10–15% of these drop attacks cause serious injury, particularly fractures. The patient may not be able to get up after a fall. The common causes of recurrent falls in each age group are listed in Table 26 (p. 374). Those associated with loss of consciousness are described on pages 192 ff and 200.

■ Hyperventilation Syndrome (Tetany)

The clinical manifestations include paresthesiae (perioral, distal symmetrical or unilateral), generalized weakness, palpitations, tachycardia, dry mouth, dysphagia, dyspnea, yawning, pressure sensation in the chest, visual disturbances, tinnitus, dizziness, unsteady gait, muscle stiffness, and carpopedal spasms. The patients report feelings of restlessness, panic, unreality, or confusion. *Psychological causes* include anxiety, hysteria, and inner conflict. *Metabolic causes* include hypocalcemia (due to hypoparathyroidism, vitamin D deficiency, malabsorption, or pancreatitis) and a wide range of other disturbances including hypercalcemia, hypomagnesemia, prolonged vomiting, pulmonary embolism, salicylate intoxication, acute myocardial infarction, severe pain, high fever due to septicemia, pneumothorax, stroke, and neurogenic pulmonary edema. *Chronic hyperventilation syndromes* are more common than acute syndromes, but also more difficult to diagnose.

■ Tonic Spasms

These are unilateral muscular spasms (often painful) that are not accompanied by loss of consciousness; they last seconds to minutes, and occur up to 30 or more times a day. They are most commonly seen in multiple sclerosis, less commonly in cerebrovascular disorders. These spasms are often triggered by movement. Some patients have paresthesiae (tingling, burning) contralateral to the affected side before the muscle spasm sets in. The underlying lesion may be in the brain stem (pons) or internal capsule.

■ Acute Dystonic Reaction

Acute dystonic reactions can occur within a few hours to one week of starting treatment with dopamine receptor antagonists, e. g., *neuroleptics* (benperidol, fluphenazine, haloperidol, triflupromazine, perphenazine), *antiemetics* (metoclopramide, bromopride), and *calcium antagonists* (flunarizine, cinnarizine). *Symptoms and signs:* focal or segmental dystonia (p. 64), sometimes painful, marked by oculogyric crisis, blepharospasm, pharyngospasm with glossospasm and laryngospasm, or oromandibular dystonia with tonic jaw and tongue movements. Generalized reactions are also seen on occasion (p. 66).

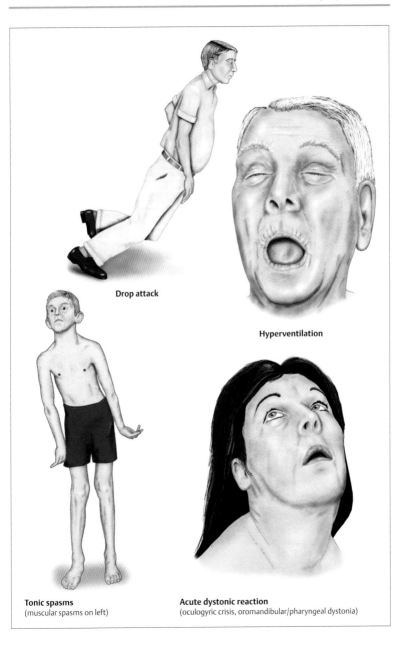

Drop attack

Hyperventilation

Tonic spasms
(muscular spasms on left)

Acute dystonic reaction
(oculogyric crisis, oromandibular/pharyngeal dystonia)

The diagnosis of Parkinson disease (PD; sometimes termed idiopathic Parkinson disease, to distinguish it from symptomatic forms of parkinsonism, and from other primary forms) is mainly based on the typical neurological findings, their evolution over the course of the disease, and their responsiveness to levodopa (L-dopa). Longitudinal observation may be necessary before a definitive diagnosis of PD can be given. PD is characterized by a number of disturbances of motor function (*cardinal manifestations*) and by other *accompanying manifestations* of different kinds and variable severity.

Cardinal Manifestations

Bradykinesia, hypokinesia, and akinesia. Motor disturbances include slow initiation of movement (*akinesia*), sluggishness of movement (*bradykinesia*) and diminished spontaneous movement (*hypokinesia*); these terms are often used nearly interchangeably, as these disturbances all tend to occur together. Spontaneous fluctuations of mobility are not uncommon. The motor disturbances are often more pronounced on one side of the body, especially in the early stages of disease. They affect the craniofacial musculature to produce a masklike facies (*hypomimia*), defective mouth closure, reduced blinking, dysphagia, salivation (drooling), and speech that is diminished in volume (hypophonia), hoarse, poorly enunciated, and monotonous in pitch (*dysarthrophonia*). The patient may find it hard to initiate speech, or may repeat syllables; there may be an involuntary acceleration of speech toward the end of a sentence (*festination*). *Postural changes* include stooped posture, a mildly flexed and adducted posture of the arms, and postural instability. *Gait disturbances* appear in the early stages of disease and typically consist of a small-stepped gait, shuffling, and limping, with reduced arm swing. Difficulty initiating gait comes about in the later stages of disease, along with episodes of "freezing"—complete arrest of gait when the patient is confronted by doorway or a narrow path between pieces of furniture. It becomes difficult for the patient to stand up from a seated position, or to turn over in bed. *Impairment of fine motor control* impairs activities of daily living such as fastening buttons, writing (*micro-*

graphia), eating with knife and fork, shaving, and hair-combing. It becomes difficult to perform two activities simultaneously, such as walking and talking.

Tremor. Only about half of all PD patients have tremor early in the course of the disease; the rest usually develop it as the disease progresses. It is typically most pronounced in the hands (pill-rolling tremor) and is seen mainly when the affected limbs are at rest, improving or disappearing with voluntary movement. Its frequency is ca. 5 Hz, it is often asymmetrical, and it can be exacerbated by even mild stress (mental calculations, etc.).

Rigidity. Elevated muscle tone is felt by the patient as muscle tension or spasm and by the examiner as increased resistance to passive movement across the joints. Examination may reveal *cogwheel rigidity*, i.e., repeated, ratchet-like oscillations of resistance to passive movement across the wrist, elbow, or other joints, which may be brought out by alternating passive flexion and extension.

Postural instability (loss of balance). Propulsion and retropulsion arise in the early stages of Parkinson disease because of generalized impairment of the postural reflexes that maintain the bipedal stance. Related phenomena include involuntary acceleration of the gait (*festination*), difficulty in stopping walking, gait instability, and frequent falls.

Accompanying Manifestations

■ **Behavioral Changes**

Depression. The range of depressive manifestations includes worry, anxiety, avoidance of social contact, general unhappiness, listlessness, querulousness, brooding, somatoform disturbances, and (rarely) suicidal ideation.

Anxiety. Tension, worry, mental agitation, lack of concentration, and dizziness are relatively common complaints.

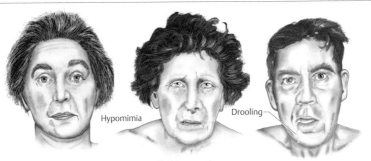

Hypomimia

Drooling

Facial expression

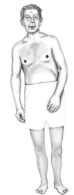

Postural change
(hypokinesia-left)

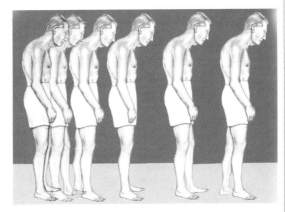

Gait impairment (postural instability, propulsion, festination)

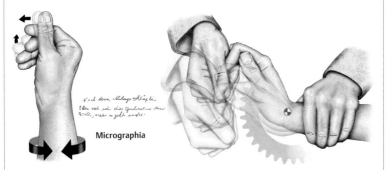

Micrographia

Resting tremor

Rigidity (cogwheel phenomenon)

Dementia. Impairment of memory and concentration in early PD-associated dementia may be difficult to distinguish from depressive manifestations. The side effects of pharmacotherapy (p. 212) must be kept in mind before treatment is initiated for patients suffering from disorientation, confusion, suspiciousness, and other emotional changes. Impaired memory is usually not a major feature of PD; as the disease progresses, about 20% of patients develop decreased flexibility of thought and action, perseveration, and increasing difficulty in planning future activities. The development of dementia in PD is correlated with an increase in the number of Lewy bodies (pp. 210).

Hallucinations. A state of excessive suspiciousness, vivid dreams, and increasing anxiety may evolve into one of severe confusion with visual hallucinations. Frank psychosis (e. g., paranoid delusions, ideas of reference, or delusional jealousy) may be due to other causes than PD, particularly an adverse effect of antiparkinsonian medication. *Dementia with Lewy bodies* (a syndrome in which the clinical features of Parkinson disease are found together with dementia, fluctuating level of consciousness, visual hallucinations, and frequent falls) is another possible cause, especially in patients who are unusually sensitive to low doses of neuroleptics (⇨ exacerbation of parkinsonism, delirium, malignant neuroleptic syndrome, p. 347).

■ **Autonomic Dysfunction**

Blood pressure changes. Hypotension is a common side effect of antiparkinsonian medications (levodopa, dopamine agonists). Marked orthostatic hypotension, if present, suggests the possible diagnosis of multisystem atrophy.

Constipation may be caused by autonomic dysfunction, as a manifestation of the disease, or as a side effect of medication (anticholinergic agents).

Bladder disorders. Polyuria, urinary urgency, and urinary incontinence occur mainly at night and in patients with severe akinesia (who have difficulty getting to the toilet). PD only rarely causes severe bladder dysfunction.

Sleep disorders. PD commonly causes disturbances of the sleep–wake cycle, including difficulty falling asleep, nocturnal breathing problems similar to sleep apnea syndrome, and shortening of the sleep cycle. Sleep may also be interrupted by nocturnal akinesia, which makes it difficult for the patient to turn over in bed.

Sexual dysfunction. Spontaneous complaints of diminished libido or impotence are rare. Increased libido is a known side effect of levodopa and dopamine agonists.

Hyperhidrosis. Mainly occurs as generalized, irregular, sudden episodes of sweating.

Seborrhea. Mainly on the forehead, nose, and scalp (greasy face, seborrheic dermatitis).

Leg edema is often the result of physical inactivity.

■ **Sensory Manifestations**

Pain in the arm or shoulder, sometimes accompanied by fatigue and weakness, may be present for years before the cardinal manifestations arise and enable a diagnosis of PD. Back pain and nuchal cramps are frequent secondary effects of parkinsonian rigidity and abnormal posture. Dystonia may also come to attention because of the pain it produces.

Dysesthesia. Heat, burning or cold sensations may be felt in various parts of the body. For *restless legs syndrome*, see p. 114.

■ **Other Motor Manifestations**

Dystonia. Tonic dorsiflexion of the big toe with extension or flexion of the other toes may occur in the early morning hours or during walking. Dystonia may be drug-induced (e. g., by levodopa) or due to the disease itself. The differential diagnosis includes dopa-responsive dystonia (a disorder of autosomal dominant inheritance) and Wilson disease (p. 307), two predominantly dystonic motor disorders with onset in childhood and adolescence.

Visual disturbances are caused by impairment of eye movement. Vertical gaze palsy is suggestive of *progressive supranuclear palsy* (p. 302). The reduced blinking rate of PD may lead to a burning sensation on the cornea, or to conjunctivitis.

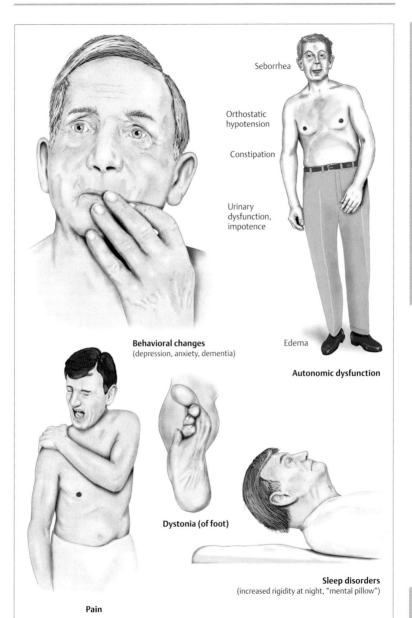

Seborrhea

Orthostatic hypotension

Constipation

Urinary dysfunction, impotence

Edema

Behavioral changes
(depression, anxiety, dementia)

Autonomic dysfunction

Dystonia (of foot)

Sleep disorders
(increased rigidity at night, "mental pillow")

Pain

Basal ganglia. The basal ganglia consist of the caudate nucleus (CN), putamen, globus pallidus (= pallidum; GPe = external segment, GPi = internal segment; putamen + pallidum = *lentiform nucleus*), claustrum, substantia nigra (SN; SNc = pars compacta, SNr = pars reticularis), and the subthalamic nucleus (STN). CN + putamen = (dorsal) *striatum*; nucleus accumbens + portions of olfactory tubercle + anterior portion of putamen + CN = limbic (ventral) striatum. *Substantia nigra* (SN): The SNr (ventral portion of SN) contains small amounts of dopamine and iron, giving it a reddish color, while the SNc (dorsal portion) contains large quantities of dopamine and melanin, making it black (whence the name, substantia nigra).

Connections. The basal ganglia are part of a number of parallel and largely distinct (segregated) neural pathways (circuits). Each circuit originates in a cortical area that is specialized for a specific function (skeletal motor, oculomotor, associative-cognitive, or emotional-motivational control), passes through several relay stations in the basal ganglia, and travels by way of the thalamus back to the cerebral cortex. Cortical projection fibers enter the basal ganglia at the striatum (*input station*) and exit from the GPi and SNr (*output station*). Input from the thalamus and brain stem also arrives at the striatum. Within the basal ganglia, there are two circuits subserving motor function, the so-called direct and indirect pathways. The *direct* pathway runs from the putamen to the GPi and SNr, while the *indirect* pathway takes the following trajectory: putamen ⇨ GPe ⇨ STN ⇨ GPi ⇨ SNr. The GPi and SNr project to the thalamus and brain stem.

Neurotransmitters. *Glutamate* mediates excitatory impulses from the cortex, amygdala, and hippocampus to the striatum. Synapses from STN fibers onto cells of the GPi and SNr are also glutamatergic. Both the excitatory and the inhibitory projections of the SNc to the basal ganglia are dopaminergic. In the striatum, *dopamine* acts on neurons bearing D_1 and D_2 receptors, of which there are various subtypes (D_1 group: d_1, d_5; D_2 group: d_2, d_3, d_4). D_1 receptors predominate in the direct pathway, D_2 receptors in the indirect pathway. Cholinergic interneurons in the striatum form a relay station within the basal ganglia (transmitter: *acetylcholine*). *Medium spiny-type*

neurons (MSN) in the striatum have inhibitory projections to the GPe, GPi, and SNr (transmitters: GABA, substance P/SP, enkephalin/Enk). Other inhibitory GABAergic projections run from the GPi to the STN, from the GPi to the thalamus (ventrolateral and ventroanterior nucleus), and from the SN to the thalamus. The thalamocortical projections are excitatory.

Motor function. The *direct pathway* is activated by cortical and dopaminergic projections to the striatum. The projection from the striatum in turn inhibits the GPi, diminishing its inhibitory output to the thalamic nuclei (i.e., causing net thalamic activation). Thalamocortical drive thus facilitates movement initiated in the cerebral cortex (voluntary movement). In the *indirect pathway*, the striatum, under the influence of afferent cortical and dopaminergic projections, exerts an inhibitory effect on the GPe and STN. The result is a diminished excitatory influence of the STN on the GPi and SNr, ultimately leading to facilitation of cortically initiated voluntary movement and inhibition of involuntary movement.

■ **Pathophysiology**

The cause of Parkinson disease is unknown. Its *structural* pathological correlate is a loss of neurons in the caudal and anterolateral parts of the SNc, with reactive gliosis and formation of *Lewy bodies* (eosinophilic intracytoplasmic inclusions in neurons) and *Lewy neurites* (abnormally phosphorylated neurofilaments) containing α-synuclein. Loss of pigment in the substantia nigra can be seen macroscopically. The most prominent *neurochemical* abnormality is a deficiency of dopamine in the striatum, whose extent is directly correlated with the severity of PD. The *physiological* effect of the lack of (mostly inhibitory) dopamine neurotransmission in the striatum is a relative increase in striatal activity, in turn causing functional disinhibition of the subthalamic nucleus via the *indirect pathway*. Meanwhile, in the *direct pathway*, decreased striatal inhibition of the GPi enhances the inhibitory influence of the GPi on the thalamus, leading to reduced activity in the thalamocortical projection. These changes in neural activity manifest themselves in the clinically observable akinesia, rigidity, and postural instability. For *tremor*, see p. 62.

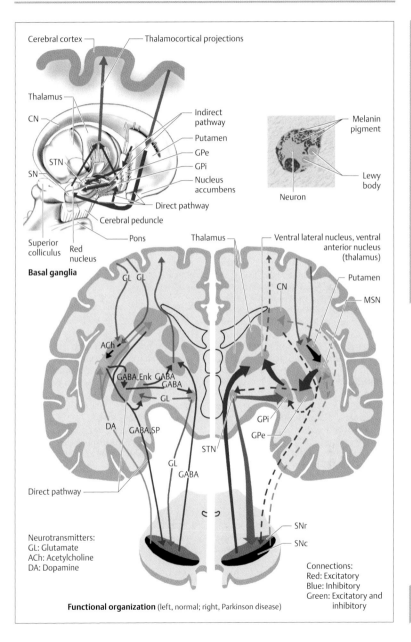

Central Nervous System

Cerebral cortex — Thalamocortical projections

Thalamus

CN

STN

SN

Superior colliculus   Red nucleus   Pons

Basal ganglia

Indirect pathway
Putamen
GPe
GPi
Nucleus accumbens
Direct pathway
Cerebral peduncle

Melanin pigment

Lewy body

Neuron

Thalamus

Ventral lateral nucleus, ventral anterior nucleus (thalamus)

Putamen

CN

MSN

ACh

GABA,Enk   GABA
GABA
GL

DA   GABA,SP

STN

GPi
GPe

GL
GABA

Direct pathway

SNr
SNc

Neurotransmitters:
GL: Glutamate
ACh: Acetylcholine
DA: Dopamine

Connections:
Red: Excitatory
Blue: Inhibitory
Green: Excitatory and inhibitory

Functional organization (left, normal; right, Parkinson disease)

Central Nervous System

The *goal of treatment* is improvement of the motor, autonomic, and cognitive symptoms of the disease. The treatment generally consists of medication along with physical, occupational, and speech therapy. Neurosurgical procedures are mostly reserved for intractable cases (see below). Pharmacotherapy is palliative, not curative. It is begun when the patient has trouble carrying out the activities of daily living and is prescribed, not according to a uniform pattern, but in relation to the needs of the individual patient.

■ **Symptomatic Treatment**

Dopaminergic agents. *Levodopa* is actively absorbed in the small intestine and rapidly distributed throughout the body (especially to skeletal muscle). Amino acids compete with the levodopa transport system at the blood–brain barrier. A decarboxylase inhibitor that does not penetrate the blood–brain barrier (benserazide or carbidopa) is administered together with levodopa to prevent its rapid breakdown in the peripheral circulation. Once it reaches the brain, levodopa is decarboxylated to dopamine, which is used for neurotransmission in the striatum. After it has been released from the presynaptic terminals of dopaminergic neurons in the striatum and exerted its effect on the postsynaptic terminals, it is broken down by two separate enzyme systems (deamination by monoamine oxidase type B, MAO-B; methylation by catechol-O-methyltransferase, COMT). Levodopa effectively reduces akinesia and rigidity, but has only a mild effect against tremor. Its long-term use is often complicated by motor fluctuations, dyskinesia, and psychiatric disturbances. *Dopamine agonists* (DAs) mimic the function of dopamine, binding to dopamine receptors. Their interaction with D_1 and D_2 receptors is thought to improve motor function, while their interaction with D_3 receptors is thought to improve cognition, motivation, and emotion. Long-term use of DAs is less likely to cause unwanted motor side effects than long-term use of levodopa. Commonly used DAs include bromocriptine (mainly a D_2 agonist), lisuride (mainly a D_2 agonist), and pergolide (a D_1, D_2, and D_3 agonist). Apomorphine, an effective D_1 and D_2 agonist, can be given by subcutaneous injection, but its effect lasts only about 1 hour. Other, recently introduced dopamine agonists are ropinirol and pramipexol (D_2 and D_3), cabergoline (D_2), and α-dihydroergocryptine (mainly D_2).
Selegiline inhibits MAO-B selectively and irreversibly (⇨ reduced dopamine catabolism ⇨ increase in striatal dopamine concentration). *Entacapone* increases the bioavailability of levodopa via peripheral inhibition of COMT.
Nondopaminergic agents. *Anticholinergic agents* (biperiden, bornaprine, metixene, trihexyphenidyl) act on striatal cholinergic interneurons. *Budipine* can relieve tremor (risk of ventricular tachycardia ⇨ ECG monitoring). *Glutamate antagonists* (amantadine, memantine) counteract increased glutamatergic activity at the N-methyl-D-aspartate (NMDA) glutamate receptor in the indirect pathway.

■ **Transplant Surgery**

Current research on intrastriatal transplantation of stem cells (derived from fetal tissue, from umbilical cord blood, or from bone marrow) seems promising.

■ **Stereotactic Neurosurgical Procedures, Deep Brain Stimulation** (for abbreviations, see p. 210)

These procedures can be used when PD becomes refractory to medical treatment. *Pallidotomy* (placement of a destructive lesion in the GPi) derives its rationale from the observed hyperactivity of this structure in PD. *Deep brain stimulation* requires bilateral placement of stimulating electrodes in the GPi or STN. High-frequency stimulation by means of a subcutaneously implanted impulse generator can improve rigor, tremor, akinesia, and dyskinesia.

■ **Genetics of PD**

A genetic predisposition for the development of PD has been postulated. Mutations in the genes for α-synuclein (AD), parkin (AR), and ubiquitin C-terminal hydrolase L1 (UCHL1; AD) have been found in pedigrees affected by the rare autosomal dominant (AD) and autosomal recessive (AR) familial forms of PD.

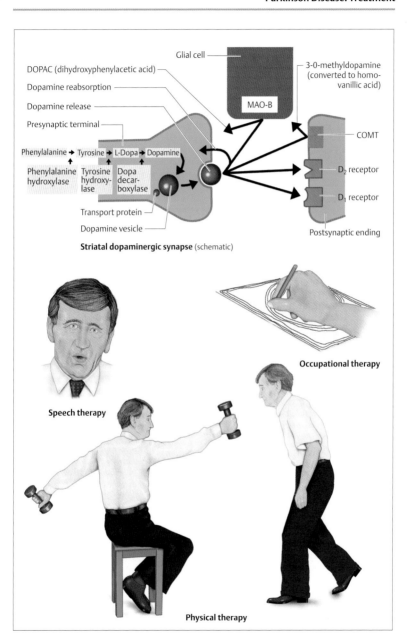

Glial cell

DOPAC (dihydroxyphenylacetic acid)

Dopamine reabsorption

Dopamine release

Presynaptic terminal

3-0-methyldopamine (converted to homo-vanillic acid)

MAO-B

COMT

Phenylalanine → Tyrosine → L-Dopa → Dopamine

Phenylalanine hydroxylase

Tyrosine hydroxy-lase

Dopa decar-boxylase

D_2 receptor

D_1 receptor

Transport protein

Dopamine vesicle

Postsynaptic ending

Striatal dopaminergic synapse (schematic)

Speech therapy

Occupational therapy

Physical therapy

Multiple sclerosis (MS) is characterized by multiple symptoms and signs of brain and spinal cord dysfunction that are disseminated in both time and space. Its pathological hallmark is inflammatory demyelination and axonal lesions; its etiology remains unknown at present despite decades of intensive investigation.

A *relapse* is the appearance of a new neurological disturbance, or the reappearance of one previously present, lasting at least 24 hours. All such disturbances arising within a one-month period are counted as a single relapse. The *relapse rate* is the number of relapses per year. Clear improvement of neurological function is termed *remission*.

The course of MS varies greatly from one individual to another, but two basic types of course can be identified: *relapsing-remitting* (66–85%; most common when onset is before age 25; well-defined relapses separated by periods of nearly complete recovery with or without residual symptoms; does not progress during remission) and *chronic progressive*. The latter can be divided into three subtypes: *primary chronic progressive* (9–37%; most common when onset is after age 40; progresses from disease onset onward); *secondary progressive* (seen in over 50% of cases 6–10 years after onset; initially remitting-relapsing, later chronically progressive; recurrences, mild remissions, and plateau phases may occur); and *progressively remitting-relapsing* (rare; complete remission may or may not occur after relapses; symptoms tend to worsen from one relapse to the next).

Clinical Manifestations

The symptoms and signs of MS reflect dysfunction of the particular areas of the nervous system involved and are not specific for this disease. Typical MS manifestations include paralysis, paresthesiae, optic neuritis (*retrobulbar neuritis*), diplopia, and bladder dysfunction.

Paresis, spasticity, fatigability. Upper-motor-neuron type paralysis of the limbs either is present at onset or develops during the course of MS. Involvement is often asymmetrical and mainly in the legs, especially in the early stage of the disease. Spasticity makes its first appearance in the form of extensor spasms; flexor spasms develop later. The latter are often painful, cause frequent falls, and, if severe and persistent, can cause flexion contractures (*paraplegia in flexion*). Many patients complain of abnormal fatigability.

Sensory manifestations. Episodic or continuous paresthesiae (sensations of tingling or numbness, tightness of the skin, heat, cold, burning, prickling) are common, particularly in the early stage of the disease, with or without other manifestations of neurological dysfunction. As the disease progresses, such positive phenomena usually recede and are replaced by sensory deficits affecting all sensory modalities. A constant or only slowly rising sensory level ("sensory transverse cord syndrome") is uncharacteristic of MS and should prompt the search for a spinal cord lesion of another kind. Many MS patients have *Lhermitte's sign* (which is actually a symptom), an electric or coldlike paresthesia traveling from the nuchal region down the spine, sometimes as far as the legs, on flexion of the neck (p. 49). If no other symptoms or signs are present, other causes should be considered (e. g., a cervical spinal cord tumor).

Pain in MS most often appears in the form of trigeminal neuralgia (p. 186), severe pain in the limbs (p. 108), tonic spasms (p. 204), or backaches, sometimes with radiation in a radicular pattern. Other painful phenomena include flexor spasms due to spasticity, contractures, and dysuria due to urinary tract infection.

Visual impairment in MS is usually due to *optic neuritis* (mostly unilateral), which also produces pain in or around the eye. The impairment begins as blurred or clouded vision and progresses to cause reading impairment and visual field defects (central scotoma or diffuse defects). *Marcus Gunn pupils* (p. 92) may be observed. Physical exercise, high ambient temperature, menstruation, or cigarette smoking can aggravate existing visual problems (*Uhthoff's phenomenon*). Optic neuritis, as an isolated finding, is not necessarily the first manifestation of MS; patients with bilateral optic neuritis have a much lower risk of developing MS than those with the unilateral form. *Diplopia* is usually due to internuclear ophthalmoplegia (p. 86). *Nystagmus* (p. 88).

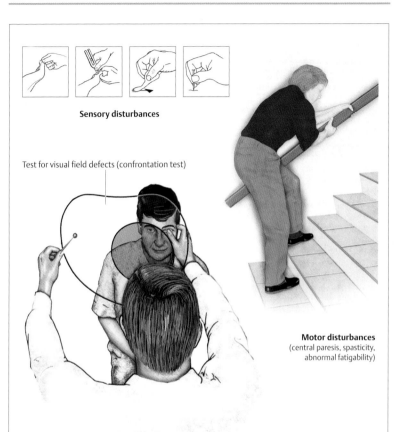

Sensory disturbances

Test for visual field defects (confrontation test)

Motor disturbances
(central paresis, spasticity,
abnormal fatigability)

Central scotoma (optic neuritis)

Atrophy

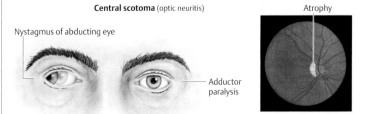

Nystagmus of abducting eye

Adductor
paralysis

Dissociated nystagmus
(internuclear ophthalmoplegia,
patient looking to right)

Temporal papillary atrophy
(after optic neuritis)

215

Incoordination. Intention tremor, dysarthria, truncal ataxia, and oculomotor dysfunction are common. Gait unsteadiness due to motor incoordination is often experienced by the patient as dizziness or lightheadedness. Acute vertigo with nausea, vomiting, and nystagmus can also occur.

Autonomic dysfunction. *Bladder dysfunction* (p. 156) frequently develops in the course of MS, causing problems such as urinary urgency, incomplete voiding, or urinary incontinence. Urinary tract infection is a not infrequent result. *Fecal incontinence* (p. 154) is rare, but constipation is common. *Sexual dysfunction* (e. g., erectile dysfunction or loss of libido) is also common and may be aggravated by spasticity or sensory deficits in the genital region. Psychological factors such as depression, insecurity, and marital conflict often play a role as well. If its cause is organic, sexual dysfunction in MS is usually accompanied by bladder dysfunction.

Behavioral changes. Mental changes (depression, marital conflict, anxiety) and cognitive deficits of variable severity can occur both as a reaction to and as a result of the disease.

Paroxysmal phenomena in MS include epileptic seizures, trigeminal neuralgia, attacks of dysarthria with ataxia, tonic spasms, episodic dysesthesiae, pain, and facial myokymia.

Differential Diagnosis

There is no single clinical test, imaging study, or laboratory finding that alone establishes the diagnosis of MS (p. 218; Table 27, p. 375). A meticulous differential diagnostic evaluation is needed in every case.

(Cerebral) Vasculitis (p. 180). Systemic lupus erythematosus, Sjögren syndrome, Behçet syndrome, granulomatous angiitis, polyarteritis nodosa, antiphospholipid syndrome, chronic inflammatory demyelinating polyradiculoneuropathy (CIDP, p. 328).

Inflammatory diseases. Neurosarcoidosis, neuroborreliosis, neurosyphilis, Whipple disease, postinfectious acute disseminated encephalomyelitis (ADEM), progressive multifocal leukoencephalopathy (PML), subacute sclerosing panencephalitis (SSPE), HIV infection, HTLV-1 infection.

Neurovascular disorders. Arteriovenous fistula of spinal dura mater, cavernoma, CADASIL (p. 172).

Hereditary/metabolic disorders. Spinocerebellar ataxias, adrenoleukodystrophy, endocrine diseases, mitochondrial encephalomyelopathy, vitamin B_{12} deficiency (funicular myelosis).

Tumors of the brain or spinal cord (e. g., lymphoma, glioma, meningioma).

Skull base anomalies. Arnold–Chiari malformation, platybasia.

Myelopathy. Cervical myelopathy (spinal stenosis).

Somatoform disturbances in the context of mental illness.

Prognosis

Favorable prognostic indicators in MS include onset before age 40, monosymptomatic onset, absence of cerebellar involvement at onset, rapid resolution of the initial symptom(s), a relapsing-remitting course, short duration of relapses, and long-term preservation of the ability to walk. A relatively favorable course is also predicted if, after the first 5 years of illness, the MRI reveals no more than a few, small lesions without rapid radiological progression and the clinical manifestations of cerebellar disease and central paresis are no more than mild. A *benign course*, defined as a low frequency of recurrences and only mild disability in the first 15 years of illness, is seen in 20–30 % of patients. The disease takes a *malignant course*, with major disability within 5 years, in fewer than 5 % of patients. Half of all MS patients have a second relapse within 2 years of disease onset.

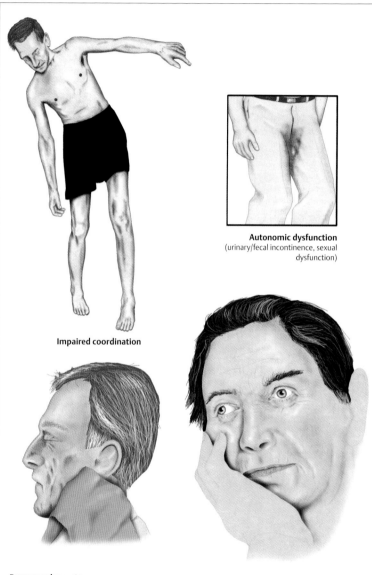

Impaired coordination

Autonomic dysfunction
(urinary/fecal incontinence, sexual dysfunction)

Paroxysmal symptoms
(trigeminal neuralgia)

Behavioral changes

Diagnosis

Patients with MS are evaluated by clinical examination, laboratory testing, neuroimaging, and neurophysiological studies. The clinical manifestations of MS and the lesions that cause them vary over the course of the disease (*dissemination in time and space*). Diagnostic classification is problematic (p. 216) if only one lesion is found (e. g., by MRI), if symptoms and signs are in only one area of the CNS (e. g., spinal cord), or if only one attack has occurred (Table 27, p 375).

■ Clinical Manifestations

Sensory deficits, upper-motor-neuron paresis, incoordination, visual impairment (field defects), nystagmus, internuclear ophthalmoplegia, and/or bladder dysfunction are common signs of MS. Complaints of pain, paresthesiae, abnormal fatigability, or episodic disturbances are often, by their nature, difficult to objectify. Clinical examination may reveal no abnormality because of the episodic nature of the disease itself.

■ Laboratory Tests and Special Studies

Evoked potentials. Visual evoked potential (VEP) studies reliably detect optic nerve lesions, but neuroimaging is better for detecting lesions of the optic tract or optic radiation. VEP reveals prolongation of the P100 latency in one eye and/or an abnormally large discrepancy between the latencies in the two eyes in roughly 40 % of MS patients without known optic neuritis, and in almost half of those with early optic neuritis. **Somatosensory evoked potential (SEP)** studies of the median or tibial nerve typically reveal prolonged latencies in MS. Low amplitude of evoked potentials, on the other hand, often indicates a pathological process of another type, e. g. tumor. SEP abnormalities are found in up to 60 % of MS patients with predominantly sensory manifestations. **Auditory evoked potential (AEP)** studies are less sensitive in MS than VEP or SEP. The most common AEP change is prolongation of latency. AEP studies are helpful for the further classification of vertigo, tinnitus, and hearing loss. **Motor evoked potential (MEP)** studies reveal prolonged central conduction times when CNS lesions involve the pyramidal pathway. The sensitivity of MEP in MS is approximately the same as that of SEP. MEP studies can provide supporting evidence for MS in patients with latent paresis, gait disturbances, abnormal reflexes, or movement disorders that are difficult to classify.

Tests of bladder function. The *residual urine volume* can be measured by ultrasound. It should not exceed 100 ml in patients with a normal bladder capacity of 400–450 ml; in general, it should normally be 15–20 % of the cystomanometrically determined bladder volume. *Urodynamic electromyography* (EMG) provides more specific data concerning bladder dysfunction.

Neuroimaging. CT may reveal other diseases that enter into the differential diagnosis of MS (e. g., brain tumor) but is insufficiently sensitive (ca. 25–50 %) to be useful in diagnosing MS itself. MRI scans reveal the characteristic foci of demyelination disseminated in the CNS (MS plaques); contrast enhancement is seen in acute but not in chronic lesions. The sensitivity of MRI for MS is greater than 90 %, but its specificity is considerably lower; thus, the MRI findings alone cannot establish the diagnosis.

CSF examination. CSF abnormalities are found in more than 95 % of MS patients. The cell count rarely exceeds 20 cells/mm³. The total protein concentration is elevated in ca. 40 % of patients, and intrathecal IgG synthesis (IgG index) in ca. 90 %. Oligoclonal IgG is found in 95 % of MS patients, and antibodies to mumps, measles and herpes zoster in 80 %.

Pathogenesis

The *early* course of MS varies among patients in accordance with the variable extent of the inflammatory lesions and disturbances of the blood–brain-barrier. The severity of *late* manifestations is correlated with the number of plaques. It is hypothesized that MS is caused by a combination of genetic (polygenic) predisposition and exogenous factors (viral or bacterial infection?) that induces an inappropriate immune response to one or more CNS autoantigens (see p. 220) that have not yet been identified.

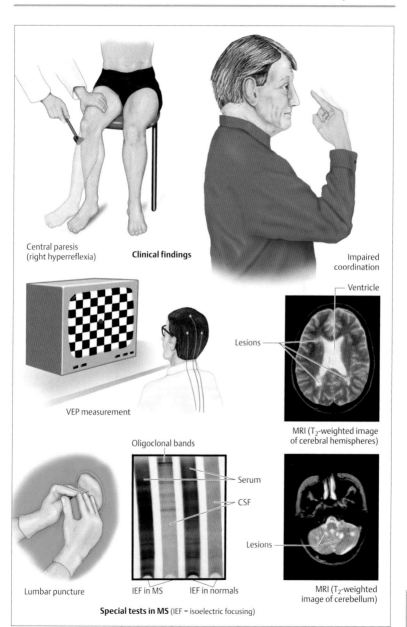

Central paresis
(right hyperreflexia)

Clinical findings

Impaired
coordination

VEP measurement

Ventricle

Lesions

MRI (T$_2$-weighted image
of cerebral hemispheres)

Oligoclonal bands

Serum

CSF

Lumbar puncture

IEF in MS   IEF in normals

Lesions

MRI (T$_2$-weighted
image of cerebellum)

Special tests in MS (IEF = isoelectric focusing)

Central Nervous System

219

Activation. Circulating autoreactive CD4+ T lymphocytes bear antigen-specific surface receptors and can cross the blood–brain barrier (BBB) when activated, e. g., by neurotropic viruses, bacterial superantigens, or cytokines. In MS, activated T lymphocytes react with MBP, PLP, MOG, and MAG. Circulating antibodies to various components of myelin can also be detected (for abbreviations, see below[1]).

Passage through the BBB. Activated lymphocytes and myelinotoxic antibodies penetrate the BBB at the venules (perivenous distribution of inflammation).

Antigen presentation and stimulation. In the CNS, antigen-presenting cells (microglia), recognition molecules (MHC class II antigens), and co-stimulatory signals (CD28, B-7.1) trigger the renewed activation and clonal proliferation of incoming CD4+ T lymphocytes into T_H1 and T_H2 cells. Proinflammatory cytokines elaborated by the T_H1 cells (IL-2, IFN-γ, TNF-α, LT)[2] induce phagocytosis by macrophages and microglia as well as the synthesis of mediators of inflammation (TNF-α, OH-, NO)[2] and complement factors. The T_H2 cells secrete cytokines (IL-4, IL-5, IL-6)[2] that activate B cells ($\Rightarrow$ myelinotoxic autoantibodies, complement activation), ultimately causing damage to myelin. The T_H2 cells also produce IL-4 and IL-10, which suppress the T_H1 cells.

Demyelination. Lesions develop in myelin sheaths (which are extensions of oligodendroglial cell membranes) and in axons when the inflammatory process outstrips the capacity of repair mechanisms.

Scar formation. The inflammatory response subsides and remyelination of damaged axons begins once the autoreactive T cells die (apoptosis), the BBB is repaired, and local anti-inflammatory mediators and cells are synthesized. Astroglia form scar tissue that takes the place of the dead cells. Axonal damage seems to be the main cause of permanent neurological deficits, as dystrophic axons apparently cannot be remyelinated.

Treatment

Relapse is treated with high-dose corticosteroids, e. g., methylprednisolone, 1 g/day for 3–5 days, which produce (unselective) immunosuppression, reduce BBB penetration by T cells, and lessen T_H1 cytokine formation. Plasmapheresis may be indicated in refractory cases.

Drugs that reduce the frequency and intensity of relapses. *Azathioprine* p.o. (immunosuppression via reduction of T cell count), interferon beta-1b and beta-1a s.c. or i.m. (cytokine modulation, alteration of T-cell activity), *glatiramer acetate* s.c. (copolymer-1; blocks/competes at binding sites for encephalitogenic peptides on MHC-II molecules), *IgG* i. v. (multiple modes of action), and *natalizumab* (selective adhesion inhibitor).

Drugs that delay secondary progression. Interferon beta-1b and beta-1a. *Mitoxantrone* suppresses B cells and decreases the CD4/CD8 ratio. *Methotrexate* and *cyclophosphamide* (different dosage schedules) delay MS progression mainly by unselective immunosuppression and reduction of the T-cell count.

Slowing of primary progression. No specific therapy is known at present.

Symptomatic therapy/rehabilitation. Medications, physical, occupational, and speech therapy, social, psychological, and dietary counseling, and mechanical aids (e. g., walking aids, wheelchair) are provided as needed. The possible benefits of oligodendrocyte precursor cell transplantation for remyelination, and of growth factors and immunoglobulins for the promotion of endogenous remyelination, are currently under investigation in both experimental and clinical studies.

[1]MBP, myelin basic protein; MOG, myelin-oligodendrocyte glycoprotein; MAG, myelin-associated glycoprotein; PLP, proteolipid protein; S100 protein, CNPase, $\alpha\beta$-crystallin, transaldolase

[2]IL, interleukin; IFN-γ, interferon-gamma; TNF-α, tumor necrosis factor-alpha; LT, lymphotoxin; OH-: hydroxyl radical; NO, nitric oxide

[3]p.o., orally; s.c., subcutaneously; i.m., intramuscularly; i. v., intravenously.

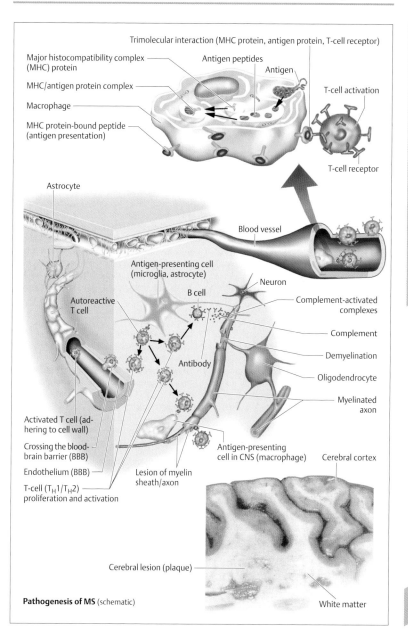

Trimolecular interaction (MHC protein, antigen protein, T-cell receptor)

Major histocompatibility complex (MHC) protein

Antigen peptides

Antigen

T-cell activation

MHC/antigen protein complex

Macrophage

MHC protein-bound peptide (antigen presentation)

T-cell receptor

Astrocyte

Blood vessel

Antigen-presenting cell (microglia, astrocyte)

Neuron

B cell

Complement-activated complexes

Autoreactive T cell

Complement

Demyelination

Antibody

Oligodendrocyte

Myelinated axon

Activated T cell (adhering to cell wall)

Crossing the blood-brain barrier (BBB)

Endothelium (BBB)

T-cell (T_H1/T_H2) proliferation and activation

Lesion of myelin sheath/axon

Antigen-presenting cell in CNS (macrophage)

Cerebral cortex

Cerebral lesion (plaque)

White matter

Pathogenesis of MS (schematic)

Syndromes

■ Localization

CNS infection may involve the leptomeninges and CSF spaces (*meningitis*), the ventricular system (*ventriculitis*), the gray and white matter of the brain (*encephalitis*), or the spinal cord (*myelitis*). A focus of bacterial infection of the brain is called a *brain abscess*, or *cerebritis* in the early stage before a frank abscess is formed. Pus located between the dura mater and the arachnoid membrane is called a *subdural empyema*, while pus outside the dura is called an *epidural abscess*.

■ Course

The clinical manifestations may be *acute* (purulent meningitis, CNS listeriosis, herpes simplex encephalitis), *subacute* (cerebral abscess, focal encephalitis, neuroborreliosis, neurosyphilis, tuberculous meningitis, actinomycosis, nocardiosis, rickettsiosis, neurobrucellosis), or *chronic* (tuberculous meningitis, neurosyphilis, neuroborreliosis, Whipple encephalitis, Creutzfeldt–Jakob disease). The epidemiological pattern of infection may be *sporadic*, *endemic* or *epidemic*, depending on the pathogen.

■ Clinical Manifestations

Meningitis and encephalitis rarely occur as entirely distinct syndromes; they usually present in mixed form (meningoencephalitis, encephalomyelitis). CSF examination establishes the diagnosis.

These disorders may present in specific ways in certain patient groups. *Neonates and children* commonly manifest failure to thrive, fever or hypothermia, restlessness, breathing problems, epileptic seizures, and a bulging fontanelle. *The elderly* may lack fever but frequently have behavioral abnormalities, confusion, epileptic seizures, generalized weakness, and impairment of consciousness ranging to coma. *Immunodeficient patients* commonly have fever, headache, stiff neck, and drowsiness in addition to the manifestations of their primary illness.

Meningitic syndrome is characterized by fever, severe, intractable headache and backache, photophobia and phonophobia, nausea, vomiting, impairment of consciousness, stiff neck, and hyperextended posture, with opisthotonus or neck pain on flexion. *Kernig's sign* (resistance to passive raising of leg with extended knee) and *Brudzinski's sign* (involuntary leg flexion on passive flexion of the neck) are signs of meningeal involvement. Painful neck stiffness is due to (lepto)meningeal irritation by infectious meningitis, septicemia, subarachnoid hemorrhage, neoplastic meningitis, or other causes. Isolated neck stiffness not caused by meningitis (*meningism*) may be due to cervical disorders such as arthrosis, fracture, intervertebral disk herniation, tumor, or extrapyramidal rigidity. Papilledema is usually absent; when present, it indicates intracranial hypertension (p. 158).

Encephalitic syndrome is characterized by headache and fever, sometimes accompanied by epileptic seizures (often focal), focal signs (cranial nerves deficits, especially of CN III, IV, VI, and VII; aphasia, hemiparesis, hemianopsia, ataxia, choreoathetosis), behavioral changes, and impairment of consciousness (restlessness, irritability, confusion, lethargy, drowsiness, coma). The neurological signs may be preceded by limb pain (myalgia, arthralgia), a slight increase in body temperature, and malaise. For *acute cerebellitis* (⇨ ataxia), see p. 276. *Brain stem encephalitis* produces ophthalmoplegia, facial paresis, dysarthria, dysphagia, ataxia, and hearing loss.

Myelitic syndrome. Myelitis presents with severe local pain, paraparesis, paresthesiae, or some combination of these. Incomplete or complete paraplegia or quadriplegia (p. 48) develops within a few hours (acute) or days (subacute). The differential diagnosis may be difficult.

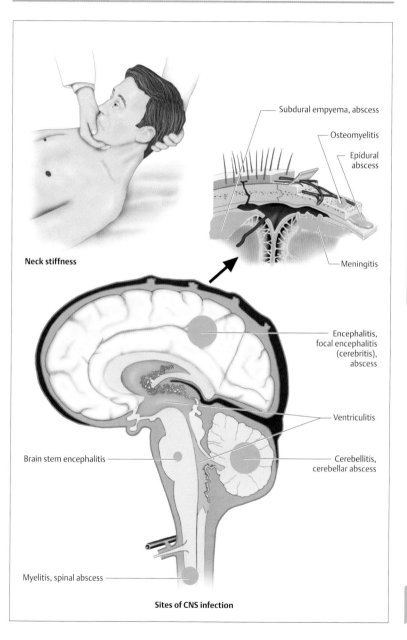

Neck stiffness

Subdural empyema, abscess

Osteomyelitis

Epidural abscess

Meningitis

Encephalitis, focal encephalitis (cerebritis), abscess

Ventriculitis

Brain stem encephalitis

Cerebellitis, cerebellar abscess

Myelitis, spinal abscess

Sites of CNS infection

Central Nervous System

Pathogenesis

Pathogens usually reach the CNS by local extension from a nearby infectious focus (e. g. sinusitis, mastoiditis) or by hematogenous spread from a distant focus. The ability of pathogens to spread by way of the bloodstream depends on their virulence and on the immune status of the host. They use special mechanisms to cross or circumvent the *blood–brain barrier* (p. 8). Some pathogens enter the CNS by centripetal travel along peripheral nerves (herpes simplex virus type I, varicella-zoster virus, rabies virus), others by endocytosis (*Neisseria meningitidis*), intracellular transport (*Plasmodium falciparum* via erythrocytes, *Toxoplasma gondii* via macrophages), or intracellular invasion (*Haemophilus influenzae*). Those that enter the *subarachnoid space* probably do so by way of the choroid plexus, venous sinuses, or cribriform plate (p. 76). Having entered the CSF spaces, pathogens trigger an *inflammatory response* characterized by the release of complement factors and cytokines, the influx of leukocytes and macrophages, and the activation of microglia and astrocytes. Disruption of the blood–brain barrier results in an influx of fluids and proteins across the vascular endothelium and into the CNS, causing vasogenic cerebral edema (p. 162), which is accompanied by both cytotoxic cellular edema and interstitial edema due to impaired CSF circulation. Cerebral edema causes *intracranial hypertension*. These processes, in conjunction with vasculitis, impairment of vascular autoregulatory mechanisms, and/or fluctuations of systemic blood pressure, lead to the development of ischemic, metabolic, and hypoxic cerebral lesions (focal necrosis, territorial infarction).

Treatment (Table 28, p. 375)

The immune system is generally no longer able to hold pathogens in check once they have spread to the CNS, as the immune response in the subarachnoid space and the neural tissue itself is less effective than elsewhere in the body. Having gained access to the CNS, pathogens meet with favorable conditions for further spread within it.

Prophylaxis. The occurrence and spread of CNS infection can be prevented by *mandatory reporting* (as specified by local law), *prevention of exposure* (isolation of sources of infection, disinfection, sterilization), and *prophylaxis in persons at risk* (active and passive immunization, chemoprophylaxis).

Treatment. Patients with bacterial or viral meningoencephalitis must be treated at once. The treatment strategy is initially based on the clinical and additional findings. Antimicrobial therapy is first given empirically in a broad-spectrum combination, then specifically tailored in accordance with the species and drug sensitivity pattern of the pathogen(s) identified. Causative organisms may be found in the CSF, blood, or other bodily fluids (e. g., throat smear, urine or stool samples, bronchial secretions, gastric juice, abscess aspirate).

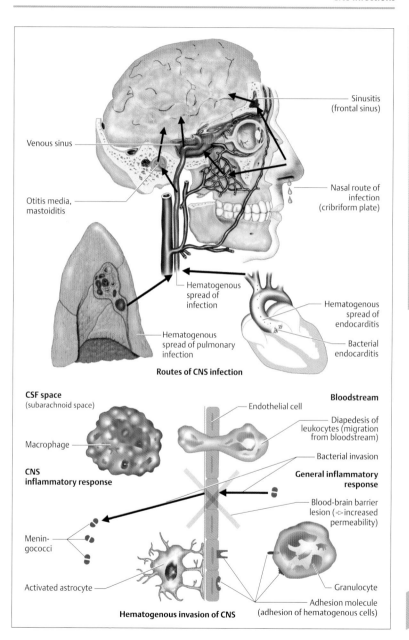

Routes of CNS infection

CSF space
(subarachnoid space)

Macrophage

CNS
inflammatory response

Meningococci

Activated astrocyte

Bloodstream

Endothelial cell

Diapedesis of leukocytes (migration from bloodstream)

Bacterial invasion

General inflammatory response

Blood-brain barrier lesion (⇨increased permeability)

Granulocyte

Adhesion molecule (adhesion of hematogenous cells)

Hematogenous invasion of CNS

Sinusitis (frontal sinus)

Venous sinus

Otitis media, mastoiditis

Nasal route of infection (cribriform plate)

Hematogenous spread of infection

Hematogenous spread of endocarditis

Bacterial endocarditis

Hematogenous spread of pulmonary infection

Bacterial Infections

■ Meningitis/Meningoencephalitis

For an overview of the most common pathogens, cf. Table 29 (p 376). *Immune prophylaxis:* Vaccines are available against *Haemophilus influenzae* type B infection (for infants, small children, and children over 6 years of age at increased risk), *Pneumococcus* (children over 2 years of age and adults with risk factors such as immunosuppression or asplenia), and *meningococcus* (travel to endemic regions, local outbreaks). *Chemoprophylaxis* is indicated for close contacts of persons infected with *Haemophilus influenzae* (rifampicin) or meningococcus (rifampicin, ciprofloxacin, or ceftriaxone).

■ Brain Abscess

Brain abscess begins as local cerebritis and is then transformed into an encapsulated region of purulent necrosis with perifocal edema. The pathogenic organisms may reach the brain by *local* or *hematogenous spread* (mastoiditis, otitis media, sinusitis, osteomyelitis; endocarditis, pneumonia, tooth infection, osteomyelitis, diverticulitis), or by *direct* inoculation (trauma, neurosurgery). The clinical manifestations include headache, nausea, vomiting, fever, impairment of consciousness, and focal or generalized epileptic seizures, neck stiffness, and focal neurological signs. The *diagnosis* is made by MRI and/or CT (which should include bone windows, as the infection may have originated in bony structures) and confirmed by culture of the pathogenic organism.

■ Bacterial Vasculitis (p. 180)

Arteries. Vessel wall inflammation in association with sepsis. Bacterial endocarditis causes cerebral abscess formation or infarction by way of infectious thromboembolism (⇨ focal inflammatory changes in the cerebral parenchyma ⇨ metastatic or embolic focal encephalitis). The syndrome is characterized by headache, fever, epileptic seizures, and behavioral changes in addition to focal neurological signs. *Meningoencephalitis* may cause arteritis by direct involvement of the vessels. Embolization of infectious material may lead to the development of *septic* ("mycotic") *aneurysms*.

Veins. Bacterial *thrombophlebitis* of the cerebral veins or venous sinuses may arise as a complication of meningitis or by local spread of infection from neighboring structures.

■ Ventriculitis

Infection of the ventricular system (perhaps in connection with an intraventricular catheter for internal or external CSF drainage). The clinical findings are often nonspecific (somnolence, impairment of concentration and memory). Abdominal complaints (peritonitis) may predominate if the infection has spread down a ventriculoperitoneal shunt to the abdomen. *Diagnosis:* CSF examination and culture.

■ Septic Encephalopathy

Bacteremia leads to the release of endotoxins, which, in turn, impair cerebral function. Septic encephalopathy can produce findings suggestive of meningoencephalitis such as impairment of consciousness, epileptic seizures, paresis, and meningismus, despite the absence of CSF inflammatory changes and a sterile CSF culture. *Diagnosis:* EEG changes consistent with the diagnosis (general changes, triphasic complexes, burst suppression) in the setting of known systemic sepsis with sterile CSF. CT and MRI are normal.

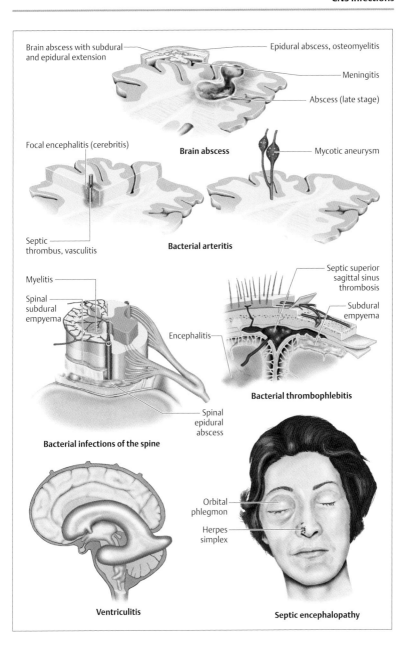

Brain abscess with subdural and epidural extension

Epidural abscess, osteomyelitis

Meningitis

Abscess (late stage)

Focal encephalitis (cerebritis)

Brain abscess

Mycotic aneurysm

Septic thrombus, vasculitis

Bacterial arteritis

Myelitis

Spinal subdural empyema

Encephalitis

Septic superior sagittal sinus thrombosis

Subdural empyema

Bacterial thrombophlebitis

Spinal epidural abscess

Bacterial infections of the spine

Orbital phlegmon

Herpes simplex

Ventriculitis

Septic encephalopathy

■ Lyme Disease (Neuroborreliosis)

Pathogenesis. The spirochete *Borrelia burgdorferi* sensu lato (Europe: *B. garinii*, *B. afzelii*; North America: *B. burgdorferi* sensu stricto) is transmitted to man by ticks (Europe: *Ixodes ricinus*; North America: *Ixodes pacificus*, *I. scapularis*). The probability of infection is low unless the infected tick remains attached to the skin for at least 24–48 hours. Only 1–2% of individuals bitten by ticks become infected. The incubation time ranges from 3–30 days. The disease occurs in three stages, as described below.

Clinical manifestations. *Stage I (localized infection).* Up to 90% of all patients develop a painless, erythematous macule or papule that gradually spreads outward from the site of the tick bite in a ringlike or homogeneous fashion (*erythema chronicum migrans*). This is commonly accompanied by symptoms due to hematogenous spread of the pathogen, such as fever, fatigue, arthralgia, myalgia, or other types of pain, which may be the chief complaint, rather than the skin rash. Regional or generalized lymphadenopathy (*lymphadenosis benigna cutis*) is a less common presentation. All of these findings may resolve spontaneously.

Stage II (disseminated infection). Generalized symptoms such as fatigue, anorexia, muscle and joint pain, and headache develop in 10–15% of patients within ca. 3–6 weeks, sometimes accompanied by mild fever and neck stiffness. *Cardiac manifestations:* Myocarditis or pericarditis with AV block. *Neurological manifestations:* Cranial nerve palsies, painful polyradiculitis and lymphocytic meningitis (*Bannwarth syndrome*, meningopolyneuritis) are commonly seen in combination. One or more cranial nerves may be affected; the most common finding is unilateral or bilateral facial palsy of peripheral type. Neuroborreliosis-related *polyradiculoneuropathy* (which may be mistaken for lumbar disk herniation) is characterized by intense pain in a radicular distribution, most severe at night, with accompanying neurological deficits (motor, sensory, and reflex abnormalities, focal muscle atrophy). Borrelia-related *meningitis* (Lyme meningitis) usually causes alternating headache and neck pain, but the headache is mild or absent in some cases. It may be worst at certain times of day. CSF studies reveal a mononuclear pleocytosis with a high plasma cell count and an elevated protein concentration, while the glucose concentration is normal. *Encephalitis* occurs relatively rarely and may cause focal neurological deficits as well as behavioral changes (impaired concentration, personality changes, depression). MRI reveals cerebral white-matter lesions, and the CSF findings are consistent with meningitis. *Myelitis*, when it occurs, often affects the spinal cord at the level of a radicular lesion.

Stage III (persistent infection). The latency from clinical presentation to the onset of stage III disease varies from 1 to 17 years (chronic Lyme neuroborreliosis). Few patients ever reach this stage, characterized by neurological deficits such as ataxia, cranial nerve palsies, paraparesis or quadriparesis, and bladder dysfunction (*Lyme encephalomyelitis*). *Encephalopathy* causing impairment of concentration and memory, insomnia, fatigue, personality changes, and depression has also been described. *Myositis* and *cerebral vasculitis* may also occur. In stage III of Lyme disease, *acrodermatitis chronica atrophicans* of the extensor surface of the limbs may be seen along with a type of polyneuropathy specific to *Borrelia afzelii*.

Diagnosis. Many patients have no memory of a tick bite. The diagnosis of Lyme disease is based on the presence of erythema chronicum migrans, the immunological confirmation of *Borrelia* infection (e. g., by ELISA, indirect immunofluorescence assay, Western blot, or specific IgG antibody–CSF-serum index) and/or the identification of the causative organism (e. g., by culture, histology, or polymerase chain reaction). By definition, the diagnosis also requires the presence of lymphocytic meningitis (with or without cranial nerve involvement or painful polyradiculoneuritis), encephalomyelitis, or encephalopathy.

Treatment. *Local symptoms:* Antibiotic such as doxycycline or amoxicillin (p.o.) for 3 weeks. *Neuroborreliosis:* Ceftriaxone or cefotaxime (i. v.) for 2–3 weeks. A vaccine has been approved for use in the United States, and another is being developed for use in Europe.

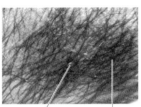

Tick — Erythema (thigh)

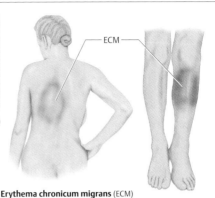

ECM

Erythema chronicum migrans (ECM)

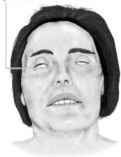

Lagophthalmos

Facial paresis (bilateral)

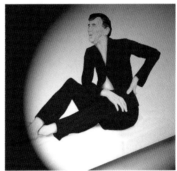

Radicular pain

Stage I	Stage II	Stage III
• Erythema chronicum migrans • General symptoms	• General symptoms • Bannwarth syndrome • Meningitis • Encephalitis • Carditis • Myelitis	• Encephalomyelitis • Encephalopathy • Myositis • Cerebral vasculitis • Acrodermatitis chronica atrophicans • Polyneuritis

Days........................Weeks..................Months................Years............

↑
Infection   **Stages of Lyme disease**

■ Neurosyphilis

Pathogenesis. Syphilis is caused by the spirochete (bacterium) *Treponema pallidum* (TP) ssp. *pallidum* and is transmitted by direct exposure to infected lesions, usually on the skin or mucous membranes, during sexual contact. Other routes of transmission, such as the sharing of needles by intravenous drug users, are much less common. The disease has three clinical stages. In the *primary and secondary stages*, nonspecific tests (VDRL and RPR) and specific tests (TPHA, FTA-ABS, and 19S-(IgM-)FTA-ABS tests) yield positive results. *Tertiary stage (currently rare):* After an asymptomatic period of a few months to years (*latent syphilis*), organ manifestations develop, such as gummata (skin, bone, kidney, liver) and cardiovascular lesions (aortic aneurysm). The first year of the tertiary stage is designated the *early latency* period and is characterized by a high likelihood of recurrence and, thus, recurrent infectivity.

Clinical manifestations. TP may invade the nervous system at any stage of syphilis without necessarily producing signs or symptoms.

Early meningitis. A variably severe meningitic syndrome may be accompanied by deficits of CN VIII (sudden hearing loss), VII (facial palsy), or II (visual impairment). Meningopolyradiculitis is rare. CSF examination reveals lymphocytic pleocytosis (up to 400 cells/µl) and an elevated protein concentration. Meningitis resolves spontaneously, but late complications may occur. *Asymptomatic meningitis* (CSF changes in the absence of a meningitic syndrome) occurs in 20–30 % of all infected persons.

Meningovascular neurosyphilis. Fluctuating symptoms such as headache, visual disturbances, and vertigo occur 5–12 years after the initial infection. Vasculitis (*von Heubner angiitis*) causes stroke, particularly in the territory of the middle cerebral artery, and may also affect small perforating vessels as well as cranial nerves (VIII, VII, V). Hydrocephalus, personality changes, epileptic seizures, and spinal cord signs (paraparesis, bladder dysfunction, anterior cord syndrome) round out the kaleidoscopic clinical picture. Gummata are rarely seen. CT and MRI findings suggest the diagnosis, and CSF examination reveals a mononuclear pleocytosis (up to 100 cells/µl), elevated protein concentra-

tion, elevated oligoclonal IgG, and VDRL positivity (up to 80 %).

Progressive paralysis. Chronic meningoencephalitis with progressive paralysis occurs 10–25 years after the initial infection. The "preparalytic" stage, characterized by personality changes and mild impairment of concentration and memory, later evolves into the "paralytic" stage, characterized by more severe cognitive changes, dysarthria, dysphasia, tremor (mimic tremor), apraxia, gait impairment, urinary incontinence, and abnormal pupillary reflexes (roughly 25 % of patients have *Argyll–Robertson pupils*, p. 92). The CSF findings resemble those of meningovascular syphilis.

Tabes dorsalis. This late meningovascular complication (25–30 years after the initial infection) produces *ocular manifestations* (Argyll–Robertson pupils, strabismus, papillary atrophy), *pain* (lightning pains = lancinating pain mainly in the legs; colicky abdominal pain), *gait impairment* (due to loss of acrognosis and proprioception), and *autonomic dysfunction* (impotence, urinary dysfunction). *Joint deformities* (Charcot joints) in the lower limbs are occasionally seen. The CSF cell count is relatively low, as in meningovascular syphilis.

Antibiotic therapy. The efficacy of treatment depends on the stage of disease in which it is instituted (the earlier, the better). Penicillin is the agent of choice.

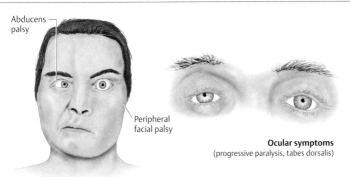

Abducens palsy

Peripheral facial palsy

Early meningitis (cranial nerve dysfunction)

Ocular symptoms
(progressive paralysis, tabes dorsalis)

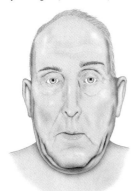

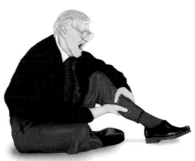

Tabes dorsalis (lancinating pain)

Progressive paralysis (behavioral changes)

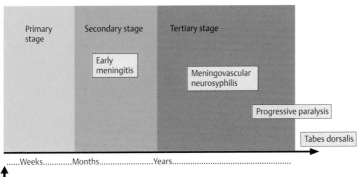

Primary stage	Secondary stage	Tertiary stage
	Early meningitis	
		Meningovascular neurosyphilis
		Progressive paralysis
		Tabes dorsalis

......Weeks............Months......................Years..

Infection   **Development of symptoms of neurosyphilis** (no fixed time course)

■ Tuberculous Meningitis

Pathogenesis. *Mycobacterium tuberculosis* transmission in man is usually by transfer of droplets from and to the respiratory tract (rarely orally or through skin lesions). The pathogen replicates in the lungs (*primary infection*), either in the lung tissue itself or within alveolar macrophages. Macrophages can only destroy tubercle bacilli after they have been activated by T cells; the course of the infection thus depends on the state of the immune system, i.e., on the ability of activated macrophages to hold the bacilli in check. The stage of primary infection lasts 2–4 weeks, is not necessarily symptomatic (if it is, then with nonspecific symptoms such as fever, anorexia, and lethargy), and cannot be detected by immune tests performed on the skin. The inflammatory process may also involve the regional (hilar) lymph nodes (*primary complex*). Calcified foci in the primary complex are easily seen on plain radiographs of the chest. The bacilli may remain dormant for years or may be reactivated when the patient's immune defenses are lowered by HIV infection, alcoholism, diabetes mellitus, corticosteroid therapy, or other factors (*reactivated tuberculosis*). Spread from the primary focus to other organs (*organ tuberculosis*) can occur during primary infection in immunocompromised patients, but only after reactivation in other patients. The bacilli presumably reach the CNS by hematogenous dissemination; local extension to the CNS from tuberculous bone (spinal cord, base of skull) is rare.

Symptoms and signs. The type and focus of CNS involvement (*neurotuberculosis*) vary, depending mainly on the age and immune status of the host.

Tuberculous meningoencephalitis. The prodromal stage lasts 2–3 weeks and is characterized by behavioral changes (apathy, depression, irritability, confusion, delirium, lack of concentration), anorexia, weight loss, malaise, nausea, and fever. Headache and neck stiffness reflect *meningeal involvement*. Finally, *cerebral involvement* manifests itself in *focal signs* (deficits of CN II, III, VI, VII, and VIII; aphasia, apraxia, central paresis, focal epileptic seizures, SIADH) and/or *general signs* (signs of intracranial hypertension, hydrocephalus). The focal signs are caused by leptomeningeal adhesions, cerebral ischemia due to vasculitis, or mass lesions (tuberculoma). *Chronic meningitis* most likely reflects inadequate treatment, or resistance of the pathogen, rather than being a distinct form of the disease. *Diagnosis:* CSF examination for initial diagnosis and monitoring of disease course. The diagnosis of tuberculous meningitis can only be confirmed by detection of mycobacteria in the CSF with direct microscopic visualization, culture, or molecular biological techniques. As the prognosis of untreated tuberculous meningitis is poor, treatment for presumed disease should be initiated as soon as the diagnosis is suspected from the clinical examination and CSF findings; the latter typically include high concentrations of protein (several grams/liter) and lactate, a low glucose concentration ($< 50\%$ of blood glucose), a high cell count (over several hundred), and a mixed pleocytosis (lymphocytes, monocytes, granulocytes).

Tuberculoma is a tumorlike mass with a caseous or calcified core surrounded by granulation tissue (giant cells, lymphocytes). Tuberculomas may be solitary or multiple and are to be differentiated from tuberculous abscesses, which are full of mycobacteria and lack the surrounding granulation tissue. *Diagnosis:* CT or MRI.

Spinal tuberculosis. Transverse spinal cord syndrome can arise because of tuberculous myelomeningoradiculitis, epidural tuberculous abscess associated with tuberculous spondylitis/discitis, or tuberculoma. *Diagnosis:* MRI.

Antibiotic treatment. One treatment protocol specifies a combination of isoniazid (with vitamin B$_6$), rifampicin (initially i.v., then p.o.), and pyrazinamide (p.o.). After 3 months, pyrazinamide is discontinued, and treatment with isoniazid and rifampicin is continued for a further 6–9 months. The treatment for HIV-positive patients includes up to five different antibiotics.

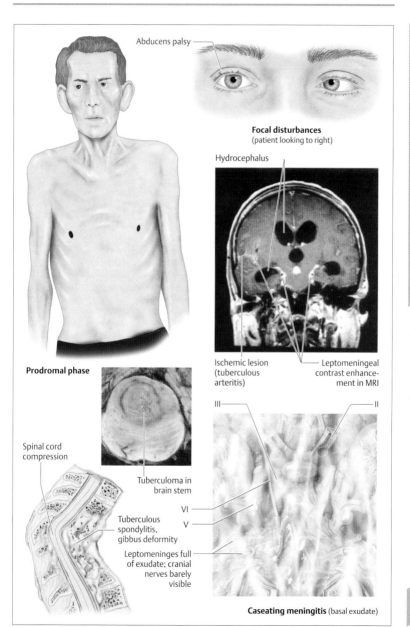

Abducens palsy

Focal disturbances
(patient looking to right)

Hydrocephalus

Ischemic lesion
(tuberculous
arteritis)

Leptomeningeal
contrast enhance-
ment in MRI

Prodromal phase

Spinal cord
compression

Tuberculoma in
brain stem

Tuberculous
spondylitis,
gibbus deformity

Leptomeninges full
of exudate; cranial
nerves barely
visible

III

II

VI

V

Caseating meningitis (basal exudate)

233

Viral Infections

■ Viral Meningoencephalitis

Aseptic meningitis is characterized by a meningitic syndrome (p. 222) that arises acutely and takes a benign course over the ensuing 1 or 2 weeks, in the absence of signs of generalized or local infection (otitis media, craniospinal abscess, sinusitis). *CSF findings:* A mild granulocytic pleocytosis is seen in the first 48 hours and is then transformed into a mild lymphomonocytic pleocytosis which can persist as long as 2 months after the clinical findings have regressed. The CSF protein and lactate concentrations are normal or only slightly elevated, while the CSF glucose concentration is normal or mildly decreased. The term "viral meningitis" is often used synonymously with aseptic meningitis, though, strictly speaking, the clinical picture of aseptic meningitis can also be produced by fungal, parasitic, or even bacterial infection (e. g., mycobacteria, mycoplasma, *Brucella*, spirochetes, *Listeria*, rickettsiae, incompletely treated bacterial meningitis). Aseptic meningitis may be *postinfectious* (HIV, rubella, measles, zoster) or *postvaccinial* or a sequela of *sarcoidosis, Behçet disease, Vogt–Koyanagi–Harada syndrome, Mollaret meningitis, connective tissue diseases*, and other, *noninflammatory disorders* (meningeal carcinomatosis, contrast agents, medications, subarachnoid hemorrhage, lead poisoning).

Pathogens. Their seasonal peak frequency is shown in the following table.

Viral meningitis. Frontal or retro-orbital headache, fever, and low-grade neck stiffness usually begin acutely and last for 1–2 weeks. The CSF findings are those of aseptic meningitis, described above; the IgG index or oligoclonal IgG may be elevated.

Viral encephalitis. The meninges are usually involved concomitantly (meningoencephalitis). Acute encephalitis mainly affects the gray matter and perivascular areas of the brain. Behavioral changes, psychomotor agitation, and focal epileptic seizures may be the leading symptoms (p. 192). The CSF findings are generally as listed above for aseptic meningitis, though pleocytosis may be absent at first. Diffuse and focal EEG changes are usually seen. CT and MRI often reveal pathological changes.

Acute demyelinating encephalomyelitis (ADEM) predominantly affects perivenous regions and the cerebral white matter (*leukoencephalitis*). The disease takes a variable course (a monophasic course with complete resolution is among the possibilities). ADEM can occur during or after a bout of infectious disease (measles, chickenpox, rubella, influenza) or after a vaccination (smallpox, measles, mumps, polio). Both encephalitic and myelitic syndromes can occur (spastic paraparesis or quadriparesis). The white-matter lesions are demonstrated best by MRI, less well by CT.

Summer, Early Spring	Autumn, Winter	Winter, Spring	All Year Round
Arboviruses, enteroviruses	Lymphocytic choriomeningitis virus	Mumps	HIV, herpes simplex virus, cytomegalovirus

The viral pathogens that most commonly cause meningitis differ from those most commonly causing encephalitis and myelitis (cf. Table 30, p. 376).

Identification of pathogen: Serologic tests or isolation of the virus from *throat smears* (poliovirus, coxsackievirus, mumps virus; ade-

novirus, HSV type 1), *stool samples* (coxsackievirus, polio virus), *CSF* (coxsackievirus, mumps, adenovirus, arbovirus, rabies, VZV, LCMV, HSV type 2), *blood* (arbovirus, EBV, LCMV, CMV, HSV type 2), *urine* (mumps, CMV), or *saliva* (mumps, rabies).

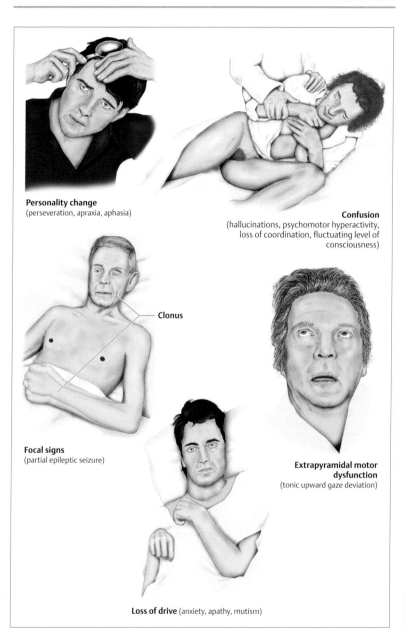

Personality change
(perseveration, apraxia, aphasia)

Confusion
(hallucinations, psychomotor hyperactivity,
loss of coordination, fluctuating level of
consciousness)

Clonus

Focal signs
(partial epileptic seizure)

**Extrapyramidal motor
dysfunction**
(tonic upward gaze deviation)

Loss of drive (anxiety, apathy, mutism)

Central Nervous System

235

■ Herpes Simplex Virus Infection

Pathogenesis. *Herpes simplex virus type 1* (HSV-1) is usually transmitted in childhood through lesions of the oral mucosa (gingival stomatitis, pharyngitis). The virus travels centripetally by way of nerve processes toward the sensory ganglia (e. g., the trigeminal ganglion), where it remains dormant for a variable period of time until reactivated by a trigger such as ultraviolet radiation, dental procedures, immunosuppression, or a febrile illness. It then travels centrifugally, again over nerve processes, back to the periphery, producing blisterlike vesicles (herpes labialis). HSV-1 also causes eye infection (keratoconjunctivitis), as well as (meningo)encephalitis when it spreads via CN I and leptomeningeal fibers of CN V. There is no association between herpes labialis and HSV-1 encephalitis. *Herpes simplex virus type 2* (HSV-2) reaches the lumbosacral ganglia by axonal transport from a site of (asymptomatic) urogenital infection. Its reactivation causes genital herpes. In adults, HSV-2 infection can cause (aseptic) *meningitis* and, occasionally, *polyradiculitis* or *myelitis*. HSV-2 virus can be transmitted to the newborn during the birth process, causing encephalitis. HSV-1 encephalitis is very rare in neonates, and HSV-2 encephalitis is very rare in adults.

Symptoms and signs. *Herpes simplex encephalitis* (HSE) in adults begins with local inflammation of the caudal and medial parts of the frontal and temporal lobes. Uncharacteristic prodromal signs such as fever, headache, nausea, anorexia, and lethargy last a few days at the most. Focal symptoms including olfactory and gustatory hallucinations, aphasia, and behavioral disturbances (confusion, psychosis) then appear, along with focal or complex partial seizures with secondary generalization. There is usually repeated seizure activity, but status epilepticus is rare. Intracranial hypertension causes impairment of consciousness or coma within a few hours. In neonates, the inflammation spreads throughout the CNS.

The diagnosis of HSE can be difficult, especially at first. The *clinical findings* include neck stiffness, hemiparesis, and mental disturbances. *CSF examination* reveals a lymphomonocytic pleocytosis (granulocytes may predominate initially) with an elevated protein concentration;

low glucose and high lactate concentrations are only rarely found. Xanthochromia and erythrocytes may be present (hemorrhagic necrotizing encephalitis). In the first 3 weeks, the virus can almost always be detected in the CSF by polymerase chain reaction; brain biopsy is only rarely needed for identification of the viral pathogen. Lumbar puncture carries a risk if intracranial hypertension is present (p. 162). EEG reveals periodic high-voltage sharp waves and 2–3 Hz slow wave complexes as a focal or diffuse finding in one or both temporal lobes. In the acute stage of HSE, CT is normal or reveals only mild temporobasal hypointensity without contrast enhancement. Hemorrhage may appear as a hyperdense area. Sharply defined areas of hypodensity appear on CT only in the later stages of HSE. T2-weighted MRI, however, already reveals inflammatory lesions in early HSE. Thus, MRI is used for early diagnosis, CT for the monitoring of encephalitic foci and cerebral edema over the course of the disease.

Meningitis. The clinical manifestations are those of aseptic meningitis (p. 234).

Myelitis. Low back pain, fever, sensory deficit with spinal level, flaccid or spastic paraparesis, bladder and bowel dysfunction. These manifestations usually regress within 2 weeks.

Radiculitis. Inflammation of the lumbosacral nerve roots produces a sensory deficit and bladder and bowel dysfunction.

Virustatic agents. HSV infection of the CNS is treated with acyclovir 10 mg/kg (i. v.) q8h for 14–21 days. Particularly in HSE, it is important to begin treatment as soon as possible.

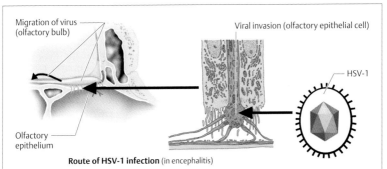

Migration of virus (olfactory bulb)

Viral invasion (olfactory epithelial cell)

HSV-1

Olfactory epithelium

Route of HSV-1 infection (in encephalitis)

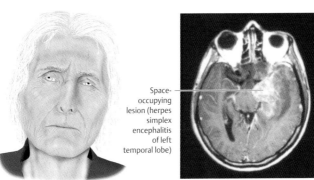

Prodromal signs, behavioral changes

Space-occupying lesion (herpes simplex encephalitis of left temporal lobe)

MRI (contrast-enhanced T_1-weighted image)

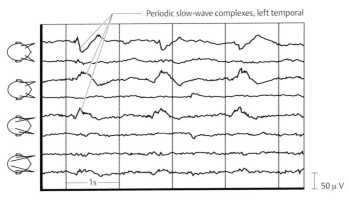

Periodic slow-wave complexes, left temporal

1 s

50 μV

EEG

Central Nervous System

■ Varicella-Zoster Virus Infection

Pathogenesis. In children, *primary infection* with varicella-zoster virus (VZV) usually causes chickenpox (varicella). The portals of entry for infection by droplets or mucus are the conjunctiva, oropharynx, and upper respiratory tract. The virions replicate locally, then enter cells of the reticulohistiocytic system by hematogenous and lymphatic spread (primary viremia). There, they replicate again and disseminate (secondary viremia). VZV infection is followed by immunity. VZV travels by centripetal axonal transport through the sensory nerve fibers of the skin and mucous membranes to the spinal and cranial ganglia and may remain latent there for years (*ganglionic latency phase*). The thoracic and trigeminal nerve ganglia are most commonly affected, but those of CN VII, IX, and X can also be involved. Spontaneous *viral reactivation* in the ganglia (ganglionitis) is most common in the elderly, diabetics, and immunocompromised persons (HIV, lymphoma, radiotherapy, chemotherapy, etc.). The reactivated virus travels over the axons centrifugally to the dermatome corresponding to its ganglion of origin, producing the typical dermatomal rash of herpes zoster. It may also spread to the CNS via the spinal dorsal roots (radiculitis), causing herpes zoster myelitis or meningoencephalitis. VZV attacks cerebral blood vessels by way of axonal transport from the trigeminal ganglion. Postherpetic neuralgia is thought to be due to disordered nociceptive processing in both peripheral and central structures.

Symptoms and signs. *Chickenpox:* After an incubation period of 14–21 days, crops of itchy efflorescent lesions appear, which progress through the sequence macule, papule, vesicle, scab within a few hours. The scabs detach in 1–2 weeks. *Immunocompromised patients* can develop severe hemorrhagic myelitis, pneumonia, encephalitis, or hepatitis. *Acute cerebellitis* in children causes appendicular, postural, and gait ataxia, less commonly dysarthria and nystagmus. CSF examination reveals mild pleocytosis and elevation of the protein concentration, or is normal, and the MRI is usually normal. VZV cerebellitis resolves slowly in most cases. *Herpes zoster* begins with general symptoms (lethargy, fever) followed by pain, itching, burning or tingling in the affected dermatome(s), which are most commonly thoracic or craniocervical (special forms: *herpes zoster ophthalmicus*, *oticus*, and *occipitocollaris*). Within a few days, groups of distended vesicles containing clear fluid appear on an erythematous base within the affected dermatome. The contents of the vesicles become turbid and yellowish in 2–3 days. The rash dries, becomes encrusted, and heals in another 5–10 days. The pain and dysesthesia of herpes zoster generally last no longer than 4 weeks. They may also occur without a rash (*herpes zoster sine herpete*).

Complications. Elderly and immunocompromised persons are at increased risk for complications. Pain that persists more than 4 weeks after the cutaneous manifestations have healed is called *postherpetic neuralgia* and is most common in the cranial and thoracic dermatomes. *Cranial nerve involvement* may cause unilateral or bilateral ocular complications (ophthalmoplegia, keratoconjunctivitis, visual impairment) or Ramsay–Hunt syndrome (facial palsy, hearing loss, tinnitus, vertigo). Other cranial nerves (IX, X, XII) are rarely affected. Further complications include Guillain–Barré syndrome, myelitis, segmental muscular paresis/atrophy, myositis, meningitis, ventriculitis, encephalitis, autonomic disturbances (anhidrosis, complex regional pain syndrome), generalized herpes zoster, and vasculitis (ICA and its branches, basilar artery). The viral pathogen is detected in CSF with the polymerase chain reaction.

Virustatic therapy. *Acyclovir:* 5 mg/kg i. v. q8h or 800 mg p.o. 5 times daily; *brivudine:* 125 mg p.o. 4 times daily; *famciclovir:* 250 mg p.o. 3 times dialy; or *valacyclovir:* 1 g p.o. 3 times daily. Treatment is continued for 5–7 days. These agents are only effective during the viral replication phase. Intrathecal administration of methylprednisolone is effective in postherpetic neuralgia.

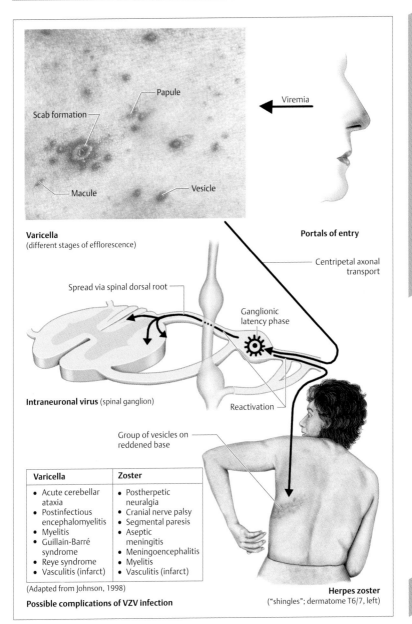

Papule

Viremia

Scab formation

Macule

Vesicle

Varicella
(different stages of efflorescence)

Portals of entry

Centripetal axonal transport

Spread via spinal dorsal root

Ganglionic latency phase

Intraneuronal virus (spinal ganglion)

Reactivation

Group of vesicles on reddened base

Varicella	Zoster
• Acute cerebellar ataxia	• Postherpetic neuralgia
• Postinfectious encephalomyelitis	• Cranial nerve palsy
• Myelitis	• Segmental paresis
• Guillain-Barré syndrome	• Aseptic meningitis
• Reye syndrome	• Meningoencephalitis
• Vasculitis (infarct)	• Myelitis
	• Vasculitis (infarct)

(Adapted from Johnson, 1998)

Possible complications of VZV infection

Herpes zoster
("shingles"; dermatome T6/7, left)

Central Nervous System

■ Human Immunodeficiency Virus (HIV) Infection

Pathogenesis. HIV type 1 (HIV-1) is found worldwide, HIV-2 mainly in western Africa and only rarely in Europe, America, and India. HIV is transmitted by sexual contact, by exposure to contaminated blood or blood products, or from mother to neonate (vertical transmission). It is not transmitted through nonsexual contact during normal daily activities, by contaminated food or water, or by insect bites. In industrialized countries, the mean incubation period for HIV is 9–12 years, and the mean survival time after the onset of *acquired immunodeficiency syndrome* (AIDS) is 1–3 years. In *primary infection* (transmitted through mucosal lesions, etc.), the free or cell-bound organisms enter primary target cells in the hematopoietic system (T cells, B cells, macrophages, dendritic cells), CNS (macrophages, microglia, astrocytes, neurons), skin (fibroblasts), or gastrointestinal tract (goblet cells). After replicating in the primary target cells, the virions spread to regional lymph nodes, CD4+ T cells, and macrophages, where they replicate rapidly, leading to a marked viremia with *dissemination* of HIV to other target cells throughout the body. About 7–14 days after this viremic phase, the *immune system* gains partial control over viral replication, and *seroconversion* occurs. The subsequent period of clinical latency is characterized by a steady rate of viral replication, elimination of HIV by the immune system, and the absence of major clinical manifestations for several years. Eventually, the immune system fails to keep up with the replicating virus, various immune functions become impaired, and the CD4+ T-lymphocyte count declines sharply. The rising viral load correlates with the progression of HIV infection to AIDS. In the nervous system, HIV initially appears in the CSF, but is later found mainly in macrophages and microglia.

Symptoms and signs. Neurological manifestations can occur at any stage of HIV infection, but usually appear only in the late stages of AIDS. One-half to two-thirds of all HIV-positive individuals develop neurological disturbances as a primary or secondary complication of HIV infection or of a concomitant disease.

Primary HIV infection. *Early manifestations* at the time of seroconversion are rare; these include acute reversible encephalitis or aseptic meningitis (p. 234), cranial nerve deficits (especially facial nerve palsy), radiculitis, or myelitis. Neurological signs are usually *late manifestations* of HIV infection. *HIV encephalopathy* progresses over several months and is characterized by lethargy, headache, increasing social withdrawal, insomnia, forgetfulness, lack of concentration, and apathy. Advanced AIDS is accompanied by bradyphrenia, impaired ocular pursuit, dysarthrophonia, incoordination, myoclonus, rigidity, and postural tremor. Incontinence and central paresis develop in the final stages of the disease. CT of the brain reveals generalized atrophy, and MRI reveals multifocal or diffuse white-matter lesions. The CSF examination may be normal or reveal a low-grade pleocytosis and an elevated protein concentration. EEG reveals increased slow-wave activity. Other neurological manifestations include HIV *myelopathy* (vacuolar myelopathy), distal symmetrical *polyradiculoneuropathies*, *mononeuritis multiplex*, and *polymyositis*.

Secondary complications of HIV infection include *opportunistic CNS infections* (toxoplasmosis, cryptococcal meningitis, aspergillosis, progressive multifocal leukoencephalopathy, cytomegalovirus encephalitis, herpes simplex encephalitis, herpes zoster, tuberculosis, syphilis), *tumors* (primary CNS lymphoma), *stroke* (infarction, hemorrhage), and *metabolic disturbances* (iatrogenic or secondary to vitamin deficiency).

Virustatic treatment. Antiretroviral combination therapy (HAART: highly active antiretroviral therapy).

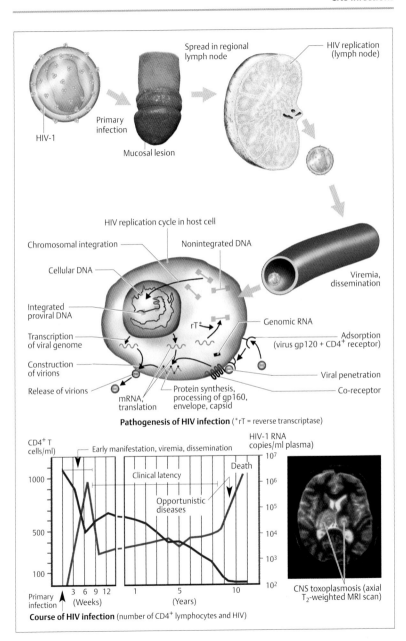

Spread in regional lymph node

HIV replication (lymph node)

Primary infection

HIV-1

Mucosal lesion

HIV replication cycle in host cell

Chromosomal integration

Cellular DNA

Nonintegrated DNA

Viremia, dissemination

Integrated proviral DNA

Genomic RNA

rT*

Transcription of viral genome

Adsorption (virus gp120 + CD4+ receptor)

Construction of virions

Viral penetration

Release of virions

Co-receptor

mRNA, translation

Protein synthesis, processing of gp160, envelope, capsid

Pathogenesis of HIV infection (*rT = reverse transcriptase)

CD4+ T cells/ml

HIV-1 RNA copies/ml plasma)

Early manifestation, viremia, dissemination

Death

Clinical latency

Opportunistic diseases

Primary infection

3 6 9 12
(Weeks)

1   5   10
(Years)

CNS toxoplasmosis (axial T2-weighted MRI scan)

Course of HIV infection (number of CD4+ lymphocytes and HIV)

■ Poliomyelitis

Pathogenesis. There are three types of poliovirus: type 1 (ca. 85% of all infections), type 2 and type 3. Like other enteroviruses (e. g., coxsackievirus, echovirus, and hepatitis-A virus), they are transmitted via the fecal–oral and oral–oral routes, and poor sanitary conditions favor their spread. Having entered the body, the virions infiltrate epithelial cells, where they replicate, and then spread to the lymphatic tissues of the nasopharynx (tonsils) and intestinal wall (Peyer's patches). A second replication phase (6–8 days) is followed by hematogenous dissemination (viremia), with nonspecific symptoms. Polioviruses reach the CNS via the bloodstream and can produce signs of poliomyelitis 10–14 days after infection. The virus is present in the saliva for 3–4 days and in the feces for 3–4 weeks. The infected individual becomes immune only to the specific type of poliovirus that caused the infection. The viral pathogen can be detected in throat smears and feces by serology or by the polymerase chain reaction.

Symptoms and signs. 90–95% of all poliovirus infections remain asymptomatic (occult immunization). Roughly 5–10% of infected persons develop abortive poliomyelitis, while only 1–2% go on to develop major spinal, bulbar, or encephalitic disease.

Minor poliomyelitis (abortive type) has nonspecific manifestations including fever, headache, sore throat, limb pain, lethargy, and gastrointestinal disturbances (nausea, anorexia, diarrhea, constipation), which resolve in 4 days at most, without CNS involvement.

Major poliomyelitis (preparalytic and paralytic types). Either immediately or after a latency period of 2–3 days, fever rises and organ manifestations appear, with a meningitic syndrome (*preparalytic stage*) that may be followed by paralysis in the later course of the disease (*paralytic stage*). The meningitis of the preparalytic stage exhibits typical features of aseptic meningitis as well as marked generalized weakness and apathy. It resolves in about one-half of cases; in the other half, increasing myalgia and stiffness herald the onset of the paralytic stage. The *spinal form* (most common) causes flaccid paresis (usually with asymmetrical proximal weakness) and areflexia, mainly in the lower limbs. The paresis may worsen over 3–5 days; its severity is highly variable. Some patients develop paresthesiae without sensory loss or autonomic dysfunction (urinary retention, hypohidrosis, constipation). Muscle atrophy develops within a week of the onset of paralysis. *Bulbar poliomyelitis* develops in some 10% of patients (in isolated form, or concurrently with spinal poliomyelitis), involving CN VII, IX, and X to produce dysphagia and dysphonia. Involvement of the brain stem reticular formation causes hemodynamic fluctuations, respiratory insufficiency or paralysis, and gastric atony. The *encephalitic form* is very rare; it may be accompanied by autonomic dysfunction (p. 222).

Postpolio syndrome. Newly arising manifestations in a patient who recovered from poliomyelitis at least 10 years earlier with stable neurological deficits in the intervening time. Postpolio syndrome is characterized by *general symptoms* (abnormal fatigability, intolerance to cold, cyanosis of the affected limbs, etc.), *arthralgias*, and increasing *neuromuscular deficits* (exacerbation of earlier weakness, weakness of previously unaffected muscles, new atrophy), sometimes accompanied by dysphagia, respiratory insufficiency, and sleep apnea.

Prevention. Subcutaneous immunization with inactivated polioviruses (e. g., Salk vaccine), followed by a first booster in 6–8 weeks and a second booster in 8–12 months.

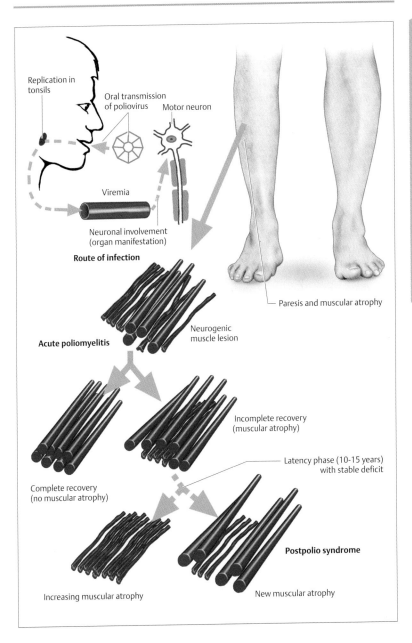

Replication in tonsils

Oral transmission of poliovirus

Motor neuron

Viremia

Neuronal involvement (organ manifestation)

Route of infection

Paresis and muscular atrophy

Neurogenic muscle lesion

Acute poliomyelitis

Incomplete recovery (muscular atrophy)

Latency phase (10-15 years) with stable deficit

Complete recovery (no muscular atrophy)

Postpolio syndrome

Increasing muscular atrophy

New muscular atrophy

Central Nervous System

■ Progressive Multifocal Leukoencephalopathy (PML)

Pathogenesis. The causative organism, JC virus, is a ubiquitous papovavirus that usually stays dormant within the body. It is reactivated in persons with impaired cellular immunity and spreads through the bloodstream to the CNS, where it induces multiple white-matter lesions.

Symptoms and signs. PML appears as a complication of cancer (chronic lymphatic leukemia, Hodgkin lymphoma), tuberculosis, sarcoidosis, immune suppression, and AIDS, producing variable symptoms and signs. The *major manifestations* in patients without AIDS are visual disturbances (visual field defects, cortical blindness), hemiparesis, and neuropsychological disturbances (impairment of memory and cognitive functions, dysphasia, behavioral abnormalities). The major manifestations of PML as a complication of AIDS are (from most to least frequent): central paresis, cognitive impairment, visual disturbances, gait impairment, ataxia, dysarthria, dysphasia, and headache. PML usually progresses rapidly, causing death in 4–6 months. The definitive *diagnosis* is by histological examination of brain tissue obtained by biopsy or necropsy. CT reveals asymmetrically distributed, hypodense white-matter lesions without mass effect or contrast enhancement; these lesions are hyperintense on T2-weighted MRI, which also demonstrates involvement of the subcortical white matter ("U fibers"). The CSF findings are usually normal, but oligoclonal bands may be found in AIDS patients.

Virustatic therapy. There is as yet no validated treatment regimen.

■ Cytomegalovirus (CMV) Infection

Pathogenesis. CMV, a member of the herpesvirus family, is transmitted through respiratory droplets, sexual intercourse, and contact with contaminated blood, blood products, or transplanted organs. It is widely distributed throughout the world, with a regional and age-dependent prevalence of up to 100%. CMV virions are thought to replicate initially in oropharyngeal epithelial cells (salivary glands) and then disseminate to the organs of the body, including the nervous system, through the bloodstream. The virus remains dormant in monocytes and lymphocytes as long as the immune system keeps it in check. Reactivation of the virus is almost always asymptomatic in healthy individuals, but severe generalized disease can develop in persons with immune compromise due to AIDS, organ transplantation, immunosuppressant drugs, or a primary malignancy.

Symptoms and signs. The *primary infection* is usually clinically silent. Intrauterine fetal infection leads to generalized fetopathies in fewer than 5% of neonates. In immunocompromised patients, particularly those with AIDS, (*reactivated*) CMV *infection* presents a variable combination of manifestations, including retinitis (partial or total loss of vision), pneumonia, and enteritis (colitis, esophagitis, proctitis). The *neurological manifestations* of CMV infection are manifold. PNS involvement is reflected as Guillain–Barré syndrome or lumbosacral polyradiculopathy (subacute paraparesis with or without back pain or radicular pain). CNS involvement produces encephalitis, meningitis, ventriculitis (inflammatory changes in the ependyma) and/or myelitis. Symptoms and signs may be absent, minor, or progressively severe, as in HIV-related encephalopathy. CMV vasculitis may lead to ischemic stroke. The diagnosis usually cannot be made from the clinical findings alone (except in the case of CMV retinitis). MRI reveals periventricular contrast enhancement in CMV vasculitis; other MRI and CT findings are nonspecific. There may be CSF pleocytosis with an elevated protein concentration. The diagnosis can be established by culture or identification by polymerase chain reaction of CMV in tissue, CSF, or urine, or by serological detection of CMV-specific antibodies.

Virustatic therapy. Ganciclovir, foscarnet, or cidofovir are given for initial treatment and secondary prophylaxis.

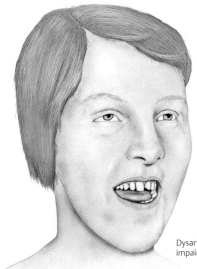

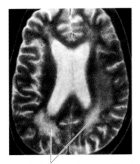

Foci of demyelination seen on MRI (no mass effect or contrast enhancement)

Dysarthria, dysphasia, cognitive impairment, behavioral changes

Progressive multifocal leukoencephalopathy

Cotton-wool spots near optic disk

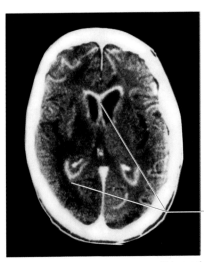

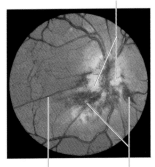

Microangiopathy   Hemorrhage

CMV retinitis

CMV ventriculitis on MRI (ependymal contrast enhancement)

Cytomegalovirus (CMV) infection

■ Rabies

Pathogenesis. Rabies virus is a rhabdovirus that is mainly transmitted by the bite of a rabid animal. The reservoirs of infection are wild animals in Europe and America (foxes, wild boar, deer, martens, raccoons, badgers, bats; *sylvatic rabies*) and dogs in Asia (*urban rabies*). The virus replicates in muscles cells near the site of entry and then spreads via muscle spindles and motor end plates to the peripheral nerves, as far as the spinal ganglia and spinal motor neurons, where secondary replication takes place. It subsequently spreads to the CNS and other organs (salivary glands, cornea, kidneys, lungs) by way of the fiber pathways of the autonomic nervous system. The limbic system (p. 144) is usually also involved. The mean incubation time is 2–3 months (range: 1 week to 1 year). Proof that the biting animal was rabid is essential for diagnosis, as rabies is otherwise very difficult to diagnose until its late clinical manifestations appear. The virus can be isolated from the patient's sputum, urine or CSF in the first week after infection.

Symptoms and signs. The course of rabies can be divided into three stages. The *prodromal stage* (2–4 days) is characterized by paresthesia, hyperesthesia, and pain at the site of the bite and the entire ipsilateral side of the body. The patient suffers from nausea, malaise, fever, and headache and, within a few days, also from anxiety, irritability, insomnia, motor hyperactivity, and depression.

Hyperexcitability stage. In the ensuing days, the patient typically develops increasing restlessness, incoherent speech, and painful spasms of the limbs and muscles of deglutition, reflecting involvement of the midbrain tegmentum. *Hydrophobia*, as this stage of the disease is called, is characterized by painful laryngospasms, respiratory muscle spasms, and opisthotonus, with tonic-clonic spasms throughout the body that are initially triggered by attempts to drink but later even by the mere sight of water, unexpected noises, breezes, or bright light. There may be alternating periods of extreme agitation (screaming, spitting, and/or scratching fits) and relative calm. The patient dies within a few days if untreated, or else progresses to the next stage after a brief clinical improvement.

Paralytic stage (*paralytic rabies*). The patient's mood and hydrophobic manifestations improve, but spinal involvement produces an ascending flaccid paralysis with myalgia and fasciculations. Weakness may appear in all limbs at once, or else in an initially asymmetrical pattern, beginning in the bitten limb and then spreading. In some cases, the clinical picture is dominated by cranial nerve palsies (oculomotor disturbances, dysphagia, drooling, dysarthrophonia) and autonomic dysfunction (cardiac arrhythmia, pulmonary edema, diabetes insipidus, hyperhidrosis).

Rabies prophylaxis. *Preexposure prophylaxis:* Vaccination of persons at risk (veterinarians, laboratory personnel, travelers to endemic areas).

Local wound treatment: Thorough washing of the bite wound with soap and water.

Postexposure prophylaxis: Vaccination and rabies immunoglobulin.

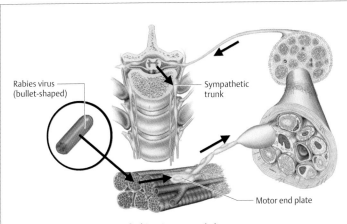

Rabies virus (bullet-shaped)

Sympathetic trunk

Motor end plate

Route of rabies virus transmission

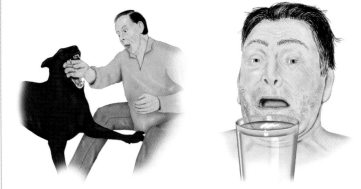

Animal bite

Excitation stage (hydrophobia)

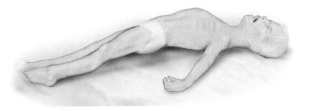

Excitation stage (spasms, opisthotonus)

Opportunistic Fungal Infections

CNS mycosis is sometimes found in otherwise healthy persons but mainly occurs as a component of an *opportunistic systemic mycosis* in persons with immune compromise due to AIDS, organ transplantation, severe burns, malignant diseases, diabetes mellitus, connective tissue diseases, chemotherapy, or chronic corticosteroid therapy. Certain types of mycosis (blastomycosis, coccidioidmycosis, histoplasmosis) are endemic to certain regions of the world (North America, South America, Africa).

■ Cryptococcus neoformans (Cryptococcosis)

Cryptococcus, a yeastlike fungus with a polysaccharide capsule, is a common cause of CNS mycosis. It is mainly transmitted by inhalation of dust contaminated with the feces of pet birds and pigeons. Local pulmonary infection is followed by hematogenous spread to the CNS. In the presence of a competent immune system (particularly cell-mediated immunity), the pulmonary infection usually remains asymptomatic and self-limited. Immune-compromised persons, however, may develop *meningoencephalitis* with or without prior signs of pulmonary cryptococcosis. Its manifestations are heterogeneous and usually progressive. Signs of subacute or chronic meningitis are accompanied by cranial nerve deficits (III, IV, VI), encephalitic syndrome, and/or signs of intracranial hypertension. *Diagnosis:* MRI reveals granulomatous cystic lesions with surrounding edema. Lung infiltrates may be seen. The nonspecific CSF changes include a variable (usually mild) lymphomonocytic pleocytosis as well as elevated protein, low glucose, and elevated lactate concentrations. An india ink histological preparation reveals the pathogen with a surrounding halo (carbon particles cannot penetrate its polysaccharide capsule). *Identification of pathogen:* demonstration of antigen in CSF and serum; tests for anticryptococcal antibody yield variable results. *Treatment:* initially, amphotericin B + flucytosine; subsequently, fluconazole or (if fluconazole is not tolerated) itraconazole.

■ Candida (Candidiasis)

Candida albicans is a constituent of the normal body flora. In persons with impaired cell-medi-

ated immunity, Candida can infect the oropharynx (*thrush*) and then spread to the upper respiratory tract, esophagus, and intestine. CNS infection comes about by hematogenous spread (*candida sepsis*), resulting in *meningitis* or *meningoencephalitis*. Ocular changes: *Candida endophthalmitis. Diagnosis:* Candida abscesses can be seen on CT or MRI. The CSF changes included pleocytosis (several hundred cells/µl) and elevated concentrations of protein and lactate. *Pathogen identification:* Microscopy, culture, or detection of specific antigens or antibodies. *Local treatment:* Amphotericin B or fluconazole. *Systemic tratment:* Amphotericin B + flucytosine.

■ Aspergillus (Aspergillosis)

The mold *Aspergillus fumigatus* is commonly found in cellulose-containing materials such as silage grain, wood, paper, potting soil, and foliage. Inhaled spores produce local inflammation in the airways, sinuses, and lungs. Organisms reach the CNS by hematogenous spread or by direct extension (e.g., from osteomyelitis of the skull base, otitis, or mastoiditis), causing encephalitis, dural granulomas, or multiple abscesses. *Diagnosis:* CT and MRI reveal multiple, sometimes hemorrhagic lesions. The CSF findings include granulocytic pleocytosis and markedly elevated protein, decreased glucose, and elevated lactate concentration. *Pathogen identification:* Culture; if negative, then lung or brain biopsy. *Treatment:* Amphotericin B + flucytosine or itraconazole.

■ Mucor, Absidia, Rhizopus (Mucormycosis)

Inhaled spores of these molds enter the nasopharynx, bronchi, and lungs, where they mainly infect blood vessels. *Rhinocerebral mucormycosis* is a rare complication of diabetic ketoacidosis, lymphoproliferative disorders, and drug abuse; infection spreads from the paranasal sinuses via blood vessels to the retro-orbital tissues (causing retro-orbital edema, exophthalmos, and ophthalmoplegia) and to the brain (causing infarction with secondary hemorrhage). *Diagnosis:* CT, MRI; associated findings on ENT examination. *Pathogen identification:* Biopsy, smears. *Treatment:* Surgical excision of infected tissue if possible; amphotericin B.

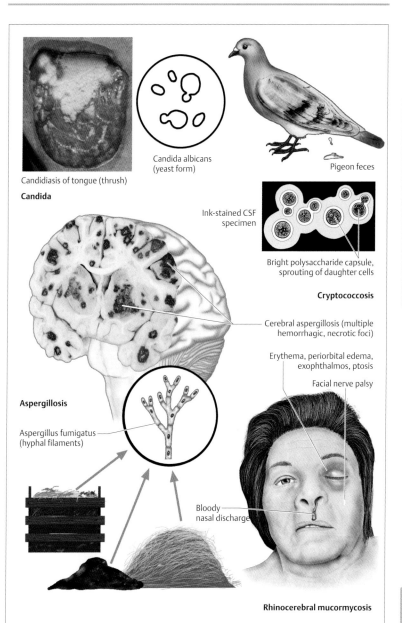

Candidiasis of tongue (thrush)

Candida

Candida albicans
(yeast form)

Pigeon feces

Ink-stained CSF
specimen

Bright polysaccharide capsule,
sprouting of daughter cells

Cryptococcosis

Cerebral aspergillosis (multiple
hemorrhagic, necrotic foci)

Erythema, periorbital edema,
exophthalmos, ptosis

Facial nerve palsy

Aspergillosis

Aspergillus fumigatus
(hyphal filaments)

Bloody
nasal discharge

Rhinocerebral mucormycosis

Protozoan and Helminthic Infections

■ Toxoplasma gondii (Toxoplasmosis)

This protozoan goes through three stages of development. *Tachyzoites* (endozoites; acute stage) are crescent-shaped, rapidly replicating forms that circulate in the bloodstream and are spread from one individual to another through contaminated blood or blood products. These develop into *bradyzoites* (cystozoites; latent stage), which aggregate to form tissue cysts (e. g., in muscle) containing several thousand organisms each. *Oocysts* are found only in the intestinal mucosa of the definitive host (domestic cat). Infectious sporozoites (sporulated oocysts) appear 2–4 days after the oocysts are eliminated in cat feces. Reuptake of the organism by the definitive host, or infection of an intermediate host (human, pig, sheep), occurs by ingestion of sporozoites from contaminated feces, or by consumption of raw meat containing tissue cysts. In the intermediate host, the sporozoites develop into tachyzoites, which then become bradyzoites and tissue cysts. Placental transmission (*congenital toxoplasmosis* ⇨ hydrocephalus, intracellular calcium deposits, chorioretinitis) occurs only if the mother is initially infected during pregnancy. In *immunocompetent* persons, acute toxoplasmosis is usually asymptomatic, and only occasionally causes symptoms such as lymphadenopathy, fatigue, low-grade fever, arthralgia, and headache. IgG antibodies can be detected in latent toxoplasmosis (bradyzoite stage). In *immunodeficient* persons (p. 240), however, latent toxoplasmosis usually becomes symptomatic on reactivation. The central nervous system is most commonly affected (mainly *encephalitis*; *myelitis* is rare); other organs that may be affected include the *eyes* (chorioretinitis, iridocyclitis), heart, liver, spleen, PNS (*neuritis*) and muscles (*myositis*). *Diagnosis:* EEG (slowing, focal signs), CT/MRI (solitary or multiple ring-enhancing abscesses), CSF (lymphomonocytic pleocytosis, mildly elevated protein concentration). *Treatment:* pyrimethamine/sulfadiazine or clindamycin/folinic acid.

■ Taenia solium (Neurocysticercosis)

Ingestion of the tapeworm *Taenia solium* in raw or undercooked pork leads to a usually asymptomatic infection of the human gut. Tapeworm segments that contain eggs (proglottids) are eliminated in the feces of pigs (the intermediate host) or humans with intestinal infection and then reingested by humans (or pigs) under poor hygienic conditions. The oval-shaped larvae pass through the intestinal wall and travel to multiple organs (including the eyes, skin, muscles, lung, and heart) by hematogenous, lymphatic, or direct spread. The CNS is often involved, though manifestations such as epileptic seizures, intracranial hypertension, behavioral changes (dementia, disorientation), hemiparesis, aphasia, and ataxia are uncommon. Spinal cysts are rare. *Diagnosis:* CT (solitary or multiple hypodense cysts with or without contrast enhancement, calcification and/or hydrocephalus), MRI (demonstration of cysts and surrounding edema), CSF examination (low-grade lymphocytic pleocytosis, occasional eosinophilia). *Treatment:* Praziquantel or albendazole; neurosurgical excision of intraventricular cysts; ventricular shunting in patients with hydrocephalus.

■ Plasmodium falciparum (Cerebral Malaria)

This protozoan is most commonly transmitted by the bite of the female anopheles mosquito. Primary asexual reproduction of the organisms takes place in the hepatic parenchyma (*pre-erythrocytic schizogony*). The organisms then invade red blood cells and develop further inside them (*intraerythrocytic development*). The repeated liberation of merozoites causes recurrent episodes of fever. *P. falciparum* preferentially colonizes the capillaries of the brain, heart, liver, and kidneys. *Pathogen identification:* Blood culture. *Treatment:* See current topical literature for recommendations.

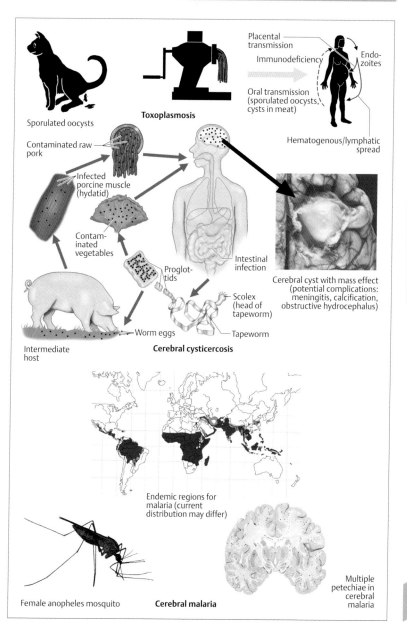

Sporulated oocysts

Toxoplasmosis

Placental transmission

Immunodeficiency

Endo-zoites

Oral transmission (sporulated oocysts, cysts in meat)

Hematogenous/lymphatic spread

Contaminated raw pork

Infected porcine muscle (hydatid)

Contaminated vegetables

Proglottids

Intestinal infection

Scolex (head of tapeworm)

Worm eggs

Tapeworm

Intermediate host

Cerebral cysticercosis

Cerebral cyst with mass effect (potential complications: meningitis, calcification, obstructive hydrocephalus)

Endemic regions for malaria (current distribution may differ)

Female anopheles mosquito

Cerebral malaria

Multiple petechiae in cerebral malaria

Transmissible Spongiform Encephalopathies

The transmissible spongiform encephalopathies (TSEs) are characterized by spongiform histological changes in the brain (vacuoles in neurons and neuropil), transmissibility to humans by way of infected tissue or contaminated surgical instruments, and, in some cases, a genetic determination. TSEs are transmitted by nucleic acid-free proteinaceous particles called prions and are associated with mutations in prion protein (PrP); they are therefore referred to as *prion diseases*.

Normal cellular prion protein (PrP^c) is synthesized intracellularly, transported to the cell membrane, and returned to the cell interior by endocytosis. Part of the PrP^c is then broken down by proteases, and another fraction is transported back to the cell surface. The physiological function of PrP^c is still unknown. It is found in all mammalian species and is especially abundant in neurons. *PRNP*, the gene responsible for the expression of PrP^c in man, is found on the short arm of chromosome 20. *PRNP* mutations yield the mutated form of PrP (ΔPrP) that causes the *genetic spongiform encephalopathies*. Another mutated form of PrP (PrP^{sc}) causes the *infectious spongiform encephalopathies*. PrP^{sc} induces the conversion of PrP^c to PrP^{sc} in the following manner: PrP^{sc} enters the cell and binds with PrP^c to yield a heterodimer. The resulting conformational change in the PrP^c molecule (α-helical structure) and its interaction with a still unidentified cellular protein (protein X) transform it into PrP^{sc} (β-sheet structure). Protein X is thought to supply the energy needed for protein folding, or at least to lower the activation energy for it. PrP^{sc} cannot be formed in cells lacking PrP^c. Mutated PrP^{sc} presumably reaches the CNS by axonal transport or in lymphatic cells; these forms of transport have been demonstrated in forms of spongiform encephalopathies that affect domestic animals, e.g., scrapie (in sheep) and bovine spongiform encephalopathy (BSE). ΔPrP and PrP^{sc} cannot be broken down intracellularly and therefore accumulate within the cells. Partial proteolysis of these proteins yields a protease-resistant molecule (PrP 27–30) that polymerizes to form amyloid, which, in turn, induces further neuropathological changes. PrP and amyloid have been found in certain myopathies (such as inclusion body myositis, p. 344); others involve an accumulation of PrP (PrP overexpression myopathy).

■ Creutzfeldt–Jakob Disease (CJD)

CJD is a very rare disease, arising in ca. 1 person per 10^6 per year. It usually affects older adults (peak incidence around age 60). 85–90% of cases are sporadic (due to a spontaneous gene mutation or conformational change of PrP^c to PrP^{sc}); 5–15% are familial (usually autosomal dominant); and very rare cases are iatrogenic (transmitted by contaminated neurosurgical instruments or implants, growth hormone, and dural and corneal grafts). It usually progresses rapidly to death within 4–12 months of onset, though the survival time in individual cases varies from a few weeks to several years. *Early manifestations* are not typically seen, but may include fatigability, vertigo, cognitive impairment, anxiety, insomnia, hallucinations, increasing apathy, and depression. The *principal finding* is a rapidly progressive dementia associated with myoclonus, increased startle response, motor disturbances (rigidity, muscle atrophy, fasciculations, cerebellar ataxia), and visual disturbances. *Late manifestations* include akinetic mutism, severe myoclonus, epileptic seizures, and autonomic dysfunction. A new variant of CJD has recently arisen in the United Kingdom; unlike the typical form, it tends to affect younger patients, produces mainly behavioral changes in its early stages, and is associated with longer survival (though it, too, is fatal). It is thought to be caused by the consumption of beef from cattle infected with BSE. *Diagnosis:* EEG (1 Hz periodic biphasic or triphasic sharp-wave complexes), CT (cortical atrophy), T2/proton-weighted MRI (bilateral hyperintensity in basal ganglia in ca. 80%), CSF examination (elevation of neuron-specific enolase, S100β or tau protein concentration; presence of protein 14–3-3).

■ Gerstmann–Sträussler–Scheinker Disease (GSS) and Fatal Familial Insomnia (FFI)

See pp. 114 and 280.

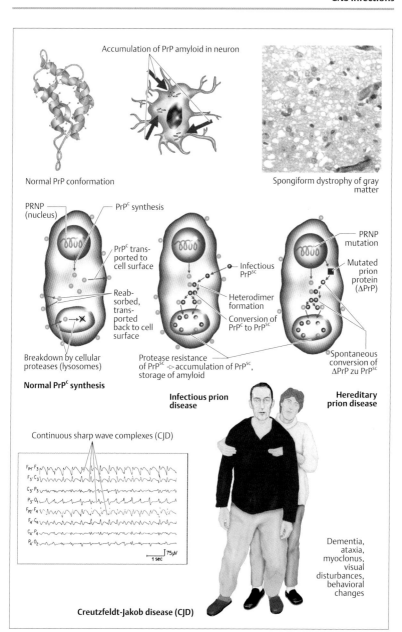

Accumulation of PrP amyloid in neuron

Normal PrP conformation

Spongiform dystrophy of gray matter

PRNP (nucleus)

PrP^c synthesis

PrP^c transported to cell surface

Reabsorbed, transported back to cell surface

Breakdown by cellular proteases (lysosomes)

Normal PrP^c synthesis

Infectious PrP^{sc}

Heterodimer formation

Conversion of PrP^c to PrP^{sc}

Protease resistance of PrP^{sc} ⇨ accumulation of PrP^{sc}, storage of amyloid

Infectious prion disease

PRNP mutation

Mutated prion protein (ΔPrP)

Spontaneous conversion of ΔPrP zu PrP^{sc}

Hereditary prion disease

Continuous sharp wave complexes (CJD)

F_{P1}-F_3
F_3-C_3
C_3-P_3
P_3-O_1
F_{P2}-F_4
F_4-C_4
C_4-P_4
P_4-O_2

75μV
1 sec

Dementia, ataxia, myoclonus, visual disturbances, behavioral changes

Creutzfeldt-Jakob disease (CJD)

Symptoms and Signs

The clinical manifestations of a brain tumor may range from a virtually asymptomatic state to a constellation of symptoms and signs that is specific for a particular type and location of lesion. The only way to rule out a brain tumor for certain is by neuroimaging (CT or MRI).

■ Nonspecific Manifestations

Tumors whose manifestations are mainly non-specific include astrocytoma, oligodendro-glioma, cerebral metastasis, ependymoma, meningioma, neoplastic meningitis, and primary CNS lymphoma.

Behavioral changes. Patients may complain of easy fatigability or exhaustion, while their relatives or co-workers may notice lack of concentration, forgetfulness, loss of initiative, cognitive impairment, indifference, negligent task performance, indecisiveness, slovenliness, and general slowing of movement. Such manifestations are often mistaken for signs of depression or stress. Apathy, obtundation, and somnolence worsen as the disease progresses. There may also be increasing confusion, disorientation, and dementia.

Headache. More than half of patients with brain tumors suffer from headache, and many headache patients fear that they might have a brain tumor. If headache is the sole symptom, the neurological examination is normal, and the headache can be securely classified as belonging to one of the primary types (p. 182 ff), then a brain tumor is very unlikely. Neuroimaging is indicated in patients with longstanding headache who report a change in their symptoms. The clinical features of headache do not differentiate benign from malignant tumors.

Nausea, vertigo, and malaise are frequent, though often vague, complaints. The patient feels unsteady or simply "different." Vomiting (sometimes on an empty stomach) is less common and not necessarily accompanied by nausea; there may be spontaneous, projectile vomiting.

Epileptic seizures. Focal or generalized seizures arising in adulthood should prompt evaluation for a possible brain tumor.

Focal neurological signs usually become prominent only in advanced stages of the disease but may be present earlier in milder form. Hemiparesis, aphasia, apraxia, ataxia, cranial nerve palsies, or incontinence may occur depending on the type and location of the tumor.

Intracranial hypertension (elevated ICP) (p. 158) may arise without marked focal neurological dysfunction because of a medulloblastoma, ependymoma of the fourth ventricle, cerebellar hemangioblastoma, colloid cyst of the 3rd ventricle, craniopharyngioma, or glioblastoma (e.g. of the frontal lobe or corpus callosum). Cervical tumors very rarely cause intracranial hypertension. Papilledema, if present, is not necessarily due to a brain tumor, nor does its absence rule one out. Papilledema does not impair vision in its acute phase.

■ Specific Manifestations

Some tumors produce symptoms and signs that are specific for their histological type, location, or both. These tumors include craniopharyngioma, olfactory groove meningioma, pituitary tumors, cerebellopontine angle tumors, pontine glioma, chondrosarcoma, chordoma, glomus tumors, skull base tumors, and tumors of the foramen magnum. In general, these specific manifestations are typically found when the tumor is relatively small and are gradually overshadowed by nonspecific manifestations (described above) as it grows.

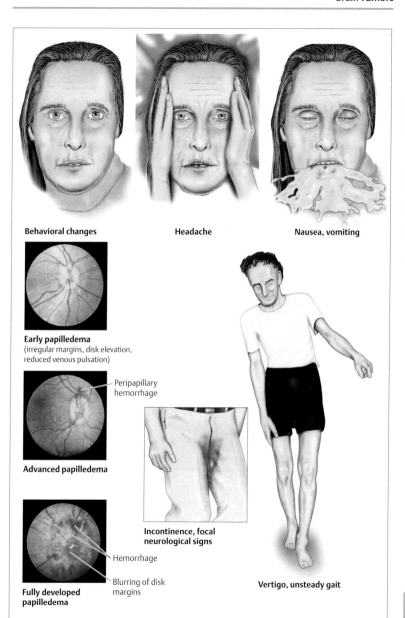

Behavioral changes

Headache

Nausea, vomiting

Early papilledema
(irregular margins, disk elevation,
reduced venous pulsation)

Peripapillary
hemorrhage

Advanced papilledema

Incontinence, focal
neurological signs

Hemorrhage

Blurring of disk
margins

**Fully developed
papilledema**

Vertigo, unsteady gait

Benign Brain Tumors

■ Astrocytoma (WHO grades I and II)

Astrocytomas arise from blastomatous astro-cytes. They are classified as benign (WHO grade I) or semibenign (WHO grade II) according to their histological features (p. 377).

Pilocytic astrocytoma (WHO grade I) is a slowly growing tumor that mainly occurs in children and young adults and usually arises in the cerebellum, optic nerve, optic chiasm, hypothalamus, or pons. It is not uncommonly found in the setting of neurofibromatosis I. There may be a relatively long history of headache, abnormal gait, visual impairment, diabetes insipidus, precocious puberty, or cranial nerve palsies before the tumor is discovered.

Low-grade astrocytoma (WHO grade II). Fibrillary astrocytoma is more common than the gemistocytic and protoplasmic types. These tumors most commonly arise in the frontal and temporal lobes and often undergo malignant transformation to grades III and IV over the course of several years. They may be calcified. They may produce epileptic seizures and behavioral changes.

Oligodendroglioma (WHO grade II) usually appears in the 4th or 5th decade of life. It tends to arise at or near the cortical surface of the frontal and temporal lobes and may extend locally to involve the leptomeninges. Oligodendrogliomas are often partially calcified. Tumors of mixed histology (oligodendrocytoma plus astrocytoma) are called *oligoastrocytomas*.

Pleomorphic xanthoastrocytoma (WHO grade II) is a rare tumor that mainly arises in the temporal lobes of children and young adults and is associated with epileptic seizures in most cases. It can progress to a grade III tumor.

■ Meningioma (WHO grade I)

Meningiomas are slowly growing, usually benign, dural-based extraaxial tumors that are thought to arise from arachnoid cells. Twelve histological subtypes have been identified. Meningiomas tend to recur if they are not totally resected. They may involve not only the dura mater but also the adjacent bone (manifesting usually as hyperostosis, more rarely as thinning) and may infiltrate or occlude the cerebral venous sinuses. They can occur anywhere in the CNS but are most often found in *supratentorial* (falx, parasagittal region, sphenoid wing, cerebral convexities), *infratentorial* (tentorium, cerebellopontine angle, craniocervical junction), and *spinal* locations. Multiple or intraventricular meningioma is less common. *Extracranial meningiomas* rarely arise in the orbit, skin, or nasal sinuses. Familial meningioma is seen in hereditary disorders such as type II neurofibromatosis.

■ Choroid Plexus Papilloma (WHO grade I)

This rare tumor most commonly arises in the (left) lateral ventricle in children and in the 4th ventricle in adults. Signs of intracranial hypertension, due to obstruction of CSF flow, are the most common clinical presentation and may arise acutely.

■ Hemangioblastoma (WHO grade I)

These solid or cystic tumors usually arise in the cerebellum (from the vermis more often than the hemispheres) and produce vertigo, headache, truncal ataxia, and gait ataxia. Obstructive hydrocephalus may occur as an early manifestation. 10 % of cases are in patients with von Hippel–Lindau disease (p. 294).

■ Ependymoma (WHO grades I–II)

Ependymomas most commonly arise in children, adolescents, and young adults. They may arise in the ventricular system (usually in the fourth ventricle) or outside it; they may be cystic or calcified. *Subependymoma* of the fourth ventricle (WHO grade I) may appear in middle age or later. Spinal ependymomas may arise in any portion of the spinal cord.

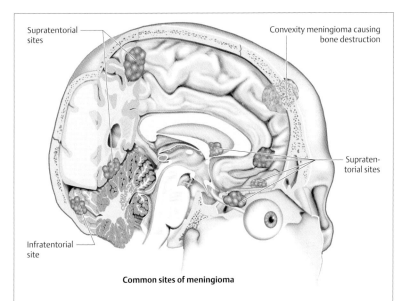

Supratentorial
sites

Convexity meningioma causing
bone destruction

Supraten-
torial sites

Infratentorial
site

Common sites of meningioma

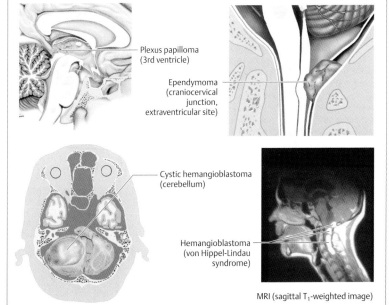

Plexus papilloma
(3rd ventricle)

Ependymoma
(craniocervical
junction,
extraventricular site)

Cystic hemangioblastoma
(cerebellum)

Hemangioblastoma
(von Hippel-Lindau
syndrome)

MRI (sagittal T_1-weighted image)

Central Nervous System

Tumors in Specific Locations

■ Supratentorial Region

Colloid cyst of 3rd ventricle. These cysts filled with gelatinous fluid are found in proximity to the interventricular foramen (of Monro). Small colloid cysts may remain asymptomatic, but large ones cause acute or chronic obstructive hydrocephalus (p. 162). Sudden obstruction of the foramen causes acute intracranial hypertension, sometimes with loss of consciousness. Symptomatic colloid cysts can be surgically removed with stereotactic, neuroendoscopic, or open techniques.

Craniopharyngioma (WHO grade I). *Adamantinomatous* craniopharyngioma is suprasellar tumor of children and adolescents that has both cystic and calcified components. It produces visual field defects, hormonal deficits (growth retardation, thyroid and adrenocortical insufficiency, diabetes insipidus), and hydrocephalus. Large tumors can cause behavioral changes and epileptic seizures. *Papillary* craniopharyngioma is a tumor of adults that usually involves the 3rd ventricle.

Pituitary adenomas (WHO grade I). Adenomas smaller than 10 mm, called *microadenomas*, are usually hormone-secreting, while those larger than 10 mm, called *macroadenomas*, are often non–hormone-secreting. In addition to possible hormone secretion, these tumors have *intrasellar* (hypothyroidism, adrenocortical hormone deficiency, amenorrhea reflecting anterior pituitary insufficiency, and, rarely, diabetes insipidus), *suprasellar* (chiasmatic lesions, p. 82, hypothalamic compression, hydrocephalus), and *parasellar* manifestations (headache, deficits of CN III–VI, encirclement of the ICA by tumor, diabetes insipidus), which gradually progress as the tumor enlarges. Hemorrhage or infarction of a pituitary tumor can cause acute pituitary failure (cf. Sheehan's postpartum necrosis of the pituitary gland). *Prolactinomas* (prolactin-secreting tumors) elevate the serum prolactin concentration above 200 µg/l, in distinction to the less pronounced secondary hyperprolactinemia (usually < 200 µg/l) associated with as pregnancy, parasellar tumors, dopamine antagonists (neuroleptics, metoclopramide, reserpine), and epileptic seizures. Prolactinomas can cause secondary amenorrhea, galactorrhea, and hirsutism in women, and headache, impotence, and galactorrhea (rarely) in men. *Growth hormone-secreting tumors* cause gigantism in adolescents and acromegaly in adults. Headache, impotence, polyneuropathy, diabetes mellitus, organ changes (goiter), and hypertension are additional features. *ACTH-secreting tumors* cause Cushing disease.

Tumors of the pineal region. The most common tumor of the pineal region is germinoma (WHO grade III), followed by pineocytoma (WHO grade I) and pineoblastoma (WHO grade IV). The clinical manifestations include Parinaud syndrome (p. 358), hydrocephalus, and signs of metastatic dissemination in the subarachnoid space (p. 262).

■ Infratentorial Region

Acoustic neuroma (WHO grade I) is commonly so called, though it is in fact a schwannoma of the vestibular portion of CN VIII. Early manifestations include hearing impairment (rarely sudden hearing loss), tinnitus, and vertigo. Larger tumors cause cranial nerve palsies (V, VII, IX, X), cerebellar ataxia, and sometimes hydrocephalus. Bilateral acoustic neuroma is seen in neurofibromatosis II.

Chordoma arises from the clivus and, as it grows, destroys the surrounding bone tissue and compresses the brain stem, causing cranial nerve palsies (III, V, VI, IX, X, XII), pituitary dysfunction, visual field defects, and headache.

Paragangliomas. This group of tumors includes *pheochromocytoma* (arising from the adrenal medulla), *sympathetic paraganglioma* (arising from neuroendocrine cells of the sympathetic system), and *parasympathetic ganglioma* or *chemodetectoma* (arising from parasympathetically innervated chemoreceptor cells). The last-named is a highly vascularized tumor that may grow invasively. It arises from the glomus body.

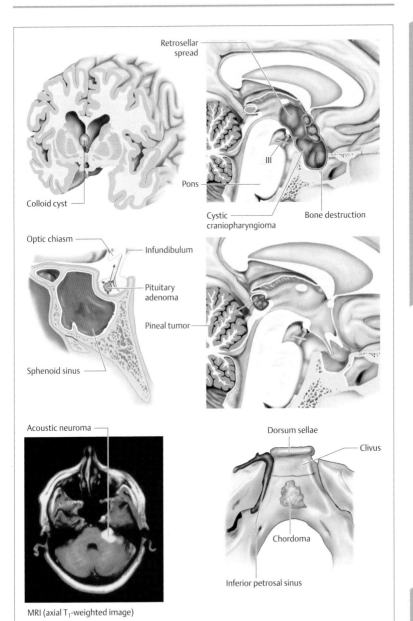

Retrosellar spread

Colloid cyst

Pons

III

Cystic craniopharyngioma

Bone destruction

Optic chiasm

Infundibulum

Pituitary adenoma

Pineal tumor

Sphenoid sinus

Acoustic neuroma

Dorsum sellae

Clivus

Chordoma

Inferior petrosal sinus

MRI (axial T₁-weighted image)

Malignant Tumors

■ **Anaplastic Astrocytoma (WHO grade III)
and Glioblastoma (WHO grade IV)**

These infiltrative, rapidly growing tumors usually arise in adults between the ages of 40 and 65. They usually involve the cerebral hemispheres, but are sometimes found in infratentorial locations (brain stem, cerebellum, spinal cord). They are occasionally multicentric or diffuse (*gliomatosis cerebri* is extremely rare). Infiltrative growth across the corpus callosum to the opposite side of the head is not uncommon (*"butterfly glioma"*). These tumors are often several centimeters in diameter by the time of diagnosis. Even relatively small tumors can produce considerable cerebral edema. Metastases outside the CNS (bone, lymph nodes) are rare. CT and MRI reveal ringlike or garlandlike contrast around a hypointense center.

■ **Primary Cerebral Lymphoma
(WHO grade IV)**

These tumors are usually non-Hodgkin lymphomas of the B-cell type and are only rarely of the T-cell type. They are commonly associated with congenital or acquired immune deficiency (Wiskott–Aldrich syndrome; immune suppression for organ transplantation, AIDS) and can arise in any part of the CNS (80 % supratentorial, 20 % infratentorial). Headache, cranial nerve palsies, polyradiculoneuropathy, meningismus, and ataxia suggest (primary) *leptomeningeal* involvement. *Ocular manifestations:* Infiltration of the uvea and vitreous body (visual disturbances; slit-lamp examination). Moreover, lymphomas may occur as solitary or multiple tumors or may spread diffusely through CNS tissue (periventricular zone, deep white matter). They produce local symptoms and also such general symptoms as psychosis, dementia, and anorexia. *CT* reveals them as hyperdense lesions surrounded by edema, usually with homogeneous contrast absorption and with little or no mass effect. *MRI* is more sensitive for lymphoma than CT; it reveals the extent of surrounding edema and is especially useful for the detection of spinal, leptomeningeal, and multilocular involvement. *CSF examination* reveals malignant cells in the early stages of the disease; the CSF protein concentration is not necessarily elevated. Biopsies and/or CSF serology for diagnosis should be performed before treatment is initiated, because some of the drugs used, particularly corticosteroids, can make the disease more difficult to diagnose.

■ **Anaplastic Oligodendroglioma
(WHO grade III)**

This rare form of oligodendroglioma responds well to chemotherapy with **p**rocarbazine, **C**CNU, and **v**incristine (PCV). As histological confirmation of cellular anaplasia (the defining criterion for grade III) can be difficult, the diagnosis must sometimes be based on the clinical and radiological findings. There may be leptomeningeal dissemination or meningeal gliomatosis.

■ **Anaplastic Ependymoma (WHO grade III)**

These tumors may have subarachnoid and (rarely) extraneural metastases, e. g., to the liver, lungs and ovaries.

■ **Primitive Neuroectodermal Tumor
(PNET; WHO grade IV)**

A PNET is a highly malignant embryonal tumor of the CNS that mainly arises in children. PNETs arising in the cerebellum, called *medulloblastomas*, are most commonly found in the vermis; they tend to metastasize to the leptomeninges and subarachnoid space (*drop metastasis*). The primary tumor and its metastases are best seen on MRI; they may appear in CT scans as areas of hyperdensity.

■ **Primary Cerebral Sarcoma (WHO grade IV)**

The very rare tumors in this group, including meningeal sarcoma, fibrosarcoma, chondrosarcoma, rhabdomyosarcoma, and malignant fibrous histiocytoma, all tend to recur locally and only rarely metastasize.

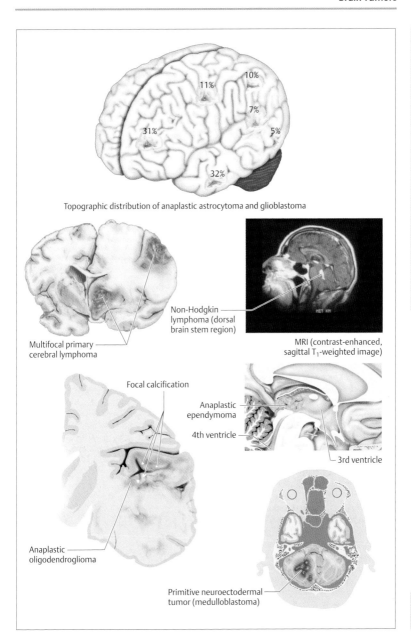

Topographic distribution of anaplastic astrocytoma and glioblastoma

Multifocal primary cerebral lymphoma

Non-Hodgkin lymphoma (dorsal brain stem region)

MRI (contrast-enhanced, sagittal T$_1$-weighted image)

Focal calcification

Anaplastic ependymoma

4th ventricle

3rd ventricle

Anaplastic oligodendroglioma

Primitive neuroectodermal tumor (medulloblastoma)

261

Metastatic Disease

Metastases spread to the nervous system through the *bloodstream* (cerebral, spinal, and leptomeningeal metastases), *lymphatic vessels* (metastases to the PNS), and *cerebrospinal fluid* (so-called drop metastases in the spinal sub-arachnoid space). Aside from direct metastatic involvement, the nervous system can also be affected by local tumor infiltration (e.g., of the brachial plexus by a Pancoast tumor), by external compression (e.g., of the spinal cord by a vertebral tumor, or of a peripheral nerve by a tumor-infiltrated lymph node), or by perineural infiltration (e.g. melanoma or salivary gland carcinoma). Only a small fraction of proliferating tumor cells are capable of metastasizing; thus, the biological behavior and drug response of metastasizing cells may differ from that of the primary tumor. Angiogenesis is essential for tumor growth and metastasis. Local invasion of surrounding tissue by the primary tumor makes it possible for tumor cells to break off and metastasize by way of the lymphatic vessels, veins, and arteries. Metastatic cells often settle in a vascular bed just downstream from the site of the primary tumor, thus (depending on its location) in the lungs, liver, or vertebral bodies. The nervous system may become involved thereafter in a second phase of metastasis (*cascade hypothesis*), or else directly, in which case the metastasizing cells must have passed through the intervening capillary bed without settling in it. Metastases may also bypass the lungs through a patent foramen ovale (*paradoxical embolism*).

■ Intracranial Metastases

Of all intracranial metastases, 85 % are supratentorial, 15 % infratentorial. The primary process in men is usually a tumor of the lung, gastrointestinal tract, or urogenital system, in women a tumor of the breast, lung, or gastrointestinal tract. Prostate, uterine, and gastrointestinal tumors metastasize preferentially to the cerebellum. The clinical manifestations of intracranial metastases are usually due to their local mass effect and surrounding cerebral edema. Brain metastases of melanoma, choriocarcinoma, and testicular cancer tend to produce hemorrhages. Metastases to the calvaria are usually asymptomatic. Skull base metastases cause pain and cranial nerve deficits. Dural-based metastases may compress or infiltrate the adjacent brain tissue, or exude fluid containing malignant cells into the subdural space. Pituitary metastases (mainly of breast cancer) cause endocrine dysfunction and cranial nerve deficits.

■ Spinal Metastases

The clinical manifestations of vertebral metastases, including vertebral or radicular pain, paraparesis/paraplegia, and gait ataxia, are mainly due to epidural mass effect. The bone marrow itself being insensitive to pain, pain arises only when the tumor compresses the periosteum, paravertebral soft tissue, nerve roots, or spinal cord. Spinal instability and pathological fractures cause additional pain. Pain in the spine may be the first sign of spinal metastasis. Subarachnoid and intramedullary metastases are rare (<5%).

■ Leptomeningeal Metastases (Neoplastic Meningeosis, "Carcinomatous Meningitis")

Seeding of the meninges may be diffuse or multifocal. Meningeal metastases may spread into the adjacent brain or spinal cord tissue, cranial nerves, or spinal nerves. *Cerebral* leptomeningeal involvement produces headache, gait ataxia, memory impairment, epileptic seizures, and cranial nerve deficits (e.g., facial nerve palsy, hearing loss, vertigo, diplopia, and loss of vision). *Spinal* involvement produces neck or back pain, radicular pain, paresthesia, paraparesis, and atony of the bowel and bladder.

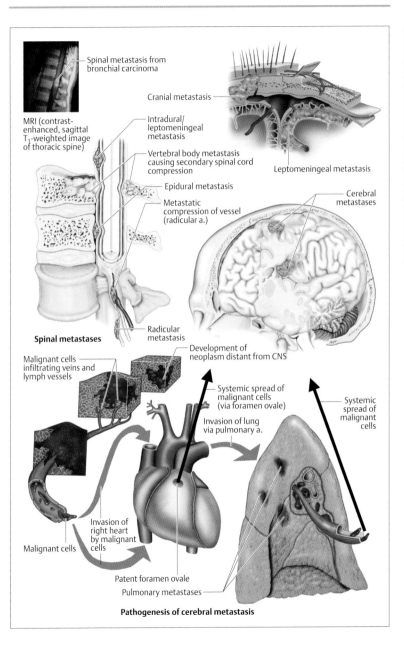

Spinal metastasis from bronchial carcinoma

Cranial metastasis

MRI (contrast-enhanced, sagittal T$_1$-weighted image of thoracic spine)

Intradural/leptomeningeal metastasis

Vertebral body metastasis causing secondary spinal cord compression

Leptomeningeal metastasis

Epidural metastasis

Metastatic compression of vessel (radicular a.)

Cerebral metastases

Radicular metastasis

Spinal metastases

Malignant cells infiltrating veins and lymph vessels

Development of neoplasm distant from CNS

Systemic spread of malignant cells (via foramen ovale)

Invasion of lung via pulmonary a.

Systemic spread of malignant cells

Invasion of right heart by malignant cells

Malignant cells

Patent foramen ovale

Pulmonary metastases

Pathogenesis of cerebral metastasis

Classification and Treatment

As the treatment and prognosis of brain tumors depend on their histological type and degree of malignancy, the first step of management is tissue diagnosis (see Table 31, p. 377). The subsequent clinical course may differ from that predicted by the histological grade because of "sampling error" (i.e., biopsy of an unrepresentative portion of the tumor). Other factors influencing prognosis include age, the completeness of surgical resection, the preoperative and postoperative neurological findings, tumor progression, and the site of the tumor.

■ **Incidence** (adapted from Lantos et al., 1997)

The most common primary intracranial tumors in patients under 20 years of age are medulloblastoma, pilocytic astrocytoma, ependymoma, and astrocytoma (WHO grade II); from age 20 to age 45, astrocytoma (WHO grade II), oligodendroglioma, acoustic neuroma (schwannoma), and ependymoma; over age 45, glioblastoma, meningioma, acoustic neuroma, and oligodendroglioma. The overall incidence of pituitary tumors (including pituitary metastases), craniopharyngioma, and intracranial lymphoma and sarcoma is low.

■ **Severity** (Table 32, p. 378)

The Karnofsky scale (Karnofsky et al., 1951) is a commonly used measure of neurological disability, e. g., due to a brain tumor. Its use permits a standardized assessment of clinical course.

■ **Treatment**

The initial treatment is often neurosurgical, with the objective of removing the tumor as completely as possible without causing a severe or permanent neurological deficit. The resection can often be no more than subtotal because of the proximity of the tumor to eloquent brain areas or the lack of a distinct boundary between the tumor and the surrounding tissue. The overall treatment plan is usually a combination of different treatment modalities, chosen with consideration of the patient's general condition and the location, extent, and degree of malignity of the tumor.

Symptomatic treatment. *Edema:* The antiedematous action of glucocorticosteroids

takes effect several hours after they are administered; thus, acute intracranial hypertension must be treated with an intravenously given osmotic agent (20% mannitol). Glycerol can be given orally to lower the corticosteroid dose in chronic therapy. *Antiepileptic drugs* (e. g., phenytoin or carbamazepine) are indicated if the patient has already had one or more seizures, or else prophylactically in patients with rapidly growing tumors and in the acute postoperative setting. *Pain* often requires treatment (headache, painful neoplastic meningeosis, painful local tumor invasion; cf. WHO staged treatment scheme for cancer-related pain). *Restlessness:* treatment of cerebral edema, psychotropic drugs (levomepromazine, melperone, chlorprothixene). *Antithrombotic prophylaxis:* Subcutaneous heparin.

Grade I tumors. Some benign tumors, such as those discovered incidentally, can simply be observed—for example, with MRI scans repeated every 6 months—but most should be surgically resected, as a total resection is usually curative. Residual tumor after surgery can often be treated radiosurgically (if indicated by the histological diagnosis). Pituitary tumors and craniopharyngiomas can cause endocrine disturbances. Meningiomas and craniopharyngiomas rarely recur after (total) resection.

Grade II tumors. Five-year survival rate is 50–80%. Complete surgical resection of grade II tumors can be curative. As these tumors grow slowly, they are often less aggressively resected than malignant tumors, so as not to produce a neurological deficit (partial resection, later resection of regrown tumor if necessary). Observation with serial MRI rather than surgical resection may be an appropriate option in some patients after the diagnosis has been established by stereotactic biopsy; surgery and/or radiotherapy will be needed later in case of clinical or radiological progression. Chemotherapy is indicated for unresectable (or no longer resectable) tumors, or after failure of radiotherapy

Grade III tumors. Patients with grade III tumors survive a median of 2 years from the time of diagnosis with the best current treatment involving multiple modalities (surgery, radiotherapy, chemotherapy). Many patients, however, live considerably longer. There are still inadequate data on the potential efficacy of chemotherapy against malignant forms of meningioma, plexus papilloma, pineocytoma, schwannoma, hemangiopericytoma, and pituitary adenoma.

Grade IV tumors. Patients with grade IV tumors survive a median of ca. 10 months from diagnosis even with the best current multimodality treatment (surgery, radiotherapy, chemotherapy). The 5-year survival rate of patients with glioblastoma is no more than 5%. PNET (including medulloblastoma) and primary cerebral lymphoma have median survival times of a few years.

Cerebral metastases: Solitary, surgically accessible metastases are resected as long as there is no acute progression of the underlying malignant disease, or for tissue diagnosis if the primary tumor is of unknown type. Solitary metastases of diameter less than 3 cm can also be treated with local radiotherapy, in one of two forms: interstitial radiotherapy with surgically implanted radioactive material (brachytherapy), or stereotactic radiosurgery. The latter is a closed technique, requiring no incision, employing multiple radioactive cobalt sources (as in the Gamma Knife and X-Knife) or a linear accelerator. Solitary or multiple brain metastases in the setting of progressive primary disease are generally treated with whole-brain irradiation. Chemotherapy is indicated for tumors of known responsiveness to chemotherapy in patients whose general condition is satisfactory. Metastatic small-cell lung cancer, primary CNS lymphoma, and germ cell tumors are treated with radiotherapy or chemotherapy rather than surgery.

Spinal metastases: Resection and radiotherapy for localized tumors; radiotherapy alone for diffuse metastatic disease.

Leptomeningeal metastases: Chemotherapy (systemic, intrathecal, or intraventricular); irradiation of neuraxis.

■ Aftercare

Follow-up examinations are scheduled at shorter or longer intervals depending on the degree of malignity of the neoplasm and on the outcome of initial management (usually involving some combination of surgery, radiotherapy, and chemotherapy), with adjustment for individual factors and for any complications that may be encountered in the further course of the disease. A single CT or MRI scan 3 months postoperatively may suffice for the patient with a completely resected, benign tumor, while patients with malignant tumors should be followed up by examination every 6 weeks and neuroimaging every 3 months, at least initially. Later visits can be less frequent if the tumor does not recur.

Central Nervous System

Traumatic Brain Injury (TBI)

The outcome of traumatic brain injury depends on the type and extent of the acute (primary) injury and its secondary and late sequelae.

Direct/indirect history. A history of the precipitating event and of the patient's condition at the scene should be obtained from the patient (if possible), or from an eyewitness, or both. Vomiting or an epileptic seizure in the acute aftermath of the event should be noted. Also important are the past medical history, current medications (particularly anticoagulants), and any history of alcoholism or drug abuse.

Physical examination. *General:* Open wounds, fractures, bruises, bleeding or clear discharge from the nose or ear. *Neurological:* Respiration, circulation, pupils, motor function, other focal signs.

Diagnostic studies. *Laboratory:* Blood count, coagulation, electrolytes, blood glucose, urea, creatinine, serum osmolality, blood alcohol, drug levels in urine, pregnancy testing if indicated.

Essential radiological studies: Head CT with brain and bone windows is mandatory in all cases unless the neurological examination is completely normal. A cervical spine series from C1 to C7 is needed to rule out associated cervical injury. Plain films of the skull are generally unnecessary if CT is performed.

Additional studies, as indicated: Cranial or spinal MRI or MR angiography, EEG, Doppler ultrasonography, evoked potentials.

In multiorgan trauma: Blood should be typed and cross-matched and several units should be kept ready for transfusion as needed. Physical examination and ancillary studies for any fractures, abdominal bleeding, pulmonary injury.

■ Primary Injury

The primary injury affects different parts of the skull and brain depending on the precipitating event. The traumatic lesion may be focal (hematoma, contusion, infarct, localized edema) or diffuse (hypoxic injury, subarachnoid hemorrhage, generalized edema). The worse the injury, the more severe the impairment of consciousness (pp. 116 ff). The clinical assessment of impairment of consciousness is described on pp. 378 f (Tables 33 and 34).

Region	Type of Injury
Scalp	Cephalhematoma (neonates), laceration, scalping injury
Skull	• *Fracture mechanism*: Bending fracture (caused by blows to the head, etc.), burst fracture (caused by broad skull compression) • *Fracture type*: Linear fracture (fissure, fissured fracture, separation of cranial sutures), impression fracture, fracture with multiple fragments, puncture fracture, growing skull fracture (in children only) • *Fracture site*: Convexity (calvaria), base of skull • *Basilar skull fracture*: Frontobasal (bilateral periorbital hematoma ("raccoon sign"), bleeding from nose/mouth, CSF rhinorrhea) or laterobasal (hearing loss, eardrum lesion, bleeding from the ear canal, CSF otorrhea, facial nerve palsy) • *Facial skull fracture*: LeFort I–III midface fracture; orbital base fracture
Dura mater	Open head trauma[1], CSF leak, pneumocephalus, pneumatocele
Blood vessels	Acute epidural, subdural, subarachnoid or intraparenchymal hemorrhage; carotid–cavernous sinus fistula; arterial dissection
Brain[2]	• Contusion • Diffuse axonal injury (clinical features: coma, autonomic dysfunction, decortication or decerebration, no focal lesion on CT or MRI) • Penetrating (open or closed[3]) injury, or perforating (open) injury • Brainstem injury

1 Wound with open dura and exposure of brain (definition). **2** Excluding cranial nerve lesions. **3** Without dural penetration (definition).

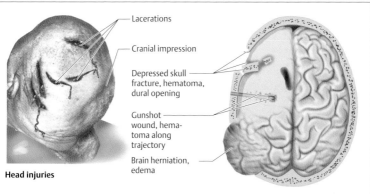

Lacerations

Cranial impression

Depressed skull fracture, hematoma, dural opening

Gunshot wound, hematoma along trajectory

Brain herniation, edema

Head injuries

Head trauma (schematic)

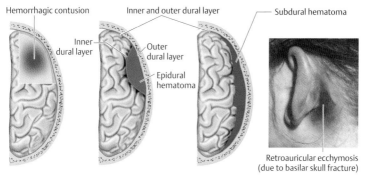

Hemorrhagic contusion

Inner and outer dural layer

Subdural hematoma

Inner dural layer

Outer dural layer

Epidural hematoma

Retroauricular ecchymosis (due to basilar skull fracture)

Traumatic intracranial hematoma

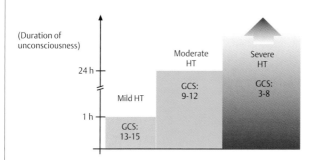

(Duration of unconsciousness)

24 h

1 h

Moderate HT

Severe HT

Mild HT

GCS: 13-15

GCS: 9-12

GCS: 3-8

Classification of head trauma (HT) **by Glasgow Coma Scale** (GCS)

Central Nervous System

Trauma

■ Secondary Sequelae of TBI

Type of Sequela	Location/Syndrome	Special Features
Neurological		
● Hematoma	⇨ Epidural	⇨ Lucid interval[1], immediate unconsciousness, or progressive deterioration of consciousness
	⇨ Subdural	⇨ May be asymptomatic at first, with progressive decline of consciousness
	⇨ Subarachnoid	⇨ Meningism
	⇨ Intraparenchymal	⇨ Intracranial hypertension, ⇧focal signs; often a severe injury
● Intracranial hypertension	● Cerebral edema, hydrocephalus, massive hematoma	● See p. 162. Risk of herniation
● Ischemia	● Vasospasm, arterial dissection, fat embolism	● Acute focal signs
● Epileptic seizure	● Focal or generalized	● Common in focal injury
● Infection	● CSF leak, open head injury	● Recurrent meningitis, encephalitis, empyema, abscess, ventriculitis
● Amnesia	● Anterograde/retrograde	● See p. 134
General		
● Hypotension, hypoxia, anemia	● Shock, respiratory failure	● Multiple trauma, pneumothorax or hemothorax, pericardial tamponade, blood loss, coagulopathy
● Fever, meningitis	● Infection	● Pneumonia, sepsis, CSF leak
● Fluid imbalance	● Hypothalamic lesion	● Diabetes insipidus[2], SIADH[3]

1 Patient immediately loses consciousness ⇨ awakens and appears normal for a few hours ⇨ again loses consciousness. **2** Polyuria, polydipsia, nocturia, serum osmolality > 295 mOsm/kg, ⇩ urine osmolality. **3** Syndrome of inappropriate secretion of ADH: euvolemia, serum osmolality < 275 mOsm/kg, excessively concentrated urine (urine osmolality > 100 mOsm/kg), ⇧urinary sodium despite normal salt/water intake; absence of adrenal, thyroid, pituitary and renal dysfunction.

For overview of late complications of head trauma, see p. 379 (Table 35).

■ Prognosis

Head trauma causes physical impairment and behavioral abnormalities whose severity is correlated with that of the initial injury.

Severity[1]	Prognosis
Mild	Posttraumatic syndrome resolves within 1 year in 85–90 % of patients. The remaining 10–15 % develop a chronic posttraumatic syndrome
Moderate	The symptoms and signs resolve more slowly and less completely than those of mild head injury. The prognosis appears to be worse for focal than for diffuse injuries. Reliable data on the long-term prognosis are not available
Severe	Age-dependent mortality ranges from 30 % to 80 %. Younger patients have a better prognosis than older patients. Late behavioral changes (impairment of memory and concentration, abnormal affect, personality changes)

1 For severity of head trauma, cf. pp. 378 f, Tables 33 and 34.

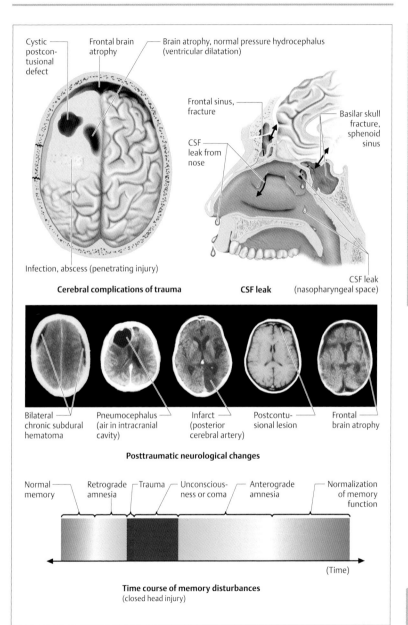

Cystic postcontusional defect

Frontal brain atrophy

Brain atrophy, normal pressure hydrocephalus (ventricular dilatation)

Frontal sinus, fracture

Basilar skull fracture, sphenoid sinus

CSF leak from nose

Infection, abscess (penetrating injury)

CSF leak (nasopharyngeal space)

Cerebral complications of trauma

CSF leak

Bilateral chronic subdural hematoma

Pneumocephalus (air in intracranial cavity)

Infarct (posterior cerebral artery)

Postcontusional lesion

Frontal brain atrophy

Posttraumatic neurological changes

Normal memory

Retrograde amnesia

Trauma

Unconsciousness or coma

Anterograde amnesia

Normalization of memory function

(Time)

Time course of memory disturbances (closed head injury)

■ Posttraumatic Headache

Posttraumatic headache may be acute (<8 weeks after head trauma) or chronic (>8 weeks). The duration and intensity of the headache are not correlated with the severity of the precipitating head trauma. It can be focal or diffuse, continuous or episodic. It often worsens with physical exertion, mental stress, and tension and improves with rest and stress avoidance. Its type and extent are highly variable. If the headache gradually increases in severity, or if a new neurological deficit arises, further studies should be performed to exclude a late posttraumatic complication, such as chronic subdural hematoma (p. 379).

■ Pathogenesis of Traumatic Brain Injury

Direct blunt or penetrating injuries of the head and acceleration/deceleration injuries can damage the scalp, skull, meninges, cerebral vasculature, ventricular system, and brain parenchyma. The term *primary injury* refers to the initial mechanical damage to these tissues. Traumatized brain tissue is more sensitive to physiological changes than nontraumatized tissue. *Secondary injury* is caused by cellular dysfunction due to focal or global changes in cerebral blood flow and metabolism. Mechanisms involved in secondary injury include disruption of the blood–brain barrier, hypoxia, neurochemical changes (increased concentrations of acetylcholine, norepinephrine, dopamine, epinephrine, magnesium, calcium, and excitatory amino acids such as glutamate), cytotoxic processes (production of free radicals and of calcium-activated proteases and lipases), and inflammatory responses (edema, influx of leukocytes and macrophages, cytokine release).
Epidural hematoma. Bleeding into the epidural space (pp. 6, 267) due to detachment of the outer dural sheath from the skull and rupture of a meningeal artery (usually the middle meningeal artery, torn by a linear fracture of the temporal bone). Epidural hematoma is less frequently of venous origin (usually due to tearing of a venous sinus by a skull fracture).
Subdural hematoma. Bleeding into the subdural space (pp. 6, 176, 267) because of disruption of larger bridging veins; often accompanied by focal contusion of the underlying brain. Frequently located in the temporal region.

Intracerebral hematoma. Bleeding into the tissue of the brain (intraparenchymal hematoma) under the site of impact, on the opposite side (*contre-coup*), or in the ventricular system (intraventricular hemorrhage) (pp. 176, 267).
Subarachnoid hemorrhage. Rupture of pial vessels.

■ Treatment

At the scene of the accident. The scene should be secured to prevent further injury to the injured person, bystanders, or rescuers. *First aid:* Evaluation and clearing of the airway; cardiopulmonary resuscitation (CPR) if necessary. Immobilization of the cervical spine with a hard collar. Recognition and treatment of hemodynamic instability (keep systolic blood pressure above 120 mmHg), fluid administration as needed ("small volume resuscitation" with hyperoncotic-hypertonic solutions'). Dressing of wounds, sedation if necessary to reduce agitation, elevation of the upper body to 30°. *Documentation:* Time and nature of accident, general and neurological findings, drugs given. *Transport:* Cardiorespiratory monitoring.
In the hospital. Systematic assessment and treatment by organ system, with documentation of all measures taken. Cardiorespiratory monitoring: monitoring of blood gases and blood pressure (cerebral perfusion pressure >60–70 mmHg, p. 162). *Respiratory system:* Supplementary oxygen, intubation, and ventilation as needed. *Cardiovascular system:* Central venous access, administration of fluids and pressors as needed. Treatment of fever or hyperthermia. Administration of anticonvulsants as needed. Evaluation of tetanus vaccination status. Immediate *neurosurgical consultation* regarding the possible need for surgery. *Treatment of intracranial hypertension:* Sedatives, analgesics; if ICP (p. 162) is above 20–25 mmHg, osmotherapy with 20% mannitol, bolus of 0.35 mg/kg over 10–15 minutes, repeated every 4–8 hours as needed; barbiturate coma (thiopental); decompressive bifrontal craniectomy may be indicated in refractory cerebral edema.

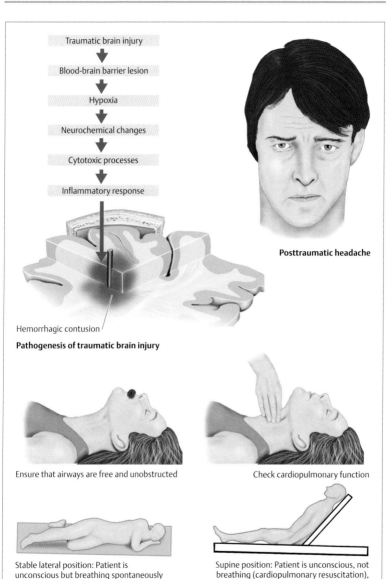

Traumatic brain injury

↓

Blood-brain barrier lesion

↓

Hypoxia

↓

Neurochemical changes

↓

Cytotoxic processes

↓

Inflammatory response

Posttraumatic headache

Hemorrhagic contusion

Pathogenesis of traumatic brain injury

Ensure that airways are free and unobstructed

Check cardiopulmonary function

Stable lateral position: Patient is unconscious but breathing spontaneously

Supine position: Patient is unconscious, not breathing (cardiopulmonary resuscitation), and may have spinal injury. Elevate upper body if there is a head injury

First-aid measures at scene of accident

Spinal Trauma

Spinal injury can involve the vertebrae, ligaments, intervertebral disks, blood vessels, muscles, nerve roots, and spinal cord. The spinal cord and spinal nerve roots may be directly injured (e. g. by gunshot or stab wounds) or secondarily affected by compression (bone fragments), hyperextension (spinal instability), and vascular lesions (ischemia, hemorrhage). *Diagnosis:* Bone injuries can be identified by radiography and/or CT; spinal cord lesions (hemorrhage, contusion, edema, transection) and soft-tissue lesions (hematoma, edema, arterial dissection) are best seen on MRI.

Cervical spine distortion (whiplash injury). *Indirect* spinal trauma (head-on or rear-end collision) leads to sudden passive retroflexion and subsequent anteflexion of the neck. The forces acting on the spine (acceleration, deceleration, rotation, traction) can produce both cervical spine injuries (spinal cord, nerve roots, retropharyngeal space, bones, ligaments, joints, intervertebral disks, blood vessels) and cranial injuries (brain, eyes, temporomandibular joint). There may be an interval of 4–48 hours until symptoms develop, rarely longer (asymptomatic period). *Symptoms and signs:* Pain in the head, neck, and shoulders, neck stiffness, and vertigo may be accompanied by forgetfulness, poor concentration, insomnia, and lethargy. The symptoms usually resolve within 3–12 months but persist for longer periods in 15–20% of patients, for unknown reasons. *Severity classification:* Grade I = no neurological deficit or radiological abnormality, grade II = neurological deficit without radiological abnormality, grade III = neurological deficit and radiological abnormality.

Vertebral fracture. It must be determined whether the fracture is stable or unstable; if it is unstable, any movement can cause (further) damage to the spinal cord and nerve roots. Thus, all patients who may have vertebral fractures must be transported in a stabilized supine position, with the head in a neutral position (e. g., on a vacuum mattress). Repositioning the patient manually with the "collar splint grip," "paddle grip," or "bridge grip" should be avoided if possible. In the assessment of stability, it is useful to consider the spinal column and intervertebral disks as composed of three columns. Involvement of only one column = stable injury; two columns = potentially unstable; three columns = unstable. For details, see p. 380 (Table 36).

Trauma to nerve roots and brachial plexus. *Nerve root lesions* usually involve the ventral roots, and thus usually produce a motor rather than sensory deficit. Nerve root avulsion may be suspected on the basis of (multi)radicular findings and/or Horner syndrome and can be confirmed by myelography (empty root sleeves, bulging of the subarachnoid space) or MRI. Downward or backward traction on the shoulder and arm (as in a motorcycle accident) can produce severe *brachial plexus injuries* accompanied by nerve root avulsion. Brachial plexus lesions can also be caused by improper patient positioning during general anesthesia, intense supraclavicular pressure (backpack paralysis), or local trauma (stab or gunshot wound, bone fragments, contusion, avulsion). These injuries more commonly affect the upper portion of the brachial plexus (pp. 34, 321).

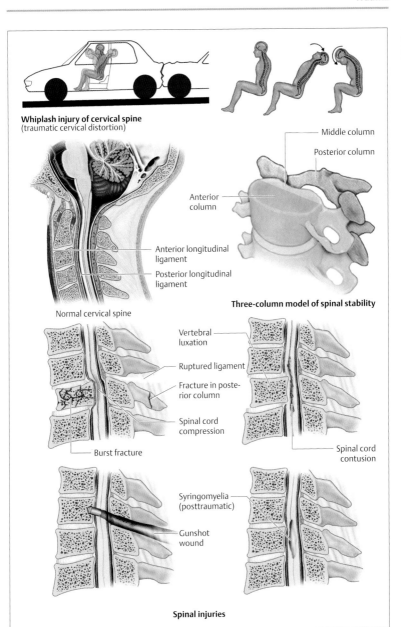

Whiplash injury of cervical spine
(traumatic cervical distortion)

Middle column

Posterior column

Anterior column

Anterior longitudinal ligament

Posterior longitudinal ligament

Three-column model of spinal stability

Normal cervical spine

Vertebral luxation

Ruptured ligament

Fracture in posterior column

Spinal cord compression

Burst fracture

Spinal cord contusion

Syringomyelia (posttraumatic)

Gunshot wound

Spinal injuries

Spinal Cord Trauma

Open spinal cord trauma, by definition, involves penetration of the dura mater by a stab wound, gunshot wound, bone fragment, or severely dislocated vertebra. *Closed* spinal cord trauma (with dura intact) is the indirect effect of a non-penetrating injury. The result may be a complete or incomplete *spinal cord transection syndrome* (p. 48; Table 37, p. 380).

Acute stage (spinal shock). The acute manifestations of spinal cord transection syndrome are seen below the level of the injury and include the total loss of voluntary and reflex *motor function* (flaccid paraplegia or quadriplegia, areflexia) and *sensation*, and *autonomic dysfunction* (urinary retention ⇨ overflow incontinence, intestinal atony ⇨ paralytic bowel obstruction, anhidrosis ⇨ hyperthermia, cardiovascular dysfunction ⇨ orthostatic hypotension, cardiac arrhythmia, paroxysmal hypertension). Patients are usually stable enough to begin rehabilitation in 3–6 weeks (rehabilitation stage, see below). For acute treatment, see p. 380 (Table 38).

Rehabilitation stage. The neurological deficits depend on the level of the lesion.

Level[1]	Motor Deficit	Sensory Deficit[2]	Autonomic Deficit[3]
C1–C3[4]	Quadriplegia, neck muscle paresis, spasticity, respiratory paralysis	Sensory level at back of head/edge of lower jaw; pain in back of head, neck, and shoulders	Voluntary control of bladder, bowel, and sexual function replaced by reflex control; Horner syndrome
C4–C5	Quadriplegia, diaphragmatic breathing	Sensory level at clavicle/shoulder	Same as above
C6–C8[5]	Quadriplegia, spasticity, flaccid arm paresis, diaphragmatic breathing	Sensory level at upper chest wall/back; arms involved, shoulders spared	Same as above
T1–T5	Paraplegia, diminished respiratory volume	Sensory loss from inner surface of lower arm, upper chest wall, back region downward	Voluntary control of bladder, bowel, and sexual function replaced by reflex control
T5–T10	Paraplegia, spasticity	Sensory level on chest wall and back corresponding to level of spinal cord injury	Same as above
T11–L3	Flaccid paraplegia	Sensory loss from groin/ventral thigh downward, depending on level of injury	Same as above
L4–S2[6]	Distal flaccid paraplegia	Sensory loss at shin/dorsum of foot/posterior thigh downward, depending on level of injury	Flaccid paralysis of bladder and bowel, loss of erectile function
S3–S5[7]	No motor deficit	Sensory loss in perianal region and inner thigh	Flaccid paralysis of bladder and bowel, loss of erectile function

1 Spinal cord level (not the same as vertebral level). **2** See p. 32 ff. **3** Disturbance of bladder, bowel, rectal, and erectile function, sweating, and blood pressure regulation; p. 140 ff. **4** High cervical cord lesion. **5** Low cervical cord lesion. **6** Epiconus. **7** Conus medullaris.

Chronic stage—late sequelae. Persistence of neurological deficits; assorted complications including venous thrombosis, pulmonary embolism, respiratory insufficiency, bowel obstruction, urinary tract infections, sexual dysfunction, cardiovascular disturbances, spasticity, chronic pain, bed sores, heterotopic ossification, and syringomyelia.

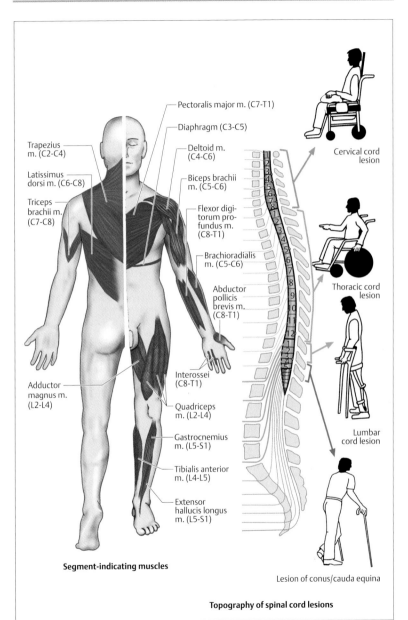

Pectoralis major m. (C7-T1)

Diaphragm (C3-C5)

Deltoid m. (C4-C6)

Biceps brachii m. (C5-C6)

Flexor digitorum profundus m. (C8-T1)

Brachioradialis m. (C5-C6)

Abductor pollicis brevis m. (C8-T1)

Interossei (C8-T1)

Quadriceps m. (L2-L4)

Gastrocnemius m. (L5-S1)

Tibialis anterior m. (L4-L5)

Extensor hallucis longus m. (L5-S1)

Trapezius m. (C2-C4)

Latissimus dorsi m. (C6-C8)

Triceps brachii m. (C7-C8)

Adductor magnus m. (L2-L4)

Segment-indicating muscles

Cervical cord lesion

Thoracic cord lesion

Lumbar cord lesion

Lesion of conus/cauda equina

Topography of spinal cord lesions

■ **Signs of Cerebellar Dysfunction**

Loss of coordination and balance. *Ataxia* is uncoordinated, irregular, and poorly articulated movement (dyssynergy). The typical patient sways while sitting (*truncal ataxia*) or standing (*postural ataxia*), undershoots or overshoots an intended target of movement (*dysmetria* = hypometria or hypermetria), and walks with quick, irregular steps in an unsteady, swaying, broad-based gait reminiscent of alcohol intoxication (*gait ataxia*, p. 54). Pointing tests are used to detect dysmetria, incoordination, and tremor that is worst as a movement approaches its target (*intention tremor*); the *finger–nose, finger–finger, and heel–knee–shin tests* should be carried out with the eyes open and closed. *Bárány's pointing test:* The patient is asked to close his or her eyes, touch the doctor's finger with his or her own index finger, then lower and raise the still outstretched arm and touch the doctor's finger again; the patient's finger deviates laterally from the target, and the direction of deviation is toward the side of the lesion. Unsteadiness of stance of cerebellar origin, which may be so severe as to make standing impossible (*astasia*), is not influenced by opening or closing the eyes (*Romberg sign*) and differs in this respect from spinal (sensory) ataxia. Stepping in place for 30–60 seconds with the eyes closed causes the body to turn to the side of the lesion. Patients with mild ataxia find it difficult or impossible to walk a straight line (*abasia*; detected by heel-to-toe walking, tandem gait). The patient may be unable to perform rapid alternating movements (*dysdiadochokinesia)*. The handwriting is enlarged (*macrographia*), coarse, and shaky, and the patient's drawing of parallel lines or a spiral is unsatisfactory.

Dysarthria. The patient's speech (p. 130) is slow, unclear (babbling, slurred), and monotonous (*dysarthrophonia*), and possibly also discontinuous (choppy, faltering, or scanning speech). There is poor coordination of breathing with the flow of speech, resulting in a sudden transition from soft to loud speech (explosive speech).

Oculomotor disturbances. Gaze-evoked nystagmus is a frequent finding in cerebellar disease. Voluntary saccades are too short or too long (*ocular dysmetria*) and are therefore followed by afterbeats. Slow pursuit movements are jerky (saccadic). Patients are frequently unable to suppress the vestibulo-ocular reflex (p. 26), i.e., the normal visual suppression of nystagmus is impaired. The result is impaired visual fixation on turning of the head.

Muscle tone. Decreased muscle tone is mainly found in patients with acute unilateral lesions of the cerebellum. The examiner can detect it by passively swinging or shaking the patient's limbs, or by testing for the *rebound phenomenon*. The patient is asked to extend the arms with the eyes closed (*posture test*) and the examiner lightly taps on one wrist, causing deflection of the arm. The rebound movement undershoots or overshoots the original arm position. Alternatively, the patient can be asked to flex the elbow against resistance. When the examiner suddenly releases the resistance, the affected arm rebounds unchecked.

■ **Topography of Cerebellar Lesions**

Lesions of the cerebellum and its afferent and efferent connections (p. 54) produce characteristic signs of cerebellar disease. Expanding lesions may go on to produce further, extracerebellar deficits (e. g., cranial nerve palsies, hemiparesis, sensory loss).

■ **Special Diagnostic Studies**

The diagnostic studies to be obtained depend on the clinical findings (to be described below) and may include imaging studies (MRI, CT), neurophysiological studies (nerve conduction studies, electromyography), ECG, pathological studies (of tissue, blood, CSF, bone marrow, muscle, or nerve biopsy specimens), and/or ophthalmological consultation (optic nerve atrophy, Kayser–Fleischer ring, tapetoretinal degeneration).

■ **Idiopathic Cerebellar Ataxia (IDCA)**

This group of disorders includes various forms of nonfamilial cerebellar ataxia of unknown cause with onset in adulthood (generally age 25 years or older). IDCA occurs as an isolated disturbance or as a component of multiple system atrophy (MSA; p. 302).

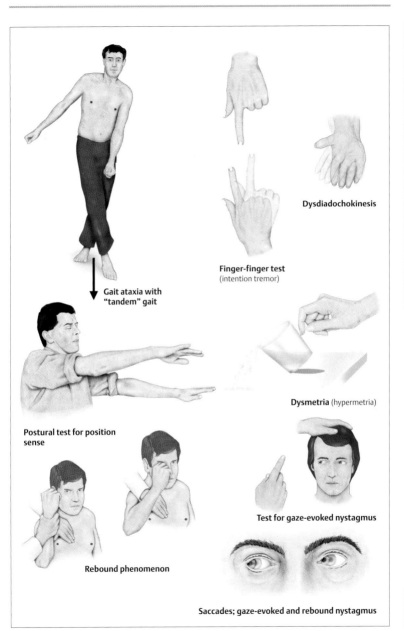

Gait ataxia with "tandem" gait

Finger-finger test (intention tremor)

Dysdiadochokinesis

Dysmetria (hypermetria)

Postural test for position sense

Rebound phenomenon

Test for gaze-evoked nystagmus

Saccades; gaze-evoked and rebound nystagmus

Acquired Cerebellar Syndromes

Onset	Etiology	Symptoms and Signs
Acute (minutes to hours)	• Infection[1]	• Viral infection: varicella-zoster virus, Epstein–Barr virus, rubella, mumps, influenza, parainfluenza, echovirus, coxsackievirus, cytomegalovirus, FSME, herpes simplex virus. Children are more commonly affected than adults. Special type: opsoclonus-ataxia syndrome[2]. • Abscess • Miller Fisher syndrome (ataxia, ophthalmoplegia, areflexia; p. 395)
	• Vascular	• Brainstem signs (pp. 70 ff., 170) predominate • Infarcts can be differentiated from hemorrhages by imaging studies • Early treatment, often neurosurgical, may be needed to prevent rapid development of life-threatening complications (p. 174 f)
	• Toxic	• Alcohol, barbiturates, phenytoin, lithium
Subacute (days to weeks)	• Tumor[3] • Paraneoplastic[4]	• Occipital pain (radiating to forehead, nuchal region, and shoulders), recurrent vomiting, stiff neck, vertigo, truncal ataxia; obstructive hydrocephalus • Cerebellar dysfunction may appear months or years before the tumor is discovered. Anti-Purkinje-cell antibodies are present in the serum and CSF of patients with neuron loss
	• Toxic • Other	• Alcohol • Medications (anticonvulsants, e. g., phenytoin; lithium, 5-fluorouracil, cytosine arabinoside) • Heavy metals (mercury, thallium, lead) • Solvents (toluene, carbon tetrachloride) • Hypoxia, heat stroke, hyperthermia
Chronic (months to years)	• Infection	• Progressive rubella panencephalitis (very rare complication of congenital rubella infection in boys; onset at age 8 to 19 years; characterized by ataxia, dementia, spasticity, and dysarthria) • Creutzfeldt–Jakob disease (p. 252)
	• Vascular • Metabolic	• Meningeal siderosis causes ataxia and partial or complete hearing loss (leptomeningeal deposition of hemosiderin in chronic subarachnoid hemorrhage ⇨ vascular malformations, oligodendroglioma, ependymoma of the cauda equina, postoperative occurrence) • Hypothyroidism, malabsorption syndrome (vitamin E deficiency), thiamin deficiency (acute ⇨ Wernicke encephalopathy) • Refsum disease[5] (↑serum phytanic acid level, p. 332) • Wilson disease[5] (ataxia, tremor, dysarthrophonia, dysphagia, dystonia, behavioral disturbances, p. 307)
Intermittent	• Metabolic[5]	• Hereditary metabolic disorders in neonates, children, and juveniles (see also pp. 306 f, 386 f) • Disorders of amino acid metabolism (hyperammonemia, Hartnup syndrome, maple syrup urine disease) • Storage diseases (metachromatic leukodystrophy, neuronal ceroid lipofuscinosis, sialidosis, GM$_2$ gangliosidosis)

1 Partial listing; numerous infections can cause ataxia as part of the syndrome of encephalomyelitis. **2** High-frequency bursts of saccades in all directions of gaze without an intersaccadic interval. **3** See p. 254 ff; cerebellar astrocytoma, medulloblastoma, ependymoma, hemangioblastoma (von Hippel–Lindau disease), meningioma of the cerebellopontine angle, metastases (lung cancer, breast cancer, melanoma). **4** Antibodies (p. 388) against Hu, Yo, TR, CV2, Ma1, CRD1, CRD2, Ma2, and mGluR1. **5** Genetic; listed here for differential diagnostic purposes.

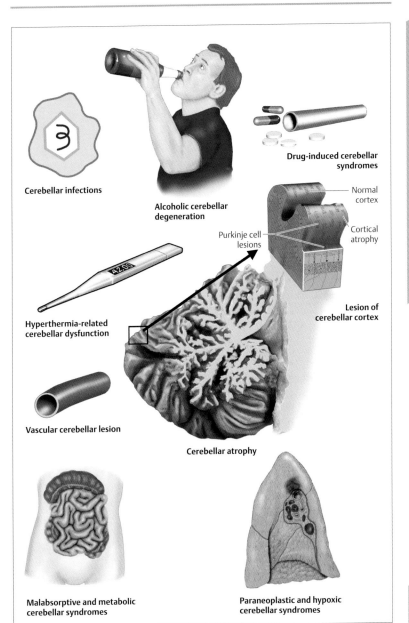

Cerebellar infections

Alcoholic cerebellar degeneration

Drug-induced cerebellar syndromes

Purkinje cell lesions

Normal cortex

Cortical atrophy

Lesion of cerebellar cortex

Hyperthermia-related cerebellar dysfunction

Vascular cerebellar lesion

Cerebellar atrophy

Malabsorptive and metabolic cerebellar syndromes

Paraneoplastic and hypoxic cerebellar syndromes

Hereditary Cerebellar Syndromes

■ Autosomal Recessive Cerebellar Syndromes (partial listing)

Syndrome	Symptoms and Signs	CL[1]/Gene Product
Friedreich ataxia[2,7]	*Usual manifestations:* • Progressive limb/gait ataxia • Age of onset < 30 years • Areflexia in legs • Neurophysiological evidence of sensory neuropathy *Variable manifestations:* • Dysarthria, distal muscular atrophy/paresis (ca. 50 %), pes cavus (ca. 50 %), scoliosis, optic nerve atrophy (ca. 25 %), nystagmus (ca. 20 %), oculomotor disturbances (p. 276), hearing loss (ca. 10 %), cardiomyopathy (ca. 65 %), diabetes mellitus (ca. 10 %)	9q13, 9p23-p11/ frataxin *Mutation:* Extended GAA-trinucleotide repeat
Ataxia with vitamin E deficiency[7] (serum: ⇓ vitamin E, ⇓ cholesterol/ triglycerides)	• Onset in childhood or adulthood • Gait ataxia • Dysarthria • Other symptoms similar to those of Friedreich ataxia	8q13.1-q13.3/α-tocopherol transfer protein
Abetalipoprotein-emia[3,7] (p. 300)	• Steatorrhea, other symptoms similar to those of Friedreich ataxia	4q24/triglyceride transfer protein
Ataxia-telangiec-tasia[4,7]	• Ataxia first seen when child learns to walk • Choreoathetosis • Oculomotor disturbances[5] • Oculocutaneous telangiectases • Immunodeficiency (frequent infections) • Increased risk of malignant tumors • Elevated serum α-fetoprotein	11q22.3/phosphatidyl-inositol-3'-kinase and rad3[6]

1 Chromosome location (CL). **2** Classic form. **3** Bassen–Kornzweig syndrome; vitamin A and E deficiency, low cholesterol/ triglyceride levels, acanthocytosis. **4** Louis-Bar syndrome. **5** Oculomotor apraxia. **6** DNA repair kinase/cell cycle control; ataxia-telangiectasia-mutated (ATM) gene. **7** A direct gene test is available.

For mitochondrial syndromes with ataxia, see p. 403.

■ Autosomal Dominant Cerebellar Syndromes (partial listing)

Syndrome	Symptoms and Signs	CL/Gene Product
Autosomal dominant cerebellar ataxia (ADCA); spinocerebellar ataxia (SCA)[1]	• ADCA1: Ataxia, ophthalmoplegia, pyramidal/extrapyramidal disturbances (p. 44); SCA1[5], SCA2[5], SCA3[2,5], SCA4, SCA8[5], SCA12, SCA13, SCA17 • ADCA2: Ataxia, retinopathy, SCA7[5] • ADCA3: Predominant cerebellar ataxia; SCA5, SCA6[5], SCA10, SCA11, SCA12[5], SCA14, SCA15, SCA16	SCA1: 6p23/ataxin1 SCA2: 12q24/ataxin2 SCA3: 14q24.3-q31/MJD1 protein SCA4: 16q22.1 SCA5: 11p11-q11 SCA6: 19p13/α-1A calcium channel SCA7: 3p21.1-p12
Episodic ataxia (EA)[3]	• EA1: Episodes of ataxia lasting seconds to minutes, 1 to 10 times daily; provoked by abrupt changes of position, emotional or physical stress, and caloric vestibular stimulation; myokymia in face and hands between attacks; continuous spontaneous activity in resting EMG	• 12p13[5]/potassium channel (point mutation)
	• EA2: Episodes of ataxia lasting minutes to hours (rarely days) of variable frequency (daily to yearly); headache, tinnitus, vertigo, ataxia, nausea, vomiting, nystagmus; induced by same stimuli as EA1; ataxia, nystagmus, and head tremor between attacks	• 19p13[5]/voltage-gated calcium channel[4] (point mutation)
Gerstmann–Sträussler–Scheinker syndrome (p. 252)	Onset between the ages 40 and 50 years; presents with cerebellar ataxia; dysarthrophonia, dementia, nystagmus, rigor, visual disturbances, and hearing loss develop in the course of the disease	20pter-p12/P102L
Fatal familial insomnia (p. 252)	Progressive insomnia, autonomic dysfunction (arterial hypertension, tachycardia, hyperthermia, hyperhidrosis), myoclonus, tremor, ataxia	20pter-p12/D178N

1 Definitive identification of the SCA types listed is possible only with molecular genetics tests (examples in right column, see OMIM for details). **2** Machado–Joseph disease (MJD). **3** Other forms: EA3 and EA4. **4** Other mutations of this gene are associated with SCA6 and familial hemiplegic migraine. **5** A direct genetic test is available.

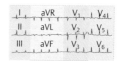

Cardiomyopathy in FA
(ECG shows repolarization
disturbances and left axis deviation)

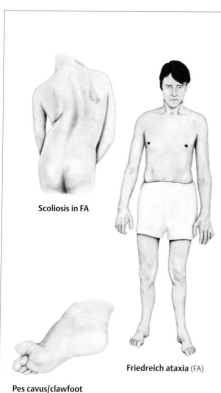

Scoliosis in FA

Pes cavus/clawfoot

Friedreich ataxia (FA)

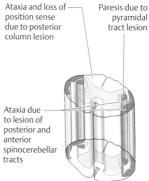

Ataxia and loss of
position sense
due to posterior
column lesion

Paresis due to
pyramidal
tract lesion

Ataxia due
to lesion of
posterior and
anterior
spinocerebellar
tracts

Spinal degeneration in FA

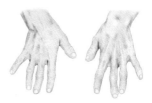

Distal muscular atrophy

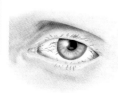

Ocular telangiectasia

Acanthocyte
(crenated erythrocyte)
in abetalipoproteinemia

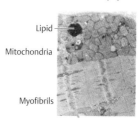

Lipid

Mitochondria

Myofibrils

Mitochondrial encephalomyopathy

Central Nervous System

281

Central Nervous System

The clinical differential diagnosis of myelopathies is based on the level of the spinal cord lesion, the particular structures affected, and the temporal course of the disorder (p. 48, Table 39, p. 381).

Acute Myelopathies

Symptoms and signs develop within minutes, hours, or days.

■ Spinal Cord Trauma
(See p. 274)

■ Myelitis

Viral myelitis (p. 234 ff). Enteroviruses (poliovirus, coxsackievirus, echovirus), herpes zoster virus, varicella zoster virus, FSME, rabies, HTLV-1, HIV, Epstein–Barr virus, cytomegalovirus, herpes simplex virus, postvaccinial myelitis.

Nonviral myelitis (p. 222 ff). Mycoplasma, neuroborreliosis, abscess (epidural, intramedullary), tuberculosis, parasites (echinococcosis, cysticercosis, schistosomiasis), fungi, neurosyphilis, sarcoidosis, postinfectious myelitis, multiple sclerosis/neuromyelitis optica (Devic syndrome), acute necrotizing myelitis, connective tissue disease (vasculitis), paraneoplastic myelitis, subacute myelo-optic neuropathy (SMON), arachnoiditis (after surgical procedures, myelography, or intrathecal drug administration).

■ Vascular Syndromes (p. 22)

Anterior spinal artery syndrome. Segmental paresthesia and pain radiating in a bandlike distribution may precede the development of motor signs by minutes to hours. A flaccid paraparesis or quadriparesis (corticospinal tract, anterior horn) then ensues, along with a dissociated sensory loss from the level of the lesion downward (spinothalamic tract ⇨ impaired pain and temperature sensation, with intact perception of vibration and position) and urinary and fecal incontinence. Often only some of these signs are present.

Posterior spinal artery syndrome is rare and difficult to diagnose. It is characterized by pain in the spine, paresthesiae in the legs, a loss of position and vibration sense below the level of the lesion, and global anesthesia with segmental loss of deep tendon reflexes at the level of the lesion. Larger lesions cause paresis and sphincter dysfunction.

Sulcocommissural artery syndrome. Segmental pain at the level of the lesion, followed by flaccid paresis of ipsilateral arm/leg; loss of proprioception, position sense, and touch perception with contralateral dissociated sensory loss (Brown–Séquard syndrome). Sphincter dysfunction is rare.

Complete spinal infarction. Acute spinal cord transection syndrome with flaccid paraplegia or quadriplegia, sphincter dysfunction, and total sensory loss below the level of the lesion. Autonomic dysfunction may also occur (e. g., vasodilatation, pulmonary edema, intestinal atony, disordered thermoregulation). The cause is often an acute occlusion of the great radicular artery (of Adamkiewicz).

Central spinal infarction. Acute paraplegia, sensory loss, and sphincter paralysis.

Claudication of spinal cord. Physical exercise (running, long walks) induces paresthesiae or paraparesis that resolves with rest and does not occur when the patient is lying down.

Cause: Exercise-related ischemia of the spinal cord due to a dural arteriovenous fistula or high-grade aortic stenosis (see also p. 284).

Dural/perimedullary arteriovenous (AV) fistula is an abnormal communication (shunt) between an artery and vein between the two layers of the dural mater. An arterial branch of a spinal artery feeds directly into a superficial spinal vein, which therefore contains arterial rather than venous blood, flowing in the opposite direction to normal. Paroxysmal stabbing pain and/or episodes of slowly progressing paraparesis and sensory loss separated by periods of remission occur in the early stage of the disorder, which usually affects men between the ages of 40 and 60. If the suspected diagnosis cannot be confirmed by MRI scans (because of low shunt volume), myelography may be helpful (⇨ dilated veins in the subarachnoid space).

Spinal hemorrhage can occur in epidural, subdural, subarachnoid, and intramedullary locations (intramedullary hemorrhage = hematomyelia). *Possible causes:* intradural/intramedullary AV malformation, cavernoma, tumor, aneurysm, trauma, lumbar puncture, and coagulopathy.

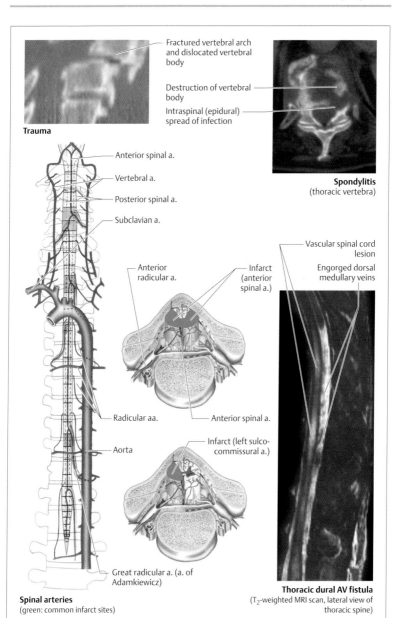

Fractured vertebral arch and dislocated vertebral body

Trauma

Destruction of vertebral body

Intraspinal (epidural) spread of infection

Spondylitis
(thoracic vertebra)

Anterior spinal a.

Vertebral a.

Posterior spinal a.

Subclavian a.

Anterior radicular a.

Infarct (anterior spinal a.)

Radicular aa.

Anterior spinal a.

Aorta

Infarct (left sulco-commissural a.)

Great radicular a. (a. of Adamkiewicz)

Spinal arteries
(green: common infarct sites)

Vascular spinal cord lesion

Engorged dorsal medullary veins

Thoracic dural AV fistula
(T$_2$-weighted MRI scan, lateral view of thoracic spine)

Central Nervous System

283

Subacute and Chronic Myelopathies

Spinal cord syndromes (p. 282) may be subacute or chronic depending on their cause. The complete clinical picture may develop over days to weeks (subacute) or months to years (chronic). For myelopathies due to developmental disorders, see p. 288 ff.

■ Mass Lesions

Syndrome	Symptoms and Signs	Causes	Diagnosis/Treatment[1]
Cervical myelopathy	Progressive paraparesis or quadriparesis, spasticity, Lhermitte's sign, reduced mobility of cervical spine; cervical radiculopathy may also occur	Spinal cord compression[2] by cervical spine lesions[3]	MRI, CT, myelography; evoked potentials, EMG for radicular lesions, plain radiograph of cervical spine. *Treatment:* Surgery for progressive impairment or severe stenosis; otherwise, symptomatic treatment
Lumbar spinal stenosis[4] (intermittent claudication)	*Early:* Paresthesiae (sensation of heaviness) occur upon standing or walking (especially down stairs) and disappear with rest. *Late:* Only partial improvement of paresthesiae with rest; reduced walking range	Compression of cauda equina by lumbar spine lesions[5]	Diagnostic testing as above. *Treatment:* Surgery for severely decreased walking range or persistent symptoms; otherwise, analgesics and physiotherapy (to strengthen trunk muscles)
Syringomyelia[6]	Pain, central cord deficits, kyphoscoliosis	Anomalous development of neural groove, obstruction of CSF flow, trauma, tumor	Diagnostic testing as above. *Treatment:* Surgery for progressive symptoms, especially pain[7]
Neoplasm	Pain, sensory loss, segmental/radicular paresis, Lhermitte's sign (cervical), incomplete or complete spinal cord transection syndrome	*Intramedullary:* Ependymoma, glioma *Extramedullary:* Meningioma, neurofibroma, vascular malformation *Extradural:* Metastasis, sarcoma	Diagnostic testing as above. *Treatment:* Surgery; radiotherapy if indicated; symptom control with corticosteroids and analgesics

1 Principles of diagnosis and treatment. 2 Symptoms arise when sagittal diameter of spinal canal is in the range of 7–12 mm (normal 17–18 mm). 3 Primary spinal canal stenosis, disk protrusion/herniation, spinal degenerative disease (spondylosis, osteochondrosis), hyperextension of cervical spine (trauma, chiropractic maneuvers, dental procedures) in patient with cervical stenosis, Paget disease, or ossification of the posterior longitudinal ligament. 4 Not a myelopathy (the cauda equina is affected); mentioned here for differential diagnostic reasons. 5 Primary spinal canal stenosis, intervertebral disk protrusion/herniation, degenerative changes in spinal column. 6 Syringobulbia ⇨ pain (V), caudal cranial nerve lesions (VIII–XII), nystagmus. 7 Suboccipital decompression in Chiari malformation (p. 292), shunt ⇨ syringotomy.

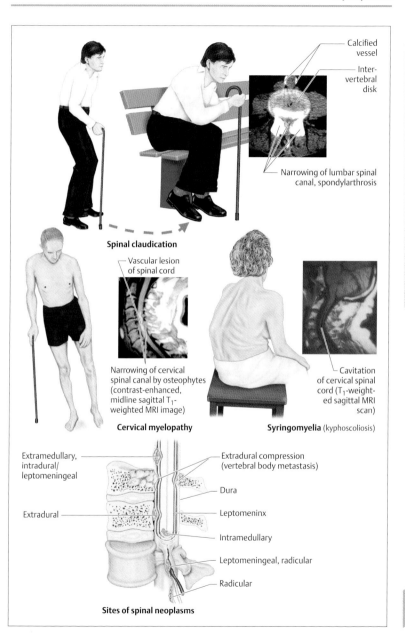

Calcified vessel

Intervertebral disk

Narrowing of lumbar spinal canal, spondylarthrosis

Spinal claudication

Vascular lesion of spinal cord

Narrowing of cervical spinal canal by osteophytes (contrast-enhanced, midline sagittal T_1-weighted MRI image)

Cervical myelopathy

Cavitation of cervical spinal cord (T_1-weighted sagittal MRI scan)

Syringomyelia (kyphoscoliosis)

Extramedullary, intradural/ leptomeningeal

Extradural compression (vertebral body metastasis)

Dura

Extradural

Leptomeninx

Intramedullary

Leptomeningeal, radicular

Radicular

Sites of spinal neoplasms

Non-Mass Lesions

Myelitis. See p. 282 for a listing of various infectious myelitides.

Subacute combined degeneration (SCD) appears in middle to old age, causing tingling and burning dysesthesiae in the limbs, gait unsteadiness, and abnormal fatigability. There may also be visual disturbances and depressive or psychotic symptoms accompanied by weight loss, glossopyrosis, and abdominal complaints. The neurological examination reveals a loss of position sensation ($\Rightarrow$ spinal ataxia), spastic paraparesis, variable abnormalities of the deep tendon reflexes, and autonomic dysfunction (bladder, bowel, sexual dysfunction). Megalocytic anemia is usually present. The cause is vitamin B_{12} deficiency, which may, in turn, be due to malabsorption, cachexia, or various medications. Folic acid deficiency produces a similar syndrome. The patient should be treated with parenteral cyanocobalamin or hydroxocobalamin as soon as possible. Neurological deficits can arise even if the hematocrit and red blood cell count are normal.

Toxic myelopathy. Most patients initially present with polyneuropathy, developing clinically apparent myelopathy only in the later stages of disease. Common causes include solvent abuse ("glue sniffing"), a high dietary intake of gross peas (lathyrism; p. 304), and consumption of cooking oil adulterated with lubricant oil (triorthocresyl phosphate poisoning).

Hereditary. The clinically and genetically heterogeneous forms of *familial spastic paraplegia* (FSP; spinal paralysis = SPG, p. 384) become symptomatic either in the first decade of life or between the ages of 10 and 40. Progressive central paraparesis with spasticity arises either in isolation (uncomplicated SPG) or accompanied by variable neurological deficits (complicated SPG). Both types can be transmitted in an autosomal dominant, autosomal recessive, or X-linked inheritance pattern. *Spinal muscular atrophy*, see p. 304. *Adrenomyeloneuropathy*, see p. 384.

Diagnostic Studies in Myelopathy[1]

Method	Information Provided
Evoked potentials	SEP[2]: conduction delay. MEP[3]: prolongation of CMT[4]
Plain radiograph	Anomalies of spinal column or craniocervical junction, degenerative changes, fractures, lytic lesions, spondylolisthesis
CT	Same as above, tumor, 3-D reconstruction
MRI	Tumor, myelitis, vascular myelopathy, (MR) myelography
Bone scan	Vertebral body lesions (trauma, neoplasm, inflammation, degeneration)
CSF analysis	Inflammatory, hemorrhagic (vascular), or neoplastic changes
Myelography[5]	Position-dependent changes (dynamic spondylolisthesis), spinal stenosis, arachnoiditis, nerve root avulsion
Spinal angiography	Arteriovenous fistula/malformation, location of source of hemorrhage

1 Urodynamic tests are used to evaluate bladder dysfunction (p. 156). **2** Somatosensory EP. **3** Motor EP. **4** Central motor conduction time (CMT). **5** Used when CT/MRI findings are ambiguous, in an emergency if CT and MRI are not available, or if position-dependent changes must be evaluated.

Treatment of Myelopathies (partial listing)

Cause	Treatment Measures
Myelitis	*HSV/VZV*[1]: acyclovir. *Bacterial infection*: antibiotics. *Unknown pathogen*: corticosteroids
Neoplasm[2]	Surgical resection of tumor and stabilization of spinal column; radiotherapy; corticosteroids; chemotherapy; hormonal therapy
Vascular lesion	*AV malformation*: Embolization, surgery. *Ischemia/hematomyelia*: symptomatic treatment, physiotherapy

1 HSV/VZV: herpes simplex virus/varicella-zoster virus. **2** Treatment depends on type and extent of neoplasm.

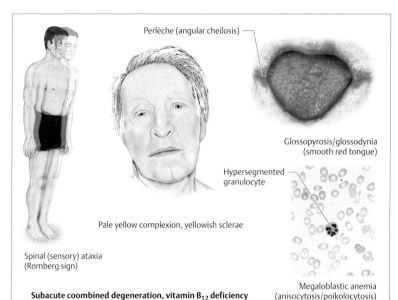

Perlèche (angular cheilosis)

Glossopyrosis/glossodynia
(smooth red tongue)

Hypersegmented
granulocyte

Pale yellow complexion, yellowish sclerae

Spinal (sensory) ataxia
(Romberg sign)

Megaloblastic anemia
(anisocytosis/poikolocytosis)

Subacute coombined degeneration, vitamin B$_{12}$ deficiency

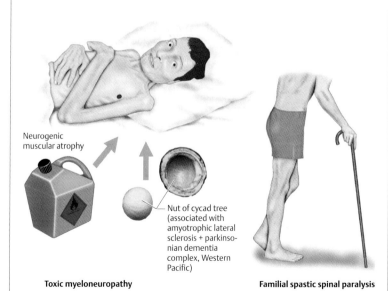

Neurogenic
muscular atrophy

Nut of cycad tree
(associated with
amyotrophic lateral
sclerosis + parkinso-
nian dementia
complex, Western
Pacific)

Toxic myeloneuropathy

Familial spastic spinal paralysis

Hereditary Diseases

Phenotype. The manner in which a hereditary disease expresses itself at a given moment in development (phenotype) is the product of both the individual's genetic makeup (genotype) and the environment in which development has taken place.

Inheritance. The human genome consists of 22 pairs of chromosomes (autosomes) and 2 sex chromosomes (either XX or XY). Individuals inherit half of their chromosomes from each parent. The chromosomes are made of DNA and bear the genes, sequences of nucleotide base pairs that encode the proteins of the body. Stretches of DNA that encode proteins are called *exons*; there are also intervening noncoding sequences, called *introns*. The inheritance pattern of hereditary diseases can be *monogenic*—the disease is due to a defect in a single (autosomal or X-chromosomal) gene, and is transmitted in a recessive or dominant manner in accordance with Mendel's laws; *polygenic*—the disease is due to defects in multiple genes; or *multifactorial*—the cause of disease is not exclusively genetic, and exogenous factors along with genetic factors determine its phenotype. Mitochondrial disorders are transmitted exclusively by maternal inheritance, as mitochondrial DNA is nonchromosomal and is inherited exclusively from the mother.

Mutation. *Alleles* are different forms of a gene. A *gene mutation* is a change in the DNA sequence of a gene and may involve a change in a single base pair (point mutation), the loss of one or more base pairs (deletion), the insertion of one or more base pairs, or unstable trinucleotide repeats. There are also *genome mutations*, which involve a change in the number of chromosomes, such as trisomy 21 (the cause of Down syndrome), as well as *chromosome mutations*, in which the chromosomal structure is altered. Mutations can occur either in the germ cells (*germ-line mutation*) or in the differentiated cells of the body (*somatic mutation*). Somatic mutations cause cancer, autoimmune diseases, and congenital anomalies.

Diagnosis. The diagnosis of hereditary diseases is by family history. Many monogenic diseases can be diagnosed by *direct* genotypic analysis (DNA sequencing). *Indirect* genotypic analysis, with investigation of the affected and nonaffected members of a single pedigree, is used in the diagnosis of disorders for which a gene locus is known but the responsible mutation(s) has not yet been determined.

Malformations and Developmental Anomalies (Table 40, p. 381)

Malformation. A malformation is a structural abnormality of an organ or part of the body in an individual whose body tissues are otherwise normal. Malformations arise during prenatal development because of primary absence or abnormality of the primordial tissue destined to develop into a particular part of the body ("anlage"). *Dysplasia* is malformation due to anomalous organization or function of tissues and tissue components; disorders involving dysplasia include tuberous sclerosis, neurofibromatosis, migration disorders, and various neoplastic diseases.

Developmental anomaly. Disruption of the growth of an organ or body part after normal (primary) primordial development can cause a secondary developmental anomaly. Mechanical influences during development can cause an anomalous position and shape (deformity) of an organ or body part.

■ Infantile Cerebral Palsy (CP) (p. 291)

Infantile cerebral palsy (cerebral movement disorder) is a manifest, but not necessarily unvarying, motor and postural disorder caused by nonprogressive damage to the brain before, during, or after birth. The underlying brain damage is usually of multifactorial origin. *Prenatal* causes include chromosomal defects, infection, hypoxia, or blood group intolerance; *perinatal* causes include hypoxia, cerebral hemorrhage, birth injury, adverse drug effects, and kernicterus; *postnatal* causes include meningoencephalitis, stroke, brain tumor, metabolic disturbances, and trauma.

Symptoms and signs. Paucity of spontaneous movement, abnormal patterns of movement, and delayed development of standing and walking are noted just after birth and as the child develops. Cerebral palsy frequently involves central paresis (hemiparesis, paraparesis, or quadriparesis), spasticity, ataxia, and choreoathetosis (p. 66). There may also be mental retardation, epileptic seizures, behavioral disturbances (restlessness, impulsiveness, lack of concentration, impaired affect control), and impairment of vision, hearing, and speech. The motor disturbances produce deformities of the bones and joints (talipes equinus, contracture, scoliosis, hip dislocation).

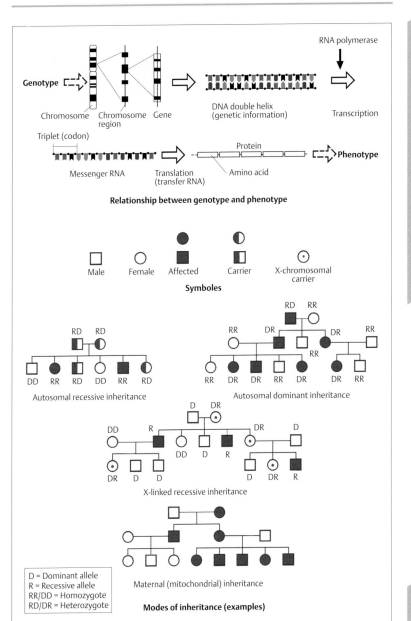

Relationship between genotype and phenotype

Symboles

Male Female Affected Carrier X-chromosomal carrier

Autosomal recessive inheritance

Autosomal dominant inheritance

X-linked recessive inheritance

Maternal (mitochondrial) inheritance

D = Dominant allele
R = Recessive allele
RR/DD = Homozygote
RD/DR = Heterozygote

Modes of inheritance (examples)

Treatment. Physical, occupational, and speech therapy and perception training should be started as soon as possible. Botulinum toxin can be useful in the treatment of spasticity at certain sites (dynamic talipes equinus, leg adductors, arm flexors). *Other measures:* Orthopedic care, seeing and hearing aids, developmental support.

■ Hydrocephalus

Hydrocephalus is dilatation of the cerebral ventricles (p. 8) due to obstruction of CSF outflow (p. 162). Common etiologies include aqueductal stenosis, Dandy–Walker and Chiari malformations, infection (toxoplasmosis, bacterial ventriculitis), hemorrhage, and obstructing tumors (colloid cyst of the third ventricle, midline tumors).

Symptoms and signs. If the cranial sutures have not yet fused, congenital obstructive hydrocephalus produces an enlarged head (macrocephaly) with a protruding forehead, the result of chronic intracranial hypertension. The head circumference should be measured regularly, as it is a more useful indicator of congenital hydrocephalus than the clinical signs of intracranial hypertension (p. 158), which are often not very pronounced in infants and may be masked by irritability, failure to thrive, crying, and psychomotor developmental delay. These signs include distended veins visible through the patient's thin scalp; bulging of the fontanelles, and vertical gaze palsy (the lower lid covers the open eye to the pupil, the upper lid reveals a portion of the sclera ⇨ "sunsetting"). Signs of intracranial hypertension are the most useful indicators of hydrocephalus once the cranial sutures have fused. A chronic form of hydrocephalus to be differentiated from NPH (p. 160) has been described as long-standing overt ventriculomegaly in adults (LOVA hydrocephalus); symptoms include macrocephaly, headache, lightheadedness, gait disturbances, and bladder dysfunction.

Treatment. *Acute hydrocephalus:* There is a limited role for medical treatment (e. g., with carbonic anhydrase inhibitors and osmodiuretic agents); neurosurgical treatment is generally needed for CSF drainage (external drainage or surgical shunt) and/or the resection of an obstructing lesion.

■ Porencephaly

Porencephaly (from Greek *poros*, "opening"), the formation of a cyst or cavity in the brain, is usually due to infarction, hemorrhage, trauma, or infection. Porencephaly in the strict sense of the term involves a communication with the ventricular system. Porencephalic cysts are only rarely associated with intracranial hypertension. Large ones reflect extensive loss of brain tissue; the extreme case is termed *hydranencephaly*. Porencephaly may be asymptomatic or may be associated with focal signs (paresis, epileptic seizures).

■ Arachnoid Cysts

An arachnoid cyst is a developmental anomaly of the leptomeninges (p. 6), usually supratentorial, and located either within the leptomeningeal membranes or between the arachnoid and pia mater. Some arachnoid cysts communicate with the subarachnoid space. Many are asymptomatic, even when large. In rare cases, they can obstruct the CSF pathways (midline or infratentorial arachnoid cysts) or cause new or progressive signs and symptoms because of intracystic hemorrhage, cyst expansion (perhaps by a one-way valve mechanism), or cyst rupture. Symptomatic arachnoid cysts are treated neurosurgically by shunting, fenestration, or excision.

■ Agenesis of the Corpus Callosum

Hypoplasia or agenesis of the corpus callosum occurs as an isolated finding or in combination with other anomalies (Chiari malformation, heterotopy, chromosomal anomaly, Aicardi syndrome ⇨ infantile spasms, micro-ophthalmia, chorioretinopathy, costovertebral anomalies). Isolated agenesis of the corpus callosum may be asymptomatic and is occasionally found incidentally on CT or MRI scans. Cystic deformities of the septum pellucidum (cavum septi pellucidi, cavum vergae) may obstruct the flow of CSF and cause intracranial hypertension.

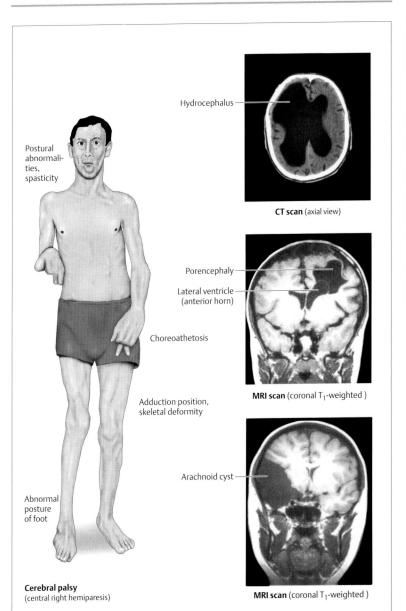

Postural abnormalities, spasticity

Hydrocephalus

CT scan (axial view)

Porencephaly

Lateral ventricle (anterior horn)

Choreoathetosis

MRI scan (coronal T$_1$-weighted)

Adduction position, skeletal deformity

Arachnoid cyst

Abnormal posture of foot

Cerebral palsy
(central right hemiparesis)

MRI scan (coronal T$_1$-weighted)

Malformations and Developmental Anomalies

■ Anomalies of the Craniocervical Junction

Syndrome	Symptoms and Signs	Causes	Diagnosis/Treatment
Platybasia	Usually asymptomatic	Flattening of the skull base	Plain radiograph[1]/None
Occipitalization of C1	Usually asymptomatic; possible signs of medullary dysfunction	Synostosis of C1 with the occiput	Plain radiograph, CT, MRI/ Surgical decompression if symptomatic
Basilar impression	Occipitocervical pain; reduced neck flexibility. Long-term: impairment of gait, urinary retention, dysarthria, dysphagia, vertigo, nausea	Underdevelopment of the occipital bone causing "elevation" of cervical spine[2]	Plain radiograph, CT, MRI/ Usually symptomatic; medullary symptoms ⇨ neurosurgical treatment
Klippel–Feil syndrome[3]	Short neck, abnormal head posture, high shoulders, headache, radicular symptoms in arm; possible spinal cord compression	Fused cervical vertebrae	Same as above/ Treatment depends on signs and symptoms

1 Angle between root of nose and clivus > 145°. **2** Congenital (Chiari malformation), acquired (Paget disease, osteomalacia). **3** Additional malformations such as syringomyelia, spina bifida, cleft palate, or syndactyly may be present.

■ Spinal Dysraphism (Neural Tube Defects)

Syndrome	Symptoms and Signs	Causes	Diagnosis/Treatment
Anencephaly	Absence of cranial vault; cerebral aplasia; normally developed viscerocranium	Nonclosure of anterior portion of neural tube	Prenatal ultrasound screening/Termination of pregnancy
Encephalocele	Protrusion of brain tissue through a midline skull defect[1]	Inhibition malformation (incomplete closure of neural tube)	Measurement of α-fetoprotein[2], prenatal ultrasound screening/Folic acid-vitamin B_{12} administration during pregnancy; surgical repair if indicated
Dandy–Walker malformation	Hydrocephalus, hypoplasia/ agenesis of vermis; cystic dilatation of 4th ventricle; variable degree of facial dysmorphism	Abnormality of embryonal development	CT, MRI/Shunt
Chiari malformation[3]	Lower cranial nerve and brainstem dysfunction (dysphagia, respiratory dysfunction); head, neck and shoulder pain; abnormal head posture, vertigo, downbeat nystagmus, hydrocephalus (type II)	Abnormality of early embryonal development (weeks 5–6 of gestation)	CT, MRI/Suboccipital decompression; shunt procedure for hydrocephalus; early surgery for myelomeningocele
Spina bifida[4]	*Spina bifida occulta*: Dermal sinus, lumbar hypertrichosis, lumbosacral fistula, leg pain, gait disturbance, foot deformities, bladder dysfunction (enuresis in children) *Other forms*: Sensorimotor paraplegia at birth; bladder/bowel dysfunction, foot deformities; hydrocephalus may occur	Inhibition malformation (incomplete closure of neural tube)	α-Fetoprotein[2], prenatal ultrasound screening, plain X-ray, CT, MRI/Folic acid administration during pregnancy; surgical treatment, physiotherapy, orthopedic therapy
Tethered cord syndrome	Same as above, with varying severity. Low-lying conus medullaris, fixed filum terminale	Traction on spinal cord and cauda equina	MRI/Surgery for symptoms and signs reflecting dysfunction of the spinal cord and/or cauda equina

1 *Meningocele*: Only the meninges protrude through the skull defect. *Meningoencephalocele*: Meninges + brain. *Meningoencephalocystocele*: meninges + brain + ventricular system. **2** In maternal serum; also in amniotic fluid in open defects. **3** Type I: unilateral or bilateral cerebellar tonsillar herniation with or without caudal displacement of medulla; hydrocephalus, syringomyelia (p. 284); there may be an accompanying anomaly of the skull base. Type II: same as type I + caudal displacement of medulla, parts of cerebellum, and fourth ventricle, with myelomeningocele. Type III: same as type II + occipital encephalocele. **4** Rachischisis = fissure of vertebral column, incomplete closure of neural tube; *spina bifida occulta* = incomplete vertebral arch (lamina) with normal position of spinal cord and meninges; *meningocele* = the arachnoid lies directly under the skin, not covered by the missing dura and bone; *myelomeningocele* = prolapse of spinal cord (or cauda equina) and arachnoid through the dural and bony defect; *diastematomyelia* = split spinal cord, with two halves separated by connective tissue or a bone spur.

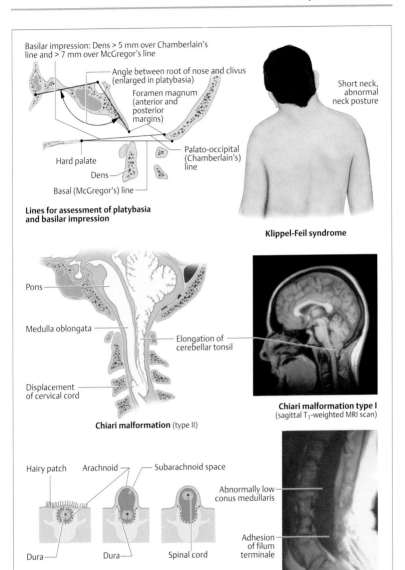

Basilar impression: Dens > 5 mm over Chamberlain's line and > 7 mm over McGregor's line

Angle between root of nose and clivus (enlarged in platybasia)

Foramen magnum (anterior and posterior margins)

Palato-occipital (Chamberlain's) line

Hard palate

Dens

Basal (McGregor's) line

Lines for assessment of platybasia and basilar impression

Short neck, abnormal neck posture

Klippel-Feil syndrome

Pons

Medulla oblongata

Elongation of cerebellar tonsil

Displacement of cervical cord

Chiari malformation (type II)

Chiari malformation type I
(sagittal T₁-weighted MRI scan)

Hairy patch   Arachnoid   Subarachnoid space

Dura   Dura   Spinal cord

Spina bifida
(left, spina bifida occulta; middle, meningocele; right, meningomyelocele)

Abnormally low conus medullaris

Adhesion of filum terminale

Tethered cord syndrome
(sagittal T₁-weighted MRI scan)

The Phakomatoses

The phakomatoses (neurocutaneous diseases) are a group of congenital diseases in which pathological changes are found in both the central nervous system and the skin. Neurofibromatosis, tuberous sclerosis, and von Hippel–Lindau disease are transmitted in an autosomal dominant inheritance pattern with high penetrance and variable phenotypic expression. These disorders are generally characterized by the formation of benign nodules (hamartoma); malignant tumors (e. g., hamartoblastomas) are rare.

■ Neurofibromatosis (NF; von Recklinghausen Disease)

The genetic locus for neurofibromatosis type 1 (NF1), the "classical" form of the disease, is on chromosome 17q11.2; that for NF type 2 (NF2) is on 22q12.2.

Symptoms and signs. The characteristic lesions of *NF1* are found in the *skin* (early stage: café-au-lait spots, axillary/inguinal freckling; later stages: neurofibromas/plexiform neurofibromas), *eyes* (Lisch nodules = whitish hamartomas of the iris, optic glioma), and *bone* (cysts, pathological fractures, skull defects, scoliosis). There may also be syringomyelia, hydrocephalus, epileptic seizures, precocious puberty, or pheochromocytoma. The hallmark of *NF2* is bilateral acoustic neuroma with progressive bilateral hearing loss. Cutaneous manifestations are rare; other nervous system tumors (neurofibroma, meningioma, schwannoma, glioma) are more common. Subcapsular cataract is a typical feature of NF2 in children.

Treatment. Symptomatic tumors are resected.

■ Tuberous Sclerosis (TSC; Bourneville–Pringle Disease)

The clinical syndrome of tuberous sclerosis is produced by a mutation at either one of two known loci (TSC1: 9q34, TSC2: 16p13.3). TSC1 and TSC2 are clinically identical.

Symptoms and signs. *Epileptic seizures* (infantile spasms and salaam seizures = West syndrome; focal, generalized) are found in association with *skin changes* (early: hypomelanotic linear spots readily visible under UV light; late signs: adenoma sebaceum, subungual angiofibroma, thick and leathery skin in the lumbar region), *ocular*

changes (retinal hamartoma), and *tumors* (cardiac rhabdomyoma, renal angiomyolipoma, cysts). There may be marked mental retardation and behavioral abnormalities (vocal and motor stereotypy, psychomotor restlessness). CT and MRI reveal periventricular calcification, cortical lesions, and tumors.

Treatment. Symptomatic (anticonvulsants).

■ Von Hippel–Lindau Disease

Gene locus. 3p25-p26.

Symptoms and signs. Cystic cerebellar hemangioblastoma causes headache, vertigo, and ataxia, and possibly hydrocephalus by compression of the 4th ventricle. Hemangioma may also occur in the spinal cord. Further lesions are often present in the *eyes* (retinal angiomatosis ⇨ retinal detachment), *kidneys* (cysts, carcinoma), *adrenal glands* (pheochromocytoma), *pancreas* (multiple cysts), and *epididymis* (cystadenoma).

Treatment. Regular screening of each potentially involved organ system is carried out so that tumors can be resected and vascular complications prevented as early as possible.

■ Cutaneous Angiomatoses with CNS Involvement

Sturge–Weber disease (encephalofacial angiomatosis). A unilateral or bilateral port wine stain (nevus flammeus) is present at birth and may be either localized (characteristically in the upper eyelid and forehead, in which case involvement of the brain is likely) or widespread (entire head or body). Not all cutaneous hemangiomas are accompanied by cerebral involvement.

Hereditary hemorrhagic telangiectasia (HHT; Osler–Weber–Rendu disease). Known genetic loci: 9q34.1 (HHT1) and 12q11–14 (HHT2). Telangiectases (vascular anomalies) of the skin, mucous membranes, gastrointestinal tract, urogenital tract, and CNS cause recurrent bleeding (nosebleed, gastrointestinal hemorrhage, hematuria, hemoptysis, cerebral hemorrhage, anemia). Arteriovenous shunting in the lung may cause cyanosis and polycythemia.

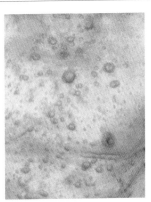

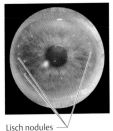

Lisch nodules

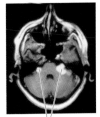

Bilateral acoustic neuroma (axial T_1-weighted MRI scan)

Neurofibroma

Periventricular calcification (axial CT scan)

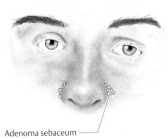

Adenoma sebaceum

Tuberous sclerosis

Hemangioblastoma of the cervical spinal cord

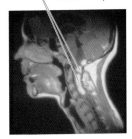

Telangiectasis

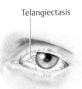

Hemangioma of upper eyelid

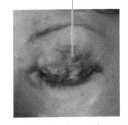

Ataxia-telangiectasia

von Hippel-Lindau syndrome
(sagittal MRI scan)

Sturge-Weber syndrome

Throughout the industrialized world, the population is becoming older. It is predicted that the percentage of persons over age 65 will rise further, while that of persons under age 15 will fall.

Aging

Aging is a biological process with a characteristic temporal course. *Senescence* refers to the physical changes associated with aging. It is still unclear whether human aging is specifically genetically predetermined or, alternatively, reflects cumulative damage incurred over time. The cellular correlates of aging include an increase in spontaneous chromosomal mutations, altered protein conformations, impairment of cell metabolism by the accumulation of free oxygen radicals, a decline of mitochondrial function with an increase in apoptosis (genetically programmed cell death), and diminished activity of regenerative processes. It is not yet known whether these processes are the cause or the effect of aging.

The current *average natural lifespan*, barring premature death from disease or external causes, is approximately 85 years. The *maximum* human lifespan (to date, at least) is approximately 120 years. *Life expectancy* is the average statistically predicted lifespan of a given population at a given point in time. Human life expectancy has risen considerably in the course of history, particularly in the 20th century. The *active life expectancy*, or the expected time during which the individual can function independently with regard to meals, dressing, personal hygiene, shopping, and finances, is of practical significance. About 35% of persons over 85 are not fully independent, and about 20% need nursing-home care.

Aging and Disease

Aging decreases physiological reserve, i.e., the ability to compensate for the effects of harmful influences, be they endogenous (e. g., diabetes mellitus, heart failure, thyroid dysfunction) or exogenous (e. g., trauma, infection, side effects of medication). Diseases therefore tend to affect the elderly with shorter latency and greater severity. Age-related changes promote the development of diseases such as Alzheimer disease or stroke, as well as accidents such as falls. Brain tumors (p. 254), particularly metastases, glioma, meningioma, acoustic neuroma, and primary cerebral lymphoma, are more common in older patients. Aging is neither a disease nor a cause of disease, but it increases the chance of becoming ill. The physician must distinguish changes due to disease from those of normal aging (see Table 41, p. 382).

Aging and Degenerative Changes

Structural changes in the brain due to aging rather than disease are referred to as *involution*. *Gross* changes include diminished brain volume, gyral atrophy, ventriculomegaly, leukoaraiosis (p. 298), parasagittal leptomeningeal fibrosis, and ventricular expansion, while *microscopic* changes include neuron and axon loss, gliosis, and the presence within neurons of lipofuscin, neuromelanin, granulovacuolar degeneration, microtubular neurofibrillary tangles (NFTs), senile plaques, Lafora bodies, and Lewy bodies. The term *abiotrophy* refers to the genetically determined, age-dependent occurrence of degenerative changes such as these. *Degenerative diseases*, on the other hand, are characterized by an abnormal accentuation of these and other morphological changes, producing typical constellations of functional disturbances (disease-specific clinical syndromes). They develop slowly, progressively, sometimes asymmetrically, and with variable intervals of relatively stable disease manifestations. Some are familial.

Alzheimer Disease (AD)

Alzheimer disease (in its sporadic form) is the most common cause of dementia in old age (p. 136). It progresses steadily or stepwise and usually leads to death in 8–10 years (range, 1–25 years). Risk factors for AD include old age, family history of AD, female sex, elevated plasma homocysteine concentration, and the presence of the allele Apo Eε4. Nonsteroidal anti-inflammatory drugs appear to lower the risk of AD. Familial AD is rare; it is transmitted in an autosomal dominant inheritance pattern.

■ **Symptoms and Signs**

Early stage. Memory impairment develops gradually and almost imperceptibly, barely differing at first from that of benign senile forgetfulness (p. 136). Ultimately, however, the cognitive deficits of AD produce noticeable changes of behavior, e. g., when the patient is working, shopping, running errands, or taking care of finances, or operating such devices as a telephone, stove, television, or computer. The patient may be aware of these deficits and become additionally anxious and depressed because of them. The distinction between AD with depressive features and primary depression with secondary cognitive changes (pseudodementia) has major implications for treatment (Table 42, p. 383).

Intermediate stage. The patient is too confused and disoriented to carry out previous occupational and social activities (p. 132) and needs help and supervision in almost all activities, but may still be able to perform habitual daily routines, carry on a simple conversation, and abide by the basic rules of etiquette. *Aphasia* (e. g., impaired comprehension of speech, word-finding difficulty, cf. p. 126) and *apraxia* (p. 128) are often present. The patient cannot do simple arithmetic or tell time. Visual agnosia is rare at this stage.

Late stage. The increasing cognitive impairment and loss of reasoning and judgment make it impossible for the patients to plan their activities. The patient's aimless wandering, undirected motor activity, and inability to recognize people—even close relatives and friends—complicate the caregiver's job, along with changes in the patient's circadian rhythm (quiet or apathetic by day, restless by night), impulsive behavior (packing suitcases or running away), delusions, hallucinations, paranoid suspicion of close relatives and friends, aggressive behavior, and neglect of personal hygiene. Patients with advanced AD need help with the simplest activities of daily living (eating, dressing, going to the toilet). They may become incontinent of urine and stool, bedridden, akinetic, and mute. Pathological reflexes (sucking and grasping) can be elicited. Auditory and tactile stimuli may trigger epileptic seizures and myoclonus (for differentiation from

Creutzfeldt–Jakob disease, see p. 252). Death is caused by secondary complications such as pneumonia and heart failure.

■ **Pathogenesis**

PET and SPECT studies in early AD reveal bilateral metabolic disturbances in the parietotemporal cortex and decreased neurotransmitter activity in cortical cholinergic fibers (acetylcholine, choline acetyltransferase, nicotinic acetylcholine receptors ⇨ nucleus basalis, medial septal region), serotonergic fibers (raphe nuclei), and noradrenergic fibers (locus coeruleus). There is probably a reduction of cortical glutamatergic activity (excitatory) with a preponderance of GABAergic activity (inhibitory). *Neuropathology:* Changes such as neuronal death, neuritic (senile) plaques (NPs), and intraneuronal neurofibrillary tangles (NFTs) are seen mainly in the entorhinal cortex, hippocampus, temporal cortex, primary/secondary visual cortex, and nucleus basalis. NPs consist of a central core containing amyloid-Aβ, apolipoprotein E (Apo E), α_1-antichymotrypsin, synuclein, and other proteins, surrounded by dead neurons, activated glial cells, macrophages, and other inflammatory cells. NFTs consist of paired helical filaments (PHFs) composed of tau proteins, which are normally an important stabilizing component of the microtubular (neurofibrillary) cytoskeleton. Increased phosphorylation of tau proteins leads to the formation of NFTs. Amyloid-Aβ (normal function unknown) is formed by proteolysis of the transmembrane amyloid precursor protein (APP), to which neurotrophic and neuroprotective properties have been ascribed. A point mutation in APP on chromosome 21q has been implicated in familial AD; patients over 40 years of age with Down syndrome (trisomy 21) also have neuropathological changes similar to those of AD. Accumulation of amyloid-Aβ in arterial walls is the basic abnormality in amyloid angiopathy (p. 178). The gene for Apo E (a lipoprotein involved in cholesterol transport) is found on chromosome 19q and has three alleles, designated ε2, ε3, and ε4; ε4 is strongly associated with both sporadic and familial AD. Other familial forms of AD have been traced to mutations of the presenilin-1 gene (*PS1* ⇨ 14q24.3 ⇨ protein S182) and the presenilin-2 gene (*PS2* ⇨ 1q31-42 ⇨ STM2 protein).

These genes encode cytoplasmic neuronal proteins whose function is as yet unknown.

■ **Treatment**

There is no specific treatment for AD. Symptomatic, social, and psychiatric measures and family assistance are the mainstays of treatment. Acetylcholinesterase inhibitors (donepezil, galantamine, rivastigmine, tacrine) or N-methyl-D-aspartate (NMDA) inhibitors (memantine) can improve cognitive function in the early stages of disease. A proposed protective effect of estrogen therapy in postmenopausal women has not been confirmed.

Pick Disease, Frontotemporal Dementia (FTD)

Pick disease causes behavioral changes (e. g., reduced interpersonal distance, apathy, abulia, obsessive-compulsive symptoms, amnestic aphasia, increased appetite) and impairment of semantic memory. CT and MRI mainly reveal asymmetric frontotemporal atrophy. *Neuropathology:* Neuron loss, gliosis, and variably severe "ballooning" of neurons (Pick cells). There are no neuritic plaques. The disease is familial in 40% of cases; familial Pick disease is transmitted in an autosomal dominant inheritance pattern and is due to a mutation on chromosome 17 (FTDP-17) that causes changes in tau protein (⇨ FTD with parkinsonian manifestations).

Vascular Dementia (Table 14, p. 367)

Cerebrovascular disturbances can produce dementia in a variety of ways. The main risk factors for cerebrovascular dementia are old age, arterial hypertension, diabetes mellitus, and generalized atherosclerosis. After AD, cerebrovascular disturbance are the second most common cause of dementia.

Multi-infarct dementia. Multiple small infarcts (lacunes) or large bilateral infarcts may produce any of a variety of focal neurological, behavioral, and cognitive disturbances, depending on their location and extent. These disturbances usually progress in stepwise fashion. CADASIL (p. 172) is a rare cerebrovascular disorder that predisposes to multi-infarct dementia.

Subcortical arteriosclerotic encephalopathy (SAE) is characterized by rarefaction of the white matter (leukoaraiosis) due to microangiopathy. *Neuropathology:* Histological examination reveals demyelination and reactive gliosis in the white matter, along with changes in the walls of small arteries (hyalinosis, fibrinoid necrosis, hypertrophy). These vascular changes are the cause of chronic ischemic and secondary metabolic damage in areas of white matter supplied by terminal branches. Behavioral changes (attention deficit, loss of cognitive flexibility, abulia, disorientation), gait disturbances, pseudobulbar palsy, urinary incontinence, and other neurological deficits develop slowly and continuously (not in stepwise fashion, as in multi-infarct dementia).

Strategic infarct dementia. Dementia can be produced by a localized infarct in a particular, "strategic" areas of the brain (e. g., limbic system, thalamus, cortical association areas).

Leukoaraiosis is characterized by white-matter lesions (WMLs) that are hypodense on CT and hyperintense on T2-weighted MRI. The extent of WMLs is correlated with the clinical severity of the disease: there may be mild or moderate cognitive impairment (cognitive slowing, memory loss) or severe dementia. WMLs are not always due to a cerebrovascular disturbance and are present in a variety of conditions other than chronic arterial hypertension (e. g., AD, multiple sclerosis, PML, Creutzfeldt–Jakob disease, ADEM, trauma, radiation therapy, chemotherapy, vitamin B_{12} deficiency, hypoxic-ischemic encephalopathy, CADASIL, central amyloid angiopathy).

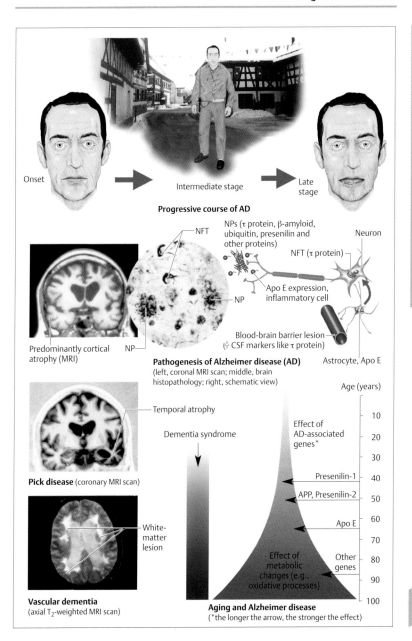

Onset → Intermediate stage → Late stage

Progressive course of AD

NFT

NPs (τ protein, β-amyloid, ubiquitin, presenilin and other proteins)

Neuron

NFT (τ protein)

Apo E expression, inflammatory cell

NP

Blood-brain barrier lesion (⇡ CSF markers like τ protein)

Predominantly cortical atrophy (MRI)   NP

Astrocyte, Apo E

Pathogenesis of Alzheimer disease (AD)
(left, coronal MRI scan; middle, brain histopathology; right, schematic view)

Temporal atrophy

Dementia syndrome

Pick disease (coronary MRI scan)

White-matter lesion

Vascular dementia
(axial T$_2$-weighted MRI scan)

Age (years)

Effect of AD-associated genes*

Presenilin-1   40
APP, Presenilin-2   50
Apo E   60

Other genes

Effect of metabolic changes (e.g., oxidative processes)

Aging and Alzheimer disease
(*the longer the arrow, the stronger the effect)

299

Huntington Disease (HD)

The first symptoms of HD typically appear between the ages of 35 and 45 years. HD appearing before age 20 (the Westphal variant of HD) is characterized by akinesia, bradykinesia, epileptic seizures, action tremor, and myoclonus. Onset before age 10 or after age 70 is rare. HD patients require total nursing care 10–15 years after the onset of this inexorably progressive, and ultimately fatal degenerative disease.

■ Symptoms and Signs

Early stage. In cases of earlier onset, akinesia and cognitive impairment tend to be more prominent than choreiform movements, while, in cases of later onset, the reverse is true. *Behavioral changes* such as depression, suicidal tendencies, paranoia, querulousness, irritability, impulsiveness, emotional outbursts, aggressive behavior, poor hygiene, loss of initiative, and inappropriate sexual behavior impair familial and social relationships and may even lead to criminal charges. Other changes include cognitive slowing, diminished tolerance for stress, and impairment of memory and concentration. The patient becomes obviously unable to perform his or her usual tasks at work or at home. *Chorea* (p. 66; Table 43, p. 383) may initially be misdiagnosed as "nervous" agitation or fidgeting. Even severe chorea disappears during sleep. Chorea may be accompanied by akinesia, dystonia, and decreased voluntary motor control. The patient's gait is impaired by poor balance and loss of postural motor control. Oculomotor disturbances are also common.

Intermediate stage. Progressive dementia (p. 136) is accompanied by loss of drive, generalized choreiform, dystonic, and bradykinetic movements, and frequent falls.

Late stage. Many patients become cachectic, with muscular atrophy (⇨ interosseous muscles of hands) and weight loss despite an adequate caloric intake. Chorea is largely replaced by akinesia in late HD. General motor control is greatly impaired. Urinary incontinence is not uncommon. These patients need full nursing care.

■ Pathogenesis (for abbreviations, see p. 211)

HD is characterized by generalized cerebral atrophy, especially of the dorsal striatum

(p. 210), and, neurochemically, by a marked deficiency of GABA and of glutamate decarboxylase (an enzyme involved in GABA synthesis). HD is transmitted in an autosomal dominant pattern with complete penetrance, that is, all persons bearing the gene eventually develop the disease. The gene for HD (*IT15*) is on the end of the short arm of chromosome 4 (4p16.3), which contains CAG repeats (the trinucleotide sequence CAG codes for glutamine; cf. p. 288). Healthy subjects have 11–34 CAG repeats at this locus, while persons with HD have more than 40. Paternal inheritance is associated with *anticipation* (increasingly early onset in subsequent generations), but maternal inheritance is not. The gene product is referred to as *huntingtin*. The pathophysiological mechanism of HD remains obscure; increased glutamatergic transmission at NMDA receptors is thought to produce neurodegenerative changes (*excitotoxicity*). There is now a direct gene test that can be performed on a peripheral blood sample to detect HD before the onset of symptoms. It may only be performed with the informed consent of a patient above the legal age of majority, after the potential social and psychiatric implications of a positive result have been explained.

Neuroacanthocytosis

Acanthocytes (crenated erythrocytes with thorny processes) make up more than 3% of all erythrocytes in fresh blood smears obtained from patients with the following neurological diseases: *abetalipoproteinemia* (Bassen–Kornzweig syndrome, p. 280, 307; ⇩ cholesterol and triglycerides), *McLeod syndrome* (X-linked recessive myopathy; absence of Kell precursor protein), and *neuroacanthocytosis* (normal lipoprotein concentrations). The mode of inheritance of neuroacanthocytosis is unknown. Its major features, orofacial dyskinesia (tonguebiting and lip-biting) and chorea, usually appear between the ages of 20 and 30 years.

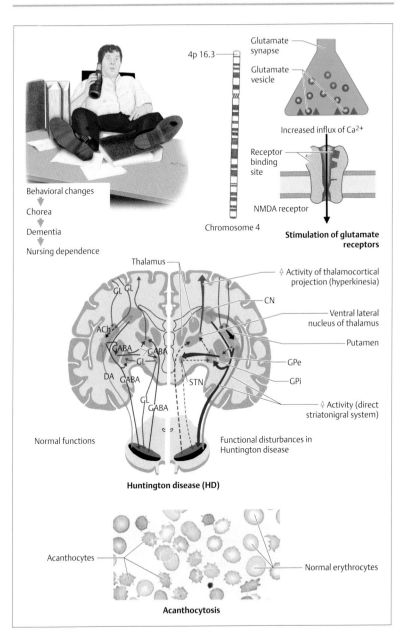

4p 16.3

Chromosome 4

Glutamate synapse
Glutamate vesicle

Increased influx of Ca²⁺

Receptor binding site

NMDA receptor

Stimulation of glutamate receptors

Behavioral changes
↓
Chorea
↓
Dementia
↓
Nursing dependence

Thalamus

⇧ Activity of thalamocortical projection (hyperkinesia)

GL GL

CN

ACh

Ventral lateral nucleus of thalamus

GABA GABA

Putamen

GL

GPe

DA GABA

GPi

GL STN

GABA

⇧ Activity (direct striatonigral system)

Normal functions

Functional disturbances in Huntington disease

Huntington disease (HD)

Acanthocytes

Normal erythrocytes

Acanthocytosis

Atypical Parkinsonian Syndromes

Roughly 80% of patients with parkinsonism suffer from *idiopathic Parkinson disease* (p. 206 ff), while the rest have either *symptomatic parkinsonism* (Table 44, p. 383) or *atypical parkinsonism* (AP) due to one of the neurodegenerative "Parkinson-plus" syndromes. The more common AP syndromes are multiple system atrophy, progressive supranuclear palsy, and corticobasal degeneration. An unequivocal differentiation of these disorders from one another, and from idiopathic Parkinson disease, may not be possible at the onset of symptoms, or even later in the course of the disease.

■ Multiple System Atrophy (MSA)

MSA is a gradually progressive, sporadic, nonfamilial disease of adults marked by autonomic and cerebellar dysfunction of variable severity, accompanied by parkinsonian manifestations that respond poorly to levodopa. The term MSA covers the earlier-described disorders olivopontocerebellar atrophy (OPCA), idiopathic orthostatic hypotension (IOH), Shy–Drager syndrome, and striatonigral degeneration (SND). The onset of symptoms is usually between the ages of 45 and 70. Autonomic dysfunction is manifested by urinary incontinence (p. 156; abnormal EMG of urethral/anal sphincter ⇨ increased polyphasic rate) and orthostatic hypotension (p. 148), and sometimes by hypertension while the patient is lying down. Cerebellar dysfunction is manifested by gait ataxia, frequent falls, dysarthria, and oculomotor disturbances. The parkinsonian manifestations include akinesia, rigidity, postural instability (p. 206), and frequent falling, but there is no resting tremor.

■ Progressive Supranuclear Palsy (PSP)

PSP (Steele–Richardson–Olszewski syndrome) is a progressive, nonfamilial disease that usually appears around the age of 40. Its major features are unsteady gait, postural instability, frequent falls (often backward), axial dystonia, rigidity, akinesia, behavioral changes (bradyphrenia, irritability, social withdrawal, abnormal fatigability, uncontrollable laughing and crying), and pseudobulbar palsy (p. 166). Paralysis of voluntary conjugate upward gaze may be present at onset, but paralysis of downward gaze is more common. Passive (reflex) vertical eye movements (doll's eye sign) are still present, i.e., the vestibulo-ocular reflex remains intact (p. 26). The fully developed clinical picture of PSP (abnormally erect posture, retrocollis, wide-open eyes, elevated forehead muscles, dysarthria, dysphagia, and frontal brain syndrome, p. 122) is practically pathognomonic, but its manifestations in the early phase can be very difficult to distinguish from those of other neurodegenerative diseases. The symptoms and signs of PSP respond poorly to levodopa, if at all.

■ Corticobasal Degeneration (CBD)

CBD is a progressive neurodegenerative disease that most often occurs in adults over the age of 60. Its major features are akinesia, rigidity, limb apraxia (p. 128), and cortical sensory deficits (astereognosis, graphanesthesia). There is a loss of motor control, so that the patient's hands (limbs) appear to move spontaneously without the patient's guiding them (*alien hand/limb phenomenon*). Gait instability is an early sign and is later accompanied by dysarthria, dysphagia, myoclonus, dystonic arm posture (wrist and elbow flexion, shoulder adduction), action/postural tremor, supranuclear oculomotor disturbances (p. 86), blepharospasm, and cognitive impairment. Levodopa is unhelpful.

■ Dementia with Lewy Bodies (DLB), Diffuse Lewy Body Disease

DLB is characterized at first by an akinetic-rigid parkinsonian syndrome (p. 208), which is later accompanied by fluctuating behavioral changes (attention deficit, disorientation, impairment of consciousness, visual hallucinations) and frequent falling for no apparent reason. Patients are hypersensitive to neuroleptics and benzodiazepines. An abundance of Lewy bodies (p. 211) can be observed, particularly in cortical neurons.

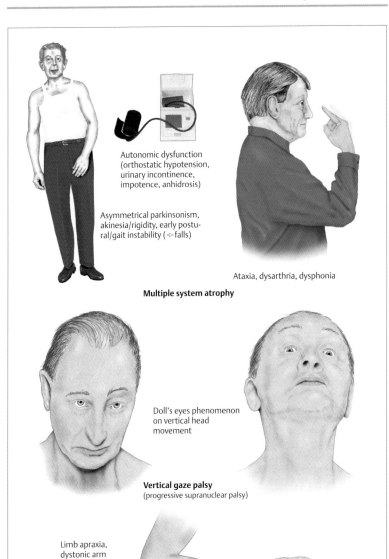

Autonomic dysfunction
(orthostatic hypotension,
urinary incontinence,
impotence, anhidrosis)

Asymmetrical parkinsonism,
akinesia/rigidity, early postu-
ral/gait instability (⇨falls)

Ataxia, dysarthria, dysphonia

Multiple system atrophy

Doll's eyes phenomenon
on vertical head
movement

Vertical gaze palsy
(progressive supranuclear palsy)

Limb apraxia,
dystonic arm
position

Myoclonus

Corticobasal degeneration

Motor Neuron Diseases

These diseases involve a degeneration of the cerebral and/or spinal motor neurons (p. 44). They present with a wide variety of neurological syndromes of varying temporal course.

■ **Upper Motor Neuron Diseases**
(p. 46; Table 45, p. 384)

Hereditary. Familial spastic spinal paralysis (p. 286), adrenomyeloneuropathy, spinocerebellar ataxia type 3 (p. 280).

Acquired. Lathyrism (central spastic paraparesis due to a neurotoxin in the pulse *Lathyrus sativus* (grass pea), a dietary staple in certain poor districts in India); konzo (= cassavaism, a toxic reaction to flour made of insufficiently processed cassava, seen in certain parts of Africa); tropical spastic paraparesis (HTLV1-associated myelopathy = HAM).

■ **Lower Motor Neuron Diseases**
(p. 50; Table 46, p. 385)

Most cases of spinal muscular atrophy are hereditary. Their clinical features vary according to the age of onset. Acquired forms are rare.

■ **Diseases Affecting Both the Upper and the Lower Motor Neuron**

Hereditary. Amyotrophic lateral sclerosis (ALS) is familial in 5–10% of cases. Familial ALS with onset in childhood and adolescence (*juvenile ALS*) is transmitted either as an autosomal recessive trait (ALS2:2q33;ALS5:15q15.1–21.1) or as an autosomal dominant trait (9q34 linkage). Adult-onset familial ALS is transmitted as an autosomal dominant trait (ALS1:21q22.1; ALS3:18q21) associated with a mutation of the gene for superoxide dismutase 1 (SOD1). SOD1 plays a role in converting cytotoxic oxygen radicals to hydrogen peroxide. It remains unknown how the SOD1 defect causes motor neuron disease. Autosomal dominant inheritance has also been found for ALS plus frontotemporal dementia (9q21–22). ALS together with parkinsonism and dementia occurs among the Chamorro people of Guam.

Acquired. Sporadic ALS usually becomes apparent between the ages 50 and 70 (Table 47, p. 386). The presentation is typically with asymmetric weakness of the limbs, either proximal (difficulty raising the arms or standing up from a sitting position) or distal (frequent falls; difficulty grasping, turning a key in a lock), or else with bulbar dysfunction (dysarthria). These deficits are often accompanied by leg cramps and continuous, marked fasciculation in the proximal limb muscles. As the disease progresses, weakness, muscular atrophy, dysphagia, and dysarthria become increasingly severe. Respiratory weakness leads to respiratory insufficiency. Spasticity, hyperreflexia, pseudobulbar palsy, emotional lability, and Babinski reflex (inconsistent) are caused by dysfunction of the first motor neuron; muscular atrophy and fasciculation are caused by dysfunction of the second motor neuron; and dysarthria, dysphagia, and weakness are caused by both. About 10% of patients have paresthesiae, and some have pain in later stages of the disease. Bladder, rectal, and sexual dysfunction, impairment of sweating, and bed sores are not part of the clinical picture of ALS. The disease progresses rapidly and usually causes death in 3–5 years.

■ **Treatment**

There is currently no effective primary treatment for motor neuron diseases. Treatment can be provided for the palliation of various disease manifestations, e. g., dysarthria (speech therapy, communication aids), dysphagia (swallowing training, percutaneous endoscopic gastrostomy, surgery), and drooling (medication to decrease salivary flow). Antispasmodic agents can be used to treat spasticity and muscle spasms, and psychiatric medications to treat emotional lability. Physical and occupational therapy are provided, including breathing exercises, contracture prophylaxis, and measures to increase mobility. Further measures include orthoses, breathing training (aspiration prophylaxis, secretolysis, ventilator for home use, tracheotomy), and psychosocial support. Riluzole (a glutamate antagonist) has been found to prolong survival in ALS.

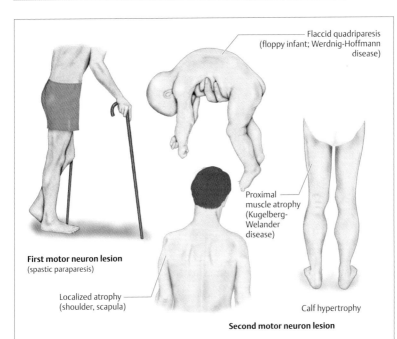

Flaccid quadriparesis
(floppy infant; Werdnig-Hoffmann
disease)

Proximal
muscle atrophy
(Kugelberg-
Welander
disease)

First motor neuron lesion
(spastic paraparesis)

Localized atrophy
(shoulder, scapula)

Calf hypertrophy

Second motor neuron lesion

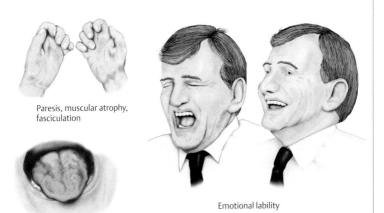

Paresis, muscular atrophy,
fasciculation

Emotional lability

Tongue muscle atrophy, dysarthria, dysphagia

Lesion of both first and second motor neurons

The term *encephalopathy* refers to a focal or generalized disturbance of brain function of noninfectious origin. Depending on their etiology, encephalopathies may be reversible, persistent, or progressive. Their clinical manifestations are diverse, depending on the particular functional system(s) of the brain that they affect.

Hereditary Metabolic Encephalopathies

These disorders frequently cause severe cognitive impairment. Most of them have an autosomal recessive inheritance pattern; a few are X-linked recessive. The underlying primary enzyme defect (enzymopathy) may be a monogenic, polygenic, or mitochondrial genetic trait, or a multifactorial disorder (see p. 288). All hereditary metabolic encephalopathies are characterized by chronic progression, recurrent impairment of consciousness, spasticity, cerebellar ataxia, extrapyramidal syndromes, and psychomotor developmental delay. The following tables contain a partial listing of hereditary metabolic encephalopathies (Lyon et al., 1996); for such disorders affecting neonates and infants, see p. 386f. Some of the diseases listed may appear earlier or later than the typical age of onset indicated.

■ **Metabolic Encephalopathies of Infancy (up to age 2 years)**

Syndrome	Defect/Enzyme Defect	Symptoms and Signs
Phenylketonuria	Phenylalanine hydroxylase deficiency	Psychomotor retardation, hyperactivity, movement disorders, stereotypic movements
Hartnup disease	Impaired renal/intestinal transport of neutral amino acids	Reddish, scaly changes of exposed skin, emotional lability, episodic cerebellar ataxia
Gaucher disease (type III, subacute neuropathic form)	See p. 387	Generalized seizures, ataxia, myoclonus, progressive mental decline, supranuclear oculomotor disturbances, splenomegaly
Niemann–Pick disease (type C)	Exact defect not known	Mental retardation, seizures, ataxia, dysarthria, vertical gaze palsy
Metachromatic leukodystrophy	Arylsulfatase A deficiency	Progressive gait impairment, spasticity, progressive dementia, dysarthria, blindness, cerebellar ataxia, polyneuropathy
Leigh disease[1]	No consistent defect[2]	Respiratory disturbances, gaze palsy, ataxia, decreased muscle tone, retinitis pigmentosa, seizures

1 Subacute necrotizing encephalomyelopathy. **2** Known defects include mitochondrial respiratory chain defects (complexes IV and V) and protein synthesis defects. The clinical features are heterogeneous. MRI scans show multiple, bilaterally symmetric lesions with sparing of the mamillary bodies. CSF lactate concentration increased. Muscle biopsy reveals no ragged red fibers.

■ **Metabolic Encephalopathies of Childhood and Adolescence (ages 3–18 years)**

Syndrome	Defect/Enzyme Defect	Symptoms and Signs
Abetalipoproteinemia	See pp. 280, 300	Gait impairment, ataxia, dysarthria, poly-neuropathy, night blindness
Progressive myoclonus epilepsy[1] with Lafora bodies[2]	Lysosomes	Epileptic seizures, myoclonus, dementia, cerebellar ataxia, epileptic visual phenomena
Wilson disease (dystonic type)	Copper transport protein[3]	Dysfunction/cirrhosis of liver, behavioral changes, facio-oropharyngeal rigidity (dysarthria, dysphagia), parkinsonism, tremor, dystonia, Kayser–Fleischer ring (p. 309)
Neuronal ceroid lipofuscinosis (Spielmeyer–Vogt syndrome)	Storage of lipid pigment in lysosomes	Visual impairment, dysarthria, dementia, epileptic seizures, myoclonus, parkinsonism
Panthothenate kinase-associated degeneration[8]	Accumulation of iron pigment in substantia nigra and globus pallidus[4]	Gait impairment, dystonia, dysarthria, behavioral changes, dementia, retinal depigmentation
Adrenoleukodystrophy[5]	Peroxisomes (p. 386)	Behavioral changes/dementia, gait impairment, cortical blindness, spastic quadriparesis, deafness, primary adrenocortical insufficiency
Homocystinuria[6]	Cystathionine β-synthase[7]	Dementia/behavioral changes, osteoporosis, ectopia lentis
Fabry disease[6]	α-Galactosidase A (⇑glycosphingolipids)	Attacks of pain in digits and abdomen; diffuse angiokeratomas; cataract
Mitochondrial syndromes	See p. 402	See p. 402

1 Other forms (p. 68) include Unverricht–Lundborg syndrome, myoclonus epilepsy with ragged red fibers (MERRF, p. 402), late forms of other lysosome defects (e. g., sialidosis type I, GM$_2$-gangliosidosis). **2** Cytoplasmic inclusion bodies containing glycoprotein mucopolysaccharides in the brain, muscles, skin, and liver (also called Lafora disease). **3** Autosomal recessive trait, mutation at 13q14.3; ⇓ serum ceruloplasmin, ⇑ hepatic copper, free serum copper, and urinary copper levels, ⇓ rate of incorporation of ^{64}Cu in ceruloplasmin, MRI signal changes (striatum, dentate nucleus, thalamus). **4** MRI shows bilaterally symmetric hypointensity of globus pallidus with central zone of hyperintensity ("tiger eye" sign). **5** Adrenomyeloneuropathy, p. 384. **6** Increased risk of stroke. **7** Most common form. **8** Formerly called Hallervorden-Spatz disease.

■ **Metabolic Encephalopathies of Adulthood**

Syndrome	Defect/Enzyme Defect	Symptoms and Signs
Metachromatic leukodystrophy	Arylsulfatase-A deficiency	Behavioral changes, gait impairment, dementia
Krabbe disease	See p. 387	Gait impairment, spastic quadriparesis, poly-neuropathy, optic nerve atrophy
Adrenoleukodystrophy	Peroxisomes	Adult form extremely rare
Neuronal ceroid lipofuscinosis (Kufs disease)	Storage of lipid pigment in lysosomes	Type A: Epilepsy, myoclonus, dementia, ataxia Type B: Behavioral changes/dementia, facial dyskinesia, movement disorders
GM$_1$ gangliosidosis	See p. 387	Progressive dysarthria and dystonia
GM$_2$ gangliosidosis[1]	See p. 387	Chronic progression (p. 387)
Wilson disease (pseudo-sclerotic type)[2]	See above	Postural/intention tremor (beginning in one arm), behavioral changes, dysarthria, dysphagia, masklike facies, parkinsonism
Gaucher disease type 3	See p. 387	Supranuclear ophthalmoplegia, epileptic seizures, myoclonus, splenomegaly
Niemann–Pick disease (type C)	See p. 387	Cerebellar ataxia, intention tremor, dysarthria, supranuclear vertical gaze palsy
Mitochondrial syndromes	See p. 402	See p. 402

1 Tay–Sachs disease. **2** Westphal–Strümpell disease.

Central Nervous System

Acquired Metabolic Encephalopathies

Hypoxic–ischemic encephalopathy. An acute lack of oxygen (Pao_2 < 40 mmHg), severe hypotension (< 70 mmHg systolic), or a combination of the two causes loss of consciousness within minutes. The most important causes of hypoxic and ischemic states are an inadequate pumping function of the heart (as in myocardial infarction, shock, and cardiac arrhythmia), suffocation, carbon monoxide poisoning, respiratory muscle paralysis (as in spinal trauma, Guillain–Barré syndrome, and myasthenia), and inadequate ventilation (as in opiate intoxication). Permanent damage usually does not occur if the partial pressure of oxygen and the blood pressure can be brought back to normal in 3–5 minutes. Longer periods of hypoxia and ischemia are rarely tolerated (except under conditions of hypothermia or barbiturate intoxication); brain damage usually ensues, and may be permanent. Persistent coma (p. 118) with absent brain stem reflexes (pp. 26, 118) once the circulation is restored indicates a poor prognosis; the probable outcome is then a persistent vegetative state or death (p. 120). Patients who regain consciousness may develop various *postanoxic syndromes*, e. g., dementia, visual agnosia, parkinsonism with personality changes, choreoathetosis, cerebellar ataxia, intention or action myoclonus (Lance–Adams syndrome), and Korsakoff syndrome. *Delayed postanoxic syndrome* occurs 1–4 weeks after the initial recovery from anoxia and is characterized by behavioral changes (apathy, confusion, restlessness) that may either regress or worsen, perhaps to coma. These changes may be accompanied by gait impairment and parkinsonism. *Hypercapnia* ($\uparrow PaCO_2$) due to chronic hypoventilation (as in emphysema, fibrosing alveolitis, or central hypoventilation) causes headache, behavioral disturbances, impairment of consciousness (p. 116 ff), asterixis (p. 68), fasciculations, and bilateral papilledema.

Hypoglycemia. If the blood glucose concentration *acutely* falls below 40 mg/dl, behavioral changes occur (restlessness, hunger, sweating, anxiety, confusion). Any further decrease leads to unconsciousness (grand mal seizure, dilated pupils, pale skin, shallow breathing, bradycardia, decreased muscle tone). Glucose must be given intravenously to prevent severe brain damage. *Subacute* hypoglycemia produces slowed thinking, attention deficits, and hypothermia. *Chronic* hypoglycemia produces behavioral changes and ataxia (p. 324); it is rarely seen (e. g., in pancreatic islet cell tumors).

Hyperglycemia (p. 324). *Diabetic ketoacidosis* is characterized by dehydration, headache, fatigue, abdominal pain, Kussmaul respiration (deep, rhythmic breathing at a normal or increased rate). Blood glucose > 350 mg/dl ($\uparrow$ pH, $\downarrow p_{CO_2}$, $\downarrow HCO_3^-$). In *hyperosmolar non-ketotic hyperglycemia*, the blood glucose concentration is > 600 mg/dl and there is little or no ketoacidosis. The persons at greatest risk are elderly patients being treated with corticosteroids and/or hyperosmolar agents to reduce edema around a brain tumor.

Hepatic/portosystemic encephalopathy occurs by an unknown pathogenetic mechanism in patients with severe liver failure (hepatic encephalopathy) and/or intrahepatic or extrahepatic venous shunts (portosystemic encephalopathy). Venous shunts can develop spontaneously (e. g., hepatic cirrhosis) or be created surgically (portocaval anastomosis, transjugular intrahepatic stent). *Clinical features* (see Table 50, p. 387): Behavioral changes, variable neurological signs (increased or decreased reflexes, Babinski reflex, rigidity, decreased muscle tone, asterixis, dysarthrophonia, tremor, hepatic coma), and EEG changes (generalized symmetric delta/triphasic waves). The diagnosis is based on the clinical findings, the exclusion of other causes of encephalopathy (such as intoxication, sepsis, meningoencephalitis, and electrolyte disorders), and an elevated arterial serum ammonia concentration.

Repeated episodes of hepatic coma may lead to *chronic encephalopathy* (head tremor, asterixis, choreoathetosis, ataxia, behavioral changes); this can be prevented by timely liver transplantation.

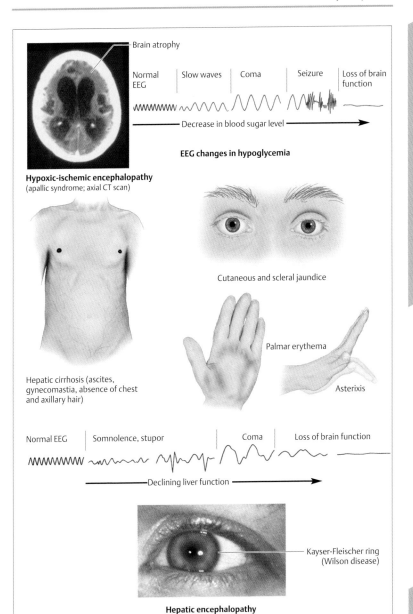

Brain atrophy

Normal EEG | Slow waves | Coma | Seizure | Loss of brain function

Decrease in blood sugar level

EEG changes in hypoglycemia

Hypoxic-ischemic encephalopathy
(apallic syndrome; axial CT scan)

Cutaneous and scleral jaundice

Palmar erythema

Asterixis

Hepatic cirrhosis (ascites, gynecomastia, absence of chest and axillary hair)

Normal EEG | Somnolence, stupor | Coma | Loss of brain function

Declining liver function

Kayser-Fleischer ring (Wilson disease)

Hepatic encephalopathy

Encephalopathies

Disorders of fluid and electrolyte balance. The regulation of water balance (*osmoregulation*) is reflected in the serum sodium concentration, [Na$^+$]. The hypothalamus, which contains osmoreceptors (p. 142), controls thirst and the secretion of ADH; these in turn determine fluid intake and urine osmolality. Sodium salts account for more than 95 % of the plasma osmolality (moles of osmotically active particles per kg of water). Hyperhydration causes a decrease in plasma osmolality (⇓ [Na$^+$]). The ensuing inhibition of thirst and of ADH secretion leads to a reduction of oral fluid intake and to the production of dilute urine (⇓ urinary [Na$^+$]), restoring the normally hydrated state. Dehydration induces the opposite changes, again resulting in restoration of the normally hydrated state.

The regulation of sodium balance (*volume regulation*) maintains adequate tissue perfusion (p. 148). Volume receptors in the carotid sinus and atria of the heart are the afferent arm of the reflex pathway controlling renal sodium excretion, whose efferent arms are the sympathetic system, the renin–angiotensin–aldosterone system (RAAS), and natriuretic peptides. *Hypovolemia and hypervolemia* usually involve combined abnormalities of water and sodium balance.

In neurological disorders (head trauma, meningoencephalitis, brain tumor, subarachnoid hemorrhage, acute porphyria), the *syndrome of inappropriate ADH secretion* (SIADH) is characterized by water retention (volume expansion), abnormally concentrated urine, and hyponatremia. The more rapidly hyponatremia develops, the more severe its clinical signs (e. g., confusion, seizures, impairment of consciousness). SIADH is to be distinguished from *central salt-wasting syndrome*, which is characterized by hypovolemia and dehydration.

Too rapid correction of hyponatremia causes most cases of *central pontine myelinolysis* (other causes are serum hyperosmolality and malnutrition). In this syndrome (p. 315), a patient with a major systemic illness (e. g., postoperative state, alcoholism) develops quadriplegia, pseudobulbar palsy, and locked-in syndrome (p. 120) over the course of a few days. A less severe form of central pontine myelinolysis is characterized by confusion, dysarthria, and gaze palsies.

Calcium/magnesium. *Hypercalcemia* causes nonspecific symptoms along with apathy, progressive weakness, and impairment of consciousness (or even coma). *Hypocalcemia* is characterized by increased neuromuscular excitability (muscle spasms, laryngospasm, tetany, Chvostek's and Trousseau's signs), irritability, hallucinations, depression, and epileptic seizures. *Hypomagnesemia* has similar clinical features.

Uremic encephalopathy arises in patients with renal failure and is characterized by behavioral changes (apathy, cognitive impairment, attention deficit, confusion, hallucinations), headache, dysarthria, and hyperkinesia (myoclonus, choreoathetosis, tremor, asterixis). Severe uremia can produce coma. The differential diagnosis of uremic encephalopathy includes cerebral complications of the primary disease, such as intracranial hemorrhage, drug intoxication because of impaired catabolism, and hypertensive encephalopathy. A similar neurological syndrome can arise during or after hemodialysis or peritoneal dialysis (*dysequilibrium syndrome*). *Dialysis encephalopathy* (dialysis dementia; now rare) is probably due to aluminum poisoning as a complication of chronic hemodialysis. Its manifestations include dysarthria with stuttering and stammering, myoclonus, epileptic seizures, and behavioral changes (p. 122 ff).

Endocrine encephalopathy is characterized by agitation with hallucinations and delirium, anxiety, apathy, depression or euphoria, irritability, insomnia, impairment of memory and concentration, psychomotor slowing, and impairment of consciousness. It may be produced (in varying degrees of severity) by Cushing disease, high-dose corticosteroid therapy, Addison disease, hyperthyroidism or hypothyroidism, and hyperparathyroidism or hypoparathyroidism.

Symptome and signs

Increase in thirst, ADH, urinary [Na$^+$], hematocrit, and total protein; decrease in blood pressure and central venous pressure; tachycardia

Water loss (dehydration) ($\Rightarrow \triangle$[Na$^+$]) (hypertonic disturbances)

```
─ 305
─ 300
─ 295
─ 290    Euhydration
          Isotonic [Na⁺] (isotonic disturbances)
─ 285
─ 280
─ 275    Water retention (hyperhydration)
          ⇨ [Na⁺] (hypotonic disturbances)¹
```

Decrease in thirst, ADH, urinary [Na$^+$], hematocrit, and total protein; increase in blood pressure and central venous pressure; edema, dyspnea

Water balance (mOsm/kg water; [1] "pseudohyponatremia" in association with hyperglycemia, hyperlipidemia, and hyperproteinemia)

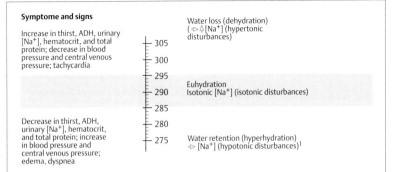

Causes [2]

Diabetes insipidus, hypothalamic dysfunction, hyperhidrosis, dysphagia, Cushing syndrome, hyperaldosteronism

Syndromes

Coma, epileptic seizure, lethargy, confusion, irritability

Hypernatremia (hypertonic)

```
─ 160
─ 155
─ 150
─ 145
─ 140    Normonatremia
          (isotonic)
─ 135
─ 130
─ 125
─ 120
```

Vomiting, diarrhea, burns, diuretics, Addison disease, SIADH, polydipsia, hyperglycemia, mannitol

Headache, nausea, vomiting, impairment of consciousness, confusion, epileptic seizure, coma

Hyponatremia (hypotonic)

Sodium balance (mmol/L; [2] examples, some with combined deficits)

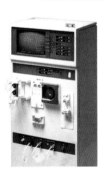

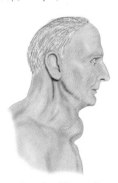

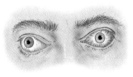

Marked endocrine orbitopathy (in Graves disease)

Dialysis for uremia   **Hypothyroidism, goiter**

Encephalopathy due to sepsis, multiple organ failure, or burns may arise within a few hours, manifesting itself as impaired concentration, disorientation, confusion, and psychomotor agitation in addition to the already severe systemic disturbances. In severe cases, there may be delirium, stupor or coma. Focal neurological signs are absent; meningismus may be present, and CSF studies do not show signs of meningoencephalitis. There are nonspecific EEG changes (generalized delta and theta wave activity). The pathogenesis of these syndromes is unclear. Their prognosis is poor if the underlying disease does not respond rapidly to treatment.

Paraneoplastic encephalopathy occurs as a complication of neoplasms outside the central nervous system. It can only be diagnosed after the exclusion of local tumor invasion or metastasis, complications of tumor treatment, or other complications of the primary disease. For paraneoplastic encephalopathy, see Table 51, p. 388; for paraneoplastic disorders affecting the PNS, neuromuscular junction, and muscle, see p. 406.

Wernicke–Korsakoff syndrome. *Wernicke encephalopathy* is characterized by gaze-evoked nystagmus or dissociated nystagmus, ophthalmoplegia (abducens palsy, conjugate gaze palsy or, rarely, miosis), postural and gait ataxia, and impairment of consciousness (p. 116; apathy, indifference, somnolence). *Korsakoff syndrome* is characterized by confabulatory amnesia (p. 134), disorientation, and decreased cognitive flexibility. Most patients have a combination of these two syndromes, which is then called *Wernicke–Korsakoff syndrome*. Polyneuropathy, autonomic dysfunction (orthostatic hypotension, tachycardia, exercise dyspnea), and anosmia may also be present. These syndromes are caused by a deficiency of thiamin (vitamin B_1) due to alcoholism or malnutrition (malignant tumors, gastroenterologic disease, thiamin-free parenteral nutrition). This, in turn, causes dysfunction of thiamin-dependent enzymes (increase in transketolase, pyruvate decarboxylase, α-ketoglutarate dehydrogenase, and serum pyruvate and lactate; decrease in transketolase activity in erythrocytes). MRI reveals lesions in paraventricular areas (thalamus, hypothalamus, mamillary bodies) and periaqueductal areas (mid brain, motor nucleus of X, vestibular nu-

clei, superior cerebellar vermis). *Treatment:* Immediate intravenous infusion of thiamin (50–100 mg) in glucose solution. *Note:* glucose infusion without thiamin in a patient with latent or unrecognized thiamin deficiency may provoke or exacerbate Wernicke encephalopathy.

Encephalopathies Due to Substance Abuse

Alcohol. Acute alcohol intoxication (drunkenness, inebriation) may be mild (blood alcohol 0.1–1.5‰ ⇨ dysarthria, incoordination, disinhibition, increased self-confidence, uncritical self-assessment), moderate (blood alcohol 1.5–2.5‰ ⇨ ataxia, nystagmus, explosive reactions, aggressiveness, euphoria, suggestibility), or severe (blood alcohol >2.5‰ ⇨ loss of judgment, severe ataxia, impairment of consciousness, autonomic symptoms such as hypothermia, hypotension, or respiratory arrest). Concomitant intoxication with other substances (sedatives, hypnotics, illicit drugs) is not uncommon. The possibility of a traumatic brain injury (subdural or epidural hematoma, intracerebral hemorrhage) must also be considered. *Pathological intoxication* after the intake of relatively small quantities of alcohol is a rare disorder characterized by intense outbursts of emotion and destructive behavior, followed by deep sleep. The patient has no memory of these events.

Alcohol withdrawal syndrome. Reduction of alcohol intake or total abstinence from alcohol after chronic alcohol abuse causes acute autonomic disturbances (sweating, tachycardia, insomnia, nausea, vomiting), tremor, impairment of concentration, and behavioral changes. This initial stage of *predelirium* is followed by a stage of *delirium* (delirium tremens), in which all of the disturbances listed worsen and are accompanied by visual hallucinations. Epileptic seizures may occur. The course of delirium tremens can be complicated by systemic diseases that are themselves complications of alcoholism (hepatic and pancreatic disease, pneumonia, sepsis, electrolyte imbalances). Auditory alcoholic hallucinosis without autonomic symptoms or disorientation is an unusual form of alcohol withdrawal syndrome.

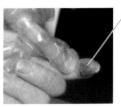

Microemboli in a patient with bacteremia (*Staphylococcus aureus*)

Sepsis

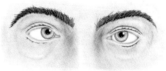

Wernicke encephalopathy (ophthalmoplegia)

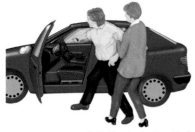

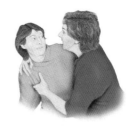

Acute alcohol intoxication (uncritical self-assessment, disinhibition)

- Decline of general health
- Loss of appetite, weight loss
- Gastrointestinal disturbances
- Behavioral changes
- Wernicke-Korsakoff syndrome
- Brain atrophy
- Head trauma
- Polyneuropathy
- Myopathy

Additional intoxication with hypnotics or other substances

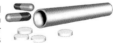

- Epileptic seizures
- Predelirium/delirium
- Alcoholic hallucinosis

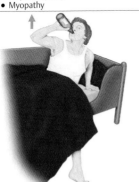

Chronic alcoholism

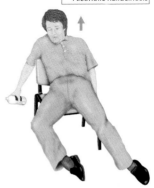

Alcohol withdrawal syndrome

Alcoholism

Late complications of alcoholism. Various disorders are associated with chronic alcohol abuse, though alcohol abuse may not be the only causative factor. *Brain atrophy* is often seen in CT or MRI scans and seems to be reversible by abstinence. In *alcoholic dementia*, brain atrophy is accompanied by cognitive impairment; most cases are probably due to Wernicke–Korsakoff syndrome (p. 312). *Cerebellar atrophy* predominantly affects the anterosuperior vermis (⇨ postural and gait ataxia). *Central pontine myelinolysis* (p. 310) and *tobacco–alcohol amblyopia* (bilateral impairment of visual acuity and visual defects, probably due to a combined deficiency of vitamins B_1, B_6, and B_{12}) are other late complications of alcoholism. *Fetal alcohol syndrome* (congenital malformations, hyperactivity, attention deficit, impaired fine motor control) is seen in the children of alcoholic mothers.

Substance abuse. Neurological signs of substance abuse are described in the table below.

Substance	Pupils	Motor Dysfunction	Reflexes[3]	Behavior/Consciousness
Cocaine[1,2]	Dilated	Chorea, tremor, dystonia, myoclonus, bruxism	⇧	Anxiety, agitation, insomnia, psychosis/hypervigilance ⇨ lethargy, coma
Amphetamines[1,2]	Dilated	Chorea, bruxism, muscle spasms, tremor	⇧	Euphoria, hyperactivity, dysphoria, hallucinations, confusion/ hypervigilance
MDMA[1,2,4]	Dilated	Tremor, rigidity	⇧	Anxiety, hyperactivity, psychosis/coma[5]
Opiates[1,6]	Pinpoint	Hypokinesia, parkinsonism	⇩	Euphoria/somnolence ⇨ coma, respiratory depression
LSD[7]	Dilated, sluggish	Tremor	⇧	Euphoria, panic, depression, hallucinations, illusions
Phencyclidine (PCP)	Miotic; nystagmus	Ataxia, tremor, increased muscle tone	⇧	Euphoria, dysphoria, psychosis, aggressiveness, hallucinations/ coma (rare)

1 Epileptic seizures may occur. **2** Cerebral infarction or hemorrhage may occur. **3** ⇩ : weak; ⇧: brisk or increased. **4** Methylenedioxymethamphetamine = "ecstasy." **5** Causes: dehydration, hyponatremia, cerebral edema, cardiovascular complications, hyperthermia, rhabdomyolysis. **6** Myelopathy, polyneuropathy, Guillain–Barré syndrome, and rhabdomyolysis may occur in chronic heroin users. **7** D-lysergic acid diethylamide.

Iatrogenic Encephalopathies

Neurological side effects of diagnostic studies and therapies must be kept in mind in the clinical decision-making process (risk/benefit analysis) and must be considered in the differential diagnosis of encephalopathy. Such side effects are easily mistaken for neurological dysfunction of another etiology. Examples are listed in Table 52 (p. 389).

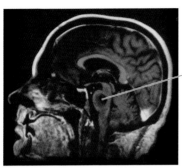

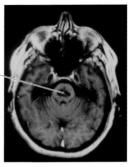

Signal
attenuation
(pons)

Central pontine myelinolysis
(sagittal/axial T$_1$-weighted MRI images)

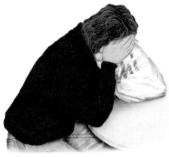

Inhalation of industrial or household chemicals
("sniffing")

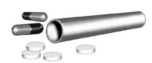

Iatrogenic encephalopathy

- Ethylene oxide (gas sterilization)
- Lead (children)
- Industrial waste
- Organic solvents (hydrocarbons, ketones, esters, alcohols)
- Organic tin compounds (wood care products, silicone rubber, thermal insulators)
- Pesticides
- Mercury
- Thallium (rat poison)

Encephalopathies caused by industrial toxins

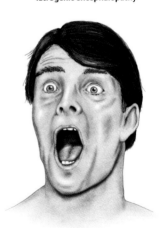

Drugs (behavioral changes)

Peripheral Nerve and Muscle

Neuropathy Syndromes

Disturbances of the peripheral nervous system may be subdivided into those affecting neuronal cell bodies (*neuronopathy*) and those affecting peripheral nerve processes (*peripheral neuropathy*). *Neuronopathies* include anterior horn cell syndromes (motor neuron lesions; p. 50) and sensory neuron syndromes (sensory neuronopathy, ganglionopathy; pp. 2, 107, 390). Motor neuron diseases are described on p. 304. *Peripheral neuropathy* is characterized by damage to myelin sheaths (myelinopathy) and/or axons (axonopathy). Neuropathies may affect a single nerve (mononeuropathy), multiple isolated nerves (mononeuropathy multiplex), all peripheral nerves generally (polyneuropathy), or all peripheral nerves generally with accentuation of one or a few (focal polyneuropathy). Polyneuropathy may be accompanied by autonomic dysfunction (p. 140). The terms polyneuropathy (PNP) and peripheral neuropathy are often used synonymously. *Radiculopathies* (nerve root lesions) are classified as either monoradiculopathies or polyradiculopathies, depending on whether a single or multiple roots are involved.

■ Symptoms and Signs

Peripheral neuropathy causes sensory, motor, and/or autonomic dysfunction. Its etiological diagnosis is based on the pattern and timing of clinical manifestations (Table 53, p. 390).

Sensory dysfunction (p. 106) is often the first sign of neuropathy. Sensory deficits have distinctive patterns of distribution: they may be predominantly proximal or distal, symmetrical (stocking/glove distribution) or asymmetrical (multiple mononeuropathy), or restricted to individual nerves (cranial nerves, single nerves of the trunk or limbs; p. 32 f). Disordered sensory processing (p. 108 f) can produce hyperalgesia (more pain than normal upon noxious stimulation), hyperesthesia (increased tactile sensation with lowering of threshold), paresthesia (spontaneous or provoked abnormal sensation), dysesthesia (spontaneous or provoked, abnormal, painful sensation), or allodynia (pain resulting from nonnoxious stimuli). Damage to rapidly conducting, thickly myelinated A-β fibers causes paresthesiae such as tingling, prickling ("pins and needles"), formication, and sensations of tension, pressure, and swelling. Damage to slowly conducting, thinly myelinated A-δ and C fibers (*small fiber neuropathy*) causes hypalgesia or analgesia with thermal hypesthesia or anesthesia, abnormal thermal sensations (cold, heat), and pain (burning, cutting, or dull, pulling pain).

Motor dysfunction (p. 50). Weakness usually appears first in distal muscles. In very slowly progressive neuropathies, muscles may become atrophic before they become weak, but weakness is usually the initial symptom, accompanied by hyporeflexia or areflexia. The cranial nerves can be affected. Hyperactivity in motor A-α fibers produces muscle spasms, fasciculations, and/or myokymia.

Autonomic dysfunction (p. 146 f) can be manifest as vasomotor disturbances (syncope), cardiac arrhythmias (tachycardia, bradycardia, fixed heart rate), urinary and gastrointestinal dysfunction (urinary retention, diarrhea, constipation, gastroparesis), sexual dysfunction (impotence, retrograde ejaculation), hyperhidrosis or hypohidrosis, pupillary dysfunction, and trophic lesions (skin ulcers, bone and joint changes).

■ Etiology (Table 54, p. 390)

Polyneuropathies can be hereditary or acquired (see Table 54).

■ Diagnosis (Table 55, p. 391)

The diagnosis of a neuropathy is based on the characteristic clinical findings and patient history. Additional diagnostic studies not indicated on the basis of the patient history and clinical findings may produce not only unjustified costs but also confounding data, leading occasionally to misdiagnosis. Studies to be performed as indicated include neurophysiological tests (nerve conduction studies, electromyography), laboratory tests (blood, CSF), tissue biopsy (nerve, skin, muscle), and genetic tests.

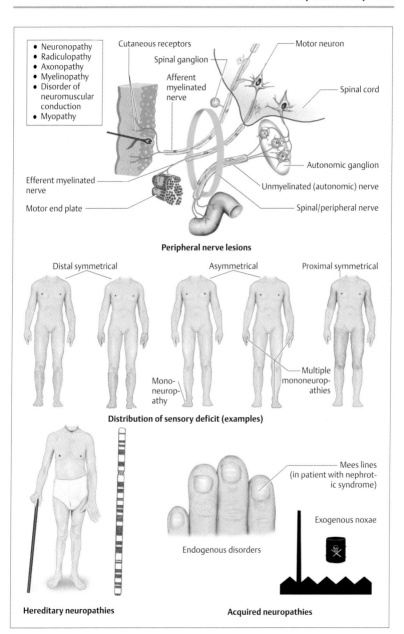

- Neuronopathy
- Radiculopathy
- Axonopathy
- Myelinopathy
- Disorder of neuromuscular conduction
- Myopathy

Cutaneous receptors

Spinal ganglion

Afferent myelinated nerve

Motor neuron

Spinal cord

Efferent myelinated nerve

Motor end plate

Autonomic ganglion

Unmyelinated (autonomic) nerve

Spinal/peripheral nerve

Peripheral nerve lesions

Distal symmetrical

Asymmetrical

Proximal symmetrical

Mono-neuropathy

Multiple mononeuropathies

Distribution of sensory deficit (examples)

Mees lines (in patient with nephrotic syndrome)

Exogenous noxae

Endogenous disorders

Hereditary neuropathies

Acquired neuropathies

Peripheral Nerve and Muscle

317

Radicular Lesions

■ Symptoms and Signs

Patients usually complain mainly of positive sensory symptoms (tingling, burning, intense pain), which, like the accompanying sensory deficit (mainly hypalgesia, see p. 104 f), are in a dermatomal distribution (p. 32 ff). Weakness, if any, is found mainly in muscles that are largely or entirely innervated by a single nerve root (pp. 32, 50); loss of the segmental deep tendon reflex (p. 40) is, however, a typical early finding. Monoradiculopathy does not cause any evident autonomic dysfunction in the limbs. Lumbar monoradiculopathy is frequently caused by lumbar disk herniation with secondary root compression; typical findings in such cases include exacerbation of radicular pain by coughing, straining at stool, sneezing, or vibration (⇨ the patient adopts an antalgic posture), as well as Lasègue's sign (radicular pain on passive raising of the leg with extended knee) and Bragard's sign (radicular pain on dorsiflexion of the foot with the leg raised and extended). Bladder, bowel, and sexual dysfunction may be caused by a lesion affecting multiple roots of the cauda equina (p. 48), or by processes affecting the spinal cord (pp. 48, 282) or sacral plexus (see below).

Pseudoradicular syndromes (including so-called myofascial syndrome, tendomyalgia, myotendinosis) are characterized by limb pain, localized muscle tenderness, and muscle guarding and disuse, without radicular findings.

■ Causes

See Table 56, p. 392, and p. 320.

Plexopathy (p. 321)

For clinical purposes the brachial plexus (p. 34) located behind the clavicle may be divided into *supraclavicular* and *infraclavicular* regions. The supraclavicular plexus consists of the primary (ventral and dorsal) roots, mixed spinal nerves, five anterior primary rami, and three trunks; the infraclavicular plexus is composed of the three cords and the terminal nerves. Lesions affecting the supraclavicular plexus can either be preganglionic (intradural, inside the spinal canal) or infraganglionic (extradural, extraforaminal, outside the spinal canal). Supraclavicular plexopathies are more common than infraclavicular ones.

■ Symptoms and Signs

Brachial plexus. Lesions affecting the *entire brachial plexus* cause anesthesia and flaccid paralysis of the entire upper limb, with muscle atrophy. Lesions of the *upper brachial plexus* (C5–C6) cause weakness of shoulder abduction and external rotation, elbow flexion, and supination, with preservation of hand movement (Erb palsy). The limb hangs straight down with the hand pronated. A sensory deficit may be found on the lateral aspect of the arm and forearm. Lesions of the *lower brachial plexus* (C8–T1) mainly cause weakness of the hand muscles (Klumpke–Dejerine palsy); atrophy of the intrinsic muscles produces a claw hand deformity. A sensory deficit is found on the ulnar aspect of the forearm and in the hand. Concomitant involvement of the cervical sympathetic pathway produces Horner syndrome. Erb palsy is more likely to recover spontaneously than Klumpke–Dejerine palsy.

Lumbosacral plexus. Lesions of the *lumbar plexus* (L1–L4) cause weakness of hip flexion and knee extension (as in a femoral nerve lesion) as well as thigh adduction and external rotation. A sensory deficit is found in the affected dermatomes (p. 36). Lesions of the *sacral plexus* (L5–S3) cause weakness of the gluteal muscles, hamstrings, and plantar and dorsiflexors of the foot and toes. A sensory deficit is found on the dorsal aspect of the thigh, calf, and foot. Lesions of the *lumbar sympathetic trunk* cause leg pain and an abnormally warm foot with diminished sweating on the sole.

■ Causes

See Table 57, p. 393.

Mononeuropathies (p. 322 f)

Lesions affecting a single nerve tend to occur at certain favored sites and are usually of mechanical origin (compression, hyperextension, transection) (Table 58, p. 394).

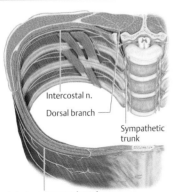

Intercostal n.

Dorsal branch

Sympathetic trunk

Anterior cutaneous branch

Segmental distribution (radicular n.)

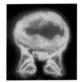

Lateral herniation

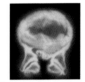

Mediolateral herniation

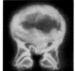

Medial herniation

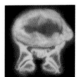

Lateral herniation (extraforaminal)

Lumbar intervertebral disk herniation (axial CT)

Peripheral Nerve and Muscle

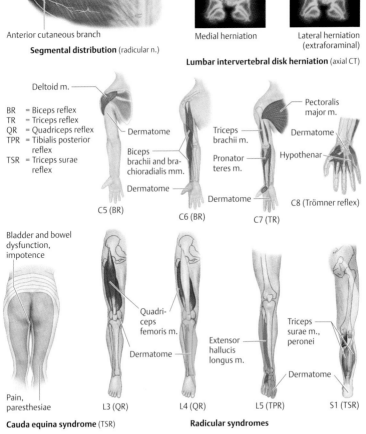

Deltoid m.

BR = Biceps reflex
TR = Triceps reflex
QR = Quadriceps reflex
TPR = Tibialis posterior reflex
TSR = Triceps surae reflex

Dermatome

Biceps brachii and brachioradialis mm.

Dermatome

C5 (BR)

C6 (BR)

Triceps brachii m.

Pronator teres m.

Dermatome

C7 (TR)

Pectoralis major m.

Dermatome

Hypothenar

C8 (Trömner reflex)

Bladder and bowel dysfunction, impotence

Pain, paresthesiae

Cauda equina syndrome (TSR)

Quadriceps femoris m.

Dermatome

L3 (QR)

L4 (QR)

Extensor hallucis longus m.

L5 (TPR)

Triceps surae m., peronei

Dermatome

S1 (TSR)

Radicular syndromes

319

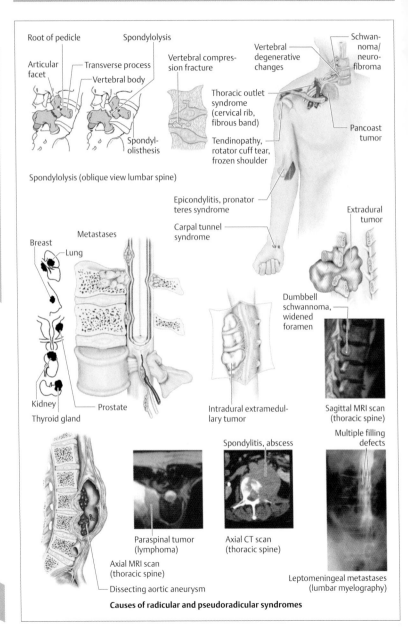

Root of pedicle

Spondylolysis

Articular facet

Transverse process

Vertebral body

Vertebral compression fracture

Vertebral degenerative changes

Schwannoma/neurofibroma

Thoracic outlet syndrome (cervical rib, fibrous band)

Pancoast tumor

Spondylolisthesis

Tendinopathy, rotator cuff tear, frozen shoulder

Spondylolysis (oblique view lumbar spine)

Epicondylitis, pronator teres syndrome

Carpal tunnel syndrome

Extradural tumor

Metastases

Breast

Lung

Dumbbell schwannoma, widened foramen

Kidney

Prostate

Thyroid gland

Intradural extramedullary tumor

Sagittal MRI scan (thoracic spine)

Multiple filling defects

Spondylitis, abscess

Paraspinal tumor (lymphoma)

Axial CT scan (thoracic spine)

Axial MRI scan (thoracic spine)

Dissecting aortic aneurysm

Leptomeningeal metastases (lumbar myelography)

Causes of radicular and pseudoradicular syndromes

Peripheral Nerve and Muscle

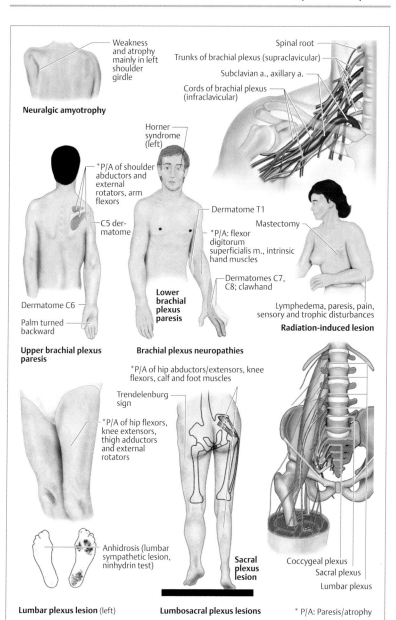

Neuralgic amyotrophy

Weakness and atrophy mainly in left shoulder girdle

Spinal root
Trunks of brachial plexus (supraclavicular)
Subclavian a., axillary a.
Cords of brachial plexus (infraclavicular)

Horner syndrome (left)

*P/A of shoulder abductors and external rotators, arm flexors

C5 dermatome

Dermatome T1

Mastectomy

*P/A: flexor digitorum superficialis m., intrinsic hand muscles

Dermatomes C7, C8; clawhand

Lower brachial plexus paresis

Lymphedema, paresis, pain, sensory and trophic disturbances

Radiation-induced lesion

Dermatome C6

Palm turned backward

Upper brachial plexus paresis

Brachial plexus neuropathies

*P/A of hip abductors/extensors, knee flexors, calf and foot muscles

Trendelenburg sign

*P/A of hip flexors, knee extensors, thigh adductors and external rotators

Anhidrosis (lumbar sympathetic lesion, ninhydrin test)

Sacral plexus lesion

Coccygeal plexus
Sacral plexus
Lumbar plexus

Lumbar plexus lesion (left)

Lumbosacral plexus lesions

* P/A: Paresis/atrophy

Peripheral Nerve and Muscle

321

Peripheral Nerve and Muscle

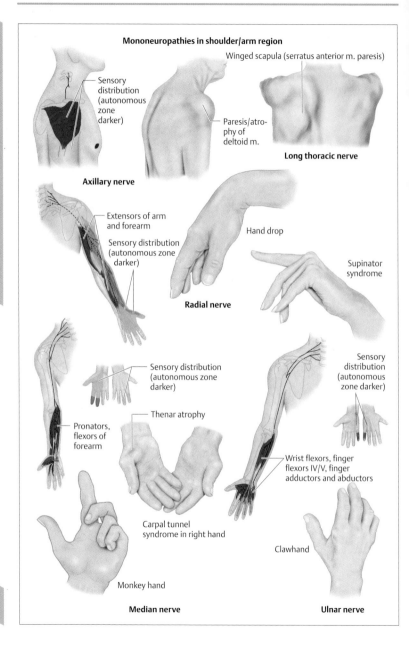

Mononeuropathies in shoulder/arm region

Winged scapula (serratus anterior m. paresis)

Sensory distribution (autonomous zone darker)

Paresis/atrophy of deltoid m.

Long thoracic nerve

Axillary nerve

Extensors of arm and forearm

Sensory distribution (autonomous zone darker)

Hand drop

Supinator syndrome

Radial nerve

Sensory distribution (autonomous zone darker)

Thenar atrophy

Pronators, flexors of forearm

Carpal tunnel syndrome in right hand

Sensory distribution (autonomous zone darker)

Wrist flexors, finger flexors IV/V, finger adductors and abductors

Clawhand

Monkey hand

Median nerve

Ulnar nerve

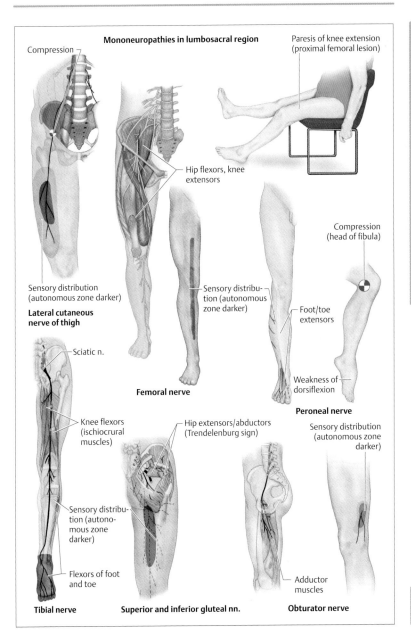

Mononeuropathies in lumbosacral region

Compression

Paresis of knee extension (proximal femoral lesion)

Hip flexors, knee extensors

Sensory distribution (autonomous zone darker)

Lateral cutaneous nerve of thigh

Sensory distribution (autonomous zone darker)

Femoral nerve

Compression (head of fibula)

Foot/toe extensors

Weakness of dorsiflexion

Peroneal nerve

Sciatic n.

Knee flexors (ischiocrural muscles)

Sensory distribution (autonomous zone darker)

Flexors of foot and toe

Tibial nerve

Hip extensors/abductors (Trendelenburg sign)

Adductor muscles

Superior and inferior gluteal nn.

Sensory distribution (autonomous zone darker)

Obturator nerve

Diabetic Neuropathies

■ Diabetes Mellitus

Diabetes mellitus (DM) is a syndrome of impaired carbohydrate metabolism due to insulin deficiency. In Type 1 DM (about 10% of cases), the insulin-secreting pancreatic cells are destroyed by an autoimmune process; Type 2 DM (the remaining 90%) is a nonautoimmune disorder typified by insulin resistance and abnormally low insulin secretion, usually in conjunction with obesity. Sequelae of DM include arteriosclerosis, microangiopathy, retinopathy, nephropathy, and peripheral neuropathy. The fasting blood glucose concentration is elevated (≥ 126 mg/dl), or else the blood glucose concentration is elevated after a standardized oral glucose load. An integrated index of elevated blood glucose concentration over time can be obtained by measuring the concentration of glycosylated hemoglobins (HBA$_1$, HBA$_{1C}$ $\Rightarrow$ 4–6 weeks) and proteins (fructosamine $\Rightarrow$ 8–14 days).

■ Syndromes

Pathogenesis. Distal symmetric polyneuropathy, a form of diabetic polyneuropathy (DPN), is due to generalized peripheral nerve damage. It is a complication of continuous hyperglycemia and the related metabolic changes ($\Rightarrow$ polyols, phospholipids, fatty acids, oxidative radicals, lack of nerve growth factors). Normalization of the blood glucose concentration by medical treatment can prevent DPN (at least partially) but, long-standing severe DPN, once established, cannot be completely reversed by euglycemia. Pathological examination reveals extensive axon loss, which is thought to be due either to the chronic hyperglycemia itself or to the resulting (perhaps inflammatory) microvascular changes. Repeated episodes of *hypoglycemia* (p. 308) can also cause neuropathy.

Symptoms and signs. DPN produces both negative neurological signs (sensory loss, sensory ataxia, thermanesthesia, hypalgesia, autonomic dysfunction, paresis) and positive neurological signs (paresthesia, dysesthesia, pain). The manifestations of DPN are classified in Table 59 (p. 395). They may be present in varying combinations.

Diagnosis. DPN is diagnosed in diabetic patients with distal, symmetric, sensorimotor poly-

neuropathy of the lower limbs, after the exclusion of other causes (e. g., diabetic lumbosacral or radicular lesions ($\Rightarrow$ Table 59), other neuropathies or primary illnesses); it is usually accompanied by diabetic retinopathy or nephropathy of comparable severity. Other neuropathic syndromes found in diabetes (some symmetric, some asymmetric) require the use of specialized tests for their differential diagnosis (p. 391).

Treatment. The main objective of treatment is normoglycemia. *Pain* (p. 108) due to diabetic neuropathy usually responds to tricyclic antidepressants (amitryptiline, clomipramine), anticonvulsants (carbamazepine, gabapentin, lamotrigine), antiarrhythmics (lidocaine, mexiletine), capsaicin (administered locally as a 0.075% cream), or transdermal clonidine. *Autonomic dysfunction* of various types is treated symptomatically. Other factors that may worsen the neuropathy should be avoided (alcohol, vitamin deficiency, medication side effects). The *complications* of DPN (diabetic foot ulcer, infection, weakness, falls) may require specific treatment.

Uremic Neuropathy

Uremic neuropathy is a distal, symmetrical, sensorimotor, axonal peripheral neuropathy that mainly affects the legs. Paresthesiae and a "restless legs" sensation are typical. Uremic neuropathy may complicate renal failure of any etiology and is treated by therapy of the underlying disease.

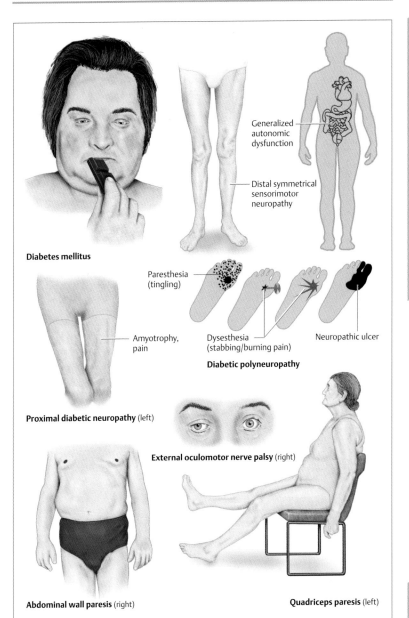

Diabetes mellitus

Generalized autonomic dysfunction

Distal symmetrical sensorimotor neuropathy

Paresthesia (tingling)

Amyotrophy, pain

Dysesthesia (stabbing/burning pain)

Neuropathic ulcer

Diabetic polyneuropathy

Proximal diabetic neuropathy (left)

External oculomotor nerve palsy (right)

Abdominal wall paresis (right)

Quadriceps paresis (left)

Peripheral Nerve and Muscle

Inflammatory Polyneuropathies

■ Guillain–Barré Syndrome

The term Guillain–Barré syndrome (GBS) covers a group of monophasic, acute, inflammatory polyneuropathies of autoimmune pathogenesis (Table 60, p. 395). Their onset is 1–4 weeks after a respiratory or gastrointestinal infection in two-thirds of all cases. The causative organism often cannot be identified. GBS is known to be associated with certain viruses (cytomegalovirus, Epstein–Barr virus, varicella-zoster virus, HIV ⇨ lymphocytic pleocytosis in CSF), bacteria (*Campylobacter jejuni*, *Mycoplasma pneumoniae*), and vaccines (rabies).

Pathogenesis. The organisms causing the preceding infection are thought to induce T-cell autoreactivity; after a latency period of days to weeks, antigen-specific T and B cells are activated. The target antigen is still unknown. IgG antibodies of various types, produced by the B cells, can be detected in serum in varying concentrations. These antibodies may block impulse conduction (⇨ acute paralysis) or activate complement and macrophages (⇨ myelin lesions). T_H1 lymphocytes release proinflammatory cytokines (IFN-γ, TNF-α; p. 220) that stimulate macrophages (⇨ peripheral nerve lesions). Once the inflammatory response has subsided, regenerative processes (axonal growth and remyelination) begin.

Symptoms and signs. GBS classically presents with an acute ascending and often rapidly progressive symmetrical weakness, areflexia, and relatively mild sensory abnormalities (paresthesiae). Pain is not uncommon, especially at onset; it is often in the back, of shocklike, tingling, aching, or myalgic quality, and may be misattributed to a herniated disk, "the flu," or "rheumatism." Cranial nerve deficits (VII, often bilateral; III, IV, VI, IX, X) are almost always present. So, too, are respiratory weakness and autonomic disturbances (bradycardia or tachycardia, hypotension or hypertension, abnormalities of fluid and electrolyte balance), all of which frequently cause complications. The sudden onset of disease with severe, ascending weakness is often a terrifying experience for patients and their families.

The clinical features and course of GBS are highly variable. Predictors of an unfavorable outcome include age over 60 years, progression to quadriplegia within one week, the need for mechanical ventilation, and a reduction of the amplitude of motor evoked potentials to less than 20 % of normal. The manifestations of less common forms of GBS are listed on p. 395.

Diagnosis (Table 61, p. 396). GBS is diagnosed from its typical clinical features. Neurophysiological findings are used to support the diagnosis, rule out alternative diagnoses, and document the type and extent of peripheral nerve damage. CSF studies are mainly useful for the exclusion of alternative diagnoses. It may be difficult to determine which specific type of GBS is present.

Treatment. Complications of GBS are mainly due to autonomic dysfunction, respiratory insufficiency, and immobility (⇨ deep venous thrombosis, pulmonary embolism, compression neuropathies, pressure sores, contractures). Patients should thus be closely monitored in an intensive care unit, especially in the acute phase. They and their relatives should be offered clear and ample information about the disease, as well as psychological counseling. GBS may be treated by intravenous gammaglobulin therapy or plasmapheresis.

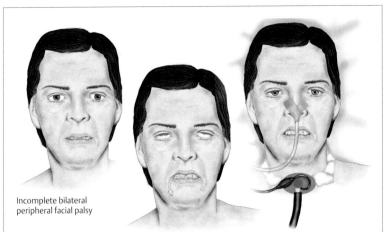

Incomplete bilateral peripheral facial palsy

Bilateral peripheral complete facial palsy, dysphagia, beginning respiratory insufficiency

Respiratory insufficiency, dysphagia, facial palsy in regression

Guillain-Barré syndrome

Initially dispersed and prolonged

Normalization (week 2)

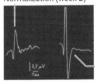

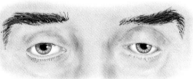

Intended gaze direction

External ophthalmoplegia

Normal findings (week 8)

Miller Fisher syndrome
(left: sensory action potentials of sural nerve)

Demyelination   Hypomyelinated fibers

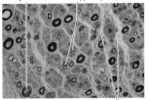

Nerve biopsy (sural n., semithin cross section)   Proliferation of connective tissue

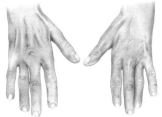

Distal symmetrical muscle atrophy

Chronic inflammatory demyelinating polyradiculoneuropathy (CIDP)

Chronic Inflammatory Demyelinating Polyradiculoneuropathy (CIDP)

CIDP differs from GBS in that it is of subacute onset (slow progression over 2 months or more) and responds readily to immune suppression (corticosteroids, azathioprine, cyclophosphamide; dose titrated to response) in combination with immunoglobulins or plasmapheresis. Its course is usually progressive or relapsing rather than monophasic. It is less commonly preceded by systemic infection than GBS but otherwise has very similar clinical features. Pain may accompany or precede an exacerbation of the illness. Neurophysiological studies reveal evidence of demyelination. The CSF protein concentration is markedly elevated, and sural nerve biopsy reveals chronic demyelination and remyelination with rare inflammatory infiltrates.

Multifocal Motor Neuropathy (MMN)

MMN is characterized by progressive asymmetrical weakness, which usually begins in the upper limbs. The underlying lesion is usually in isolated peripheral nerves (most often radial, median, ulnar, and common peroneal). Muscle spasms and fasciculations are common. Sensory loss, if any, is mild, and muscle atrophy is mild or absent even if weakness is marked. The reflexes may be absent, diminished, or (rarely) brisk. Nerve conduction studies reveal a motor conduction block. There may be an elevated serum concentration of IgM antibodies to GM_1. Repeated intravenous administration of immunoglobulin or cyclophosphamide is an effective treatment. The differential diagnosis includes amyotrophic lateral sclerosis, distal spinal muscular atrophy (p. 385), and CIDP.

Paraproteinemic Polyneuropathies

These disorders are most commonly due to non-malignant monoclonal gammopathies, usually of IgM type, rarely IgG or IgA, though there is progression to plasmocytoma or Waldenström macroglobulinemia in some 20% of cases. The main features of *monoclonal gammopathy of undetermined significance* (MGUS) include: κ-type, M protein <25 g/l, Bence Jones proteinuria (rare), no skeletal or organ involvement, normal blood smear. The clinical manifestations are of slowly progressive, distal, symmetrical, sensorimotor polyneuropathy, which is sometimes painful. Serum antibodies to myelin-associated glycoprotein (MAG) may be present, and the CSF protein concentration may be elevated. The treatment is by immune suppression, but the ideal type of agent, timing, and dosage have not yet been determined. *POEMS syndrome* (PNP + organomegaly + endocrinopathy + M protein + skin changes; *Crow–Fukase syndrome*) is a rare systemic manifestation of osteosclerotic myeloma.

Neuropathy of Infectious Origin

Leprosy, HIV infection, herpes zoster infection, borreliosis, tetanus, botulism, diphtheria, or other infectious diseases may cause neuropathy. Leprosy is the most common cause of peripheral neuropathy around the world. Its pathogenic organism (*Mycobacterium leprae*) attacks peripheral nerves in the cooler parts of the body, such as the skin, nose, anterior portion of the eye, and testes. There is segmental thickening of peripheral nerves (elbow, wrist, ankle). Areas of skin become depigmented and anhidrotic, with dissociated sensory loss. There are different types of leprosy, each of which is associated with a characteristic type of neuropathy.

Neuralgic Amyotrophy

This disorder involves acute, usually nocturnal attacks of severe pain in the shoulder for several days or weeks, followed by weakness and muscle atrophy. Sensory deficits are rare (axillary nerve distribution). The symptoms usually resolve spontaneously.

Vasculitic Neuropathy

Peripheral neuropathy due to connective tissue disease is usually multifocal, rarely symmetric (p. 180). Early treatment by immune suppression improves the outcome. Various connective tissue diseases can produce an isolated sensory trigeminal neuropathy.

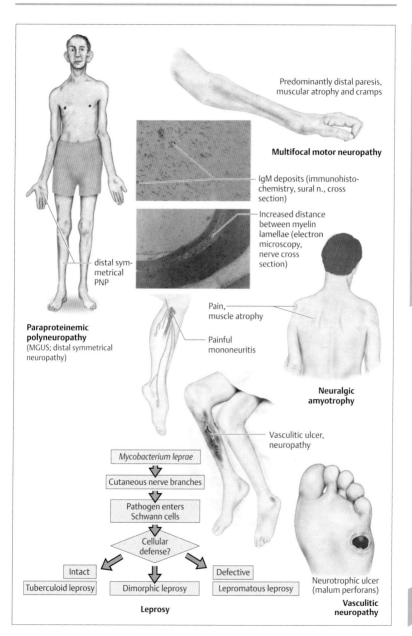

Predominantly distal paresis, muscular atrophy and cramps

Multifocal motor neuropathy

IgM deposits (immunohisto-chemistry, sural n., cross section)

Increased distance between myelin lamellae (electron microscopy, nerve cross section)

distal sym-metrical PNP

Paraproteinemic polyneuropathy
(MGUS; distal symmetrical neuropathy)

Pain, muscle atrophy

Painful mononeuritis

Neuralgic amyotrophy

Vasculitic ulcer, neuropathy

Mycobacterium leprae

Cutaneous nerve branches

Pathogen enters Schwann cells

Cellular defense?

Intact

Tuberculoid leprosy

Dimorphic leprosy

Defective

Lepromatous leprosy

Neurotrophic ulcer (malum perforans)

Leprosy

Vasculitic neuropathy

329

Peripheral Nerve Injuries

Peripheral nerves can be temporarily or permanently damaged by pressure, transection, crushes, blows, or traction.

Type of Lesion	Selected Causes/Features	Classification[1]/Prognosis
Local conduction block, with normal conduction distal to the lesion	Local demyelination due to compression Conduction blockade without EMG evidence of degeneration	*Neurapraxia* Resolution within a few weeks in most cases
Damage to axon and myelin sheath with preservation of enveloping structures (Schwann cell basal membrane and endoneurium); wallerian degeneration distal to the lesion	Crushing of nerve Regeneration occurs from proximal to distal along the enveloping structures, taking weeks, months, or years, depending on whether the damage is partial or complete[2]	*Axonotmesis* EMG evidence of reinnervation is seen first in muscle groups proximal to the lesion, and later in distal groups
Damage to axon, myelin sheath, and enveloping structures; wallerian degeneration distal to the lesion	Excessive traction, open incision wound Axon regeneration greatly limited; anomalous regeneration and neuroma development are common	*Neurotmesis* Full recovery is unusual

1 Seddon (1943). **2** Axons regenerate at 1–2 mm/day proximally, more slowly distally.

■ Pathogenesis

Local *nerve compression* displaces the axoplasm laterally from the site of compression. This causes invagination and subsequent demyelination at the nodes of Ranvier, so that saltatory impulse conduction is blocked. Compression preferentially impairs conduction in large-caliber fibers. *Crushing of a nerve* destroys the axoplasm but not the basal lamina. Schwann cells and axon processes regenerate in the damaged region and distally along the intact enveloping structures until they reach the effector muscle. *Nerve transection* is followed by axonal and Schwann cell proliferation, which may lead to the formation of a neuroma at the proximal nerve stump. Suturing the proximal and distal stumps together enables the regenerating fibers to enter the distal enveloping structures and regenerate further, but the function of the nerve is usually not fully restored to its original state.

■ Treatment

Type of Lesion	Treatment
Nerve root avulsion	Surgery (e. g., tenodesis, tendon-muscle transfer), treatment of pain
Brachial plexus injury	• Open ⇨ primary nerve suture • Closed ⇨ surgical exploration if there is no reinnervation in 3–5 months; if function fails to improve, other surgical procedures for restoration of function can be considered
Neurapraxia or axonotmesis (nontransecting injury)	• Diagnosed from clinical findings, EMG, and nerve conduction studies at presentation and 3 weeks later; treated with physical therapy • Clinical and neurophysiological re-assessment every 2–5 months • Clinical and neurophysiological improvement ⇨ further physical therapy • No clinical or neurophysiological improvement ⇨ corrective surgery 2–3 weeks after local injury (e. g., gunshot wound) or 4–5 months after extensive injury (e. g., traction injury)
Neurotmesis (nerve transection)	• Primary suture of nerve cut by knife, glass, etc. • Secondary suture 2–4 weeks after crushing injury and/or destruction of epineurium

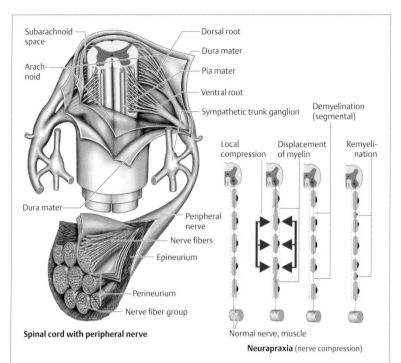

Subarachnoid space

Arach-noid

Dorsal root

Dura mater

Pia mater

Ventral root

Sympathetic trunk ganglion

Dura mater

Peripheral nerve

Nerve fibers

Epineurium

Perineurium

Nerve fiber group

Spinal cord with peripheral nerve

Demyelination (segmental)

Local compression

Displacement of myelin

Remyeli-nation

Normal nerve, muscle

Neurapraxia (nerve compression)

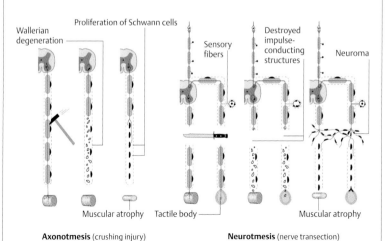

Wallerian degeneration

Proliferation of Schwann cells

Muscular atrophy

Axonotmesis (crushing injury)

Sensory fibers

Destroyed impulse-conducting structures

Neuroma

Tactile body

Muscular atrophy

Neurotmesis (nerve transection)

Nonmetabolic Hereditary Neuropathies
(Tables 62 and 63, p. 396 f)

For neuropathies associated with systemic disease, see p. 280.

■ Hereditary Motor–Sensory Neuropathy (HMSN)

These are the most common among the hereditary neuropathies, all of which are rare.

HMSN type I is characterized by high pedal arches (pes cavus), hammer toes (digitus malleus), distal weakness and atrophy, loss of vibration sense with preservation of position sense, areflexia, and unsteady gait (p. 60; frequent stumbling, steppage gait). Some peripheral nerves are palpably thickened in half of the cases (e. g., the greater auricular, ulnar, or common peroneal nerve), and tremor is present in one-third. The clinical picture is highly variable. The type I phenotype is produced by three different genotypes: CMT1 (autosomal dominant), CMT4 (autosomal recessive), and CMTX (X-linked).

HMSN type II. CMT2A and B resemble HMSN type I but begin later, with only rare areflexia and no palpable thickening of peripheral nerves. CMT2C is characterized by vocal cord paralysis (hoarseness, inspiratory stridor), proximal and distal weakness, distal muscle atrophy, and areflexia.

HMSN type III. This rare polyneuropathy (eponym: Dejerine–Sottas disease) becomes manifest at birth or in childhood with generalized weakness, areflexia, and palpable nerve thickening. Hearing loss, skeletal deformity, and sensory deficits (⇨ataxia) ensue as the disease progresses.

■ Hereditary Neuropathy with Pressure Palsies (HNPP)

HNPP is characterized by recurrent, transient episodes of weakness and sensory loss after relatively mild compression of a peripheral nerve (ulnar, peroneal, radial, or median nerve). There may be evidence of a generalized polyneuropathy or a painless plexopathy. The "sausagelike" pathological changes seen on sural nerve biopsy are the origin of the alternative name, *tomaculous neuropathy* (from Latin *tomaculum*, "sausage").

Metabolic Hereditary Neuropathies

Other members of this class are listed in the section on metabolic diseases (p. 306 ff).

■ Porphyria

Among the known porphyrias, four hepatic types are associated with encephalopathy and peripheral neuropathy: variegate porphyria, acute intermittent porphyria, hereditary coproporphyria, and δ-aminolevulinic acid dehydrase deficiency (autosomal recessive; the others are autosomal dominant). The porphyrias are hereditary enzymopathies affecting the biosynthesis of heme. Severe peripheral neuropathy is seen during attacks of acute porphyria, which are most often precipitated by medications and hormonal influences (also fasting, alcohol, and infection). The manifestations of porphyria include colicky abdominal pain, pain in the limbs, paresthesiae, tachycardia, and variable degrees of weakness. Encephalopathy is manifest as confusion, lack of concentration, somnolence, psychosis, hallucinations and/or epileptic seizures. The diagnosis of porphyria is based on the demonstration of porphyrin metabolites in the urine and feces.

■ Neuropathy Due to Hereditary Disorders of Lipid Metabolism

Polyneuropathy occurs in metachromatic leukodystrophy (p. 306), Krabbe disease (p. 307), abetalipoproteinemia (p. 300), adrenomyeloneuropathy (p. 384), Tangier disease (tonsillar hypertrophy, hepatosplenomegaly, low serum cholesterol, serum HDL deficiency), Fabry disease (punctate red angiokeratoma on buttocks and in the genital and periumbilical areas, retinovascular changes, corneal deposits, nephropathy, painful neuropathy; glycosphingolipid deposition due to α-galactosidase deficiency), and Refsum disease. The last is an autosomal recessive disorder of phytanic acid metabolism in which phytanic acid accumulation leads to tapetoretinal degeneration, night blindness, and a distal, symmetric polyneuropathy with peripheral nerve thickening. The CSF protein concentration is markedly elevated, but the CSF cell count is normal. The serum phytanic acid concentration is elevated.

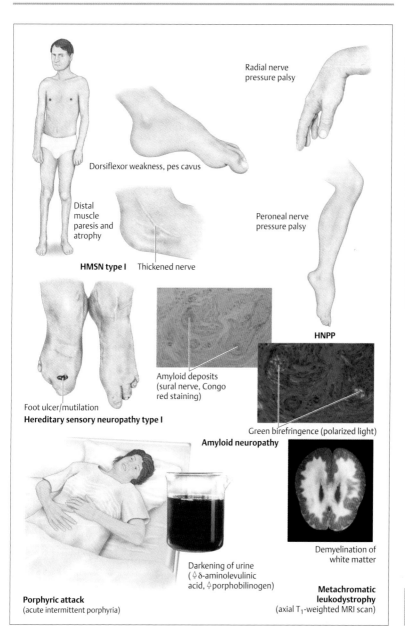

Radial nerve pressure palsy

Dorsiflexor weakness, pes cavus

Distal muscle paresis and atrophy

Peroneal nerve pressure palsy

HMSN type I   Thickened nerve

HNPP

Amyloid deposits (sural nerve, Congo red staining)

Foot ulcer/mutilation
Hereditary sensory neuropathy type I

Green birefringence (polarized light)
Amyloid neuropathy

Darkening of urine (↓ δ-aminolevulinic acid, ↓ porphobilinogen)

Demyelination of white matter

Porphyric attack
(acute intermittent porphyria)

Metachromatic leukodystrophy
(axial T_1-weighted MRI scan)

Myopathic Syndromes

Myopathies are diseases of muscle. Many different hereditary and acquired diseases attack muscle, sometimes in combination with other organs. The diagnosis and classification of the myopathies have been transformed in recent years by the introduction of molecular biological tests for the hereditary myopathies, but their treatment remains problematic. The management of the hereditary myopathies currently consists mainly of genetic counseling and the attempt to provide an accurate prognosis.

■ Symptoms and Signs (Table 64, p. 397)

Weakness (p. 52) is the most common sign of myopathy; it may be of acute, rapidly progressive, or gradual onset, fluctuating, or exercise-induced. It may be local (restricted to the muscles of the eye, face, tongue, larynx, pharynx, neck, arms, legs, or trunk), proximal, or distal, asymmetric or symmetric. *Myalgia, muscle stiffness, and muscle spasms* are less common. There may be muscle *atrophy* or *hypertrophy*, often in a typical distribution, whose severity depends on the type of myopathy. Skeletal deformity and/or abnormal posture may be a primary component of the disease or a consequence of weakness. Other features include acute paralysis, myoglobulinemia, cardiac arrhythmia, and visual disturbances.

■ Causes

For a list of causes of hereditary and acquired myopathies, see Tables 65 and 66, p. 398.

■ Diagnosis (Table 67, p. 399)

The myopathies are diagnosed primarily by history and physical examination (p. 52). Pharmacological tests are used for the differential diagnosis of myasthenia. Neurophysiological studies are used to rule out neuropathy (p. 391), to determine the specific type of acute muscle change, or to identify disturbances of muscular impulse generation and conduction. Various laboratory tests are helpful in myopathies due to biochemical abnormalities; imaging studies of muscle aid in the differential diagnosis of atrophy and hypertrophy. Muscle biopsy is often needed for a definitive diagnosis. Molecular biological studies are used in the diagnosis of hereditary myopathies.

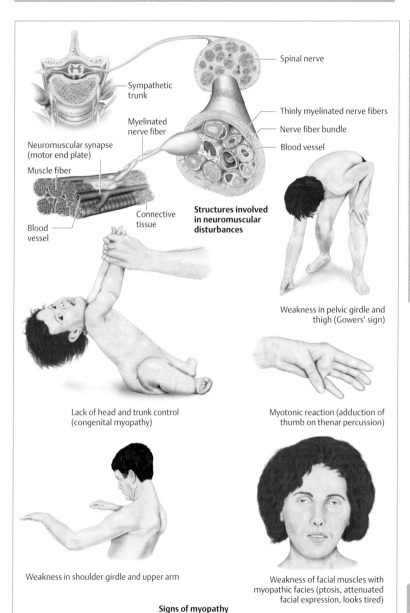

Structures involved
in neuromuscular
disturbances

Spinal nerve

Thinly myelinated nerve fibers

Nerve fiber bundle

Blood vessel

Sympathetic
trunk

Myelinated
nerve fiber

Neuromuscular synapse
(motor end plate)

Muscle fiber

Blood
vessel

Connective
tissue

Weakness in pelvic girdle and
thigh (Gowers' sign)

Lack of head and trunk control
(congenital myopathy)

Myotonic reaction (adduction of
thumb on thenar percussion)

Weakness in shoulder girdle and upper arm

Weakness of facial muscles with
myopathic facies (ptosis, attenuated
facial expression, looks tired)

Signs of myopathy

Muscular Dystrophies

The muscular dystrophies—myopathies characterized by progressive degeneration of muscle—are mostly hereditary.

■ **Pathogenesis** (Table 65, p. 398)

Dystrophinopathies are X-linked recessive disorders due to mutations of the gene encoding dystrophin, a protein found in the cell membrane (sarcolemma) of muscle fibers. Such mutations cause a deficiency, alteration, or absence of dystrophin. The functional features of dystrophin are not fully understood; it is thought to have a membrane-stabilizing effect. Some forms of *limb girdle dystrophy* (e.g., sarcoglycanopathy) are due to mutation of genes encoding dystrophin-associated glycoproteins, while others are due to mutation of genes encoding intracellular enzymes such as calpain-3. *Emery–Dreifuss muscular dystrophy* is due to a mutation of the gene for emerin, a nuclear membrane protein whose exact function is unknown.

■ **Symptoms and Signs**

Muscular dystrophies may be characterized by atrophy, hypertrophy, or pseudohypertrophy and are further classified by their mode of inheritance, age of onset, and distribution. Other features such as myocardial involvement, contractures, skeletal deformity, endocrine dysfunction, and ocular manifestations may point to one or another specific type of muscular dystrophy. Each type has a characteristic course (Table 68, p. 400).

■ **Diagnosis**

The history and physical examination are supplemented by additional diagnostic studies including ECG, creatine kinase fractionation (CK-MM), EMG, and DNA studies. If DNA analysis fails to reveal a mutation, immunohistochemical techniques, immune blotting, or the polymerase chain reaction can be used to detect abnormalities of dystrophin and sarcoglycan (e.g., in muscle biopsy samples) and thereby distinguish between Duchenne and Becker muscular dystrophy, or between dystrophinopathies and other forms of muscular dystrophy. DNA tests are used for the identification of asymptomatic female carriers (in whom muscle biopsy is hardly ever necessary), and for prenatal diagnosis.

■ **Treatment**

The goal of treatment is to prevent contracture and skeletal deformity and to keep the patient able to sit and walk for as long as possible. The patient's diet should be monitored to prevent obesity. The most important general measures are genetic counseling, social services, psychiatric counseling, and educating the patient on the special risks associated with general anesthesia. The type of schooling and employment must be appropriately suited to the patient's individual abilities and prognosis. Physical therapy includes measures to prevent contractures, as well as breathing exercises (deep breathing, positional drainage, measures to counteract increased inspiratory resistance). Patients with alveolar hypoventilation may need intermittent ventilation with continuous positive airway pressure (CPAP) at night. Orthoses may be helpful, depending on the extent of weakness (night splints to prevent talipes equinus, seat cushions, peroneal springs, orthopedic corsets, leg orthoses). Home aids may be needed as weakness progresses (padding, eating aids, toilet/bathing aids, stair-lift, mechanized wheelchair, specially adapted automobile). Surgery may be needed to correct scoliosis, prevent contracture about the hip joint (iliotibial tract release), and correct winging of the scapula (scapulopexy/scapulodesis) and other deformities and contractures. Intracardiac conduction abnormalities (e.g., in Emery–Dreifuss muscular dystrophy) require timely pacemaker implantation. Heart transplantation may be needed when severe cardiomyopathy arises in conjunction with certain types of muscular dystrophy (Becker, Emery–Dreifuss; Table 68, p. 400).

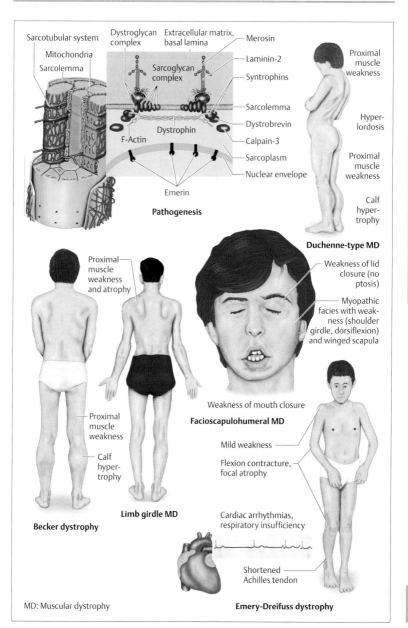

Sarcotubular system
Mitochondria
Sarcolemma

Dystroglycan complex
Extracellular matrix, basal lamina — Merosin
Sarcoglycan complex
Laminin-2
Syntrophins
Sarcolemma
Dystrophin
Dystrobrevin
F-Actin
Calpain-3
Sarcoplasm
Nuclear envelope
Emerin

Pathogenesis

Proximal muscle weakness

Hyper-lordosis

Proximal muscle weakness

Calf hyper-trophy

Duchenne-type MD

Proximal muscle weakness and atrophy

Weakness of lid closure (no ptosis)

Myopathic facies with weakness (shoulder girdle, dorsiflexion) and winged scapula

Proximal muscle weakness

Calf hyper-trophy

Weakness of mouth closure

Facioscapulohumeral MD

Mild weakness

Flexion contracture, focal atrophy

Limb girdle MD

Becker dystrophy

Cardiac arrhythmias, respiratory insufficiency

Shortened Achilles tendon

MD: Muscular dystrophy

Emery-Dreifuss dystrophy

The Myotonias (Table 69, p. 401)

■ Pathogenesis

Point mutations in ion channel genes cause channel defects that render the muscle cell membrane electrically unstable (Table 65, p. 398), leading to involuntary muscle contraction.

■ Symptoms and Signs

The transient, involuntary muscle contractions are perceived as stiffness. Depolarizing muscle relaxants used in surgery can trigger severe myotonia in susceptible patients. Acute, generalized myotonia can also be induced by tocolytic agents such as fenoterol.

■ Diagnosis

Myotonia is diagnosed from the observation of involuntary muscle contraction after voluntary muscle contraction (action myotonia) or percussion (percussion myotonia), along with the characteristic EMG findings. Specific forms of myotonia are diagnosed by their mode of inheritance and clinical features, and molecular genetic analysis. The serum creatine kinase concentration is usually not elevated, and there is usually no muscle atrophy, except in myotonic dystrophy. Muscle hypertrophy is present in myotonia congenita. Myotonic cataract is found in myotonic dystrophy and proximal myotonic myopathy; slit-lamp examination is indicated in patients with these disorders.

■ Treatment

Membrane-stabilizing drugs such as mexiletine alleviate myotonia; cardiac side effects may be problematic, particularly in myotonic dystrophy. Cold exposure should be avoided.

Episodic Paralyses (Table 69, p. 401)

■ Pathogenesis

Hyperkalemic and normokalemic paralysis, potassium-aggravated myotonia (PAM = myotonia fluctuans), and paramyotonia congenita are due to *sodium channel* dysfunction, while hypokalemic paralysis is due to *calcium channel* dysfunction.

■ Symptoms and Signs

In hypokalemic and hyperkalemic myotonia, there are irregularly occurring episodes of flaccid paresis of variable duration and severity, with no symptoms in between. The anal and urethral sphincters are not affected. In *paramyotonia congenita*, muscle stiffness increases on exertion (paradoxical myotonia) and is followed by weakness. Cold exposure worsens the stiffness.

■ Diagnosis

The diagnosis can usually be made from the personal and family history, abnormal serum potassium concentration, and molecular genetic findings (mutation of the gene for a membrane ion channel). If the diagnosis remains in question, provocative tests can be performed between attacks. The induction of paralytic attacks by administration of glucose and insulin indicates hypokalemic paralysis, while their induction by potassium administration and exercise (e. g. on a bicycle ergometer) indicates hyperkalemic paralysis. The diagnosis of paramyotonia congenita is based on the characteristic clinical features (paradoxical myotonia, exacerbation by cold exposure), autosomal dominant inheritance, and demonstration of the causative point mutation of the sodium channel gene.

■ Treatment

Acute attacks. Milder episodes of weakness in *hypokalemic* disorders need no treatment, while more severe episodes can be treated with oral potassium administration. Milder episodes of weakness in *hyperkalemic* disorders also need no treatment; more severe episodes may require calcium gluconate i. v., or salbutamol by inhaler.

Prophylaxis. *Hypokalemic paralysis:* Low-salt, low-carbohydrate diet, avoidance of strenuous exercise; oral acetazolamide or spironolactone. *Hyperkalemic paralysis:* high-carbohydrate diet; avoidance of strenuous exercise and cold; oral hydrochlorothiazide or acetazolamide.

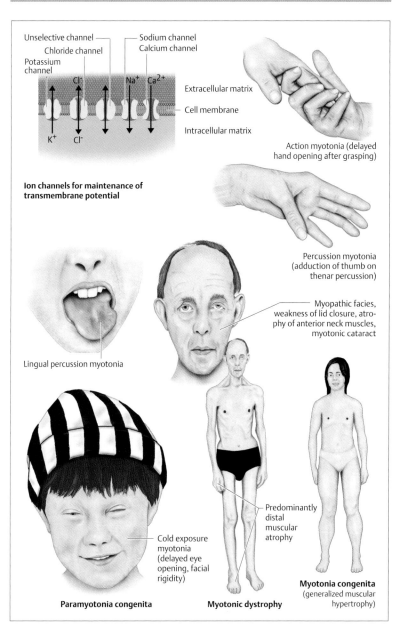

Unselective channel
Chloride channel
Potassium channel

Sodium channel
Calcium channel

K⁺   Cl⁻

Extracellular matrix

Cell membrane

Intracellular matrix

Ion channels for maintenance of transmembrane potential

Action myotonia (delayed hand opening after grasping)

Percussion myotonia (adduction of thumb on thenar percussion)

Myopathic facies, weakness of lid closure, atrophy of anterior neck muscles, myotonic cataract

Lingual percussion myotonia

Predominantly distal muscular atrophy

Cold exposure myotonia (delayed eye opening, facial rigidity)

Paramyotonia congenita

Myotonic dystrophy

Myotonia congenita (generalized muscular hypertrophy)

Congenital Myopathies

The typical pathological findings on muscle biopsy distinguish this group of disorders both
from the congenital muscular dystrophies and
from muscle changes secondary to peripheral
neuropathy. Some congenital myopathies have
distinctive clinical features. Proximal flaccid
weakness is usually present at birth (floppy
baby); skeletal deformities may also be seen
(e. g., high palate, hip luxation, pes cavus, chest
deformities). Many congenital myopathies progress slowly, causing little or no disability; the
CK and EMG may be only mildly abnormal, or
not at all. Some types can be diagnosed by
genetic analysis (Table 70, p. 402).

Metabolic Myopathies

In most metabolic myopathies (Table 71, p. 402
f), exercise induces myalgia, weakness, and
muscle cramps, and myoglobinuria. Progressive
proximal weakness is seen in myopathy due to
acid-maltase deficiency (glycogen storage disease type II), debrancher deficiency (glycogen
storage disease type III), or primary myopathic
carnitine deficiency.

Mitochondrial myopathies. Pyruvate and fatty
acids are the most important substrates for mitochondrial ATP synthesis, which occurs by oxidative phosphorylation, a function of the respiratory chain enzymes (found on the inner mitochondrial membrane). β-oxidation occurs in the
mitochondrial matrix. The respiratory chain
enzymes are encoded by both mitochondrial
and nuclear DNA (mtDNA, nDNA).

The mitochondrial myopathies are a heterogeneous group of disorders whose common feature is dysfunction of the respiratory chain, β-
oxidation, or both. These disorders have varying
clinical and biochemical features (Table 71,
p. 402 f); their inheritance is either maternal or
sporadic; non-heritable cases also occur
through mtDNA mutations. These disorders may
affect multiple organ systems, e. g.:

- Muscle (reduced endurance, pain, cramps, myoglobinuria)
- CNS (seizures, headache, behavioral abnor-malities)
- Eye (ptosis, external ophthalmoplegia, tape-toretinal degeneration)

- Ear (hearing loss)
- Heart (arrhythmia, heart failure)
- Gastrointestinal system (diarrhea, vomiting)
- Endocrine system (diabetes mellitus, hy-pothyroidism)
- ANS (impotence, sweating)

The diagnosis is based on the clinical features,
laboratory tests (elevated lactate concentration
at rest in serum, sometimes also in CSF, with
sustained increase after exercise), muscle biopsy (ragged red fibers, sometimes with cy-
tochrome-c oxidase deficiency), and molecular
studies (mtDNA analysis of muscle, platelets,
leukocytes). There is no etiological treatment for
the mitochondrial myopathies at present; a low-
fat, carbohydrate-rich diet is recommended in
disorders with defective β-oxidation, and carnitine supplementation in those with systemic
carnitine deficiency. Coenzyme Q_{10}, vitamin K_3,
vitamin C, and/or thioctic acid supplements are
recommended in disorders with impaired respiratory chain function.

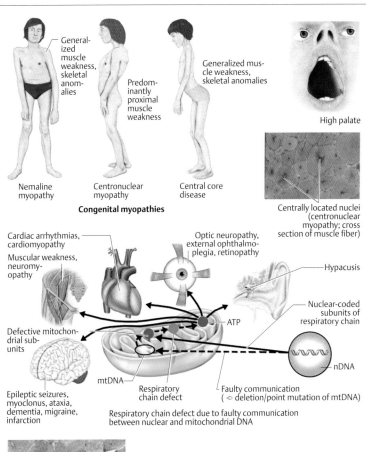

Generalized muscle weakness, skeletal anomalies

Predominantly proximal muscle weakness

Generalized muscle weakness, skeletal anomalies

High palate

Nemaline myopathy

Centronuclear myopathy

Central core disease

Congenital myopathies

Centrally located nuclei (centronuclear myopathy; cross section of muscle fiber)

Cardiac arrhythmias, cardiomyopathy

Muscular weakness, neuromyopathy

Optic neuropathy, external ophthalmoplegia, retinopathy

Hypacusis

Nuclear-coded subunits of respiratory chain

ATP

Defective mitochondrial subunits

Epileptic seizures, myoclonus, ataxia, dementia, migraine, infarction

mtDNA

Respiratory chain defect

Faulty communication (⇨ deletion/point mutation of mtDNA)

nDNA

Respiratory chain defect due to faulty communication between nuclear and mitochondrial DNA

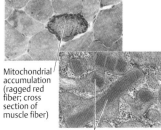

Mitochondrial accumulation (ragged red fiber; cross section of muscle fiber)

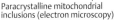

Paracrystalline mitochondrial inclusions (electron microscopy)

Tapetoretinal degeneration (CPEO)

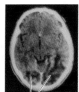

Occipital infarcts (MELAS syndrome, axial CT scan)

Mitochondrial myopathies

Myasthenic Syndromes

■ Myasthenia Gravis (MG)

Pathogenesis. The exercise-induced weakness that typifies MG is due to impaired transmission at the neuromuscular junction, which is, in turn, due to an underlying molecular lesion affecting the nicotinic acetylcholine receptor (AChR) in the postsynaptic membrane of the muscle cell. Circulating IgG autoantibodies to this receptor impair its function, speed its breakdown, and induce complement-mediated damage to the muscle cell membrane. Recently the anti-MuSK (receptor tyrosine kinase) antibody has been detected in about half of patients who are seronegative for AChR antibodies. The thymus plays an important role in this autoimmune disorder (it is normally a site of maturation and removal of autoreactive T lymphocytes). MG is usually acquired late in life; there are also rare congenital and familial forms.

Symptoms and signs. MG is characterized by asymmetric weakness and fatigability of skeletal muscle that worsens on exertion and improves at rest. Weakness often appears first in the extraocular muscles and remains limited to them in some 15% of cases (ocular myasthenia), but progresses to other muscles in the rest (generalized myasthenia). The facial and pharyngeal muscles may be affected, resulting in a blank facial expression, dysarthria, difficulty in chewing and swallowing, poor muscular control of the head, and rhinorrhea. Respiratory weakness leads to impairment of coughing and an increased risk of aspiration. It may become difficult or impossible for the patient stand up, remain standing, or walk, and total disability may ensue. Myasthenia can be aggravated by certain medications (Table 72, p. 403), infections, emotional stress, electrolyte imbalances, hormonal changes, and bright light (eyes), and is often found in association with hyperthyroidism, thyroiditis, rheumatoid arthritis, and connective tissue disease. Myasthenic or cholinergic crises can be life-threatening (Table 73, p. 404).

Diagnosis. The diagnosis is based on the characteristic history and clinical findings, supported by further tests that are listed in Table 74 (p. 404).

Treatment. Ocular MG is treated symptomatically with an acetylcholinesterase (AChE) inhibitor, such as pyridostigmine bromide; if the response is insufficient, corticosteroids or azathioprine can be added. Generalized MG is treated initially with AChE inhibitors and, if the response is insufficient, with corticosteroids, azathioprine, intravenous gammaglobulin, or plasmapheresis; once the patient's condition has stabilized, thymectomy is performed. Further treatment depends on the degree of improvement achieved by these measures. The mortality of MG with optimal management is less than 1%. Most patients can lead a normal life but need lifelong immunosuppression. Specific measures are needed to manage respiratory crises, thymoma, and pregnancy in patients with MG, and for the treatment of neonatal, congenital, and hereditary forms of MG.

■ Lambert–Eaton Myasthenic Syndrome (LEMS)

LEMS is caused by autoantibodies directed mainly against voltage-gated calcium channels in the presynaptic terminal of the neuromuscular junction; diminished release of acetylcholine from the presynaptic terminal is the result. LEMS is often a paraneoplastic manifestation of bronchial carcinoma, sometimes appearing before the tumor becomes clinically evident. It is characterized by proximal (leg) weakness that improves transiently with exercise but worsens shortly afterward. There are also autonomic symptoms (dry mouth) and hyporeflexia. EMG reveals a diminished amplitude of the summated muscle action potential, which increases on high-frequency serial stimulation. The treatment is with 3,4-diaminopyridine (which increases acetylcholine release) and AChE inhibitors. Immune suppression and chemotherapy of the underlying malignancy can also improve LEMS.

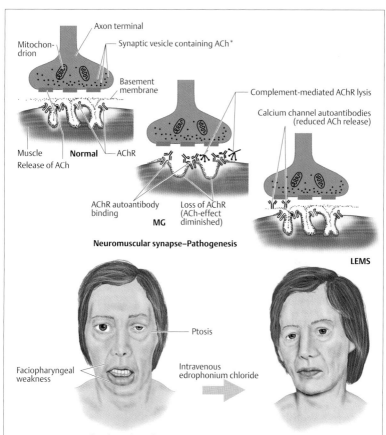

Axon terminal

Mitochon-drion

Synaptic vesicle containing ACh*

Basement membrane

Complement-mediated AChR lysis

Calcium channel autoantibodies (reduced ACh release)

Muscle

Release of ACh

Normal

AChR

AChR autoantibody binding

Loss of AChR (ACh-effect diminished)

MG

LEMS

Neuromuscular synapse–Pathogenesis

Ptosis

Faciopharyngeal weakness

Intravenous edrophonium chloride

Exercise-induced muscle weakness

Normal muscle strength (after edrophonium chloride)

Myasthenia gravis

Amplitude reduction (decrement from 1st to 5th stimulus)

Repeated low-frequency stimulation (3 Hz, trapezius m., MG)

Increase in amplitude (increment > 3.5 times higher than baseline)

Low starting amplitude

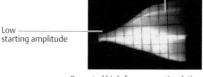

Repeated high-frequency stimulation (20 Hz, abductor digiti quinti m., LEMS)

*ACh = acetylcholine **Repetitive nerve stimulation**

Myositis

The myositides (inflammatory myopathies) are a heterogeneous group of disorders, causing three distinct clinical syndromes: polymyositis (PM), dermatomyositis (DM), and inclusion body myositis (IBM).

■ Pathogenesis

Most myositides found in the temperate zones are autoimmune diseases of unknown cause, characterized histologically by muscle inflammation and fibrosis and loss of muscle fibers. In *PM*, cytotoxic CD8+ T cells penetrate and damage muscle fibers (⇨ intramuscular cellular infiltrates). CD8+ T cell activation is induced by abnormal expression of class I HLA antigens on the surface of the muscle fibers, which are normally HLA-negative. *DM* is thought to be largely due to antibodies against blood vessels within muscle, which activate the complement system (membrane attack complex). Vascular endothelial damage ultimately leads to ischemia and death of muscle tissue (⇨ perifascicular atrophy). Inflammatory T cells and macrophages migrate into muscle and cause further damage. *IBM* is of unknown pathogenesis. *Infectious myositis* may be due to bacteria, viruses, parasites, or fungi.

■ Syndromes

Polymyositis (PM) begins with weakness of the proximal muscles of the lower limbs, which then progresses and slowly spreads to the upper limbs. The deltoid and neck flexor muscles are commonly involved. Dysphagia may be present. The involved muscles eventually become atrophic. In *overlap syndrome*, myositis appears together with another autoimmune disease, e. g., progressive systemic sclerosis, systemic lupus erythematosus, rheumatoid arthritis, polyarteritis nodosa, polymyalgia rheumatica, or Sjögren syndrome. Myalgia is often the major symptoms in patients with PM, as also in patients with hypereosinophilia syndrome (Churg–Strauss syndrome) or eosinophilic fasciitis (Shulman disease).

Dermatomyositis (DM) progresses more rapidly than PM and is distinguished from it mainly by the bluish-red or purple (heliotrope) rash found on exposed areas of the skin (eyelids, cheeks, neck, chest, knuckles, and extensor surfaces of the limbs). Small hemorrhages and telangiectasias are found in the nailbeds; affected children may have subcutaneous calcium deposits. Cancer accompanies DM six times more frequently than PM; DM is also associated with scleroderma and mixed connective tissue disease.

Inclusion body myositis (IBM) is characterized by distal (sometimes asymmetric) weakness and muscle atrophy, mainly in the lower limbs (plantar flexors), with early loss of the quadriceps reflexes. There are both sporadic and hereditary forms of IBM (see also p. 252).

■ Diagnosis

The myositides are diagnosed by history and physical examination, elevated serum concentration of sarcoplasmic enzymes (particularly CK-MM), and characteristic findings on EMG and muscle biopsy. Muscle atrophy can also be assessed with various imaging techniques (CT, MRI, ultrasonography). The presence of antibodies in association with a connective tissue disease may be relevant to the diagnosis (p. 180).

■ Treatment

PM and DM are treated by immune suppression, e. g., with corticosteroids, azathioprine, or intravenous gammaglobulin (ivig). Physical therapy is begun once the patient's condition has stabilized. IBM may respond to intravenous immunoglobulin therapy.

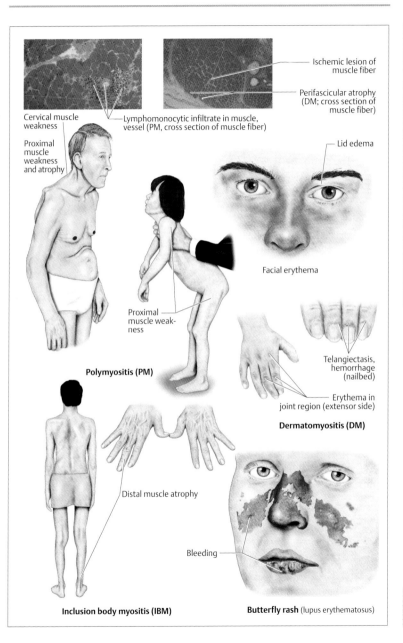

Ischemic lesion of muscle fiber

Perifascicular atrophy (DM; cross section of muscle fiber)

Cervical muscle weakness

Proximal muscle weakness and atrophy

Lymphomonocytic infiltrate in muscle, vessel (PM, cross section of muscle fiber)

Lid edema

Facial erythema

Proximal muscle weakness

Polymyositis (PM)

Telangiectasis, hemorrhage (nailbed)

Erythema in joint region (extensor side)

Dermatomyositis (DM)

Distal muscle atrophy

Bleeding

Inclusion body myositis (IBM)

Butterfly rash (lupus erythematosus)

Muscle Pain (Myalgia)

Myalgia is an aching, cramping, or piercing pain in muscle. It is triggered by stimulation of nociceptors (p. 108). Pressure or traction on a muscle causes myalgia that subsides once the mechanical stimulus is removed, while inflammatory and other lesions in muscle cause persistent and gradually increasing myalgia. Muscle ischemia and/or metabolic dysfunction are reflected by myalgia occurring only during muscle activity. Myalgia includes *allodynia,* which is defined as pain induced by normally nonpainful stimuli and is explained by the sensitization of nociceptors by pain-related substances such as bradykinin, serotonin, and prostaglandin. A "charleyhorse" is a type of myalgia that normally begins 8–24 hours after muscle overuse (simultaneous stretching and contraction) and lasts 5–7 days. It is caused by an inflammatory reaction to muscle fiber damage. Myalgia can be triggered by disorders whose primary pathology lies anywhere in the nervous system (peripheral nerve, spinal cord, brain).

■ **Causes of Myalgia**

Type of Myalgia	Selected Causes
Localized myalgia	
• Hematoma	• Trauma, coagulopathy
• Myositis	• *Infectious:* Streptococcal infection, trichinosis, influenza, epidemic pleurodynia. *Noninfectious:* Nodular focal myositis, eosinophilic fasciitis, sarcoidosis, myositis ossificans
• Ischemic	• Arteriosclerosis (intermittent claudication), embolism
• Toxic-metabolic	• Acute alcoholic myopathy, metabolic myopathy (pp. 402, 405)
• Overactivity	• Stiff-man syndrome, neurogenic myotonia, tetanus, strychnine poisoning, amyotrophic lateral sclerosis, tetany
• Exercise-induced	• Metabolic myopathy, arteriosclerosis, physical exertion
• Parkinsonian	• Rigidity
• Muscle spasm	• Polyneuropathy, metabolic disorder (electrolyte imbalance, uremia, thyroid dysfunction)
• Pain at rest	• Restless legs syndrome, painful legs and moving toes syndrome
Generalized myalgia	
• Myositis	• Polymyositis/dermatomyositis (p. 344)
• Toxic-metabolic	• Hypothyroidism, medications[2], mitochondrial myopathy (pp. 340, 402, 405)
• Other	• Polymyalgia rheumatica, amyloidosis, osteomalacia, Guillain–Barré syndrome, porphyria, hypothyroidism, corticosteroid withdrawal, fibromyalgia

(Adapted from Layzer, 1994)

1 E.g., emetine, lovastatin, and ε-aminocaproic acid.

Rhabdomyolysis

Local or generalized damage to skeletal muscle can cause myoglobinuria and an elevated serum concentration of creatine kinase, usually accompanied by the acute onset of proximal or diffuse weakness, with myalgia, muscle swelling, and general manifestations including nausea, vomiting, headache, and sometimes fever. The urine may be discolored at the onset of symptoms or several hours later. Rhabdomyolysis can be caused by certain types of myopathy (e. g., polymyositis, central core disease, metabolic myopathies; pp. 402, 405), by muscle strain or trauma (long-distance walking or running, heat stroke, delirium tremens, status epilepticus), by toxic substances (see below), and by infectious disease (bacterial sepsis, influenza, coxsackievirus or echovirus infection).

Malignant Hyperthermia (MH)

This life-threatening disorder of skeletal muscle function is characterized by hyperthermia, muscle rigidity, hyperhidrosis, tachycardia, cyanosis, lactic acidosis, hyperkalemia, massive elevation of the serum creatine kinase concentration, and myoglobinuria. It is induced by anesthetic agents such as halothane and succinylcholine. The predisposition to MH is inherited as an autosomal dominant trait (gene loci: 19q13.1, 17q11–24, 7q12.1, 5p, 3q13.1, 1q32). The creatine kinase level may be chronically elevated in susceptible individuals, who can be identified with an in vitro contracture test performed in specialized laboratories. Persons suffering from central core disease, multicore disease, and King–Denborough syndrome (dwarfism, skeletal anomalies, ptosis, high palate) are also at risk for MH. *Treatment:* dantrolene.

Malignant neuroleptic syndrome clinically resembles MH; unlike MH, however, it is usually of subacute onset (days to weeks), it is not hereditary, and it is triggered by psychotropic drugs (haloperidol, phenothiazines, lithium). Malignant neuroleptic syndrome can also be induced by abrupt withdrawal of dopaminergic agents in patients with Parkinson disease.

Toxic Neuromuscular Syndromes

The muscle fiber lesions regress if the responsible substance is eliminated in timely fashion (Table 75, p. 405).

Myopathy in Endocrine Disorders

Hyperthyroidism or hypothyroidism, hyperparathyroidism, Cushing syndrome, steroid myopathy, and acromegaly all cause proximal weakness, while Addison disease and primary hyperaldosteronism usually cause generalized weakness. Timely correction of the endocrine disorder or withdrawal of steroid drugs is usually followed by improvement.

Critical Illness Polyneuropathy (CIP) and Critical Illness Myopathy (CIM)

Sepsis is the most common cause not only of encephalopathy (see p. 312) but also of CIP and CIM. CIP is an acute, reversible, mainly axonal polyneuropathy. It causes distal, symmetric weakness with prominent involvement of the muscles of respiration, resulting in prolonged ventilator dependence and delayed mobilization. CIM causes generalized weakness. The clinical differentiation of CIM and CIP is difficult and often requires muscle biopsy.

Paraneoplastic Syndromes
(Table 76, p. 406)

Distant neoplasms can affect not only the CNS (see p. 388) but also the PNS and skeletal muscle. Remarkably, paraneoplastic syndromes sometimes appear months or years before the underlying malignancy becomes clinically manifest. Paraneoplastic neuromuscular syndromes typically present with marked weakness of subacute onset (i.e., developing over several days or weeks).

Peripheral Nerve and Muscle

4 Diagnostic Evaluation

- History and Physical Examination
- Additional Studies

A detailed description of diagnostic evaluation procedures can be found in the textbooks listed on p. 409. The goals of history-taking, physical examination, and additional testing (if necessary) are:

- Data collection (manifestations of disease)
- Localization of the lesion
- Provision of an etiological diagnosis

■ **Data Collection**

The diagnostic process begins with the history and physical examination. The history provides information about the patient's experience of illness, the temporal course of symptom development, and potentially relevant familial, social, occupational, and hereditary factors. An inaccurate or incomplete history is a frequent cause of misdiagnosis.

History. The physician engages the patient in a structured conversation about the manifestations of the illness. The physician must remember that the patient is the "expert" in this situation, as the patient alone knows what is troubling him (though perhaps helpful information can also be obtained from a close relative or friend). The physician aims to obtain accurate information on the nature, location, duration, and intensity of the symptoms by listening patiently and asking directed questions in an atmosphere of openness and trust. Questionnaires, computer programs, and ancillary personnel cannot be used for primary history-taking, as they do not enable the construction of a trusting physician–patient relationship (though they may provide useful additional information at a later stage). Some important elements of the case history are as follows.

- *Nature of symptoms.* The physician must ascertain, by detailed questioning if necessary, that he understands the patient's complaints in the same sense that the patient means to convey. "Blurred vision" may mean diplopia, "dizziness" may mean gait ataxia, "headache" may mean hemicrania, "numbness" may mean paresthesia—but patients may use all of these terms with other meanings as well.
- *Severity of symptoms.* Quality and intensity of symptoms, activities with which they interfere.

- *Onset of symptoms.* When, where, and over what interval of time did the symptoms arise?
- *Time course of symptoms.* How did they develop? Are they constant or variable? Are there any exacerbating or alleviating factors?
- *Accompanying symptoms,* if present.
- *Past history* of similar symptoms.
- *Previous illnesses* and their outcome.
- *Social, occupational,* and *family history.*
- *Medications, smoking, alcohol abuse, substance abuse, toxic exposures.*
- *Previous diagnostic studies* and *treatment.*
- *Information from third parties* may be needed for patients with aphasia, confusion, dementia, or impairment of consciousness.

Physical examination. The general and neurological physical examination may yield important clues to the disease process, but only if the examiner has the requisite knowledge of the underlying principles of (neuro-)anatomy, (neuro-)physiology, and (neuro-)pathology. The examination is guided by the case history, i.e., the patient's complaints and general physical condition determine what the examiner looks for in the examination. The unselective, "shotgun" application of every possible technique of neurological examination in every patient is not only a waste of time and money; it generally only creates confusion rather than clarifying the search for the diagnosis. The neurological examination of small children, patients with personality changes or mental illness, and unconscious patients poses special challenges.

Important elements of the neurological examination include:

- *Inspection.* Dress, appearance, posture, movements, speech, gestures, facial expression.
- *Mental Status.* Orientation (to person, place, and time), attention, concentration, memory, thought processes, language function, level of consciousness.
- *Cranial nerves.* Olfaction, pupils, visual fields, eyegrounds, eye movements, facial movement, facial sensation, hearing, tongue movements, swallowing, speaking, reflexes.
- *Motor function.* Muscular atrophy/hypertrophy, spontaneous movements, coordination, paresis, tremor, dystonia, muscle tone.

- *Reflexes* (p. 40).
- *Sensory function.* The findings of sensory testing are heavily influenced by the patient's "sensitivity" and ability to cooperate. Vague sensory abnormalities without other neurological deficits are difficult to classify; their interpretation requires a good knowledge of the underlying neuroanatomy (pp. 32 ff, 106 f).
- *Posture, station, and gait.* The observation and testing of posture, station, and gait provides important information about a possible motor deficit (p. 42 ff).
- *Autonomic function.* The patient is questioned about bladder function, bowel movement/control, sexual function, blood pressure, cardiac function, and sweating, and is examined as needed.

■ Localization of the Lesion

The findings of the history and physical examination findings are then related to dysfunction of a particular neuroanatomical structure(s) (p. 2 ff) or neurophysiological process (p. 40 ff); the site of the patient's problem is thus localized (topical diagnosis).

■ Provision of an Etiological Diagnosis

Once the site of the problem is localized, it must be determined whether it is due to a structural lesion (e. g., hemorrhage, nerve compression, or infection) or a functional disturbance (e. g.,

epileptic seizure, migraine, or Parkinson disease). The line between structural and functional pathology is not perfectly defined, as there is constant interaction between these two levels; at the same time, considerations of etiology and pathogenesis also influence data interpretation. The diagnostic process ideally ends in the diagnosis of a specific disease entity (nosological diagnosis).

Additional Diagnostic Studies

The clinical diagnosis may be considered firmly established by the history and physical examination alone in many cases, e. g., migraine or Parkinson disease. Additional diagnostic studies are merely confirmatory and are generally not needed unless doubt arises as to the diagnosis, e. g., if an epileptic seizure or new type of headache should appear.

Additional studies are needed, however, if there is no other way to decide among several diagnostic possibilities remaining after thorough history-taking and physical examination. The number and type of studies needed differ from case to case. Studies that are costly or fraught with non-negligible risk should never be ordered except to answer a clearly stated diagnostic question. The potential benefits of a proposed study must always be weighed against its risks and cost.

■ Laboratory Tests

Table 77, p. 407

Diagnostic Evaluation

Neurophysiological and Neuropsychological Tests

■ Neurophysiological Tests

Test/Purpose	Risks	Comments
Electroencephalography: To assess electrical activity of the brain[1]	Surface electrodes: none Needle electrodes: infection Induction of seizures by provocative methods[2]	Sphenoid, subdural or depth recording[3] for special questions relevant to the (preoperative) diagnostic evaluation of epilepsy
Evoked potentials (EPs): ● VEPs[4]: Study of optic nerve, optic chiasm and optic tract ● AEPs[5]: Study of peripheral and central segments of the auditory pathway[6] ● SEPs[7]: Study of somatosensory systems[8] ● MEPs[9]: Study of corticospinal motor pathway	● None ● None ● None ● May induce epileptic seizures. Contraindications: cardiac pacemakers, metal prostheses in the target area, pregnancy, unstable fractures	● Used mainly to diagnose prechiasmatic lesions ● Used mainly for diagnosis of multiple sclerosis, tumors of the posterior cranial fossa, brain stem lesions causing coma or brain death, and intraoperative monitoring ● Used to assess proximal peripheral nerve lesions (plexus, roots) and spinal cord or parietal lobe lesions ● Pyramidal tract lesions, motor neuron lesions, root compression, plexus lesions, stimulation of deep nerves, differential diagnosis of psychogenic paresis
Electromyography: Study of electrical activity in muscle	Contraindication: coagulopathy. Risk of injury in special studies[11]	Provides information on motor unit disorders in patients with peripheral nerve lesions or myopathies. Not disease-specific. Disposable needles should be used to prevent spread of infectious disease[10]
Electroneurography: Measurement of motor and sensory conduction velocities.	Needle recordings contraindicated in patients with coagulopathy	Localization (proximal, distal, conduction block) and classification (axonal, demyelinating) of peripheral nerve lesions[12]
Electro-oculography: To record and assess eye movements and/or nystagmus	Caloric testing with water contraindicated in patients with perforated eardrums	Diagnosis and localization of peripheral and central vestibular lesions. Differentiation of saccades

1 For assessment of epilepsy, localized pathology (neoplasm, trauma, meningoencephalitis, infarct) or generalized pathology (intoxication, hypoxia, metabolic encephalopathy, Creutzfeldt–Jakob disease, coma, brain death), for sleep analysis (polysomnography), or to monitor the course of such conditions. **2** Photostimulation, hyperventilation, sleep, sleep withdrawal. **3** For diagnostic assessment before epilepsy surgery, in specialized centers. **4** Visual EPs. **5** Acoustic EPs. **6** Peripheral nerve and cochlear lesions are mainly studied audiometrically, and peripheral and central disorders by electro-oculography or posturography. **7** Somatosensory EPs. **8** Functional assessment of sensory pathways (p. 104) by tibial, median, ulnar, and trigeminal nerve stimulation. **9** Motor EPs. **10** Particularly Creutzfeldt–Jakob disease, hepatitis, AIDS. **11** *Examples*: Pneumothorax in study of the serratus anterior m., perforation of the rectal wall in study of the anal sphincter. **12** F-wave measurement for localization of proximal nerve damage, H-reflex in S1 syndrome.

■ Neuropsychological Tests

Comprehensive testing of cognitive function, behavior, and affective processes, perhaps in collaboration with a neuropsychologist, is required when the history and physical examination suggest the possibility of mental illness or of mental dysfunction due to neurological disease. *Objectives:* Accurate detection and effective monitoring, prognostication, identification of etiology, and treatment of mental disorders (p. 122 ff).

Cerebrovascular Ultrasonography, Diagnostic Imaging, and Biopsy Procedures

Aspect To Be Tested	Questions/Tests
• Attention (p. 116)	• Awake, somnolent, stuporous, comatose? Arousability, attention span, perception
• Orientation	• Personal data (name, age, date/place of birth), orientation ("where are we?", place of residence); time (day of the week, date, month, year); situation (reason for consultation, nature of symptoms)
• Memory, recall	• The patient should be able to name the months of the year backward, spell a word backward, repeat random series of numbers between 1 and 9. Can the patient recall 3 objects mentioned 3 minutes ago, recall figures, name famous people? Tests of general knowledge
• Serial subtraction	• Serial subtraction of 3s (or 7s), starting from 100
• Frontal lobe function	• Perseveration[1]; hand sequence test[2]; proverb interpretation
• Language (pp. 124, 128)	• Following commands, naming, repetition, writing, reading aloud, simple arithmetic
• Praxis	• See p. 128
• Spatial orientation, visual perception	• See p. 132. Naming of colors and objects

(After Schnider, 1997)

1 Drawing of simple figures (Luria's loops). **2** Command sequence: "Make a fist—open the hand to the side—open the hand flat."

Diagnostic Evaluation

■ Cerebrovascular Ultrasonography

Ultrasound can be used to assess the extracranial and intracranial arteries. The transmitter emits ultrasonic waves in two modes, continuous wave (CW; cross-sectional data, but no depth information) and pulse wave (PW; flow information at different levels). The reflected waves are recorded (echo impulse signal) and analyzed (frequency spectrum analysis, color coding). The flow velocity of blood particles can be determined according to the Doppler principle. As the flow velocity is correlated with the diameter of a blood vessel, its measurement reveals whether a vessel is stenotic. In direct vessel recordings, CW Doppler can be used to determine the direction of flow and the presence or absence of stenosis or occlusion. In *duplex sonography*, the PW Doppler and ultrasound images (echo impulse) are combined for simultaneous demonstration of blood flow (color-coded flow image) and tissue structures (tissue image). This permits visualization and quantitation of stenosis, dissection, extracranial vasculitis, and vascular anomalies. *Transcranial Doppler* (TCD) and *duplex sonography* are used to study the intracranial arteries, e. g., for stenosis, occlusion, collateral flow, vasospasm (after subarachnoid hemorrhage), shunting (arteriovenous malformation or fistula), and hemodynamic reserve.

■ Neuroimaging

The neuroradiologist can demonstrate structural changes associated with neurological disease with a number of different imaging techniques. When a patient is sent for a neuroimaging study, the reason for ordering the study and the question(s) to be answered by it must be clearly stated. Interventional procedures in the neuroradiology suite are mainly performed to treat vascular lesions (embolization of an arteriovenous malformation, fistula, or aneurysm; thrombolysis; angioplasty; devascularization of neoplasms; stent implantation).

Cerebrovascular Ultrasonography, Diagnostic Imaging, and Biopsy Procedures

Imaging Study	Indication/Objective[1]
Conventional radiography[2] Skull, spine	Metallic foreign bodies, air-filled cavities, fractures, skull defects, bony anomalies, osteolysis, spinal degenerative disease
Computed tomography (CT) Head, spine, spinal canal, CT-guided diagnostic interventions, 3-D reconstruction	Assessment of skeleton (anomalies, fractures, osteolysis, degenerative changes, spinal canal stenosis), metastases, trauma, intracranial hemorrhage, cerebral ischemia, hydrocephalus, calcification, intervertebral disk disease, contrast studies[3] (brain, spinal canal, CT angiography)
Magnetic resonance imaging (MRI)[4] • Head, spine, spinal canal	• Tumors (brain, spine, spinal cord), infection (encephalitis, myelitis, abscess, AIDS, multiple sclerosis), structural anomalies of the brain (epilepsy), leukodystrophy, MR angiography (aneurysm, vascular malformation), ischemia of the brain or spinal cord, spinal trauma, hydrocephalus, myelopathy, intervertebral disk disease
• Skeletal muscle	• Muscular atrophy, myositis
Angiography[3,5] Cerebral, spinal; preinterventional or preoperative study[6]	High-grade arterial stenosis, aneurysm, arteriovenous malformation/ fistula, sinus thrombosis, vasculitis
Myelography[3,7]	Largely replaced by CT and, especially, MRI. Used to clarify special diagnostic questions in spinal lesions
Diagnostic nuclear medicine • Skeletal scintigraphy ("bone scan") • CSF scintigraphy • Emission tomography[8]	• Tumor metastasis, spondylodiscitis • Intradural catheter function test, CSF leak • Cerebral perfusion, cerebral metabolic disorders, degenerative diseases, diagnosis of epilepsy

1 Examples. **2** Plain radiographs, X-ray tomography. **3** Risks: allergy (⇨ intolerance), latent hyperthyroidism (⇨ thyrotoxicosis), thyroid carcinoma (⇨ radioiodine therapy cannot be performed for a long time afterward), renal failure, left heart failure (⇨ pulmonary edema), plasmacytoma (⇨ renal failure). **4** *Gadolinium* contrast agent can be used to show blood–brain barrier lesions (e. g., acute multiple sclerosis plaques). *T1-weighted scans*: CSF/ edema dark (hypointense), diploe/fat light (hyperintense), white matter light; gray matter dark. *T2-weighted scans*: CSF/edema light, scalp dark, diploe/fat light, muscle dark, white matter dark; gray matter light. *Contraindications*: Cardiac pacemaker, mobile ferromagnetic material. **5** Contraindicated in patients with coagulopathy. **6** Endovascular or surgical therapy. **7** Rare complications: generalized epileptic seizures, meningitis, post–lumbar puncture headache; acute transverse cord syndrome possible in patients with spinal tumors. Coagulopathy is a contraindication. **8** SPECT = single-photon emission computed tomography, PET = positron emission tomography.

■ Tissue Biopsy

In certain cases, the provision of a definitive diagnosis requires biopsy of nerve (usually the sural nerve, p. 391), muscle (a moderately affected muscle in myopathy, p. 399), or blood vessels (e. g., the temporal artery in suspected temporal arteritis). These biopsies can usually be carried out under local anesthesia. Spinal tumors can be biopsied under CT or MRI guidance, and brain tumors and abscesses can be biopsied with stereotactic technique.

5 Appendix

- Supplementary tables
- Detailed information
- Outlines
- Working aids

Appendix

Table 1 Cranial nerves (p. 28)

Pathway	Cranial Nerve (CN)/Nucleus		Functions
Somatosensory (afferent)	II	Retina	Vision
	III	Proprioceptors of extraocular mm.[1]	Proprioception[2]
	IV	Proprioceptors of extraocular mm.	Proprioception
	V	Semilunar ganglion, proprioceptors of masticatory, tensor veli palatini, and tensor tympani muscles	Sensation in face, nose, nasal cavity, oral cavity; proprioception, dura mater (pp. 6, 94)
	VI	Proprioceptors of extraocular mm.	Proprioception
	VII	Geniculate ganglion	External ear, parts of auditory canal, outer surface of eardrum (sensation)
	VIII	Vestibular ganglion; spiral ganglion	Balance/equilibrium; hearing
	IX	Superior ganglion	Middle ear, auditory tube (sensation)
	X	Superior ganglion	External auditory canal/dura mater of posterior fossa (p. 5)
Visceral (afferent)	I	Olfactory cells of nasal mucosa	Smell
	VII	Geniculate ganglion	Taste on anterior 2/3 of tongue (chorda tympani), taste on inferior surface of soft palate (greater petrosal n.)
	IX	Inferior and superior ganglia	Taste/sensation on posterior 1/3 of tongue, pharyngeal mucosa, tonsils, auditory tube (sensation)
	X	Inferior ganglion	Abdominal cavity (sensation), epiglottis (taste)
Motor (efferent)	III	Oculomotor nucleus[3]	Extraocular mm. (except those supplied by CN IV, VI), raise eyelid (levator palpebrae superioris m.)
	IV	Trochlear nucleus	Oblique eye movements (superior oblique m.)
	V	Motor nucleus of trigeminal n.	Mastication,[4] tensing of palate[5] and tympanic membrane[6]
	VI	Abducens nucleus	Lateral eye movements (lateral rectus m.)
	VII	Facial nucleus	Facial muscles, platysma, stylohyoid and digastric muscles
	IX	Nucleus ambiguus	Pharyngeal mm., stylopharyngeus m.
	X	Nucleus ambiguus	Swallowing (pharyngeal mm.), speech (superior laryngeal nerve)
	XI	Nucleus ambiguus, motor cells of anterior horn of cervical spinal cord	Muscles of pharynx and larynx, sternocleidomastoid m.[7] trapezius m.[8]
	XII	Hypoglossal nucleus	Muscles of tongue
Visceral (efferent)	III	Parasympathetic, Edinger–Westphal nucleus	Pupillary constriction (sphincter pupillae m.), accommodation (ciliary m.)
	VII	Parasympathetic, superior salivatory nucleus	Secretion of mucus, tears, and saliva (sublingual and submandibular glands)
	IX	Parasympathetic, inferior salivatory nucleus	Secretion of saliva (parotid gland)
	X	Parasympathetic, dorsal nucleus of vagus nerve	Lungs, heart, intestine to left colonic flexure (motor); glandular secretion (respiratory tract, intestine)

1 Eye muscles. **2** See p. 104. **3** Nucleus. **4** Masseter, temporalis, lateral pterygoid, and medial pterygoid muscles. **5** Tensor veli palatini m. **6** Tensor tympani m. **7** Shoulder elevation, scapular fixation, accompanying movements of cervical spine. **8** Neck flexion and extension, head rotation.

Table 2 Segment-indicating muscles (p. 32)

Segment	Segment-indicating Muscle(s)
C4	Diaphragm
C5	Rhomboids, supraspinatus, infraspinatus, deltoid
C6	Biceps brachii, brachioradialis
C7	Triceps brachii, extensor carpi radialis, pectoralis major, flexor carpi radialis, pronator teres
C8	Abductor pollicis brevis, abductor digiti quinti, flexor carpi ulnaris, flexor pollicis brevis
L3	Quadriceps femoris, iliopsoas; adductor longus, brevis et magnus
L4	Quadriceps femoris (vastus medialis m.)
L5	Extensor hallucis longus, tibialis anterior, tibialis posterior, gluteus medius
S1	Gastrocnemius, gluteus maximus

Tables 3 Types of tremor (p. 62)

Type	Features
Physiological tremor (PT)	Normal. Discrete, usually asymptomatic tremor of unclear significance. Isometric tremor may occur, e. g., when holding a heavy object.
Exaggerated PT, toxic or drug-induced tremor	Amplitude > PT, frequency = PT. Absent at rest. Mainly PosT.[1] *Stress* (anxiety, fatigue, excitement, cold). *Metabolic disturbances* (hyperthyroidism, hypoglycemia, pheochromocytoma). *Drugs/toxins* (alcohol or drug withdrawal; mercury, manganese, lithium, valproic acid, cyclosporine A, amiodarone, flunarizine, cinnarizine, tricyclic antidepressants, neuroleptics ⇨ tardive tremor)
Essential tremor (ET)	*Classical ET*: PosT > KT[2]. Approx. 60% autosomal dominant, rest sporadic. Hands > head > voice > trunk. Often improved by alcohol. *Orthostatic tremor*: Occurs only when standing ⇨ unsteadiness, hard to stand still. *Task-specific tremor*
Parkinsonian tremor	RT[3] See p. 206. Postural and kinetic tremor may also be present.
Cerebellar tremor	IT[4] reflecting cerebellar dysfunction. Postural tremor and head/trunk tremor may be seen when the patient is standing (alcohol intoxication).
Holmes tremor (rubral, midbrain tremor, myorhythmia)	RT + PosT + IT, mainly proximal, disabling. Associated with lesions of nigrostriatal and cerebello-thalamic pathways (multiple sclerosis, infarct)
(Poly-)neuropathic tremor	RT, PosT, or IT, predominantly either proximal or distal. 3–10 Hz[5]
Palatal tremor	Symptomatic (medullary lesion due to encephalitis, multiple sclerosis, brain stem infarct) or essential; clicking noise in ear
Psychogenic tremor	Migrates from one part of the body to another. Accompanied by muscle contraction (co-contraction)

1 PosT = postural tremor. **2** KT = kinetic tremor. **3** RT = resting tremor. **4** IT = intention tremor. **5** Occurs in hereditary sensorimotor neuropathy type I, chronic demyelinating polyradiculitis, paraproteinemic neuropathy, diabetic neuropathy, and uremic neuropathy.

Appendix

Table 4 Midbrain syndromes (p. 71)

Anterior Midbrain Lesions (Peduncle, Weber Syndrome)

Cause. Infarct. Less commonly caused by hemorrhage, tumor (germinoma, teratoma, pineocytoma, pineoblastoma, astrocytoma, tentorial edge meningioma, lymphoma), or multiple sclerosis.

Structure Affected	Symptoms and Signs
Intramesencephalic fibers of oculomotor n.	Ipsilateral oculomotor paralysis + parasympathetic dysfunction (pupil dilated and unreactive to light)
Pyramidal tract	Contralateral central paralysis + face (⇨ supranuclear facial palsy) + spasticity. Dysarthria (supranuclear hypoglossal palsy)
Substantia nigra	Rigidity (rare)

Medial Midbrain Lesions (Tegmentum, Benedikt Syndrome)

Cause. Same as in anterior lesions.

Structure Affected	Symptoms and Signs
Intramesencephalic fibers of oculomotor n.	Ipsilateral oculomotor paralysis + parasympathetic dysfunction (see above)
Medial lemniscus	Contralateral impairment of touch, position, and vibration sense
Red nucleus	Contralateral tremor (myorhythmia ⇨ red nucleus syndrome, Holmes tremor)
Substantia nigra	Rigidity (variable)
Superior cerebellar peduncle	Contralateral ataxia (⇨ Claude syndrome)

Dorsal Midbrain Lesions (Tectum, Parinaud Syndrome)

Cause. Tumor of third ventricle, infarct, arteriovenous malformation, multiple sclerosis, large aneurysm of posterior fossa, trauma, shunt malfunction, metabolic diseases (Wilson disease, Niemann–Pick disease), infectious diseases (Whipple disease, AIDS)

Structure Affected	Symptoms and Signs
Oculomotor nuclei	Pathological lid retraction (Collier's sign) due to overactivity of levator palpebrae superioris m. Over the course of the disease, accommodation is impaired; the pupils become moderately dilated and unreactive to light, but they do constrict on convergence (light-near dissociation)
Medial longitudinal fasciculus	Supranuclear palsy of upward conjugate gaze (vertical gaze palsy ⇨ the eyes move upward on passive vertical deflection of the head, but not voluntarily). Convergence nystagmus with retraction of the eyeball on upward gaze (retraction-convergence nystagmus)
Trochlear nucleus	Trochlear nerve palsy
Aqueduct (compressed)	Hydrocephalus (headache, papilledema)

Table 4 Midbrain syndromes (continued)

Top of the Basilar Artery Syndrome

Cause. Large aneurysm of the basilar tip, thromboembolism in the upper basilar territory, vasculitis, complication of angiography. (Central paralysis is not found.)

Site of Lesion	Symptoms and Signs
Midbrain	Unilateral or bilateral vertical gaze palsy; impaired convergence; retraction nystagmus. Sudden oscillations (sensation of movement of surroundings when walking or when moving head). Collier's sign. Strabismus with diplopia. Pupils may be constricted and responsive or dilated and unresponsive to light.
Thalamus, parts of temporal and occipital lobes	Visual field defects (homonymous hemianopsia, cortical blindness). Variable features: Somnolence, peduncular hallucinations (dreamlike scenic hallucinations), memory impairment, disorientation, psychomotor hyperactivity

Table 5 Pontine syndromes (p. 72)

Anterior Pontine Lesions (Ventral Pons)

Cause. Basilar artery thrombosis, hemorrhage, central pontine myelinolysis, brain stem encephalitis, tumors, trauma. Arterial hypertension (lacunar infarct).

■ **Mid Ventral Pons**

Structures Affected	Symptoms and Signs
Pyramidal tract	Contralateral central paralysis sparing the face
Intrapontine fibers of trigeminal nerve	Ipsilateral facial hypesthesia, peripheral-type weakness of muscles of mastication
Middle cerebellar peduncle	Ipsilateral ataxia

■ **Lacunar Syndromes[1]**

Structures Affected	Symptoms and Signs
Pyramidal tract	Contralateral central paralysis, sometimes more pronounced in legs, with or without facial involvement
Middle cerebellar peduncle	Ipsilateral ataxia, which may be accompanied by dysarthria and dysphagia, depending on the site of the lesion (dysarthria—clumsy hand syndrome)

[1]Similar syndromes can also occur in patients with supratentorial lacunas (internal capsule, thalamocortical pathways).

■ **Locked-in Syndrome** (p. 120)

Structures Affected	Symptoms and Signs
Ventral pons (corticobulbar and corticospinal tracts) bilaterally, abducens nucleus, pontine paramedian reticular formation, fibers of trigeminal nerve	Quadriplegia, aphonia, inability to swallow, horizontal gaze palsy (including absence of caloric response), absence of corneal reflex (risk of corneal ulceration)

Eyelid and vertical eye movements (supranuclear oculomotor tracts), sensation, wakefulness (reticular ascending system), and spontaneous breathing remain intact.

Table 5 Pontine syndromes (continued)

Dorsal Pontine Lesions (Pontine Tegmentum)

Cause. Same as in lesions of ventral pons.

■ **Oral (Superior) Pontine Tegmentum (Raymond–Céstan Syndrome)**

Structures Affected	Symptoms and Signs
Trigeminal nucleus/fibers	Ipsilateral facial hypesthesia, peripheral paralysis of muscles of mastication
Superior cerebellar peduncle	Ipsilateral ataxia, intention tremor
Medial lemniscus	Contralateral impairment of touch, position, and vibration sense
Spinothalamic tract	Contralateral loss of pain and temperature sensation
Paramedian pontine reticular formation (PPRF, "pontine gaze center")	Ipsilateral loss of conjugate movement (loss of optokinetic and vestibular nystagmus ⇨ PPRF lesion with intact vestibulo-ocular reflex (VOR, p. 84))
Pyramidal tract	Contralateral central paralysis sparing the face

■ **Caudal Pontine Tegmentum**

Structures Affected	Symptoms and Signs
Pyramidal tract	Contralateral central paralysis sparing the face
Nucleus/fibers of the facial n.	Ipsilateral (nuclear = peripheral) facial palsy (⇨ Millard–Gubler syndrome)
Fibers of abducens nerve	Ipsilateral abducens paralysis (⇨ Foville syndrome, eyes drift "away from the lesion"; loss of VOR)
Central sympathetic pathway	Ipsilateral Horner syndrome
PPRF	Loss of ipsilateral conjugate movement
Medial and lateral lemniscus	Contralateral impairment of touch, position, and vibration sense
Lateral spinothalamic tract	Contralateral impairment of pain and temperature sensation

Table 6 Medullary syndromes (p. 73)

Medial Medullary Lesions

Cause. Occlusion of the anterior spinal artery or vertebral artery.

Structures Affected	Symptoms and Signs
Hypoglossal n. nucleus/fibers	Ipsilateral peripheral (nuclear) hypoglossal paralysis
Pyramidal tract	Contralateral central paralysis sparing the face (flaccid, in isolated pyramidal tract lesions)
Medial lemniscus	Contralateral impairment of touch, position, and vibration sense (pain and temperature sensation intact)
Medial longitudinal fasciculus	Upbeat nystagmus

Lateral Medullary Lesions (Dorsolateral Medullary Syndrome, Wallenberg Syndrome)

Cause. Occlusion of posterior inferior cerebellar artery (PICA) or vertebral artery. Less common causes: tumor, metastases, hemorrhage due to vascular malformations, multiple sclerosis, vertebral artery dissection (after chiropractic maneuvers), trauma, gunshot wounds, cocaine intoxication.

Site of Lesion	Symptoms and Signs
Spinal nucleus of trigeminal nerve	Ipsilateral analgesia/thermanesthesia of the face and absence of corneal reflex with or without facial pain
Cochlear nucleus	Ipsilateral hearing loss
Nucleus ambiguus	Ipsilateral paralysis of the pharynx and larynx (hoarseness, paralysis of the soft palate), dysarthria, and dysphagia. Tongue movement remains intact
Solitary nucleus	Ageusia (impaired sense of taste)
Dorsal nucleus of vagus n.	Tachycardia and dyspnea
Inferior vestibular nucleus	Nystagmus away from the side of the lesion, tendency to fall toward the side of the lesion, nausea and vomiting
Central tegmental tract	Ipsilateral myorhythmia of the soft palate and pharynx
Central sympathetic pathway	Ipsilateral Horner syndrome
Reticular formation	Singultus
Inferior cerebellar peduncle	Ipsilateral ataxia and intention tremor
Anterior spinocerebellar tract	Ipsilateral hypotonia
Lateral spinothalamic tract	Contralateral loss of pain and temperature sensation with sparing of touch, position, and vibration sense (sensory dissociation)

Involvement of the lower pons produces diplopia. Occipital pain in Wallenberg syndrome is most commonly due to vertebral artery dissection.

Appendix

Table 7 Syndromes affecting the facial muscles (p. 98)

Syndrome	Etiology
Hypomimia or amimia	Basal ganglia dysfunction (p. 206), depression
Blepharospasm, Meige syndrome, lid-opening apraxia, oromandibular dystonia, tics (p. 64ff.)	Basal ganglia dysfunction
Melkersson–Rosenthal syndrome (recurrent swelling of face/lips, peripheral facial palsy, and fissured tongue)	Unknown
Heerfordt syndrome (fever, uveitis, parotitis, peripheral facial palsy)	Occasional manifestation of sarcoidosis, lymphoma. Cryptogenic
Bilateral peripheral facial paralysis	Neuroborreliosis, Guillain–Barré syndrome, Fisher syndrome, botulism
Möbius syndrome	Congenital bilateral facial palsy and cranial nerve involvement (bilateral: VI; unilateral: XII, IV, VIII, IX)
Synkinesis (involuntary co-movement of facial muscles, e. g., narrowing of palpebral fissure when the lips are pursed); hemifacial spasm	Faulty regeneration of CN VII after facial palsy. Nerve root compression and segmental demyelination in hemifacial spasm
Pseudobulbar palsy	Multiple bilateral supratentorial or pontine vascular lesions
Myopathic facies	Myopathic disorders (myotonic dystrophy, myasthenia, facial-scapular-humeral muscular dystrophy)
Gustatory sweating (Frey syndrome) or lacrimation ("crocodile tears")	Faulty regeneration of the auriculotemporal/facial nerve
Progressive facial hemiatrophy	Unknown

Table 8 Neurological Causes of Dysphagia (p. 102)

Symptoms and Signs	Site of Lesion	Cause
Oral phase impaired and swallowing reflex delayed (slightly) because of paralysis	Supratentorial Unilateral	Cerebral infarct, tumor or hemorrhage
Delayed swallowing reflex, aspiration (especially of fluids), prolonged oral phase (pseudobulbar palsy, akinesia, dysarthria, dysphonia, salivation, oromandibular dystonia)	Supratentorial Bilateral	Vascular lesions (single or multiple infarcts, hemorrhage), trauma, tumor, multiple sclerosis, encephalitis, parkinsonism, multiple system atrophy, Alzheimer disease, Creutzfeldt–Jakob disease, hydrocephalus, dystonia (toxic/drug-induced), chorea, intoxication, cerebral palsy
Loss of swallowing reflex, impaired pharyngeal phase, impaired cough reflex (bulbar palsy, dysarthria, respiratory disturbances), risk of aspiration	Brain stem, cerebellum	Vascular lesions, multiple sclerosis, tumor, trauma, amyotrophic lateral sclerosis, syringobulbia, poliomyelitis, Arnold–Chiari malformation, central pontine myelinolysis, listerial meningitis, spinobulbar muscular atrophy, spinocerebellar degeneration
Weakness of muscles of mastication, impaired oral phase, impaired lip closure, nasal drip; impaired pharyngeal phase (dysarthria) may occur: depending on which nerve/muscle is affected	Cranial nerves	Facial paralysis, Guillain–Barré syndrome, diabetic neuropathy, amyloidosis, base of skull syndrome (p. 74)
Same as above (generalized myopathy, dysphonia)	Neuromuscular	Myasthenia, amyotrophic lateral sclerosis, Lambert–Eaton syndrome, botulism, polymyositis/dermatomyositis, scleroderma, hyperthyroidism, oculopharyngeal muscular dystrophy, myotonic dystrophy, facial–scapular-humeral muscular dystrophy, nemaline myopathy, inclusion-body myositis

Table 9 Classification of pain[1,2] (p. 108)

Type	Clinical Features	Etiology (examples)
Nociceptive pain (somatic, p. 110)[3]	Paresthesia, allodynia,[4] loss of sensation, readily localizable	Meralgia paresthetica, carpal tunnel syndrome, skin lesion
Neuropathic pain, neuralgia (pp. 186, 318 ff.)	Severe pain in nerve distribution, paresthesiae, allodynia, sensory loss, pain on nerve pressure, readily localizable	Mononeuritis, polyneuropathy, trauma, nerve compression, trigeminal neuralgia, neuroma
Radicular pain (p. 319 f)	Same as above + aggravated by stretching (e. g., Lasègue sign) or movement	Herniated intervertebral disk, polyradiculitis, leptomeningeal metastases, neurofibroma/schwannoma
Referred pain	See p. 110	See p. 110
Deafferentation pain, anesthesia dolorosa	Pain in an anesthetic or analgesic nerve territory	Plexus lesion, radicular lesion, trigeminal nerve lesion
Phantom limb pain	Pain felt in an amputated limb	Limb amputation
Central pain	Burning, piercing pain in the region of a neurological deficit; imprecisely localizable; frequently accompanied by sensory dissociation, dysesthesia, paresthesia; triggered by stimuli	Cerebral infarct, hemorrhage, or tumor (cortex, thalamus, white matter, internal capsule), brain stem, spinal cord; syrinx, trauma, multiple sclerosis (brain stem, spinal cord)
Chronic pain ("pain disease")	Pain that lasts > 6 months, impairs social contacts, emotional state, and physical activity	Sensitization of nociceptors? Transsynaptic neuropeptide induction (calcitonin gene-related peptide = CGRP, substance P = SP, neurokinin A = NKA)?
Psychogenic pain	Discrepancy between symptoms and organ findings and/or syndrome classification	Mental illness

1 Selected types. **2** Features may overlap. **3** = nociceptor pain. **4** Pain evoked by a normally nonpainful stimulus.

Table 10 Sleep Characteristics Observed in Sleep Studies (p. 112)

Stage	EEG[1]	EOG[2]	EMG[3]
Awake	α activity (8–13 Hz)	Blinks, saccades	High muscle tone, movement artifact
NREM stage 1	Increasing θ activity (2–7 Hz), vertex waves[4]	Slow eye movements[5]	Slight decrease in muscle tone
NREM stage 2	θ activity, sleep spindles,[6] K-complexes[7]	No eye movement until stage 4, EEG artifact	Further decrease in muscle tone until stage 4
NREM stage 3	Groups of high-amplitude δ waves (0.5–2 Hz, amplitude > 0.75 µV)		
NREM stage 4	Groups of high-amplitude δ waves		
REM sleep	θ activity, saw-tooth waves[8] may be observed	Conjugate, rapid eye movements (episodic)	Low to medium muscle tone

(Berger, 1992)

1 Electroencephalogram (EEG). **2** Electro-oculogram (EOG). **3** Electromyogram (EMG). **4** Steep parasagittal waves of not more than 200 µV. **5** Slow eye movements (SEM). **6** Fusiform 11.5–14 Hz waves lasting 0.5–1.5 seconds and occurring 3–8 times/second. **7** Biphasic, initially negative δ waves appearing spontaneously or in response to acoustic stimuli. **8** Grouped, regular θ activity with a saw-toothed appearance.

Appendix

Table 11 Diagnostic criteria for death ("brain death") (recommendations of the Scientific Advisory Council of the Federal Chamber of Physicians (Germany), 1998, p. 120)

Prerequisites	Acute, severe brain damage (either primary or secondary) Exclusion of other causes[1]
Clinical criteria	**Coma** Absent light reflex, moderately to maximally dilated pupils[2] Absent oculocephalic reflex[3] Absent corneal reflex[3] Absent response to painful stimulation in trigeminal distribution Absent pharyngeal and tracheal reflexes[3] Absence of spontaneous breathing[4]
Proof of irreversible brain damage	**Required time of observation[5]** *Supratentorial primary brain damage* Adults and children over 2 years of age ⇨ at least 12 hours Children under 2 years of age ⇨ at least 24 hours[6] Neonates ⇨ at least 72 hours[6] *Infratentorial primary brain damage* Same as supratentorial damage, but with at least 1 additional examination[6] *Secondary brain damage* Adults and children over 2 years of age ⇨ at least 72 hours **Supplementary criteria[7]** Isoelectric EEG Absence of evoked potentials[8] Absence of cerebral blood flow

1 Intoxication, pharmacological sedation, neuromuscular blockade, primary hypothermia, circulatory shock or coma secondary to endocrine, metabolic or infectious disease. **2** Not due to mydriatic agents. **3** See p. 26. **4** As shown by apnea test. **5** The clinical findings at the beginning and end of the observation period must be identical. **6** At least one of the following supplementary criteria must be observed twice: isoelectric EEG, loss of early acoustic evoked potentials, demonstration of absent cerebral blood flow (by Doppler ultrasound or perfusion scintigram); standardized examination procedures must be strictly followed. **7** Once the prerequisites and clinical criteria have been met, the diagnosis of brain death can be made as soon as one of the supplementary criteria has been met. **8** Early auditory, somatosensory cerebral or high cervical components of evoked potentials.

Table 11 a Apnea test

Steps	Measures/Objective	Parameters To Be Measured
Prerequisites	Body core temperature $\geq 36.5\,°C$[1] Systolic blood pressure ≥ 90 mmHg[2] Positive fluid balance for more than 6 hours	
Preparation	Oxygenation: Inspiratory O_2 concentration 100% Tidal volume: 10 ml/kg body weight	$PO_2 \geq 200$ (to 400) mmHg (54 kPa)[3] $pCO_2 \leq 40$ mmHg (5.3 kPa)
Procedure[4]	Disconnect ventilator ⇨ administer 100% O_2 at rate of 6 to 8 l/min via thin catheter (tip at carina)	Monitor heart rate, blood pressure, SpO_2, respiratory rate; observe for chest or abdominal movement; check ABG every 2–3 minutes
Termination	If no respiratory activity/movement is observed in 8 minutes[5]	$pCO_2 \geq 60$ mmHg (8 kPa) or pCO_2 rises by more than 20 mmHg (2.7 kPa)[6]

(Wijdicks, 2001)

1 Because hypothermia impairs CO_2 production and O_2 release from oxyhemoglobin. **2** Raise with 5% albumin solution or increase intravenous dopamine when administered, if necessary. **3** Arterial blood gas (ABG) analysis. **4** If blood pressure < 90 mmHg, O_2 saturation < 80%, and there is severe cardiac arrhythmia, stop the apnea test and put patient back on ventilator. **5** Reconnect ventilator, ventilate at 10/min. **6** If pCO_2 baseline value of ≤ 40 mmHg cannot be achieved (e. g., in patient with pulmonary disease).

Table 12 Sites and manifestations of lesions causing dysarthria (p. 130)

Site of Lesion	Manifestations	Causes[1]
Periphery[2]	Slurred speech (impaired labial/lingual articulation, rhinolalia = "speaking through nose," unclear differentiation of vowels and consonants), dyspnea, whispering (recurrent laryngeal nerve paralysis), hoarseness (laryngitis, vocal cord polyp, extubation)	Facial nerve palsy, myasthenia, amyotrophic lateral sclerosis, diphtheria, Guillain–Barré syndrome, syringobulbia, tumor
Cerebellum/ brain stem (pp. 54, 70)	Ataxic dysarthria (clipped, scanning speech), articulation problems. Hoarse, deep voice (vagus nerve lesion)	See p. 278 f, multiple sclerosis, infarction
Basal ganglia (nonpyramidal dysarthria)	Hypophonia (p. 206, monotonous, soft, slurred). Spasmodic dysphonia (p. 64). Hyperkinetic speech (p. 66; explosive, loud, uncoordinated, clipped speech)	Parkinsonism, dystonia, chorea, tic, myoclonus
White matter/ cortex	Monotonous, slow, hoarse, pressured speech. Deep, variable pitch. Poor articulation	Bilateral white-matter lesions (pseudobulbar palsy, lacunar infarcts, multiple sclerosis), unilateral infarct
Diffuse	Slurred, effortful, slow speech	Intoxication, metabolic disturbances

1 Examples; see also p. 64. **2** Pontine (bulbar paralysis), nuclear (2nd motor neuron), peripheral nerve or muscle lesion.

Table 13 Types and causes of amnesia (amnesia, p. 134)

Type of Amnesia	Manifestations	Causes[1]/Site of Lesion
Transient global amnesia[2]	Acute onset, limited duration. Patient repeats questions (e. g., "What am I doing here?"), is helpless, anxious; can perform everyday activities. Anterograde/retrograde amnesia	Ischemia (venous)? Migraine? Resolves completely or nearly so
Acute transient amnesia	Anterograde/retrograde amnesia; manifestations of underlying disease	Complex partial seizures (focal epilepsy). Posttraumatic phenomenon
Acute persistent amnesia	Anterograde/retrograde amnesia; manifestations of underlying disease	Bilateral infarction (hippocampus, thalamus, anterior cerebral artery). Trauma (orbitofrontal, mediobasal, diencephalic). Hypoxia (cardiopulmonary arrest, carbon monoxide poisoning)
Subacute persistent amnesia	Many patients are initially confused, with anterograde/retrograde amnesia; manifestations of underlying disease	Wernicke–Korsakoff syndrome. Herpes simplex encephalitis. Basilar meningitis (tuberculosis, sarcoidosis, fungi)
Chronic progressive amnesia	Anterograde amnesia; retrograde amnesia develops in the course of the condition; manifestations of underlying disease	Tumor (3rd ventricle, temporal lobe). Paraneoplastic "limbic" encephalitis (lung cancer). Alzheimer disease. Pick disease

1 Examples. **2** Also called *amnestic episode*.

Appendix

Table 14 Classification of dementia (p. 136)

Cause	Diagnostic criteria[1]
Alzheimer disease (p. 297 f)	Mainly temporal and parietal lobe degeneration. Rarely hereditary (autosomal dominant). No focal neurological deficit. *CSF:* increased acetylcholine, Aβ-amyloid, and τ protein levels. *Cognitive deficits:* Anterograde amnesia, amnestic aphasia, acalculia, impaired visuospatial performance. *Behavioral changes:* Hardly any at first; later anosognosia or dissimulation, paranoia, disturbance of sleep–wake cycle.
Vascular dementia (p. 298)	Subcortical vascular demyelination due to multiple infarcts, lacunes, vasculitis or CADASIL. Fluctuating course. *Focal neurological signs:* Hemiparesis, aphasia, apraxia, gait impairment, bladder dysfunction, Babinski sign. Pseudobulbar palsy (bilateral lesion of the corticobulbar tracts ⇨ dysarthrophonia or anarthria, dysphagia, lingual/facial paralysis, loss of emotional control with outbursts of laughing or crying). *Cognitive deficits:* Memory deficit ("forgetting to remember"), frontal brain dysfunction (p. 122). *Behavioral changes:* Sluggishness, reduced drive, disturbance of sleep–wake cycle
Depression	Psychomotor slowing, reduced drive, and anxiety suggest dementia, which is not, in fact, present (*pseudodementia*). See Table 42, p. 383
Alcohol	Korsakoff syndrome: Disorientation/amnesia, confabulation
Hydrocephalus	Normal pressure hydrocephalus (p. 160)
Metabolic/endocrine disorders	Wilson disease, hypothyroidism, hypopituitarism, hepatic/uremic encephalopathy, hypoglycemia, vitamin B_{12} deficiency, Wernicke encephalopathy, pellagra, hypoxia, hypoparathyroidism or hyperparathyroidism, adrenocortical insufficiency, Cushing syndrome, acute intermittent porphyria (p. 332)
Tumor	See p. 254 ff
Degenerative diseases	Parkinson disease (p. 206 ff), atypical parkinsonism (p. 302), Huntington disease (p. 300), frontotemporal dementia (p. 298), hereditary ataxia (p. 280), motor neuron disease (p. 304), multiple sclerosis
Infectious diseases (p. 222 ff)	HIV and other viral encephalitides, prion diseases, neurosyphilis, Whipple disease, brain abscess, neurosarcoidosis, subacute sclerosing panencephalitis
Trauma	Chronic subdural hematoma, posttraumatic phenomenon, punch-drunk syndrome (dementia pugilistica)
Toxic	Drugs, substance abuse, heavy metal poisoning, organic toxins

1 Mainly early manifestations are listed; these usually worsen and are accompanied by other manifestations as the disease progresses.

Table 15 The hypothalamic-pituitary regulatory axis (p. 142)

Controlled Variable(s)	Hormones	Stimulus	Effect	Comments
Water balance and blood pressure	ADH	↓ BP[1] ↑ Plasma osmolality	Renal water reabsorption and arterial vasoconstriction (at higher ADH levels)	↓ ADH: Diabetes insipidus; ↑ADH: ectopic production, SIADH (p. 310)
Triiodothyronine (T_3), thyroxine (T_4)	TRH, TSH	↓ / ↑ T_3/T_4	TRH[2] increase/decrease ⇒ TSH[3]	↑TSH (basal) usually found in primary hypothyroidism; ↓ TSH usually found in hyperthyroidism
Cortisol	CRH, ACTH[4]	↓ / ↑ Cortisol	CRH[5] increase/decrease	↑ACTH: Cushing syndrome; ↓ ACTH: secondary adrenocortical insufficiency
Testosterone (man)	GnRH, LH, FSH[6]	↓ / ↑ Testosterone	GnRH[7] increase/decrease	↓ Testosterone: Decrease in muscle mass, loss of libido, hypospermia, impotence
Estradiol, progesterone (woman)	GnRH, LH, FSH	↓ / ↑ Estradiol, progesterone	GnRH increase/decrease	↓ LH/FSH: menstrual disturbances, breast/uterine atrophy, osteoporosis, atherosclerosis
Prolactin (PRL)	PRL	↑ PRL ↓ PRL	↓ Dopamine[8] ↓ VIP[9], TRH	↑PRL: galactorrhea, amenorrhea, headaches
Growth (somatomedins)	GHRH, GH[10]	Various stimuli	GHRH[11] Somatostatin[12]	Somatomedins mediate the effect of GH. ↑GH: acromegaly; ↓ GH: dwarfism (children), weight gain, muscle atrophy
Endogenous opioid peptides	β-endorphin (pituitary gland)	Various stimuli	Analgesia, food intake, thermoregulation, learning, memory	

1 Blood pressure. **2** Thyrotropin-releasing hormone. **3** Thyroid-stimulating hormone of the anterior pituitary = thyrotropin. **4** Adrenocorticotropic hormone of the anterior pituitary = corticotropin. **5** Corticotropin-releasing hormone. **6** LH = luteinizing hormone, FSH = follicle-stimulating hormone (both anterior pituitary hormones); both are called *gonadotropins*. **7** Gonadotropin-releasing hormone. **8** Released from the hypothalamus; inhibits prolactin release via pituitary D_2 receptors. **9** Vasoactive intestinal peptide (anterior pituitary). **10** GH = human growth hormone. **11** Growth hormone-releasing hormone (stimulatory). **12** Released from hypothalamus (inhibitory).

Appendix

Table 16 Limbic syndromes (p. 144)

Syndrome	Symptoms and Signs	Site of Lesion[1]
Delirium, acute confusional state	Disturbances of consciousness, attention, perception, memory, sleep–wake cycle, and cognition. Visual hallucinations. Fluctuating motor hypoactivity and hyperactivity. Affective disturbances (anxiety, depression, irritability, euphoria, helplessness)	Bilateral mediobasal temporal lobe (hippocampus, amygdala), hypothalamus
Pathological laughing and crying	Uncontrollable emotional outbreaks. Seen in central paralysis (pseudobulbar palsy, amyotrophic lateral sclerosis, multiple sclerosis) and focal epilepsy (gelastic seizures). Stroke prodrome	Internal capsule, basal ganglia, thalamus, corticonuclear tract
Aggressive, violent behavior; fits of rage	Aggression with minimal or no provocation, seen in focal epilepsy, head trauma, hypoxic encephalopathy, brain tumor, herpes simplex encephalitis, rabies, cerebral infarction or hemorrhage, hypoglycemia, intoxication (drugs, alcohol)	Mediobasal temporal lobe (amygdala)
Indifference, apathy, akinetic mutism	Usually due to a primary illness such as Alzheimer or Pick disease, herpes simplex or AIDS encephalitis, hypoxic encephalopathy, cerebral infarction or hemorrhage	Bilateral septal area, cingulate gyrus
Memory deficit, transitory global amnesia (p. 134, Table 13)	Korsakoff syndrome: impairment of short-term memory and sense of time. Other cognitive functions and consciousness are unimpaired	Both mamillary bodies, mediobasal temporal lobe
Disturbed sexuality	Hypersexual behavior: after head trauma or stroke, or as a side effect of dopaminergic antiparkinsonian medication. Diminished libido: depression, medications	Septal area, hypothalamus

1 The specified lesions do not always produce these syndromes, and the location and extent of the causative lesion is often not known with certainty.

Appendix

Table 17 Tests for autonomic circulatory dysfunction (p. 148)

Dizziness, syncope, lack of concentration, forgetfulness or tinnitus should not be attributed to circulatory dysfunction unless thorough diagnostic evaluation reveals a circulatory cause (see p. 166 ff).

Test	Method	Normal Findings
Tests of sympathetic function		
Schellong test (orthostasis test)	Measure heart rate and blood pressure once per minute for 10 minutes with the patient supine, then 5 minutes with the patient erect (tilt table if necessary)	Heart rate rises by no more than 20 beats/min; systolic blood pressure drops no more than 10 mmHg, diastolic no more than 5 mmHg
Valsalva maneuver (VM)	The patient inspires deeply and tries to exhale against resistance (up to 40 mmHg) for 10–15 seconds. The blood pressure is measured before, during and after the VM, or continuously	During VM, the blood pressure does not drop below 50% of initial value; after VM, the blood pressure rebounds above the initial value (+ reflex bradycardia)
Hand grip test	Isometric muscle contraction (hand grip) 30% of maximal force for 3 minutes	Diastolic blood pressure > 15 mmHg
Tests of parasympathetic function		
Schellong test with 30/15 quotient	Continuous ECG recording	Quotient of R-R interval of 30th and 15th heart beat after standing up is > 1
Respiratory sinus arrhythmia (respiratory test)	ECG recorded with patient supine and breathing maximally deeply at 6/min for a total of 8 cycles. Repeat after a period of rest	The quotient of the longest (expiration) and shortest R-R intervals is normally > 1.2 (age-dependent)
VM with ECG	Continuous ECG recording	Quotient of longest and shortest R-R interval is > 1 (age-dependent)
Carotid sinus massage[1]	Perform unilateral carotid sinus massage for 10–20 seconds while continuously monitoring blood pressure and ECG with emergency resuscitation equipment ready	Reflex decrease in heart rate and blood pressure

(Low, 1997)

1 Contraindicated in carotid stenosis. Risk of cardiac arrest and ischemic stroke.

Appendix

Table 18 Respiratory disturbances in neurological disease (p. 150)

Hypoventilation	
Site of lesion	Causes
Brain stem, upper cervical spinal cord	Tumor, infarction, hemorrhage, meningoencephalitis (*Listeria*, poliomyelitis), trauma, multiple sclerosis, intoxication, parkinsonism (rigidity of respiratory muscles)
Motor anterior horn cell	Amyotrophic lateral sclerosis, tetanus, poliomyelitis, post-polio syndrome
Peripheral nerve	Guillain–Barré syndrome, phrenic nerve lesion
Neuromuscular	Myasthenia gravis, botulism, Lambert–Eaton syndrome, muscular dystrophy, polymyositis, acid maltase deficiency, electrolyte imbalance (Na↓, K↓, Ca↓, phosphate↓, Mg↓)

Hyperventilation	
Possible metabolic changes	
Ca²⁺ ↓ ⇨ carpopedal spasm, paresthesiae, tetany; *Phosphate* ↓ ⇨ weakness; pH↑⇨ dizziness, visual disturbances, syncope, seizures	Pneumonia, pulmonary embolism, asthma, acidosis (diabetic, renal, lactate↑), meningoencephalitis, brain tumor, fever, sepsis, salicylates, anxiety, pain, psychogenic

Table 19 Neurological causes of gastrointestinal dysfunction (p. 154)

GI Syndrome[1]	Manifestations	Causes[2]
Dysphagia	See p. 102	Table 8
Gastroparesis	Delayed gastric emptying ⇨ nausea, vomiting, anorexia, bloating	Diabetes mellitus, amyloidosis, paraneoplastic syndrome, dermatomyositis, Duchenne-type muscular dystrophy
Intestinal pseudo-obstruction	Impaired intestinal motility ⇨ nausea, vomiting, bloating, weight loss, impairment of peristalsis	Parkinson disease, multiple sclerosis, transverse spinal cord syndrome, Guillain–Barré syndrome, diabetes mellitus, botulism, amyloidosis, paraneoplastic syndrome, drugs (tricyclic antidepressants, codeine, morphine, clonidine, phenothiazines, anticholinergics, vincristine), Hirschsprung disease
Constipation[3]	Highly variable. Infrequent hard stools, straining, bloating, sensation of incomplete defecation, pain, flatulence, belching	Lack of exercise, dysphagia, poor nutrition, transverse spinal cord syndrome, head trauma, brain stem lesions, Parkinson disease, multiple system atrophy, multiple sclerosis, diabetes mellitus, porphyria, drugs (morphine, codeine, tricyclic antidepressants)
Diarrhea[4]	↑Defecation rate, liquid stools, tenesmus	Diabetes mellitus, amyloidosis, HIV infection, drugs, Whipple disease
Vomiting[5]	Gagging, yawning, nausea, hypersalivation, pale skin, outbreaks of sweating, apathy, low blood pressure, tachycardia	Intracranial hypertension (p. 158), vertigo (p. 58), migraine, infectious and neoplastic meningitis, drugs (digitalis, opiates, chemotherapeutic agents), intoxication
Anal incontinence	Complete or partial loss of control of defecation	Diabetes mellitus, multiple sclerosis, spinal cord lesions, lesion of the conus medullaris or cauda equina, dementia, frontal lobe lesions (tumor, infarction)

1 Gastrointestinal syndrome. **2** Neurological diseases often associated with gastrointestinal syndromes or neurogenic causes of such syndromes. **3** Normal frequency of defecation is ca. 3 times a week (variable). **4.** Upper limit of normal frequency of defecation, ca. 3 times/day. In *diarrhea*, the stool weight is > 200 g/day. In *pseudodiarrhea*, the defecation rate in increased but the stool weight is not. Diarrhea must be differentiated from anal incontinence. **5** Vomiting is regulated by a "vomiting center" in the reticular formation, which lies between the olive and solitary tract. *Input*: Chemoreceptors of the area postrema (p. 140), vestibular system, cortex, limbic system, gastrointestinal and somatosensory afferents. *Output*: Phrenic nerve (diaphragm), spinal nerve roots (respiratory and abdominal musculature), vagus nerve (larynx, pharynx, esophagus, stomach).

Table 20 Neurogenic bladder dysfunction (p. 156)

Site of Neuro-logical Lesion	Neurological Condition	Type of Bladder Dysfunction
Supratentorial	Stroke (frontal cortex, motor pathway)	Frequency ⇧, urge ⇧[1], urge incontinence[2], detrusor hyperreflexia
	Parkinson disease	Detrusor hyperreflexia, bladder hypocontractility
	Frontal brain tumor	Frequency ⇧, urge ⇧, urge incontinence
	Dementia	Usually a late manifestation: frequency ⇧, urge incontinence
Supratentorial and infraten-torial	Multiple sclerosis[3] (variable disturbances depending on site of plaques)	Frequency ⇧, urge ⇧, imperative urinary urge, urge incontinence, detrusor hyperreflexia, DSD[4]
	Amyotrophic lateral sclerosis	Frequency ⇧, urge incontinence, detrusor hyperreflexia
	Multiple system atrophy	Nocturia, frequency ⇧, urge incontinence, impairment of voluntary voiding
Spinal cord[5]	Trauma, tumor, ischemia, myelitis, multiple sclerosis, cervical myelopathy, spinal arteriovenous fistula	Lesion above S2 ("reflex bladder") ⇒ hyperreflexia, residual urine, DSD Lesion of sacral micturition center ("autonomic bladder") ⇒ residual urine, detrusor areflexia, impaired bladder reflex
Cauda equina, peripheral nerves	Autonomic neuropathy (e. g., diabetes mellitus, paraneoplastic syndrome, Guillain–Barré syndrome, drugs, toxins), trauma, lumbar canal stenosis, myelodysplasia, tumor, herpes zoster, arachnoiditis, disk herniation	Residual urine, detrusor areflexia, impaired bladder reflex, impaired filling sensation, frequency ⇩

1 Pollakisuria. **2** Urge incontinence ⇒ involuntary passage of urine on strong (imperative) urinary urge. **3** Urinary tract infections are frequent. **4** Detrusor-sphincter dyssynergy. **5** Spinal shock with detrusor areflexia (bladder atony, "shock bladder") and residual urine formation (overflow incontinence). Overdistention of the bladder can lead to a sharp rise in blood pressure accompanied by headache, dizziness, and hyperhidrosis above the level of the spinal lesion.

Table 21 Causes of intracranial hypertension (p. 158)

Pathogenetic Mechanism	Causes
Mass lesion	Hematoma (epidural, subdural, intracerebral), brain tumor/metastasis, brain abscess
CSF outflow obstruction	Hydrocephalus
Increased brain volume	Pseudotumor cerebri, infarct, global hypoxia or ischemia, hepatic encephalopathy, acute hyponatremia
Increased brain volume and increased intravascular blood volume	Head trauma, meningitis, encephalitis, eclampsia, hypertensive encephalopathy, venous sinus thrombosis

Appendix

Table 22 Causes of intracranial hypotension (p. 160)

Pathogenetic Mechanism	Findings	Causes
Impaired spinal CSF circulation[1]	Absence of pressure rise in Queckenstedt test	Tumor, arachnoiditis, herniated intervertebral disk
CSF leak	Spinal dural defect, rhinorrhea, otorrhea	Prior LP[2], trauma, neurosurgical procedures, tumor, osteomyelitis
Dehydration	Thirst, dry skin, fatigue, low blood pressure, lightheadedness or unconsciousness	*Isotonic, hypotonic*: Vomiting, diarrhea, diuretics. *Hypertonic*: Thirst, profuse sweating, mannitol administration
Spontaneous	Low ICP	Spinal CSF fistula (?)

1 In a complete blockade, the pressure decreases sharply when small volumes of fluid are removed. In that case, there is a risk of aggravation of spinal compression syndrome due to incarceration.
2 Lumbar puncture.

Table 22 a Causes of transient monocular blindness (amaurosis fugax, p. 168)

Site and Type of Lesion	Cause
Retinal vessels—embolic	Atheroembolic/thromboembolic (e. g., internal carotid artery dissection/stenosis), cardioembolic (right–left shunt, e. g., in patent foramen ovale, thrombus in atrial fibrillation, mitral valve defect, acute myocardial infarction, endocarditis, artificial heart valve)
Retinal vessels—ischemic	*Low perfusion pressure* (orthostatic hypotension, arteriovenous shunt, intracranial hypertension, glaucoma); *high perfusion resistance* (migraine, glaucoma, malignant arterial hypertension, increased blood viscosity, retinal venous thrombosis, vasospasm)
Retina	Retinal detachment, paraneoplastic (p. 388), chorioretinitis, blow to eye
Orbit/eyeball	Tumor, subluxation of lens, vitreous body hemorrhage
Optic nerve	Vascular (ischemia, arteritis [p. 180], malignant arterial hypertension), papilledema, retrobulbar neuritis (Uhthoff sign, p. 216)
Unknown	Blowing the nose, malaria, pregnancy, hypersensitivity to cold, interleukin-2, acute stabbing pain, sinus lavage

(Gautier, 1993; Warlow et al., 2001)

Appendix

Table 23 Causes of chronic daily headache (p. 182)

Type of Headache	Symptoms and Signs/Syndromes
Primary headache	
Chronic tension headache	See p. 182
Migraine	Mild to severe, often unilateral pain (transformed migraine). Additional migraine attacks (p. 184)
Atypical facial pain	Unilateral or bilateral pain, often predominantly felt in the nasolabial or palatal region, often very severe. Unresponsive to a wide variety of medical and surgical therapies. Normal findings on a wide variety of diagnostic tests ("diagnosis of exclusion")
Secondary headache	Posttraumatic, drug-induced, vascular (p. 182), intracranial mass, hydrocephalus, sinusitis, parkinsonism, cervical dystonia, myoarthropathy of the masticatory apparatus,[1] mental illness (depression, schizophrenia, hypochondria), cervical spine lesions (degenerative lesions, fractures, Klippel–Feil syndrome), Down syndrome, basilar impression, osteoporosis, skull metastasis, spondylitis, rheumatoid arthritis, lesions of cervical spinal cord/meningismus (tumor, hemorrhage, syringomyelia, cervical myelopathy, von Hippel–Lindau syndrome, meningitis, carcinomatous meningitis, intracranial hypotension)

1 Temporomandibular joint dysfunction, oromandibular dysfunction.

Table 24 Prognostic factors in epilepsy (p. 198)

Favorable Prognostic Factors	Unfavorable Prognostic Factors
One seizure type	Multiple seizure types
No interictal neurological deficit	Interictal neurological deficit
Older age of onset	Younger age of onset
Seizures secondary to a treatable disease	Spontaneous seizures
Individual seizures of short duration	Status epilepticus
Frequent seizures	Infrequent seizures
Good response to anticonvulsants	Poor response to anticonvulsants

(Neville, 1997)

Table 25 Causes of syncope (p. 200)

Cause	Underlying Condition/Trigger
Cardiac	Arrhythmia (bradyrhythmia, tachyrhythmia, or reflex arrhythmia), heart disease (e. g., cardiomyopathy, myxoma, mitral stenosis, congenital malformation, pulmonary embolism)
Hemodynamic	Hypovolemia, hypotension (vasovagal as an emotional reaction to pain, anxiety, sudden shock, sight of blood; hypotension from prolonged standing, heat, exhaustion, alcohol; multiple system atrophy; polyneuropathies, e. g., amyloid, hereditary, toxic; polyradicular neuropathies/Guillain–Barré syndrome; antihypertensive agents, nitrates, other drugs; postural orthostatic tachycardia syndrome = POTS; paraplegia above T6)
Cerebrovascular	Subclavian steal syndrome, basilar migraine, Takayasu disease
Metabolic	Hypoglycemia, hyperventilation, anemia, anoxia, postprandial (older individuals)
Miscellaneous	Coughing fit (cough syncope = tussive syncope = laryngeal syncope), micturition (micturition syncope), defecation, prolonged laughing ("laughing fit", geloplegia), glossopharyngeal neuralgia, affect-induced respiratory convulsion in childhood (breath-holding spells), pop concerts (teenage females), lying in supine position during pregnancy (supine syndrome)

(Bruni, 1996; Lempert, 1997)

Table 26 Causes of sudden falling without loss of consciousness (p. 204)

Type of Fall/Pathogenesis	Cause	Features
Drop attack	TIA[1] in vertebrobasilar territory	Usually accompanied by dizziness, diplopia, ataxia, or paresthesias
	TIA in anterior cerebral artery territory	Seen when the two anterior cerebral arteries arise from a common trunk
	Colloid cyst of 3rd ventricle	Position-dependent headache
	Posterior fossa tumor	Sudden fall after flexion of neck
Parkinsonism	Parkinson disease, multiple system atrophy	See p. 206 f
Muscle weakness	Myopathy, Guillain–Barré syndrome, polyneuropathy, spinal lesions	See p. 50 f
Spinal or cerebellar ataxia, gait apraxia	Funicular myelosis, cerebellar lesions, metabolic encephalopathies, hydrocephalus, lacunar state, cervical myelopathy, multiple sclerosis	See specific diseases
Cryptogenic	Unknown	Occurs in women over 40 while walking
Vestibular disorder	Ménière disease (vestibular drop attack ⇨ Tumarkin otolithic crisis); occasionally due to otitis media, toxic or traumatic causes	Dizziness, nausea, nystagmus, tinnitus. Vestibular drop attacks may occur in isolation
Cataplexy	Loss of muscle tone triggered by emotional stimuli (fright, laughter, anger)	Alone or with narcolepsy

1 Transient ischemic attack.

Table 27 Diagnostic criteria for multiple sclerosis (pp. 216, 218)

Manifestations	Additional Information Needed for Diagnosis
Two or more episodes; objective evidence[1] of 2 or more lesions	None
Two or more episodes; objective evidence of 1 lesion	Disseminated lesions (MRI[2]) or two or more MS-typical lesions (MRI and positive CSF tests[3]) or relapse[4]
One episode; objective evidence of 2 or more lesions	Dissemination of lesions over time (MRI[5]) or relapse
One episode; objective evidence of 1 lesion (monosymptomatic syndrome)	Disseminated lesions (MRI[2]) or two or more MS-typical lesions (MRI + positive CSF findings[3]) + dissemination of lesions over time (MRI[5]) or relapse
Gradual worsening of neurological manifestations suggestive of MS	Positive CSF findings[3] + disseminated lesions[6] or pathological VEP + 4–8 cerebral lesions[7] + dissemination of lesions over time (MRI[5]) or continuous progression for 1 year

(McDonald et al., 2001)

1 MRI, CSF, visual evoked potentials (VEP). **2** For special criteria, see McDonald et al., 2001. **3** Oligoclonal immunoglobulin, elevated IgG index. **4** Topographic-anatomic classification differs from that of previous episodes. **5** Follow-up examination after an interval of at least 3 months; for special criteria, see McDonald et al., 2001. **6** Nine or more cerebral lesions or two or more spinal lesions or 4–8 cerebral lesions + 1 spinal lesion. **7** In patients with fewer than 4 cerebral lesions, at least 1 additional spinal lesion must be observed by MRI.

Table 28 Therapeutic guidelines for meningoencephalitis (p. 224)

Clinical Features	Additional Findings	Treatment[1]
Previously healthy patient	Gram-positive cocci in CSF	Vancomycin + cephalosporin
	Gram-negative cocci in CSF	Penicillin G
	Gram-positive bacilli in CSF	Ampicillin or penicillin G + aminoglycoside[3]
	Gram-negative bacilli in CSF	Cephalosporin[2] + aminoglycoside[3]
Previously healthy patient	Negative CSF Gram stain[5]	*Bacterial infection* suspected: cephalosporin[2]. Age > 50 years + ampicillin *Viral infection* suspected: influenza A, amantadine or rimantadine; herpes simplex (p. 236); cytomegalovirus (p. 244); poliovirus (p. 242); HIV (p. 241); varicella zoster (p. 239)
Septic focus (e. g., mastoiditis), neurosurgery, head trauma	Supportive evidence from imaging study, e. g., CT with bone windows	Vancomycin + cephalosporin[2]
Immune deficiency/immunosuppressant therapy[4]	(possible) Brain stem signs, Gram-negative bacilli in CSF	Ampicillin + ceftazidime
Nosocomial infection	(possible) Gram-negative bacilli in CSF	Cephalosporin[2] + e. g., oxacillin or fosfomycin + aminoglycoside[3]
Focal neurological signs	Temporal lobe process demonstrated by EEG, CT and/or MRI	Acyclovir (p. 236)
Spinal and radicular pain	Spinal epidural abscess confirmed by imaging study (MRI, myelography, or CT)	Cephalosporin[2] + (e. g.) oxacillin or fosfomycin + aminoglycoside[3]. Surgery
Neonate (< 3 months of age)	Negative CSF Gram stain	Ampicillin + cephalosporin[2]

1 Drugs recommended by Quagliariello and Scheld (1997). **2** E.g., cefotaxime or ceftriaxone. **3** Gentamycin or tobramycin. **4** Predisposes to tubercular, fungal, and other opportunistic infections (pp. 233, 245 f). **5** Aseptic/viral meningitis, p. 234.

Appendix

Table 29 Bacteria commonly causing meningitis and meningoencephalitis (p. 226)

Pathogen	Portal of Entry/Focus	Clinical Features
Pneumococcus (S. pneumoniae/ Gram$^+$ extracellular diplococcus) ⇨ adults[1]	Nasal and pharyngeal mucosa, head trauma, neurosurgical procedures, external CSF drainage	Meningitis may be accompanied or preceded by sinusitis, otitis media or pneumonia. Posttraumatic meningitis may occur several years after trauma; recurrent meningitis (CSF leak? Immunodeficiency?). Course may be hyperacute (nonpurulent meningitis[2]), acute or subacute (days to weeks). Epileptic seizures. Risk of brain abscess, subdural empyema or cerebral vasculitis
Meningococcus (N. meningitidis[3]/Gram$^-$ intracellular diplococcus) ⇨ children and adolescents[4]	Nasopharynx	Hyperacute course with sepsis, adrenocortical insufficiency and consumption coagulopathy (Waterhouse–Friderichsen syndrome). Petechial or confluent cutaneous hemorrhages. Myocarditis/pericarditis
Haemophilus influenzae (Gram-bacillus) ⇨ children and adolescents	Nasal and pharyngeal mucosa	Usually type B. May be accompanied or preceded by sinusitis, otitis media, or pneumonia
Listeria (L. monocytogenes/ Gram$^+$/organism difficult to identify) ⇨ neonates[5], adults >50 years of age	Gastrointestinal tract (contaminated food, e. g., dairy products or salads)	Focal neurological deficits, particularly brain stem encephalitis (rhombencephalitis), are commonly seen. Predisposing factors: pregnancy, old age, alcoholism, immune suppression, primary malignancy. CSF findings are extremely variable ("mixed cell picture")
Staphylococcus (S. aureus/ Gram$^+$) ⇨ neonates and adults Enterobacter (Gram$^-$/bacilli) ⇨ neonates	Endocarditis, head trauma, external CSF drainage, lumbar puncture, urinary tract, spondylodiskitis	In association with sepsis, i. v. drug use, alcoholism, diabetes mellitus, primary malignancy
M. tuberculosis (acid-fast bacillus)	Extracerebral organ tuberculosis	See p. 232

Gram$^+$ = Gram-positive; Gram$^-$ = Gram-negative.
1 Age >18 years. **2** Very rapidly progressive meningitis, low cell count and high total protein and lactate levels in CSF, and CSF smear culture containing large quantities of bacteria. **3** Group A, Central Africa, South America; Group B, Europe; Group C, North America; type may change. **4** Age 3 months to 18 years. **5** Age ≤3 months.

Table 30 Viruses causing CNS infection (p. 234)

Common	Occasional	Rare
Meningitis		
Enteroviruses[1,3], arboviruses[2,3], HIV[5], HSV type 2[4]	HSV type 1[4], LCMV[3], mumps virus[3]	Adenoviruses[4], CMV[4], Epstein–Barr virus (EBV)[4], influenza virus A+B[3], measles virus[3], parainfluenza virus[3], rubella virus[3], varicella-zoster virus (VZV)[4]
Encephalitis, myelitis		
Arboviruses, enteroviruses, HSV type 1, mumps virus	CMV, EBV, HIV, measles virus[3], VZV	Adenoviruses, influenza A, LCMV, parainfluenza virus, rabies virus[3], rubella virus, HTLV-I[5,6]

1 Poliovirus 1–3, coxsackievirus (B5, A9, B3, B4, B1, B6), echovirus (7, 9, 11 30, 4, 6, 18, 2, 3, 12, 22), enterovirus (70, 71). **2** Arthropod-borne viruses, including alphaviruses, flaviviruses, pestiviruses, bunyaviruses, and orbiviruses. **3** RNA virus. **4** DNA virus. **5** Retrovirus. **6** Human T-cell lymphotropic virus type I causes myelitis.

Appendix

Table 31 Grades of malignancy of brain tumors (p. 264)

Tumor	Grade I (benign)	Grade II (semi-benign)	Grade III (malignant)	Grade IV (malignant)
Neuroepithelial tumors				
Astrocytoma				
• Fibrillary, protoplasmic, gemistocytic astrocytoma		+++	++	
• Anaplastic astrocytoma			+++	
• Glioblastoma (= glioblastoma multiforme)				+++
• Pilocytic astrocytoma	+++		+	
• Pleomorphic xanthoastrocytoma		+++	++	
Oligodendroglioma				
• Oligodendroglioma		+++		
• Anaplastic oligodendroglioma			+++	
Ependymoma				
• Ependymoma (cellular, papillary, epithelial)	++	+++	++	
• Anaplastic ependymoma			+++	
Mixed glioma				
• Oligoastrocytoma		+++		
• Anaplastic oligoastrocytoma			+++	
Choroid plexus tumors				
• Plexus papilloma	+++			
• Plexus carcinoma			+++	++
Neuronal/mixed neuronal-glial tumors				
• Gangliocytoma	+++			
• Ganglioglioma		+++		
• Anaplastic ganglioglioma			+++	
Pineal tumors				
• Pineocytoma	+++	++		
• Pineoblastoma (PNET)				+++
Embryonal tumors				
• Primitive neuroectodermal tumor (PNET), see p. 260				+++
• Neuroblastoma				+++
Cranial nerve tumors				
• Schwannoma	+++			
Meningeal tumors				
• Meningioma	+++			
• Anaplastic meningioma			+++	
Blood vessel tumors				
• Hemangiopericytoma		+++	++	
• Glomus tumor	+++			
Lymphoma				
• Primary CNS lymphoma			++	+++
Germ cell tumors				
• Germinoma			+++	
Intra- and suprasellar tumors				
• Pituitary adenoma	+++		+	
• Craniopharyngioma	+++			
Metastatic tumors				+++

(Kleihues et al., 1993 and Krauseneck, 1997)

+++, Common; ++, Rare; +, Very rare.

Table 32 Karnofsky performance scale for quantification of disability (p. 264)

General Condition	%	Comments
Patient can perform normal daily activities and work without impairment	100	Normal; no complaints; no evidence of disease
No specific treatment required	90	Able to carry on normal activity; minor impairment
	80	Normal activity with effort; some impairment is clearly evident
Patient cannot work; can meet most personal needs, but needs some degree of assistance; can be cared for at home	70	Cares for self; cannot perform normal activities or work
	60	Needs occasional assistance, but can meet most personal needs
	50	Needs considerable assistance and frequent medical care
Patient cannot care for self; needs to be cared for in a hospital, nursing home, or at home by a nurse/family members. Disease may progress rapidly	40	Disabled; requires special care and assistance; home nursing care still possible
	30	Severely disabled; hospitalization indicated although death not imminent
	20	Gravely ill; hospitalization necessary
	10	Moribund

Table 33 Glasgow coma scale (p. 266)

I Eye Opening	Score	II Best Verbal Response	Score	III Best Motor Response (arms)	Score
				Obeys commands	6
		Oriented	5	Selectively avoids painful stimuli	5
Spontaneous	4	Confused	4	Withdraws limb from painful stimuli	4
To speech	3	Single words	3	Flexes limb in response to painful stimuli	3
To pain	2	Meaningless utterances	2	Extends limb in response to painful stimuli	2
No response	1	No response	1	No response	1

(Teasdale, 1995)

The scores in columns I, II, and III are summed to yield the overall value.
GCS 13–15 = mild head trauma; GCS 9–12 = moderate head trauma; GCS 3–8 = severe head trauma.

Table 34 Criteria for assessment of head trauma (p. 266)

Severity (GCS)[1]	Risk of Secondary Injury[2]	Symptoms and Signs [3]
Mild (13–15)	Low	**Impairment of consciousness lasting < 1 hour** Asymptomatic (or, at most: headache, dizziness, bruises, and lacerations)
Moderate (9–12)	Moderate	**Impairment of consciousness at time of accident or thereafter, lasting between 1 and 24 hours** Increasingly severe headache Alcohol/drug intoxication No reliable description of accident. Multiple trauma, severe facial injuries, basilar skull fracture, suspicion of depressed skull fracture or open head injury. Posttraumatic ⇨ epileptic seizure, vomiting, amnesia Age < 2 years (except in minor accidents), possibility of child abuse
Severe (3–8)	High	**Impairment of consciousness lasting < 24 hours + brain stem syndrome** or **Impairment of consciousness lasting > 24 hours** or **Posttraumatic psychosis lasting > 24 hours** Impairment of consciousness not due to alcohol/substance abuse/medications, and not a postictal or metabolic phenomenon Focal neurological signs Depressed skull fracture, open head injury

(White and Likavec, 1992)

1 Glasgow Coma Scale. **2** Patients with one or more manifestations from the list at right belong to the corresponding risk group. **3** Criteria for assessment of severity are in **bold type**.

Table 35 Late complications of head trauma (p. 268)

Complications	Clinical Features	Remarks
Posttraumatic syndrome	Headache, nausea, vertigo, orthostatic hypotension, depressed mood, irritability, fatigue, insomnia, impaired concentration	Usually follows mild head trauma; may cause significant psychosocial impairment
Chronic subdural hematoma (SDH)	Headache, behavioral change, focal signs	Usually follows mild trauma (predisposing factors: old age, brain atrophy, alcoholism)
Subdural hygroma	Same as in chronic SDH	Symptoms may improve when the patient is lying down and worsen on standing
CSF leak	Drainage of CSF from the nose or ear; risk of recurrent meningitis, brain abscess	CSF rhinorrhea worsens on head flexion. CSF otorrhea indicates a laterobasal skull fracture
Hydrocephalus	Headache, behavioral change, urinary incontinence	Normal pressure hydrocephalus, venous sinus thrombosis
Epilepsy	Focal/generalized seizures	May arise years after head trauma
Encephalopathy	Behavioral changes	See p. 122 ff. Types include septic encephalopathy, punch-drunk encephalopathy (p. 302, Table 44)
Critical illness neuropathy and myopathy	Prolonged ventilator dependence, weakness	Associated with sepsis and multiple organ failure
Heterotopic ossification (myositis ossificans)	Restricted mobility of joints, pain	Due to muscle trauma
Complications of immobility	Bed sores, peripheral nerve lesion, joint malposition	Ensure proper positioning and frequent changes of position (especially of paralyzed limbs)

Appendix

Table 36   Spinal fractures (p. 272)

Fracture/Dislocation	Pathogenesis	Stability[1]
Cervical spine		
• Atlantoaxial dislocation	• Dislocation between C1 and C2	• Unstable
• Jefferson's fracture[2]	• Axial trauma	• Unstable
• Dens fracture	• Hyperflexion	• Unstable[3]
• Bilateral axis arch fracture[4]	• Hyperflexion and distraction	• Unstable
• Dislocation fracture of C3–7	• Hyperflexion	• Unstable
• Lateral compression fracture	• Flexion and axial compression	• Stable
Thoracic spine, lumbar spine		
• Compression fracture	Fall (back, buttocks, extended legs), direct trauma. These fractures may be pathological (osteoporosis, myeloma, metastasis)	• Stable
• Burst fracture		• Stable
• Dislocation fracture		• Unstable

(Ogilvy and Heros, 1993; Sartor 2001)

1 At the time of injury. **2** Fracture of the ring of C1 due to compression between the occiput and C2. **3** May be overlooked if the dens is not displaced; sometimes stable. **4** Hangman's fracture.

Table 37   Classification of traumatic transverse spinal cord syndrome (p. 274)

Loss of Function	Category	Features
Complete	A	No sensory or motor function, including in S4–5
Incomplete	B	No motor function. Sensory function intact below level of lesion, including in S4–5
Incomplete	C	There is motor function below level of lesion; most segment-indicating muscles have strength <3
Incomplete	D	There is motor function below level of lesion; most segment-indicating muscles have strength ≥ 3
None	E	Normal motor and sensory function

(American Spinal Cord Injury Association Impairment Scale; Ditunno et al., 1994)

Table 38   Treatment of spinal trauma (p. 274)

Result of Trauma	Treatment Measures
Neck sprain/whiplash injury	Analgesics, application of heat/cold, immobilization (as brief as possible). Early initiation of active exercise therapy. Measures to prevent chronification
Fracture	Stable ⇨ conservative (extension/fixation). Unstable ⇨ surgery
Arterial dissection	Anticoagulation
Spinal cord trauma	Methylprednisolone (i. v.) within 8 hours of trauma (bolus of 30 mg/kg over 15 min, then 5.4 mg/kg/h for 23 hours). Monitor respiratory and cardiovascular function, bladder/bowel function; thrombosis prophylaxis, pain therapy, careful patient positioning and pressure sore prevention. Transfer to specialized center for rehabilitation of paraplegic patients (as indicated)

Table 39 Clinical manifestations of spinal cord lesions (p. 282)

Features	Site of Lesion	Clinical Manifestations
Spinal cord transection (p. 48)	• Cervical spinal cord • Thoracic spinal cord • Lumbar/sacral spinal cord	• Quadriplegia • Paraplegia • Paraplegia/conus syndrome with paralysis of bladder/rectum and saddle anesthesia
Lesion affecting a portion of the spinal cord (pp. 32, 50)	• Anterior root • Posterior root • Incomplete transverse cord syndrome • Complete transverse cord syndrome	• Flaccid paralysis, muscle atrophy, hyporeflexia (⇨ segment-indicating muscles, see Table 2, p. 357) • Localized/radicular/referred pain, sensory deficit in corresponding dermatome • Brown–Séquard syndrome, posterior column syndrome, anterior horn syndrome, posterior horn syndrome, central cord syndrome, anterior spinal syndrome • See p. 48
Temporal course	• Acute • Chronic	• Spinal shock • Spasticity, sensory and autonomic dysfunction

Table 40 Malformations and developmental anomalies (p. 288)

Feature	Syndrome[1]	Comments[2]
Macrocephaly (abnormally large head)	Hydrocephalus (p. 290), hydranencephaly, megalencephaly (massively enlarged brain)	4th week/ 2nd to 4th month
Craniostenosis (premature ossification of cranial sutures, p. 4)	Turricephaly (⇨ lambdoid and coronal suture; oxycephaly), scaphocephaly (⇨ sagittal suture; dolichocephaly, "long head"), brachycephaly (⇨ coronal suture; "short head")	Before 4th year of life
Migration disorder (defective migration of neuroblasts into cortex)	Schizencephaly (presence of cysts or cavities in the brain), agyria (lissencephaly[3], few or no convolutions), pachygyria (broad, plump convolutions), heterotopia/dystopia (ectopic gray matter)	2nd to 5th month
Microcephaly (abnormally small head)	Micrencephaly (abnormally small brain)	5th week (primary), peri- or postnatal (secondary)
Dysraphism (neural tube defect)	See p. 292	3rd to 4th week/ 4th to 7th week
Chromosomal anomaly	Down syndrome (trisomy 21, mongolism), Patau syndrome (trisomy 13), Edwards syndrome (trisomy 18), cri-du-chat syndrome (deletion, short arm of chromosome 5), Klinefelter syndrome (XXY), Turner syndrome (XO), fragile-X syndrome	Genome mutation
Phakomatosis	See p. 294	
Prenatal or perinatal infection	Rubella, cytomegalovirus, congenital neurosyphilis, HIV/AIDS, toxoplasmosis	
Mental retardation	A component of many syndromes (e. g., microcephaly, hydrocephalus, Down syndrome, perinatal or prenatal infection)	
Cerebral lesion	Ulegyria (postanoxic corticomedullary scarring), porencephaly (p. 290), hemiatrophy, infantile cerebral palsy (p. 288 f)	Prenatal, perinatal or postnatal

Appendix

1 (Selected). **2** The times specified refer to the gestational and neonatal ages, respectively. **3** There are two forms of lissencephaly: type 1, Miller–Dicker syndrome (craniofacial deformity), and type 2 (pronounced heterotopia with Fukuyama muscular dystrophy).

Table 41   Age-related changes (p. 296)

Change	Sequelae	Elevated risk[1] of
↓ Accommodation	Presbyopia	
Miosis	↓ Light/convergence reaction	
Cataract	Glare, ↓ visual acuity	Blindness
↓ Hearing (inner ear)	Presbycusis	Deafness
↓ Sense of smell/taste	Impaired sense of smell/taste	
↑ Body fat	↑ volume of distribution for fat-soluble drugs[2]	Obesity
↓ Total body water, ↓ Thirst	↓ volume of distribution for water-soluble drugs[2]	Dehydration, hydropenia
Arteries	Atherosclerosis, impairment of cerebral autoregulation and blood-brain barrier, decrease in cerebral blood flow, reduced tolerance of brain tissue to ischemia and metabolic changes	Stroke[3], leukoaraiosis[4], subcortical arteriosclerotic encephalopathy (p. 172), cerebral amyloid angiopathy[5], atrial fibrillation, myocardial infarction
Motor function	↓ Mobility, ↓ reactivity, ↓ coordination, ↓ fine motor control, muscle atrophy (especially thenar, dorsal interosseous, and anterior tibial muscles), ↓ muscle force, ↑ leg muscle tone, hypokinesis of arms, gait impairment (p. 60)	Falls (p. 204), osteoporosis, fear of falling/inactivity (avoidance of social contact, isolation)
Reflexes	↓ Reflex movements (p. 42), palmomental reflex, snout reflex, grasp reflex	Falls
Sensation	Pallhypesthesia in toe/knuckle region, ↓ position sense	Polyneuropathy, ataxia, falls
Brain atrophy	Senile forgetfulness[6] (impairment of episodic memory, p. 134)	Alzheimer disease, leukoaraiosis[4]
↓ Cerebral dopamine synthesis	Stooped posture	Parkinsonism
↓ Cerebral norepinephrine		Depression
↓ Non-REM stage 4 (p. 112)	Early awakening, insomnia	Sleep apnea syndrome

(Resnick, 1998)

1 Risk of developing condition in old age. **2** Increased risk of drug side effects. **3** Especially due to border zone infarction, subdural hematoma (after relatively minor trauma). **4** Rarefaction of white matter seen as bilateral, usually symmetrical hypodensity on CT and as hyperintensity on T2-weighted MRI (FLAIR = fluid-attenuated inversion recovery sequence). **5** Increased risk of spontaneous intracranial hemorrhage (p. 176). **6** Benign senescent forgetfulness, age-associated memory impairment (AAMI).

Appendix

Table 42 Criteria for differentiation between dementia and depression (p. 297)

Dementia	Depression
Patients seem indifferent to memory impairment; semantic paraphasia	Patients describe memory impairment precisely and in detail
Tests reveal cognitive deficit	Tests reveal minimal or no cognitive deficit
Depressive manifestations develop slowly (secondary)	Depressive manifestations prominent on presentation (brooding, anxiety, early awakening, loss of appetite, self-doubt)
Rare past history of depression	Frequent past history of depression

Table 43 Criteria for differentiation between different types of hyperkinesia (p. 300)

Syndrome	Features
Chorea (p. 66)	Overshooting, spontaneous, abrupt, alternating, irregular movements. Prominence varies from restlessness with little gesticulation, fidgety hand movements and hesitant, dance-like gait impairment to continuous, flowing, violent, disabling hyperkinesias
Dystonia (p. 64)	Involuntary, continuous and stereotyped muscle contractions that lead to rotating movements and abnormal posture
Athetosis (p. 66)	Localized peripheral dystonic movements
Ballismus (p. 66)	Violent, mainly proximal flinging movements of the limbs
Tics (p. 68)	Repetitive, stereotyped, localized twitches that can be voluntarily suppressed, but with a build-up of inner tension
Myoclonus (p. 68)	Brief, sudden, shocklike muscle twitches occurring repetitively in the same muscle group(s)

(Harper, 1996)

Table 44 Symptomatic forms of parkinsonism (p. 302)

Cause	Examples
Infectious disease	Encephalitis lethargica[1] (von Economo postencephalitic parkinsonism), measles, tick-borne encephalitis, poliomyelitis, cytomegalovirus, influenza A, herpes simplex
Intoxication	MPTP[2], manganese (miners, industrial workers), carbon monoxide, methanol
Drugs[3]	Neuroleptics (phenothiazines[4], butyrophenones[5], thioxanthenes[6], benzamide[7]), reserpine, calcium channel blockers (cinnarizine, flunarizine)
Other diseases[8]	Multiple brain infarcts/subcortical arteriosclerotic encephalopathy[9], punch-drunk encephalopathy (dementia pugilistica), normal pressure hydrocephalus (p. 160), brain tumor (frontal), subdural hematoma, calcification of basal ganglia[10], neuroleptic malignant syndrome[11]

1 In the aftermath of the influenza pandemic that followed the First World War (now only of historical interest). **2** 1-Methyl-4-phenyl-1,2,3,6-tetrahydropyridine. MPTP is converted into MPP$^+$, which accumulates in dopaminergic neurons and interferes with electron transfer in the mitochondrial respiratory chain, leading to an accumulation of free radicals and neuronal death. An outbreak of MPTP-induced parkinsonism occurred in California in the early 1980s, when this substance appeared as a contaminant of opiate drugs synthesized in clandestine laboratories for illegal use. **3** Parkinsonoid. **4** Fluphenazine, levomepromazine, perazine, perphenazine, promazine, triflupromazine, etc. **5** Benperidol, fluspirilene (diphenylbutylpiperidine), haloperidol, etc. **6** Chlorprothixene, clopenthixol, fluanxol. **7** Metoclopramide. **8** Includes the terms pseudoparkinsonism, hypokinetic-rigid syndrome, and hypertonic-hyperkinetic syndrome. **9** Lower-body parkinsonism. **10** Autosomal recessive (Fahr disease), associated with hypoparathyroidism and pseudohypoparathyroidism. **11** Parkinsonian hyperthermia syndrome: rigidity, hyperthermia, impairment of consciousness; induced by neuroleptic drugs or by the use or withdrawal of levodopa or other dopaminergic agonists.

Appendix

Table 45 Diseases affecting the first (upper) motor neuron (p. 304)

Syndrome	Features
Hereditary	
Familial spastic paraplegia (SPG, p. 286)	*Uncomplicated SPG*[1,2]: SPG2[6] (X/Xq22/PLP = proteolipid protein), SPG3A (AD/14q11.2–24.3/atlastin), SPG4[6] (AD/2p22-p21/spastin), SPG5A (AR/8p12-q13/?), SPG6 (AD/15q11.1/?), SPG7[6] (AR/16q24.3/paraplegin), SPG8/AD/8q23–24/?), SPG10 (AD/12q13/?), SPG11 (AR/15q13–15/?), SPG12 (AD/19q13/?), SPG13 (AD/2q24–34/?) *Complicated SPG*[3]: SPG1[6] (X/Xq28/L1-CAM = L1 cell adhesion molecule), SPG2[6] (X/Xq22/PLP), SPG7[6] (AR/16q24.3/paraplegin), SPG9 (AD/10q23.3–24.1/?), SPG14 (AR/3q27–28/?), SPG16 (X/Xq11.2/?)
Adrenomyeloneuropathy[4]	X-linked recessive, onset usually after age 20. Progressive spastic paraparesis, polyneuropathy, urinary incontinence, sometimes hypocortisolism. A similar syndrome develops in 20% of all female heterozygotes (carriers)
Spinocerebellar ataxia type 3	See p. 280
Acquired	
Primary lateral sclerosis	Onset usually after age 50. Slowly progressive symmetrical paraspasticity without marked weakness, dysarthria. More common in men than in women
Lathyrism (p. 304)	Onset usually before age 50. Subacute or chronic development of gait disturbances (tip-toe/scissors gait, dorsal tilting of trunk), leg cramps, paresthesiae, urinary retention
Tropical spastic paraparesis (TSP)[5]	Onset: Slow up to age 60. Back pain, dysesthesiae, spastic paraparesis, urinary retention, impotence

1 Abbreviations: AD = autosomal dominant, AR = autosomal recessive, X = X-chromosome/gene locus/gene product (? = unknown). **2** Isolated progressive spastic paraparesis. **3** As in uncomplicated SPG with additional manifestations including cerebellar ataxia, dystonia, optic neuropathy, tapetoretinal degeneration, muscle atrophy, dysarthria, deafness, sensory neuropathy, ichthyosis, dementia. **4** Impaired β-oxidation of very long chain fatty acids (VLCFA; C_{24-26}) due to defective peroxisomal transport ⇨ accumulation of VLFCA in nervous system, adrenal cortex, plasma. **5** HTLV-I-associated myelopathy (= HAM, human T-cell/lymphotropic virus type I); Jamaica, Japan, Caribbean. **6** Molecular genetic tests are available.

Appendix

Table 46 Diseases affecting the second (lower) motor neuron (p. 304)

Syndrome[1]	Features
Hereditary	
Proximal[2] (SMA)[3]	SMA I[4]: onset < 3 months. AR. Flaccid quadriparesis[5]. Triangular mouth shape, paradoxical respiratory movements, impaired sucking ability, unable to sit SMA II: onset < 5 years. AR. The children learn to sit independently, but never to stand/walk. Scoliosis, joint contractures SMA III[6]; SMA IIIa: onset 3 years. AR. Delayed motor development. Children learn to stand/walk SMA IIIb: onset 3–30 years. AR. Development normal. Calf (pseudo)hypertrophy. Absence of bulbar muscle involvement. CK[7] sometimes elevated SMA IV: onset > 30 years. AR
Nonproximal[8] SMA	Distal SMA[9]: forms with different ages of onset (infantile, juvenile, adult). Usually slow course, sometimes stabilizing after a few years, sometimes progressive. May be accompanied by myoclonus, deafness, dysphonia, dysarthria, and/or ataxia. Scapuloperoneal muscular atrophy[10]: Onset: Adolescence or adulthood. Weakness ⇨ foot dorsiflexors, shoulder girdle, arm Progressive bulbar palsy[11]: Onset in adulthood[12]. Progressive weakness of bulbar muscles. Muscular atrophy and respiratory muscle involvement develop as the disease progresses
Spinobulbar muscular atrophy (Kennedy type)	Onset: 20–70 years. Gynecomastia, gradual progression of muscular atrophy (legs > arms, proximal > distal, asymmetrical; dysarthria, dysphagia, tongue atrophy). Slight elevation of CK. Gene locus Xq12
Acquired	
Acute viral infection	Poliomyelitis (p. 242), other enteroviruses (e. g., echovirus, coxsackievirus, enterovirus type 70/71 ⇨ acute hemorrhagic conjunctivitis), mumps virus
Postpolio syndrome	See p. 242
Lymphoma	Accompanies Hodgkin and non-Hodgkin lymphomas. Elevation of CSF protein, oligoclonal IgG in CSF
Radiation-induced	Develops months to years after irradiation of para-aortic lymph nodes (testicular tumors, uterine carcinoma). May progress rapidly

(Tandan, 1996; Rudnik-Schöneborn, Mortier and Zerres, 1998)

AR = autosomal recessive, AD = autosomal dominant; XR = X-linked recessive.
1 Selected syndromes. **2** Proximal muscle involvement. **3** SMA = spinal muscular atrophy; gene locus for SMA I to III: 5q12.2–q13.3. **4** AR; infantile SMA, Werdnig–Hoffmann disease. **5** Floppy baby syndrome, froglike posture in supine position; lack of head control. **6** AR > AD; juvenile SMA; Kugelberg–Welander disease. **7** Creatine kinase (CK). **8** Distal or localized (monomelic segmental SMA) muscle groups, symmetrical or asymmetrical involvement. **9** AR > AD. **10** AD ⇨ Onset age 30–50 years, slowly progressive; AR ⇨ onset < 5 years; may progress slowly. **11** AD/AR. **12** Fazio–Londe type with onset at age 2–13 years, rapidly progressive

Appendix

Table 47 Diseases affecting both the first (upper) and the second (lower) motor neurons (p. 304)

Diagnostic Categories[1]	
Definite ALS[2]	Evidence of first + second motor neuron lesion in 3 regions of the body[3]
Probable ALS	Evidence of first + second motor neuron lesion in 2 regions of the body
Possible ALS	Evidence of first + second motor neuron lesion in 1 region of the body or evidence of first motor neuron lesion in 2 to 3 regions of the body
Suspected ALS	Evidence of second motor neuron lesion in 2 to 3 regions of the body
Diagnostic features	Progressive symptoms of a first (p. 46) and second motor neuron lesion (p. 50). Fasciculation in more than one region of the body. Neurogenic EMG findings, normal nerve conduction velocity/absence of motor conduction block. Absence of sensory deficits, sphincter dysfunction, visual disturbances, autonomic dysfunction, parkinsonism, and Alzheimer, Pick or Huntington disease
Syndromes with manifestations similar to those of ALS	Cervical radicular syndromes, cervical myelopathy, monoclonal gammopathy. Multifocal motor neuropathy (GM_1 antibodies). Lymphoma; paraneoplastic syndrome; hyperthyroidism, hyperparathyroidism; diabetic amyotrophy; postpolio syndrome; hexosamidinase A deficiency. Radiation-induced lesion. Toxicity (lead, mercury, manganese). Myopathy (inclusion body myositis, polymyositis, muscular dystrophy). Spinal muscular atrophy. Creutzfeldt–Jakob disease

1 According to Leigh and Ray-Chaudhuri (1994). **2** ALS = amyotrophic lateral sclerosis. **3** Brain stem, proximal/distal arm, chest, proximal/distal leg.

Table 48 Neonatal metabolic encephalopathies (from birth to 28 days, p. 306)

Syndrome	Defect/Enzyme Defect	Symptoms and Signs
Galactosemia	Galactose-1-phosphate uridyltransferase[1]	Milk intolerance, apathy, jaundice, anemia, cataract, psychomotor retardation
Nonketotic hyperglycinemia	Defective conversion of glycine to serine	Hypotonia, dyspnea, myoclonus, generalized seizures
Hyperammonemia	Urea cycle[2]	Crisislike episodes of vomiting, sucking weakness, somnolence, coma, seizures, hyperpnea, hyperpyrexia
Maple syrup urine disease	Defective breakdown of branched-chain amino acids	Hypotonia, seizures, coma, ketoacidosis
Zellweger syndrome	Peroxisomes[3]	Hypotonia, sucking weakness, nystagmus, seizures, craniofacial dysmorphism

1 Multiple types ⇨ high galactose-1-phosphate levels. **2** Defects of all six enzymes of the urea cycle are known. Adult onset is rare. Hyperammonemia in defects of carbamoyl-phosphate synthetase, ornithine carbamoyltransferase, argininosuccinic acid synthetase (citrullinemia), argininosuccinase. Arginase defect leads to argininemia. **3** Cytoplasmic organelles that mediate fatty acid oxidation, biliary acid and cholesterol synthesis, pipecolic and phytanic acid metabolism, and plasmalogen (myelin) synthesis. Other peroxisomal syndromes: neonatal adrenoleukodystrophy, infantile Refsum disease, hyperpipecolatemia.

Appendix

Table 49 Metabolic encephalopathies of infancy (first year of life, p. 306)

Syndrome	Defect/Enzyme Defect	Symptoms and Signs
Tay–Sachs disease[1]	Hexosaminidase A ($\Rightarrow$ accumulation of ganglioside GM_2)	Abnormal acoustic startle reaction, delayed development. Begins with muscular hypotonia, followed by spasticity, seizures, blindness, dementia, and optic nerve atrophy[2]
Gaucher disease[3] (type II, acute neuropathic)	Glucocerebrosidase ($\Rightarrow$ lipid storage)	Loss of motor control, apathy, dysphagia, retroflexion of the head, strabismus, splenomegaly
Niemann–Pick disease[4] (type A)	Sphingomyelinase deficiency (sphingomyelin storage $\Rightarrow$ Niemann–Pick cells)	Enlargement of spleen, liver and lymph nodes; pulmonary infiltrates, spasticity, muscular axial hypotonia, blindness, nystagmus, macular cherry red spot
GM_1 gangliosidosis	β-Galactosidase	Craniofacial dysmorphism. Initial flaccid paralysis that later becomes spastic; loss of visual acuity, nystagmus, strabismus, hepatomegaly
Krabbe disease (globoid cell leukodystrophy)	β-Galactocerebrosidase (galactocerebroside ?)	General muscular hypertonia, vomiting, opisthotonus, spasticity, blindness, deafness
Pelizaeus–Merzbacher disease[5]	Proteolipid protein synthesis	Nystagmus, ataxia, psychomotor retardation, choreoathetosis

1 GM_2 gangliosidosis. **2** Cherry red spot in optic fundus is found in over 90 % of cases. **3** Glucocerebrosidase; three known subtypes $\Rightarrow$ type 1: nonneuropathic (juvenile) form with hematological changes and bone fractures; type 3: see p. 307. **4** Different types (A, B, C) exist. Type B does not produce neurological symptoms. **5** Other sudanophil (orthochromatic) forms of leukodystrophy are known.

Table 50 Stages of hepatic/portosystemic encephalopathy (p. 308)

Stage	Behavior[1]	Motor function	EEG[2]
I	Attention deficit, impaired concentration, euphoria or depression, dysarthria, insomnia	Handwriting illegible, asterixis +/–	Usually normal to θ waves
II	Sleepy, marked behavioral changes (confusion, disorientation, apraxia)	Asterixis	Pathological (δ waves)
III	Severely confused, somnolent to soporific	Asterixis	Pathological (δ/triphasic waves)
IV	Coma	Presence (stage IVa) or absence (stage IVb) of motor responses to pain	Pathological (triphasic/arrhythmic δ/sub-δ waves)

(Adams and Foley, 1952)

1 Earlier stages are assessed with psychometric methods, e. g., number connection test (time required for patient to connect 25 numbered circles in numerical order), ability to draw a five-pointed star. **2** Nonspecific changes; actual findings may differ.

Table 51 Paraneoplastic syndromes of the CNS (p. 312)

Site	Syndrome ⇒ Time course	Symptoms and Signs	Common Tumors	Lesions/Antibodies
Cerebrum	Photoreceptor/retinal degeneration ⇒ weeks to months	Progressive blindness without pain	Small-cell lung cancer	Loss of photoreceptors/anti-CAR[1]
	Limbic encephalitis ⇒ weeks to months	Restlessness, confusion, memory impairment	Small-cell lung cancer	Neuronal loss, perivascular and meningeal lymphocytic infiltrates ⇒ medial temporal lobe, limbic system/ANNA-1[2]
Cerebellum, brain stem	Brain stem encephalitis ⇒ days to weeks	Dysphagia, dysarthria, nystagmus, diplopia, ataxia, dizziness	Small-cell lung cancer	Neuronal loss, inflammatory infiltrates in the brain stem
	Subacute cerebellar degeneration ⇒ weeks to months	Cerebellar ataxia, dysarthria, nystagmus, diplopia, vertigo	Small-cell lung cancer, carcinoma of ovary/breast, Hodgkin disease	Death of Purkinje cells/APCA[3]
	Opsoclonus-myoclonus ⇒ weeks	Abrupt, irregular eye and muscle movements, cerebellar ataxia, encephalopathy	Neuroblastoma (children); breast cancer/lung cancer (adults)	Neuronal loss in dentate nucleus (adults)/ANNA-2[4]
Spinal cord	Necrotizing myelopathy ⇒ hours, days to weeks	Flaccid para-/ quadriparesis, bladder/bowel dysfunction, segmental sensory loss	Small-cell lung cancer, lymphoma	Necrosis of white and gray matter of spinal cord
	Stiff man syndrome[5] ⇒ days to weeks	Painful muscular rigidity initially triggered by emotional, acoustic and/or tactile stimuli; autonomic dysfunction	Small-cell lung cancer, Hodgkin lymphoma, breast cancer, pharyngeal carcinoma	Transitory high-cervical lesions may be seen in MRI scans/ anti-GAD[6]

(Brown, 1998)

1 CAR = cancer-associated retinopathy. **2** ANNA-1 = antineural nuclear antibody type 1 = anti-Hu. **3** APCA = anti-Purkinje cell cytoplasmic antibody = anti-Yo. **4** ANNA-2 = antineural nuclear antibody type 2 = anti-Ri. **5** Manifestations variable (e. g., axial or distal muscle may be more prominent); attributed to diminished supraspinal inhibition of motor neurons, leading to continuous contraction of agonists and antagonists. **6** Anti-GAD = glutamic acid decarboxylase antibodies; antibodies directed against amphiphysin (terminal synaptic protein) have also been found.

Table 52   Iatrogenic encephalopathies (p. 314)

Substance	Adverse Effects[1]
Neuroleptics	Drug-induced parkinsonism (p. 383, Table 44), early/late dyskinesia (p. 66), akathisia[2], low seizure threshold
Antidepressants	Somnolence, increased drive, confusion, akathisia, low seizure threshold, tremor, serotonin syndrome[3]
Aspirin[4]	Tinnitus, dizziness
Baclofen	Fatigue, depression, headaches, low seizure threshold
Levodopa, dopamine agonists	Confusion, hallucinations, psychosis, insomnia, hyperkinesia
Corticosteroids, ACTH	Depression, increased drive, mania, insomnia, headaches, dizziness, sweating, low seizure threshold, tremor
Antibiotics	*Aminoglycosides*: Tinnitus, hearing impairment. *Quinolone derivatives*: Insomnia, hallucinations, headaches, low seizure threshold, dizziness, somnolence, tinnitus. *Tetracyclines*: Pseudotumor cerebri (children), abducens paralysis (adults)
Glycosides	Visual disturbances, somnolence, hallucinations, seizures, delirium
Calcium antagonists	Fatigue, insomnia, headaches, depression. *Flunarizine/cinnarizine*: Drug-induced parkinsonism
Coumarins	Intracranial hemorrhage (2–12 %/year)
Radiotherapy[5]	*Acute* (< 1 week): Headaches, nausea, somnolence, fever. *Subacute*: (2–16 weeks): Somnolence, focal neurological deficits, leukoencephalopathy, brain stem syndrome (rare). *Late* (> 4 months): radiation necrosis[6], leukoencephalopathy, dementia, secondary tumor
Chemotherapy[7]	*Acute*: Insomnia, confusion, restlessness, stupor, generalized seizures, myoclonus. *Late*: Apathy, dementia, insomnia, incontinence, gait impairment, ataxia

(Biller, 1998; Diener and Kastrup, 1998; Keime-Guibert et al., 1998)

1 Common adverse effects. **2** Inability to sit still with tormenting sensations in the legs that improve briefly when the patient moves about. **3** Characterized by confusion, fever, restlessness, myoclonus, diaphoresis, tremor, diarrhea, and ataxia; usually due to drug interactions, e. g., fluoxetine + sertraline, serotonin reuptake inhibitor + tryptophan, MAO inhibitors, carbamazepine, lithium, or clomipramine. **4** Acetylsalicylic acid (ASA). **5** Syndromes also occur in combination with chemotherapy. **6** One to two years after percutaneous radiotherapy, ca. 6 months after interstitial radiotherapy. Focal neurological deficits. **7** Methotrexate (high-dose i. v., intrathecal) cisplatin, vincristine, asparaginase, procarbazine, 5-fluorouracil, cytosine arabinoside, nitrosourea compounds (high-dose), ifosfamide, tamoxifen, etoposide (high-dose).

Appendix

Table 53 Neuropathy syndromes (p. 316)

Syndrome	Causes
Predominantly symmetrical motor deficits	Amyotrophic lateral sclerosis (ALS), multifocal motor neuropathy, Guillain–Barré syndrome, CIDP[1], acute porphyria, hereditary sensorimotor neuropathy
Predominantly asymmetrical or focal motor deficits	*Neuronopathy*: ALS, poliomyelitis, spinal muscular atrophy *Radicular lesion*: Root compression (herniated intervertebral disk, tumor), herpes zoster, carcinomatous meningitis, diabetes mellitus *Plexus lesion*: Neuralgic amyotrophy of shoulder, tumor infiltration, diabetes mellitus, tomaculous neuropathy, compression (positional) *Multiple mononeuropathy*: Vasculitis, diabetes mellitus, multifocal motor neuropathy, neuroborreliosis, sarcoidosis, HIV, tomaculous neuropathy, leprosy, neurofibromatosis, cryoglobulinemia, HNPP (p. 332), neoplastic infiltration *Mononeuropathy*: Compartment syndrome (median n., ulnar n.), compression (anterior interosseous n., peroneal n.), lead poisoning, diabetes mellitus
Predominantly autonomic disturbances	Diabetes mellitus, amyloidosis, Guillain–Barré syndrome, vincristine, porphyria, HIV, idiopathic pandysautonomia, botulism, paraneoplastic neuropathy
Predominant pain	Diabetes mellitus, vasculitis, Guillain–Barré syndrome, uremia, amyloidosis, arsenic, thallium, HIV, Fabry disease, cryptogenic neuropathy
Predominantly sensory disturbances	Diabetes mellitus, alcohol, ethambutol, vitamin B_{12} deficiency, folic acid deficiency, overdosage of vitamin B_6, paraneoplastic, metronidazole, phenytoin, thalidomide, leprosy, cytostatic agents (e. g., vincristine, vinblastine, vindesine, cisplatin, paclitaxel), amyloidosis (dissociated sensory loss), hereditary sensory neuropathy, monoclonal gammopathy, tabes dorsalis, Friedreich ataxia (p. 280)
Ganglioneuropathy[2] (ataxia)	Paraneoplastic, Sjögren syndrome, cisplatin, vitamin B_6 intoxication, HIV, idiopathic sensory neuronopathy

(Barohn, 1998)

1 Chronic inflammatory demyelinating polyneuropathy. **2** Asymmetrical proprioceptive loss without paralysis.

Table 54 Acquired and hereditary neuropathies (p. 316)

Cause	Examples
Acquired	
• Metabolic disorder	• Diabetes mellitus, uremia, hypothyroidism, acromegaly
• Dietary deficiency	• Vitamin deficiency (B_1 = beriberi, B_6, B_{12}, E), malabsorption
• Immune-mediated	• Guillain–Barré syndrome, Fisher syndrome, chronic inflammatory demyelinating polyneuropathy (CIDP), multifocal motor neuropathy, pandysautonomia, neuralgic amyotrophy of shoulder[1], vasculitis, connective tissue disease, plasmocytoma, benign monoclonal gammopathy, Churg–Strauss syndrome, cryoglobulinemia, rheumatoid arthritis
• Infection	• Herpes zoster, leprosy, Lyme disease, HIV, neurosyphilis, diphtheria, typhus, paratyphus
• Drugs	• Carbimazole, cisplatin, cytarabine, enalapril, ethambutol, etoposide, gentamicin, gold, imipramine, indomethacin, INH, paclitaxel, phenytoin, procarbazine, suramine, thalidomide, vinca alkaloids, vitamin B_6
• Toxins (environmental, industrial)[2], drugs[2]	• Alcohol, arsenic, benzene, lead, heroin, hexachlorophene, pentachlorophenol, polychlorinated biphenyls, mercury, carbon tetrachloride, thallium, triarylophosphate
• Neoplasm	• *Paraneoplastic*: Lung, stomach, or breast cancer; Hodgkin disease, leukemia. *Infiltration*: Hodgkin disease, leukemia, carcinomatous meningitis, polycythemia
• Mechanical	• Compression, trauma, distortion
• Unknown	• Critical illness polyneuropathy
Hereditary	See pp. 332 and 396 f

(Barohn, 1998)

1 Causes not confirmed. **2** A large number of substances can lead to polyneuropathy (PNP). Only some of them are listed.

Table 55 Additional diagnostic studies for neuropathies (p. 316)

Method	Information/Parameters
Neurography	*Motor neuron lesion*: Normal (consider conduction block) *Ganglionopathy*: MSAP[1] normal to⇩ , SNAP[2] normal to⇩ , (dermatomal) SEP[3]⇩ *Radiculopathy*: H reflex: Lateral inequality/absence[4]; F waves: some prolonged; (dermatomal) SEP ⇩ *Axonal lesion*: Motor NCV[5]: Normal; MSAP⇩ , SNAP⇩ *Demyelination*: DML[6] ⇧ NCV:⇩ or local conduction block (localize by inching); MSAP⇩ /dispersed; F waves: Prolongation or absence; SNAP: normal/dispersed in motor neuropathy, ⇩ in sensory neuropathy
Needle electro-myography	*Motor neuron lesion*: Fibrillation, positive waves, fasciculation. Amplitude, poly-phasia rate, MAP[7] duration ⇧ *Ganglionopathy*: MAP: Low-grade neurogenic changes may be observed *Radiculopathy*: Pathological spontaneous activity in paravertebral muscles/seg-ment-indicating muscles (p. 357); MAP[8]: neurogenic changes *Axonal lesion*: Pathological spontaneous activity (fibrillation, fasciculation); MAP: neurogenic changes *Demyelination*: Absence of pathological spontaneous activity, maximum innerva-tion with thinning pattern
Laboratory tests[9]	*Standard tests*: Erythrocyte sedimentation rate, differential blood count, blood glucose (diurnal profile), C-reactive protein, calcium, sodium potassium, alkaline phosphatase, SGOT[10], SGPT[11], CK[12], γ-GT[13], electrophoresis, rheumatoid factors, vitamin B_{12}/ folic acid, *Borrelia*/HIV antibodies, basal TSH[14], triglycerides, cholesterol, urine status, blood culture *Special tests*: CSF, homocysteine, hemoglobin A_{1c}, syphilis serology, parathyroid hormone, antinuclear antibodies (e. g., Sm, RNP, Ro SS-A, La SS-B, Scl-70, Jo-1, Pm-Scl), antineuronal antibodies (ANNA-1, anti-Hu), myelin-associated glyco-protein (MAG), ganglioside antibodies (GM_1, GD_{1a}, GD_{1b}, GQ_{1b}), heavy metals (blood, urine), porphyrins, cryoglobulins, serum phytanic acid, very long chain fatty acids (VLCFA, C_{24-26}), molecular genetic testing
Sural nerve biopsy[15]	Vasculitis, amyloid neuropathy, neuropathy with sarcoidosis, leprosy, chronic neu-ropathy (HMSN III/metachromatic leukodystrophy, with or without other forms of hereditary neuropathy ⇨ p. 332; chronic inflammatory neuropathy, polyglucosan body neuropathy), tumor (neurofibroma/schwannoma, neoplastic infiltration; par-aneoplastic neuropathy), neuropathy with monoclonal gammopathy, if applicable
Diagnostic imaging	Guided by clinical findings (spinal, radicular, plexus, distal peripheral lesions?), plain radiographs, ultrasound, CT, MRI, myelography, skeletal scintigraphy and/or angiography

⇧= elevated, prolonged; ⇩ = diminished, absent
1 Summated muscle action potential (evoked). **2** Amplitude of sensory nerve action potential. **3** Somatosensory evoked action potential amplitude reduced or absent. **4** For technical reasons, can only be determined for S1. **5** Nerve conduction velocity. **6** Distal motor latency. **7** Muscle action potential. **8** After 2 weeks, at earliest. **9** Par-tial list. **10** Serum glutamic–oxaloacetic transaminase. **11** Serum glutamate–pyruvate transaminase. **12** Creatine kinase. **13** γ-Glutamyl transpepsidase. **14** Thyrotropin. **15** Muscle biopsy may also be helpful in some cases.

Appendix

Table 56 Causes of radicular syndromes (p. 318)

Cause	Comments
Degenerative changes • Intervertebral disk herniation • Spondylosis deformans • Spinal canal stenosis • Spondylolisthesis	• Symptoms usually resolve with conservative treatment[1] • Torus-, buckle- or spur-shaped spondylophytes form due to degenerative changes in the intervertebral disks • See p. 284 • Slippage of a vertebra with respect to the next lower vertebra because of bilateral spondylolysis[2]
Trauma	See p. 272
Neoplasm	Primary spinal tumor (p. 284), metastatic tumor/neoplastic meningeosis (p. 262)
Infection/inflammation	See p. 222 ff. herpes zoster, borreliosis, epidural abscess, spondylitis, sarcoidosis, arachnopathy
Vascular	See p. 282
Metabolic	Diabetes mellitus (p. 324; Table 59, p. 395)
Inflammatory rheumatic	Ankylosing spondylitis, rheumatoid arthritis
Malformation	See p. 288 ff
Iatrogenic	Injection, lumbar puncture, surgery
Radiotherapy	Radiation-induced amyotrophy (cauda equina)[3]
Pseudoradicular syndrome[4], nonradicular pain	• *Arm*: Carpal tunnel syndrome, stiff shoulder, humeroscapular periarthropathy, syringomyelia • *Leg*: Facet syndrome, sacroiliac joint syndrome, coccygodynia, coxarthrosis, heterotopic ossification • *General*: Polyradiculitis, connective tissue diseases, rheumatoid diseases, malformations, myopathy/muscle trauma, strain, arthropathy, endometriosis, osteomyelitis, osteoporosis, arterial dissection, prostatitis, cystitis, Paget disease, somatization disorder

(Mumenthaler et al., 1998)

1 Absolute indications for surgery: Massive lumbar disk herniation with sphincter dysfunction, cervical disk herniation with spinal cord compression, severe weakness. Relative indications: Persistent radicular pain, frequent recurrence of radicular symptoms. **2** Defect in the pars interarticularis of the vertebral arch. **3** Development of following manifestations months to years after radiotherapy (para-aortic irradiation): malignant testicular tumor, lymphoma; progressive flaccid paraparesis without major sensory loss. **4** To be considered in the differential diagnosis.

Table 57 Causes of plexus lesions (p. 318)

Cause	Comments
Neoplasm	• Upper limb: neurofibroma/schwannoma, metastatic tumor, breast/lung cancer (Pancoast tumor) • Lower limb: urogenital tumors, cancer of the rectum, lymphoma
Vascular	• Lower limb: psoas hematoma due to anticoagulation, hemophilia, aneurysm
Metabolic	• Lower limb: diabetes mellitus (p. 395, Table 59)
Inflammatory	• Upper limb: neuralgic shoulder amyotrophy (p. 328) • Lower limb: neuropathy of lumbosacral plexus, vasculitis
Trauma	• Upper limb: stab or gunshot wound, strain, contusion (trauma, birth), cervical nerve root avulsion (p. 272) • Lower limb: pelvic fracture, sacral fracture
Compression	• Upper limb: carrying heavy loads (backpack paralysis), thoracic outlet syndrome (T1–C8)[1], costoclavicular syndrome, hyperadduction syndrome
Infection	• Lower limb: psoas abscess
Iatrogenic	• Upper limb: positioning, retraction (heart surgery), plexus anesthesia • Lower limb: hip surgery, vascular surgery, hysterectomy, adverse positioning
Pregnancy	• Lower limb: end of pregnancy, delivery
Radiotherapy	• Upper limb: brachial plexus paralysis months to years after radiotherapy • Lower limb: due to radiotherapy of neoplasms in pelvic region

1 Thoracic outlet compression may be caused by a cervical rib, fibrous band or narrow scalene gap.

Table 58 Common sites of mononeuropathy (pp. 318 and 312 f)

Nerve	Lesion ⇨ Syndrome	Cause[1]
Axillary nerve	Abduction paralysis, deltoid atrophy	Dislocation of shoulder
Long thoracic nerve	Winging of scapula; no sensory deficit, weakness of arm elevation	Compression ("backpack" paralysis), neuralgic shoulder amyotrophy, postinfectious
Radial nerve	• UA[2] ⇨ hand drop with sensory ⇩ in radial back of hand; prominent between 1st and 2nd finger • PFA[4] ⇨ supinator syndrome[5]	• Compression[3]/fracture of shaft of humerus • Fractured head of radius
Median nerve	• UA ⇨ monkey hand[6] • PFA ⇨ pronator teres syndrome, anterior interosseous syndrome[8] • DLA[9] ⇨ carpal tunnel syndrome, brachialgia, nocturnal paresthesia[10]	• Compression, fracture • Strain, compression, fracture • Compression, arteriovenous fistula/uremia, rheumatoid arthritis, pregnancy, diabetes mellitus, hypothyroidism, monoclonal gammopathy
Ulnar nerve	• UA ⇨ clawhand • PFA ⇨ clawhand • DLA ⇨ different types of paralysis	• Supracondylar process • Trauma, compression, arthrosis, habitual • Compression, habitual
Lateral femoral cutaneous nerve	• Meralgia paresthetica[12]	• Compression
Femoral nerve	• Proximal lesion ⇨ paralysis of knee extensors • Intrapelvic lesion ⇨ additional paralysis of hip flexors (gait disturbance)	• Psoas hematoma/abscess • Surgery (hip surgery, hysterectomy), trauma
Sciatic nerve	• Peroneal + tibial (partial) lesion	• Trauma, hip surgery, intragluteal injection
Common peroneal nerve	• Lesion at head of fibula ⇨ paralysis of dorsiflexors of foot (step gait)	• Compression, fracture, sprain, compartment syndrome
Tibial nerve	• Popliteal lesion ⇨ paralysis of all flexor muscles (foot, toes), sensory loss on back of calf and sole of foot; pain, absence of ankle jerk reflex • Lesion of lower leg ⇨ clawed toes; preservation of reflex • Tarsal tunnel syndrome[13], pain. • Calf, ankle, sole of foot. Clawed toes	• Fracture, compression • Compression • Compression, trauma

1 Selection. **2** Lesion at level of upper arm. **3** "Park bench paralysis", tourniquet (ischemia). **4** Lesion at level of elbow, proximal forearm. **5** Deep branch lesion: Pain on extensor surface of forearm, no sensory deficit, paralysis of long finger/thumb extensors with preservation of (radial) lifting of hand. **6** Paralysis of radial hand/finger flexors, pronators, thenar atrophy; sensory ⇩ in first 3½ fingers, trophic disturbances. **7** Pain on outer surface of forearm. **8** Lesion: anterior interosseous n.; no sensory deficit; flexor weakness in distal segments of thumb, index and middle finger. **9** Lesion of distal forearm, wrist. **10** Painful nocturnal/morning paresthesia (in arm) with sensory loss, thenar atrophy, and paralysis as the condition progresses. **11** Overextension of finger at metacarpophalangeal joint, flexion of middle and distal phalanges, sensory deficit in ulnar 1½ fingers. **12** Paresthesiae, pain in outer surface of thigh. **13** Lesion behind medial malleolus.

Table 59 Diabetic polyneuropathy syndromes (p. 324)

Syndrome	Features
Symmetric distribution • Diabetic polyneuropathy (DPN)[1]	• Distal, primarily sensory, with or without pain. NCV[2] ⇩ and/or respiration-dependent change in heart rate (p. 370) ⇩. Areflexia[3], pall-hypesthesia or pallanesthesia in toes, either initially or over time. Progression: increased sensory loss, impairment of position sense (sensory ataxia), paresthesiae, trophic changes, and paralysis. Autonomic dysfunction
• Diabetic pandysautonomia	• Cardiovascular[4], gastrointestinal[5], urogenital[6], and skin[7] changes. Usually associated with DPN, but isolated occurrence is possible
• Small-fiber polyneuropathy (PNP) with weight loss	• Painful (burning, dull dragging pain, more prominent at night). Autonomic dysfunction. Relatively mild impairment of somatic sensation, vibration and position sense, muscle strength and reflexes
• Hypoglycemic PNP	• Seen in insulinoma. May also be caused by recurrent hypoglycemia
Asymmetric distribution • Lumbosacral radicular neuropathy/plexus neuropathy[8,9]	• Rarely symmetrical. Intense pain radiating from low back to upper thigh. Weakness and atrophy of muscles innervated by the femoral nerve. Loss of quadriceps reflex. Minimal sensory loss
• Thoracolumbar radiculoneuropathy[9]	• Segmental beltlike pain distribution, sensory deficit, abdominal wall paralysis
• Compression syndromes	• Carpal tunnel syndrome (Table 58), ulnar lesion at level of elbow
• Cranial mononeuropathy[9,10]	• III ⇨ acute, painful[11] ophthalmoplegia, usually without pupillary involvement. VII ⇨ acute, often painful paralysis of the peripheral type

(Taylor and Dyck, 1999)

1 Cannot be clinically distinguished from uremic neuropathy. **2** Nerve conduction velocity (sensory/motor). **3** Mainly the gastrocnemius reflex. **4** Resting tachycardia, fixed heart rate. **5** Gastroparesis, diarrhea, constipation, biliary stasis, fecal incontinence. **6** Urinary retention, erectile dysfunction, retrograde ejaculation. **7** Hypohidrosis, hyperkeratosis. **8** Also referred to as proximal diabetic neuropathy, diabetic amyotrophy, and femoral neuropathy. **9** Indicative of favorable prognosis (partial or complete remission). **10** Local infection (rhinocerebral mucormycosis, p. 246, otitis externa circumscripta) can cause cranial nerve deficits in patients with diabetes mellitus. **11** Periorbital, retro-orbital, frontotemporal, hemispheric.

Table 60 Clinical spectrum of Guillain–Barré syndrome (p. 326)

Syndrome	Features[1]
Acute inflammatory demyelinating polyradiculoneuropathy (AIDP)[2]	Perivenous lymphocytic infiltrates and demyelination. IgM/IgG antibodies[3] against GM_1
Acute motor-sensory axonal neuropathy (AMSAN)[4]	Pronounced paralysis, early muscular atrophy. Axonal degeneration. IgG antibodies directed against GM_1
Acute motor-axonal neuropathy (AMAN)[4]	Pure motor neuropathy with axonal degeneration. IgG antibodies directed against GM_1, GD_{1a}, GD_{1b}
Miller Fisher syndrome (MFS)	Diplopia (usually external ophthalmoplegia), ataxia, areflexia. IgG antibodies to GQ_{1b}[5]

(Hahn, 1998)

1 The most common manifestations are listed. Other motor, sensory, or autonomic disturbances may also occur. **2** The most common form in Europe, North America, and Australia. **3** Ganglioside antibodies. **4** Commonly occur in North China, Japan, and Mexico; rarely in Western countries. **5** Detected in over 95% of all patients; correlated with the course of the disease.

Appendix

Table 61 Diagnostic criteria: Guillain–Barré syndrome (GBS) (p. 326)

Necessary[1]	Supportive[1]	Doubtful[1]	Exclusion [1]
• Progressive paralysis in more than one limb • Hyporeflexia or areflexia	• Progression lasting days to 4 weeks • Symmetry (relative) of involvement • Mild sensory disturbances • Cranial nerve involvement, especially VII • Resolution 2–4 weeks after end of progression • Autonomic dysfunction • Initial absence of fever • CSF protein ⇧[2] • Typical neurophysiological findings[3]	• Markedly asymmetrical involvement • Initial or persistent bladder/bowel dysfunction • Granulocytes in CSF; cell count > 50 mononuclear cells/ mm[3] • Sharply localized sensory loss in the trunk region	• Diagnosis of myasthenia, botulism, poliomyelitis, toxic neuropathy • Porphyria • Recent diphtheria • Isolated sensory disturbances without paralysis

(Asbury and Cornblath, 1990)

1 "Necessary" = prerequisite for diagnosis of GBS; "supportive" = supports the diagnosis; "doubtful" = GBS unlikely; "exclusion" = excludes the diagnosis of GBS. **2** May be normal initially, then rise in the course of the disease to several g/l; blood–brain barrier dysfunction; cell count < 10 mononuclear cells/mm[3]. **3** *Early phase*: Partial conduction block with reduced amplitude of evoked motor response potentials (proximal stimulation), loss of reflex and F-wave responses due to a proximal lesion; EMG recordings show reduced number of activatable motor units. *Later stages*: Variably reduced motor response potential; EMG shows mild to marked denervation (the less marked, the better the prognosis).

Table 62 Genetic features of hereditary polyneuropathy (p. 332)

Syndrome	Mode of Inheritance[1]/ Gene Locus
HMSN type I	
CMT1A[2]	AD/17p11.2–12[3]
CMT1B	AD/1q22–23[4]
CMT1C	AD/?
CMT4A	AR/8q
CMT4B	AR/11q23
CMT4C	AR/5q
CMTX1	XD/Xq13.1[5]
CMTX2	XR/Xp22.2
CMTX4	XR/Xq26
HMSN type II	
CMT2A	AD/1p36
CMT2B	AD/3q13–22
CMT2C	AD/?
CMT2D	AD/7p14
HMSN type III	
CMT3A	AD/17p11.2–12[3]
CMT3B	AD/1q22–23[4]
CMT3C	AD/8q
HNPP	AD/17p11.2–12[3]

(Mendell, 1998; Schaumburg et al., 1992; Schöls, 1998)

1 AD = autosomal dominant, AR = autosomal recessive, XR = X-linked recessive; XD = X-linked dominant. **2** CMT = Charcot–Marie–Tooth. **3** Gene: PMP22 (PMP = peripheral myelin protein). **4** Gene: P_0 (point mutation). **5** Gene: connexin 32 (point mutation).

Table 63 Features of rare nonmetabolic neuropathies (p. 332)

Syndrome	Inheritance/ Gene Locus	Clinical Features/NCV[1]
Giant axon neuropathy (GAN)	AR/16q24.1	PNP syndrome, fair, frizzy hair, gait impairment, NCV slightly ⇩
HSN[2] type I	AD/9q22.1–22.3	Sensory and autonomic neuropathy, reflexes ⇩, sensory loss in feet, restless legs, perforating foot ulcers, hearing loss, lancinating pain in limbs, deforming arthropathy, normal motor NLV
FAP[3]	AD	Autonomic PNP (⇨ autonomic dysfunction), dissociated sensory loss, pain, trophic disturbances, vitreous opacity, cardiomyopathy, nephropathy, hepatopathy

1 Nerve conduction velocity. **2** Hereditary sensory neuropathy. **3** Familial amyloid polyneuropathy (PNP). There are different subtypes with variable serum protein changes (transthyretin, apolipoprotein A1, gelsolin) that give rise to extracellular amyloid (AF) deposits. Liver transplantation can be performed to remove the amyloid precursors and bring about degeneration of the amyloid deposits.

Table 64 Myopathy syndromes (p. 334)

Features	Potential causes
Acute generalized weakness	Myasthenia gravis, botulism, periodic paralysis[1], polymyositis/dermatomyositis, acute rhabdomyolysis, critical illness myopathy, toxic or drug-induced myopathy[2], hypermagnesemia
Subacute or chronic, mainly proximal weakness	Myasthenia gravis, Lambert–Eaton syndrome, muscular dystrophy, congenital myopathy, polymyositis/dermatomyositis, metabolic myopathy, mitochondriopathy, electrolyte imbalance, endocrine disorder[3], toxic or drug-induced myopathy
Subacute or chronic, mainly distal weakness	Inclusion body myositis, myotonic dystrophy, facioscapulohumeral muscular dystrophy, nemaline myopathy, central core disease, scapuloperoneal syndrome, Welander myopathy[4], oculopharyngodistal myopathy
Periodic weakness	Myasthenia gravis, Lambert–Eaton syndrome, dyskalemic paralysis, paramyotonia congenita, neuromyotonia, Conn syndrome, thyrotoxicosis
Asymmetric or localized weakness	Facioscapulohumeral muscular dystrophy, myasthenia gravis, ischemic muscular necrosis, local myositis, muscle rupture/trauma
Multiple system involvement	Mitochondriopathy, critical illness myopathy, myotonic dystrophy, proximal myotonic myopathy, dermatomyositis
Dysphagia	Myasthenia gravis, polymyositis, myotonic dystrophy, oculopharyngeal muscular dystrophy, inclusion body myositis, mitochondriopathy
Myalgia	Viral/bacterial/parasitic/granulomatous/interstitial myositis, dermatomyositis/ polymyositis, vasculitis, eosinophilic fasciitis, polymyalgia rheumatica, fibromyalgia. Alcohol, drugs, hypothyroidism. Metabolic myopathies. Muscle strain. Neuromyotonia. Stiff-man syndrome
Muscle cramps	Idiopathic, exercise-induced, pregnancy, uremia, hypothyroidism, electrolyte imbalance
Muscle hypertrophy	Muscular dystrophy (Duchenne/Becker: calves, deltoid), myotonia congenita, amyloidosis, cysticercosis, acromegaly, glycogen storage disease type II (Pompe)
Cardiomyopathy	Duchenne/Becker muscular dystrophy, Emery–Dreifuss muscular dystrophy, myotonic dystrophy, centronuclear myopathy, nemaline myopathy, glycogen storage disease type II
CK-emia[5]	Physical stress, muscle trauma (fall, injection, epileptic seizure), toxins/drugs (alcohol), hypothyroidism, female carrier of trait (Duchenne/Becker muscular dystrophy), incipient myopathy (muscular dystrophy, myositis, glycogen storage disease), hereditary

1 Hypokalemic or hyperkalemic form. **2** Table 66. **3** Hypothyroidism or hyperthyroidism, acromegaly, Cushing disease, hyperparathyroidism, Conn syndrome, Cushing syndrome. **4** Myopathia distalis tarda hereditaria. **5** Elevation of creatine kinase (CK) levels in serum without clinical evidence of myopathy; risk of malignant hyperthermia (related to general anesthesia, see p. 346).

Appendix

Table 65 Some hereditary myopathies (p. 334)

Type	Myopathy	Inh.[1]	Gene locus	Gene product
Dystrophinopathy	Duchenne MD[2]	XR[3]	Xp21.2	Dystrophin
	Becker MD	XR	Xp21.2	Dystrophin
Sarcoglycanopathy	LGMD2D[4]	AR[5]	17q21	α-Sarcoglycan[6]
	LGMD2E	AR	4q12	β-Sarcoglycan
	LGMD2C	AR	13q12	γ-Sarcoglycan
	LGMD2F	AR	5q33	δ-Sarcoglycan
Other LGMDs	LGMD2A	AR	15q15.1–21.1	Calpain-3
	LGMD2B	AR	2p13.3–13.1	Dysferlin
	LGMD1A	AD	5q31	Myotilin
	LGMD1B	AD	1q11–21	Lamin A/C
	LGMD1C	AD	3p25	Caveolin-3
Other MDs	Facioscapulohumeral MD	AD	4q35	?
	Oculopharyngeal MD	AD	14q11.2-q13	PABP2[7]
	Myotonic MD[8]	AD	19q13	DMPK[9]
	Emery–Dreifuss MD	XR	Xq28	Emerin
Channel diseases				
Chloride channel	Thomsen MC[10]	AD	7q35	Chloride channel
	Becker MC	AR	7q35	Chloride channel
Sodium channel	Hyperkalemic PP[11]	AD	17q23.1–25.3	Sodium channel
	Paramyotonia congenita	AD	17q23.1–25.3	Sodium channel
	PAM[12]	AD	17q23.1–25.3	Sodium channel
Calcium channel	Hypokalemic PP[13]	AD	1q32	Calcium channel[14]
	Malignant hyperthermia	AD	1q31–32	Calcium channel[14]
	Malignant hyperthermia	AD	19q13.1	Calcium channel[15]
	Central core disease	AD	19q13.1	Calcium channel[15]
Mitochondriopathies	Mitochondrial myopathy[16]		Mitochondrial DNA[17]	

(Gene loci as specified by OMIM)

1 Mode of inheritance. **2** Muscular dystrophy. **3** X-linked recessive. **4** LGMD = limb girdle muscular dystrophy. **5** Autosomal recessive. **6** Adhalin-7-poly(A) binding protein-2. **7** Poly(A) binding protein-2. **8** Unstable trinucleotide repeat (CTG). **9** Myotonin-protein kinase. **10** Myotonia congenita. **11.** Hyperkalemic periodic paralysis. **12.** Potassium-sensitive myotonia (myotonia fluctuans). **13.** Hypokalemic periodic paralysis. **14.** Dihydropyridine receptor. **15.** Ryanodine receptor. **16** Mainly systemic diseases, usually maternally inherited or sporadic. **17.** Nuclear DNA mutations are rare.

Table 66 Some acquired myopathies (p. 334)

Type	Myopathy
Neuromuscular end plate dysfunction	Myasthenia gravis, Lambert–Eaton syndrome, botulism
Endocrine myopathy	Hyperthyroidism, hypothyroidism, Cushing syndrome, acromegaly, Conn syndrome, primary hyperparathyroidism
Inflammatory myopathy	Polymyositis, dermatomyositis, myositis with vasculitis, Churg–Strauss syndrome, granulomatous myositis, inclusion body myositis, myositis induced by pathogens (e. g., bacteria, viruses, parasites)
Toxic/drug-induced myopathy[1]	Alcohol, corticosteroids, lovastatin, simvastatin, cocaine, emetin, diazocholesterol

1 Rarely caused by other drugs or toxins (not listed).

Appendix

Table 67   Additional diagnostic studies for myopathy (p. 334)

Method	Information Supplied/Parameters
Pharmacological tests	Edrophonium chloride (p. 404) *In vitro* testing for malignant hyperthermia.
Neurography/Stimulation electromyography	Used to exclude peripheral neuropathy (p. 404). Serial stimulation: Evidence of neuromuscular conduction disturbances
Needle electromyography[1]	• *Muscular dystrophy*: Possible findings include fibrillation, positive waves, pseudomyotonic discharges. Brief, low-amplitude MAPs, polyphasia rate ⬆, rapid and dense interference pattern • *Myositis*: Fibrillation, positive waves, pseudomyotonic discharges. Polyphasia rate ⬆, narrow and low-amplitude MAPs • *Myotonia/paramyotonia*: Myotonic discharges, MAPs resembling those of muscular dystrophy
Laboratory tests	• *Creatine kinase*[2]: > 10 000 in acute rhabdomyolysis, myositis, toxic myopathy, Duchenne/Becker muscular dystrophy (early stage) • 4000–10 000 in Duchenne/Becker type muscular dystrophy (later stages), myositis • 1000–4000 in muscular dystrophies, hypokalemic or hypothyroid myopathy, congenital myopathy, female carrier (muscular dystrophy) • ≤ 1000 in spinal muscular atrophy, amyotrophic lateral sclerosis, inclusion body myositis, chronic/infectious myositis • *Myoglobin*: Severe muscle degeneration ⇨ myoglobinuria[3] • *Serum lactate/pyruvate* (venous): Elevated at rest or after light physical exercise ⇨ mitochondriopathies, respiratory chain defects. Absence of rise in disorders of glycolysis and glycogenolysis[4] • *Molecular genetics*: Depends on results of immunohistochemistry (dystrophies) and biochemical muscle analysis (mitochondriopathies). Used to supplement clinical findings if necessary (channel diseases) • *Other tests*[5]: Erythrocyte sedimentation rate, hepatitis antigen, ANCA[6] (vasculitis). Eosinophilia (eosinophil fasciitis, Churg–Strauss syndrome). Sarcoplasmic enzymes incl. SGOT, SGPT, lactate dehydrogenase, aldolase, γ-GT (elevated in PROMM[7]). Basal TSH. Rheumatoid factor (myositis). Antibodies: AChR[8] (myasthenia), Jo-1 (myositis, antisynthetase syndrome), Pm-Scl (myositis with systemic sclerosis), SS-A (Ro) (myositis with Sjögren syndrome), U₁RNP (mixed connective tissue disease)
Diagnostic imaging	Ultrasound, CT/MRI: Distribution of atrophy, fat and connective tissue. Supportive evidence when selecting site of biopsy. Localization of local muscle changes (tumor, hemorrhage, pyomyositis/ossification ⇨ scintigraphy)
Muscle biopsy	Mainly used for definitive proof of an inflammatory, vasculitic or metabolic myopathy. Also used for clarification of diseases not clearly classifiable as "myogenic" or "neurogenic." Sporadic cases of muscular dystrophy

1 For abbreviations, see p. 391. **2** U/l of CK-MM; selected examples. **3** Alcohol, barbiturates, acute myositis, malignant hyperthermia, carnitine palmitoyl transferase deficiency, glycogen storage disease type V/VII, posttraumatic, postictal, idiopathic. **4** Determined by stress testing (ischemia ⇨ risk of rhabdomyolysis). **5** Selected examples, see also p. 391. **6** Antineutrophil antibodies. **7** Proximal myotonic myopathy. **8** Acetylcholine receptor. **9** Specimens taken from muscle moderately affected by disease process. Two specimens are deep-frozen in an isopentane–nitrogen mixture (for histochemistry, immunohistochemistry; biochemical diagnosis, etc.). One specimen is fixed in glutaraldehyde for electron-microscopic study.

Table 68 Clinical features of selected muscular dystrophies[1] (p. 336)

Criteria	Duchenne MD[2]	Becker MD	Limb girdle MD	Facioscapulo-humeral MD	Myotonic MD
Mean age at onset (years)	2	12	Adolescence/ adulthood	Adolescence/ adulthood	Adolescence/ adulthood
Sex[3]	M	M	M/F	M/F	M/F
Site of onset	Pelvic girdle	Pelvic girdle	Pelvic girdle (often)	Face, shoulder girdle	Head, shoulder girdle, arms, dorsiflexors of foot
Facial muscle involvement	No	No	No	Yes	Yes (cataract)
(Pseudo) Hypertrophy	Calf, deltoid, gluteal muscles	Calf muscles	Calf muscles (rarely)	None	None
Cardiac involvement	Common	Rare	Occasional	None	Common (pacemaker)
Inheritance	X-linked recessive	X-linked recessive	Usually autosomal recessive	Autosomal dominant	Autosomal dominant
CK level[4]	50 (to 300) times higher than normal	20 (to 200) times higher than normal	< 10 times higher than normal	Normal to 4 times higher than normal	Normal to 3 times higher than normal
Dystrophin	Absent	Deficient	Normal	Normal	Normal
Myotonia	No	No	No	No	Yes
Prognosis	Age (years) 3–6, gait disturbance; 5–6, hypertrophy; 6–11, increasing weakness and contractures; death often at age 15–30	Slow progression. Unable to walk by ca. age 20. Mean age at death, 42 years (range, 23–89)	Mainly slow. Life span usually only slightly decreased	Slow progression. Ability to walk is preserved. Normal life span	Ability to walk is preserved. Life span shortened only in severe cases

1 Very rare syndromes (prevalence < 1/10[6]) such as Emery–Dreifuss MD, oculopharyngeal MD, distal myopathies, proximal myotonic MD, and congenital MD are not listed here. **2** MD = muscular dystrophy. **3** M = male; F = female. **4** CK = creatine kinase.

Table 69 Myotonia and periodic paralysis (p. 338)

Criterion	Hyperkalemic paralysis	Paramyotonia congenita	Myotonia fluctuans	Myotonia congenita Thomsen	Myotonia congenita Becker	Proximal myotonic myopathy[1]	Myotonic dystrophy
Periodic paralysis	Yes	Yes	No	No	Yes	No	No
Cold-induced paralysis	No	Yes	No	No	No	No	No
Potassium-induced paralysis	Yes	Sometimes	No	No	No	No	No
Paradoxical myotonia[2]	Sometimes	Yes	No	No	No	No	No
Additional organ involvement[3]	No	No	No	No	No	Yes	Yes
Inheritance	AD[4]	AD	AD	AD	AR[5]	AD	AD
Defect	Sodium channel	Sodium channel	Sodium channel	Chloride channel	Chloride channel	?	Protein kinase
Features	Duration of paralytic attacks varies (≤ 4 hours)	Attacks of muscle stiffness and weakness can last up to 1 day	Myotonia of variable severity	Generalized myotonia, no weakness	Myotonia more severe than in Thomsen type. Transient weakness	Proximal muscle weakness, cataract, muscle pain, mild muscular atrophy	Weakness, especially of craniocervical muscles, less pronounced in limbs (mainly distal). Cataract. Defective cardiac impulse conduction

(Ptacek et al., 1993)

1 Unlike in myotonic dystrophy, there is no cytosine–thymine–guanine (CTG) repeat. **2** In this case, myotonia generally subsides after repeated voluntary muscle contraction ("warm-up"), whereas it increases in paradoxical myotonia. **3** I.e., extramuscular involvement. **4** Autosomal dominant. **5** Autosomal recessive.

Table 70 Selected forms of congenital myopathy (p. 340)

Myopathy	Gene Locus/Gene	Comments
Central core disease	AD[1]: 19q13.1/Ryanodine receptor	Neonatal hypotonia. Slow progression. Attenuated muscles, skeletal anomalies[2], hyporeflexia or areflexia; exercise-induced muscle stiffness; risk of malignant hyperthermia
Nemaline myopathy (NEM1)	AD: 1q22–23/Tropomyosin-3	Neonatal hypotonia; nonprogressive; high palate
Nemaline myopathy (NEM2)	AR[3]/2q22/Nebulin	Delayed motor development. Attenuated muscles, thin extremities; dysplasia[4]. Respiratory disturbances (paretic diaphragm muscles), recurrent pneumonia, dysphagia, dysarthria; hyporeflexia or areflexia
Centronuclear (myotubular) myopathy	XR[5]: Xq28/Myotubularin	Neonatal hypotonia, facial muscle weakness, external ophthalmoplegia, hyporeflexia, respiratory disturbances, dysphagia, high palate

1 Autosomal dominant. **2** Congenital hip dislocation, chest deformity, kyphoscoliosis, pes cavus. **3** Autosomal recessive. **4** Elongated and oval face, open mouth, micrognathia, high palate, kyphosis, hyperlordosis, pes cavus, cardiomyopathy, heart failure. **5** X-linked recessive; autosomal recessive and autosomal dominant inheritance are also found, with less severe manifestations.

Table 71 Metabolic myopathies (p. 340)

Myopathy/Gene Locus	Defect/Inheritance	Features
Carbohydrate metabolism		
• Acid maltase deficiency[1] (type II, Pompe)/17q25.2–25.3	• 1,4-Glucosidase/ • Autosomal recessive	• Slowly progressive proximal myopathy, respiratory disturbances (nocturnal hypoventilation)
• Muscle phosphorylase deficiency[1] (type V, McArdle)/11q13	• Myophosphorylase/ • Autosomal recessive	• Exercise-induced muscle pain and stiffness, contractures that subside at rest, rhabdomyolysis
• Phosphofructokinase deficiency (type VII, Tarui)/12q13.3	• Phosphofructokinase/ • Autosomal recessive	• Similar to McArdle type
Fat metabolism		
• Carnitine deficiency myopathy/?	• Carnitine/Autosomal recessive?	• Symmetrical, proximal, slowly progressive myopathy, CK ⇑
• CPT-I deficiency[2]/11q13	• CPT I/Autosomal recessive	• Exercise and cold-induced muscle pain and weakness, rhabdomyolysis, hypoglycemia, hyperammonemia
• CPT-II deficiency/1p32	• CPT II/Autosomal recessive	• Exercise/fasting-induced muscle pain, rhabdomyolysis

(continued next page)

Table 71 Metabolic myopathies (p. 340) (continued)

Myopathy/Gene Locus	Defect/Inheritance	Features
Mitochondria		
• CPEO[3]	• mtDNA deletion in ca. 50% of cases	• Ptosis, external ophthalmoplegia, tapetoretinal degeneration, cardiac arrhythmias, proximal myopathy
• KSS[4]	• mtDNA deletion/ • duplication	• Onset before 13th year of life, ataxia, hearing impairment, ⇑CSF protein, endocrine disturbances, otherwise identical to CPEO
• MERRF[5]	• mtDNA point mutation	• Myoclonus, ataxia, seizures
• MELAS[6]	• mtDNA point mutation	• Episodic vomiting, focal seizures, dwarfism, proximal muscle weakness
• LHON[7]	• mtDNA point mutation	• Acute/subacute bilateral loss of vision, eye pain
• MILS[8]	• mtDNA point mutation[9]	• Developmental delay, ataxia, dystonia, visual disturbances, respiratory disturbances[10]

1 Adult type. **2** Carnitine palmitoyl transferase; defect located on outer mitochondrial membrane in type I, and on inner membrane in type II. **3** Chronic progressive external ophthalmoplegia. **4** Kearns–Sayre syndrome; cardiac pacemaker implantation may be necessary in patients with cardiac arrhythmias. **5** Myoclonus epilepsy with ragged red fibers. **6** Myopathy, encephalopathy, lactic acidosis, and "strokelike episodes". **7** Hereditary hepatic-optic neuropathy. **8** Maternally inherited Leigh syndrome. **9** Autosomal recessive and sporadic forms are also found. **10** T2-weighted MRI reveals bilateral symmetric lesions (brain stem, periaqueductal region, cerebellum, basal ganglia)

Table 72 Drugs that can aggravate myasthenia gravis (p. 342)

Drugs That Can Aggravate Myasthenia Gravis	Alternatives
Antibiotics: tetracyclines, aminoglycosides, polymyxins, gyrase inhibitors, penicillins	Cephalosporins, chloramphenicol
Psychoactive drugs: benzodiazepines, barbiturates, tricyclic antidepressants, chlorpromazine, haloperidol, droperidol, lithium	Promethazine, thioridazine. Chlordiazepoxide, maprotiline, mianserin or carbamazepine can be used at low doses and with careful monitoring
Anticonvulsants: phenytoin, ethosuximide, barbiturates	Carbamazepine
Cardiovascular agents: Quinidine, ajmaline, procainamide, lidocaine, ganglioplegics, nifedipine, β-blockers[1]	Digitalis, reserpine, methyldopa, tocainide, verapamil (low-dose)
Miscellaneous: ACTH, corticosteroids[2], D-penicillamine, morphine and derivatives, magnesium, general anesthesia (muscle relaxants)	Aspirin, gold, indometacin, acetaminophen, diclofenac, local/regional anesthesia, spinal anesthesia, inhalant anesthetics/deeper general anesthesia

(Selected drugs from McNamara and Guay, 1997)

1 Mask symptoms of myasthenia. **2** High starting dose.

Appendix

Table 73 Myasthenia-related crises (p. 342)

Syndrome	Symptoms and Signs	Precipitating Factors
Myasthenic crisis	Restlessness, anxiety, confusion, respiratory weakness, weak cough, dysphagia, dysarthria, mydriasis, ptosis, tachycardia, pallor	Infectious diseases, surgical interventions, anesthesia, drugs, psychosocial stress, impaired drug uptake (vomiting, diarrhea), disease progression, previously undetected myasthenia (and previously mentioned factors)
Cholinergic crisis	Restless, anxiety, confusion, respiratory weakness, weak cough, dysphagia, dysarthria, miosis, bradycardia, skin reddening, muscle fasciculation/spasms, salivation, tenesmus, diarrhea	Overdosage (relative) of AChE inhibitors; acetylcholine poisoning

Table 74 Ancillary tests in myasthenia gravis (p. 342)

Test	Objective	Interpretation of Results
Edrophonium chloride test[1] (Tensilon, Camsilon)	Increase in muscle strength (with improvement of ptosis, eye movements, speech, and swallowing)	Marked improvement (beginning 30 seconds after administration and lasting roughly 5 minutes) ⇨ unequivocal response. Sensitivity for OMG[2]: ca. 86%, for GMG[3]: ca. 95%
Electromyography (EMG)[4]	Documentation of impaired neuromuscular conduction (decrement in amplitude seen with serial stimulation; jitter may be observed in single-fiber EMG)	A decrement of 10% or more is pathological. Sensitivity of serial stimulation in OMG: ca. 34%; in GMG: up to 77%. Prior muscle exercise ⇨ more pronounced decrement. Sensitivity of single-fiber EMG: ca. 92%
Serum acetylcholine receptor antibody titer	Documentation of presence of acetylcholine receptor antibodies	Sensitivity: 50% in OMG, ca. 90% in GMG. False-positive results may occur in Lambert–Eaton syndrome, rarely in amyotrophic lateral sclerosis
Diagnostic imaging[5]	Measurement of thymus	Thymic enlargement due to thymoma or hyperplasia

(Phillips and Melnick, 1990)

1 Short-term inhibition of cholinesterase, given intravenously for diagnostic purposes. **2** Ocular myasthenia gravis. **3** Generalized myasthenia gravis. **4** Example: Repeated stimulation of accessory nerve (3/sec for 3 seconds) and recording of activity in trapezius muscle. **5** CT (contrast-enhanced) or MRI (younger patients, better differentiation of thymic hyperplasia).

Table 75 Toxic myopathies (p. 347)

Syndrome	Substances (selected)
Muscle weakness with or without pain; rhabdomyolysis may occur	Alcohol, chloroquine, cimetidine, clofibrate, cocaine, colchicine, ciclosporin, disulfiram, emetine, ergotamine, gemfibrozil, induced hypokalemia (diuretics, licorice), imipramine, isoniazide, lithium, lovastatin, meprobamate, niacin, pentazocine, thyroid hormones, vincristine, zidovudine
Myalgia	Alcohol, allopurinol, cimetidine, clofibrate, clonidine, dihydroergotamine, ergotamine, methyldopa, succinylcholine, vincristine, zidovudine
Polymyositis, pseudo-lupus erythematosus	Bezafibrate, chlorpromazine, cimetidine, clofibrate, D-penicillamine, etofibrate, etofyllin clofibrate, fenofibrate, gold, hydralazine, isoniazide, L-tryptophan, penicillin, phenytoin, procainamide, tetracyclines, zidovudine
Myotonia	Ciclosporin, 20,25-diazocholesterol, diuretics, D-penicillamine, fenoterol, pindolol, propranolol
Local muscle lesions (pain, swelling, local muscular atrophy)	Heroin, insulin, meperidine, pentazocine

Table 76 Neuromuscular paraneoplastic syndromes (pp. 347, 388)

Site of Lesion	Syndrome ⇨ Manifestation	Symptoms and Signs	Common Tumors	Lesions/ Antibodies
Motor neuron	Subacute muscular atrophy (hands, bulbar muscles) ⇨ weeks to months	Asymmetrical paralysis, muscle atrophy (p. 304)	Small-cell lung cancer, lymphoma, renal cell carcinoma	Motor neurons/ Anti-Hu[1]
Spinal posterior root, ganglion	Subacute sensory neuronopathy ⇨ weeks to months	Marked sensory loss, areflexia, ataxia, paresthesiae, pain	Small-cell lung cancer, other lung tumors	Spinal ganglia
Proximal peripheral nerve	• Acute polyradiculopathy ⇨ hours to days • Chronic polyradiculopathy[3] ⇨ weeks to months	• Ascending sensorimotor deficits[2] • Chronic progressive/recurrent sensorimotor deficits	• Hodgkin disease • Small-cell lung cancer, lymphoma, myeloma	Segmental demyelination, neuritis
Distal peripheral nerve	• Paraproteinemic polyneuropathy ⇨ weeks to months • Sensorimotor polyneuropathy ⇨ weeks to months • Neuromyotonia	• See p. 328 • Distal symmetrical polyneuropathy • Muscle stiffness, cramps	• Plasmacytoma • Small-cell lung cancer, other cancers • Thymoma, lung cancer	• Segmental demyelination • Mainly axonal lesions • Distal motor nerve/Anti-VGPC[4]
End-plate region	• Lambert–Eaton syndrome ⇨ weeks to months • Myasthenia gravis ⇨ weeks to months	• See p. 342 • See p. 342	• Small-cell lung cancer; breast, prostate or stomach cancer • Thymoma	• See p. 343/ Anti-VGCC antibodies[5] • See p. 343/ Skeletal muscle antibodies
Skeletal muscle	• Polymyositis/ dermatomyositis ⇨ months to years • Rhabdomyolysis ⇨ days to weeks	• See p. 344 • Rapidly progressive paralysis, dysphagia	• Various cancers (breast, lung or ovarian cancer, lymphoma) • Various cancers	• Myonecrosis, lymphomonocytic infiltrates • Myonecrosis, rare inflammatory infiltrates

(Brown, 1998)

1 In small-cell lung cancer. **2** Similar to Guillain–Barré syndrome (p. 326). **3** Similar to CIDP (p. 328). **4** VGPC = voltage-gated potassium channel; EMG shows high-frequency discharges (150–300 Hz). **5** VGCC = voltage-gated calcium channel.

Table 77   Laboratory tests (p. 351)

Test/Objective	Risks	Comments
Antiepileptic drugs • Verify drug compliance • Assess for drug resistance • Avoid underdosage or over-dosage • Assess for drug interactions	• Laboratory error • Misuse of measured values (the physician should be guided by the clinical objective of a seizure-free state, rather than by "therapeutic levels")	Time of sample collection is determined by the pharmacokinetics of the antiepileptic drug in question
Lumbar puncture • Measure CSF pressure • Obtain CSF sample for analysis • Intrathecal drug administration • Diagnosis (contrast agent[1], radioactive substances[2])	• Increased intracranial pressure[3] • Intraspinal mass[4] • Postpuncture headache • Intraspinal hemorrhage (coagulopathy) • Meningitis • Discitis	Suboccipital or lateral cervical puncture is very rarely indicated (e. g. if a CSF sample is required, but cannot be obtained by lumbar puncture, or for myelography above a spinal lesion). Myelography and MRI have rendered Queckenstedt's test[5] obsolete

1 For myelography. **2** For scintigraphy. **3** Risk of transtentorial/cerebellar herniation. **4** Risk of acute spinal decompensation with paraplegia. **5** Compression of jugular vein to test for patency of subarachnoid space, which may be blocked, for example, by a spinal tumor.

References

Suggested Reading

Aminoff, M. J. (ed.): Neurology and general medicine. Churchill Livingstone, New York, Edinburgh, London, Philadelphia, 2001.

Berg, B. O. (ed.): Principles of child neurology. McGraw–Hill, New York, 1996.

Bernstein, M., M. S. Berger: Neuro-oncology. Thieme Medical Publishers, New York, 2000.

Bradley, W. G., R. B. Daroff, G. M. Fenichel, C. D. Marsden (eds.): Neurology in clinical practice (Volumes 1 and 2). Butterworth–Heinemann, Boston, Oxford, Singapore, Melbourne, Toronto, Munich, Tokyo, New Delhi, 2000.

Brazis, P. W., J. C. Masdeu, J. Biller: Localization in clinical neurology. Little, Brown and Company, Boston, 1996.

Brooke, M. H.: A clinician's view of neuromuscular diseases. Williams & Wilkins, Baltimore, 1986.

Compston, A., G. Ebers, H. Lassmann, I. McDonald, B. Matthews, H. Wekerle: McAlpine's multiple sclerosis. Churchill Livingstone, Edinburgh, London, Melbourne, New York, 1998.

Dyck, P. J., P. K. Thomas, J. W. Griffin, P. A. Low, J. F. Poduslo (eds.): Peripheral neuropathy (Volumes 1 and 2). W. B.Saunders, Philadelphia, 1993.

Engel, A. G., C. Franzini-Armstrong (eds.): Myology. McGraw-Hill, New York, 1994.

Engel, J., T. A. Pedley (eds.): Epilepsy: a comprehensive textbook. Lippincott-Raven, Philadelphia, New York, 1998.

Graham, D. I., P. L. Lantos (eds.): Greenfields's neuropathology (Volumes 1 and 2). Arnold, London, Sydney, Auckland, 2002.

Haerer, A. F.: DeJongs The neurologic examination. J.B. Lippincott, Philadelphia, New York, London, Hagerstown, 1992.

Hardman, J. G., L. E. Limbird, A. G. Gilman (eds.): Goodman & Gilman's The pharmacological basis of therapeutics. McGraw, Hill, New York, 2001.

Hirsch, M. C., T. Kramer: Neuroanatomy. Springer-Verlag, Berlin, Heidelberg, New York, 1999.

Kandel, E. R., J. H. Schwartz, T. M. Jessell: Principles of neural science. McGraw-Hill, New York, 2000.

Katirji, B., H. J. Kaminski, D. C. Preston, R. L. Ruff, B. E. Shapiro: Neuromuscular disorders in clinical practice. Butterworth-Heinemann, Boston, Oxford, Auckland, Johannesburg, Melbourne, New Dehli, 2002.

Low, P. A.: Clinical autonomic disorders. Lippincott-Raven, Philadelphia, New York, 1997.

Lyon, G., R. D. Adams, E. H. Kolodny: Neurology of hereditary metabolic diseases of children. McGraw-Hill, New York 1996.

Polman, C. H., A. J. Thompson, T. J. Murray, W. I. McDonald: Multiple sclerosis: the guide to treatment and management, 5th edition. Demos Medical Publishing, New York, 2001.

Rosenberg, R. N., S. B. Prusiner, S. DiMauro, R. L. Barchi, E. Nestler: The molecular and genetic basis of neurologic and psychiatric disease. Butterworth-Heinemann, Boston, 2003.

Sadock, B. J.,V.A. Sadock: Kaplan and Sadocks's Synposis of psychiatry. Lippincott Williams & Wilkins, Baltimore, 2002.

Shapiro, C. M.: ABC of sleep disorders. BMJ Publishing Group, London, 1993.

Spillane, J. D., J. A. Spillane: An atlas of clinical neurology. Oxford University Press, Oxford, 1982.

Swaiman, K. F., S. Ashword: Pediatric neurology. Mosby, St. Louis, 1999.

Van Allen, M. W., R. L. Rodnitzky: Pictorial manual of neurological tests. Year Book Medical Publishers, Chicago, London, 1981.

Victor, M., A. H. Ropper: Adams & Victor's Principles of neurology. McGraw-Hill, New York, 2002.

Warlow, C. P., M. S. Dennis, J. van Gijn, G. J. Hankey, P. A. G. Sandercock, J. M. Bamford, J. M. Wardlaw: Stroke—a practical guide to management. Blackwell Science Ltd., Oxford, 2001.

Watts, R. L., W. C. Koller: Movement disorders: neurologic principles and practice. McGraw-Hill, New York, 1997.

Wiebers, D. O., A. J. D. Dale, E. Kokmen, J. W. Swanson (eds.): Mayo Clinic examinations in neurology. Mosby, St. Louis, 1998.

References

(numbers in brackets refer to appropriate pages)

Ackerman, M. J., D. E. Clapham: Ion channels—basic science and clinical disease. N. Engl. J. Med. 1997;336:1575–1585. [339]

Adams, R. D., J. M. Foley: The neurological disorders associated with liver disease. Proc. Assoc. Res. Nerv. Ment. Dis. 1952;32:198–237. [387]

Asbury, A. K., D. R. Cornblath: Assessment of current diagnostic criteria for Guillain Barré syndrome. Ann. Neurol. 1990;27(Suppl.):S21–S24. [396]

Bain, P. G.: The management of tremor. J.Neurol.Neurosurg.Psychiatry 2002;72(Suppl.1):13–19. [62]

Barohn, R. J.: Approach to peripheral neuropathy and neuronopathy. Semin. Neurol. 1998;18: 7–18. [390]

Behin, A., K. Hoang-Xuan, A. F. Carpentier, J.-Y. Delattre: Primary brain tumours in adults. Lancet 2003;361:323–331. [264f]

Berger, M. (ed.): Handbuch des normalen und gestörten Schlafs. Springer-Verlag, Berlin, Heidelberg, 1992. [113, 363]

Biller, J. (ed.): Iatrogenic neurology. Butterworth-Heinemann, Boston, 1998. [314, 389]

Bogousslavsky, J., L. Caplan (eds.): Stroke syndromes. Cambridge University Press, Cambridge, 1995. [166ff]

Brandt, T.: Vertigo: its multisensory syndromes. Springer-Verlag, London, 1991. [89]

Brott, T., J. Bogousslavsky: Treatment of acute ischemic stroke. N. Engl. J. Med. 2000;343:710–722. [174]

Brown, R. H.: Paraneoplastic neurologic syndromes. In: Fauci, A. S., E. Braunwald, K. J. Isselbacher, J. D. Wilson, J. B. Martin, D. L. Kasper, S. L. Hauser, D. L. Longo (eds.): Harrison's Principles of internal medicine. McGraw-Hill, New York, St. Louis, San Francisco, Colorado Springs, Auckland, 1998. Chapter 103. [388, 406]

Bruni, J.: Episodic impairment of consciousness. In: Bradley, W. G., R. B. Daroff, G. M. Fenichel, C. D. Marsden (eds.): Neurology in clinical practice. Butterworth-Heinemann, Boston, Oxford, Singapore, Melbourne, Toronto, Munich, Tokyo, New Delhi, 1996. 11–21. [200]

Compston, A., A. Coles: Multiple sclerosis. Lancet 2002;359:1221–1231. [214f]

Compston, A., G. Ebers, H. Lassmann, I. McDonald, B. Matthews, H. Wekerle (eds.): McAlpine's Multiple sclerosis. Churchill Livingstone, Edinburgh, London, Melbourne, New York, 1998. [220]

Conrad, B., A. O. Ceballos-Baumann (eds.): Bewegungsstörungen in der Neurologie. Georg Thieme Verlag, Stuttgart, New York, 1996. [64,68]

Deuschl, G.: New treatment options for tremors. N. Engl. J. Med. 2000;342:505–507. [62, 357]

Dichgans, J., T. Klockgether: Krankheiten des Kleinhirns. In: Kunze, K. (eds.): Praxis der Neurologie. Georg Thieme Verlag, Stuttgart, New York, 1999. 411–443. [55]

Diener, H. C., O. Kastrup: Nebenwirkungen medikamentöser Therapie in der Neurologie. In: Brandt, T., J. Dichgans, H. C. Diener (eds.): Therapie und Verlauf neurologischer Erkrankungen. W. Kohlhammer, Stuttgart, Berlin, Köln, 1998. 1275–1289. [389]

Ditunno, J. F., W. Young, W. H. Donovan, G. Creasey: The international standards booklet for neurological and functional classification of spinal cord injuries. Paraplegia 1994;32:70–80. [380]

Donnan,G.A., S.M. Davis, B.R. Chambers, P.C. Gates: Surgery for prevention of stroke. Lancet 1998;351:1372–1373. [174]

Dubowitz, V.: Atlas der Muskelerkrankungen im Kindesalter. Hippokrates Verlag, Stuttgart, 1991. [53, 305, 335, 339, 341, 345]

Duus, P.: Neurologisch-topische Diagnostik. Georg Thieme Verlag, Stuttgart, New York, 1995. [57, 79,85, 87, 111, 358–361]

Dyck, P. J., P. K. Thomas (eds.): Diabetic neuropathy. W. B. Saunders, Philadelphia, London, Toronto, Montreal, Sydney, Tokyo, 1999. [325]

Ebe, M., I. Homma: Leitfaden für die EEG-Praxis. Gustav Fischer Verlag, Stuttgart, Jena, New York, 1992. [309]

Elble, R. J.: Origins of tremor. Lancet 2000;355: 1113–1114. [62]

Fauci, A. S., H. C. Lane: Human immunodeficiency virus (HIV) disease: AIDS and related disorders. In: Fauci, A. S., E. Braunwald, E. M. Isselbacher, J. D. Wilson, J. B. Martin, D. L. Kasper, S. L. Hauser, D. L. Longo (eds.): Harrison's Principles of internal medicine. McGraw-Hill, New York, St. Louis, San Francisco, Colorado Springs, Auckland, 1998. Chapter 308. [241]

Ferro, J. M.: Cardioembolic stroke: an update. Lancet Neurology 2003;2:177–188. [172]

Fischbach, G. D., G. M. McKhann: Cell therapy for Parkinson's disease. N. Engl. J. Med. 2001;344:763–765. [212]

Fishman, R. A.: Cerebrospinal fluid in diseases of the nervous system. W. B. Saunders, Philadelphia, London, Toronto, Montreal, Sydney, Tokyo, 1992. [9, 163]

Fleetwood, I. G., G. K. Steinberg: Arteriovenous malformations. Lancet 2000;359:863–873. [178]

Frick, H., H. Leonhardt, D. Starck: Allgemeine Anatomie—Spezielle Anatomie I. Georg Thieme Verlag, Stuttgart, New York, 1992. [141]

Frisoni, G. B.: Structural imaging in the clinical diagnosis of Alzheimer's disease: problems and tools. J.Neurol.Neurosurg.Psychiatry 2001;70: 711–718. [297]

Gautier, J. C.: Amaurosis Fugax. N. Engl. J. Med. 1993;329:426–428. [168]

Goadsby, P. J., R. B. Lipton, M. D. Ferrari: Migraine— current understanding and treatment. N. Engl. J. Med. 2002;346:257–270. [184]

Glaser, J.S. (ed.): Neuro-ophthalmology. J. B. Lippincott, Philadelphia, 1990. [81, 159]

Gram, L.: Epileptic seizures and syndromes. Lancet 1990;336:161–163. [192, 194]

Grumme, T., W. Kluge, K. Kretzschmar, A. Roesler: Zerebrale und spinale Computertomographie. Blackwell Wissenschafts-Verlag, Berlin, Wien, 1998. [269]

Hacke, W., M. Hennerici, H. J. Gelmers, G. Krämer: Cerebral ischemia. Springer-Verlag, Berlin, Heidelberg, New York, 1991. [171]

Hahn, A. F.: Guillain Barré syndrome. Lancet. 1998;352:635–641. [395]

Hakim, A. M.: Ischemic penumbra. Neurology 1998;51(Suppl. 3):S44–S46. [175]

Hardman, J. G., L. E. Limbird, P. B. Molinoff, R. W. Ruddon, A. G. Gilman (eds.): Goodman & Gilman's The pharmacological basis of therapeutics. McGraw-Hill, New York 1996. [199]

Harms, L.: Tuberkulöse Meningitis. In: Henkes, H., H. W. Kölmel (eds.): Die entzündlichen Erkrankungen des Zentralnervensystems. ecomed, Landsberg/Lech, 1993. II-10/1–II-10/66. [233]

Harper, P. S. (eds.): Huntington's disease. W. B. Saunders, London, Philadelphia, Toronto, Sydney, Tokyo, 1996. [383]

Hartje, W., K. Poeck: Klinische Neuropsychologie. Georg Thieme Verlag, Stuttgart, New York, 1997. [124, 126, 128, 132]

Henkes, H., H.W. Kölmel (eds.): Die entzündlichen Erkrankungen des Zentralnervensystems. ecomed, Landsberg/Lech, 1993. [233, 249,251]

Hichman, S. J., A. J. Lindahl: Minerva. BMJ 1999;318:408. [267]

Hoppenfeld, S.: Orthopädische Neurologie. Ferdinand Enke Verlag, Stuttgart, 1980. [320]

Huber, A., D. Kömpf (eds.): Klinische Neuroophthalmologie. Georg Thieme Verlag, Stuttgart, New York, 1998. [83]

Huber, G., M. Voges: Andere Mißbildungen und Entwicklungsstörungen. In: Sartor, K. (eds.): Neuroradiologie. Georg Thieme Verlag, Stuttgart, New York, 1996. 48–53. [48–53]

Huber, P.: Zerebrale Angiographie für Klinik und Praxis. Georg Thieme Verlag, Stuttgart, New York, 1979. [11–19, 169, 171]

Hudson, L. D., C. M. Lee: Neuromuscular sequelae of critical illness. N. Engl. J. Med. 2003;348:745–747. [347]

International Statistical Classification of Diseases and Related Health Problems (ICD-10). 1989 Revision, World Health Organization, Geneva, 1992.

Inzitari, D., M. Eliasziw, P. Gates, B. L. Sharpe, R. K. T. Chan, H. E. Meldrum, H. J. M. Barnett, the North American Symptomatic Carotid Endarterectomy Trial Collaborators: The causes and risk of stroke in patients with asymptomatic internal-carotid-artery stenosis. N. Engl. J. Med. 2000;342:1693–1701. [174]

Jankovic, J.: Extrapyramidal disorders. In: Wyngaarden, J. B., L. H. South, J. C. Bennett (eds.): Cecil Textbook of medicine. W. B. Saunders, Philadelphia, London, Toronto, Montreal, Sydney, Tokyo, 1991. 2129–2130. [211, 301]

Jankovic, J.: Tourette's Syndrome. N. Engl. J. Med. 2001;345:1184–1192. [68]

Jeffcoate, W. J., K. G. Harding: Diabetic foot ulcers. Lancet 2003;1–7. [324]

Jerusalem, F., S. Zierz: Muskelerkrankungen: Klinik—Therapie—Pathologie. Georg Thieme Verlag, Stuttgart, New York, 1991. [397]

Johns, D. R.: Mitochondrial DNA and disease. N. Engl. J. Med. 1995;333:638–644. [341]

Johnson, R. T.: Viral infections of the nervous system. Lippincott-Raven, Philadelphia, New York, 1998. [234, 239, 253]

Kahle, W.: Nervensystem und Sinnesorgane. Georg Thieme Verlag, Stuttgart, 1979. [7, 9, 34–37, 55, 57, 71ff, 81, 95, 97]

Kandel, E. R., J. H. Schwartz, T. M. Jessell (eds.): Principles of neural science. Prentice-Hall International, London, 1991. [43, 77, 85, 147, 301]

Kapoor, W. N.: Syncope. N. Engl. J. Med.. 2000;343:1856–1862. [200]

Karnofsky, D. A., J. H. Burchenal, G. C. Armistead, C. M. Southam, J. L. Bernstein, L. F. Craver, C. P. Rhoads: Triethylene melamine in the treatment of neoplastic diseases. Arch. Intern. Med. 1951;87:477–516. [264, 378]

Kaye, A. H., E. R. Laws Jr. (eds.): Brain tumors. Churchill Livingstone, Edinburgh, Hongkong, London, Madrid, Melbourne, New York, Tokyo, 1995. [257–261]

Keime-Guibert, F., M. Napolitano, J.-Y. Delattre: Neurological complications of radiotherapy and chemotherapy. J. Neurol. 1998;245:695–708. [389]

Kleihues, P., P. C. Burger, B. W. Scheithauer: The new WHO classification of brain tumors. Brain Pathol. 1993;3:255–268. [377]

Kolb, B., I. Q. Whishaw: Neuropsychologie. Spektrum Akademischer Verlag, Heidelberg, Berlin, New York, 1996. [123, 125]

Krauseneck, P.: Neoplasien. In: Jörg, J. (eds.): Neurologische Therapie. Springer-Verlag, Berlin, Heidelberg, 1997. 242–293. [264f, 377]

Kretschmann, H.-J., W. Weinrich: Klinische Neuroanatomie und kranielle Bilddiagnostik: Computertomographie und Magnetresonanztomographie. Georg Thieme Verlag, Stuttgart, New York, 1991. [13, 17, 169]

Krstic, R. V.: Die Gewebe des Menschen und der Säugetiere. Springer-Verlag, Berlin, Heidelberg, New York, 1978. [3, 317, 331, 335, 337]

Kuhlenbäumer, G., P. Young, G. Hünermund, B. Ringelstein, F. Stögbauer: Clinical features and molecular genetics of hereditary peripheral neuropathies. J.Neurol. 2002;249:1629–1650. [332]

Lance, J. W.: Mechanism and management of headache. Butterworth-Heinemann, Oxford, 1993. [183,189]

Lantos, P. L., S. R. Vandenberg, P. Kleihues: Tumors of the nervous system. In: Graham, D., P. L. Lantos: Greenfield's Neuropathology. Arnold, London, Sydney, Auckland, 1997, 583–879. [264]

Layzer, R. B.: Muscle pain, cramps, and fatigue. In: Engel, A. G., C. Franzini-Armstrong (eds.): Myology. McGraw-Hill, New York, St. Louis, San Francisco, Colorado Springs, Auckland, 1994. 1754–1768. [346]

Leigh, P. N., K. Ray-Chaudhuri: Motor neuron disease. J. Neurol. Neurosurg. Psychiatry 1994;57:886–896. [386]

Lempert, Th.: Synkopen–Phänomenologie und Differenzierung von epileptischen Anfällen. Nervenarzt 1997;68:620–624. [200, 394]

Levin, H. S., A. L. Benton, R. G. Grossman: Neurobehavioral consequences of closed head injury. Oxford University Press, New York, 1982. [269]

Louis, E. D.: Essential tremor. N. Engl. J. Med. 2001;345:887–891. [62]

Low, P. A. (eds.): Clinical autonomic disorders. Lippincott-Raven, Philadelphia, New York, 1997. [149, 151, 153, 155, 157, 370]

Lücking, C. H., C.-W. Wallesch: Phänomenologie und Klinik der Bewußtseinsstörungen. In: Hopf, H. C., K. Poeck, H. Schliack (eds.): Neurologie in Praxis und Klinik. Georg Thieme Verlag, Stuttgart, New York, 1992. 2.1–2.18. [116, 119]

Ludin, H.-P., W. Tackmann (eds.): Polyneuropathien. Georg Thieme Verlag, Stuttgart, New York, 1984. [317]

Lyon, G., R. D. Adams, E. H. Kolodny: Neurology of hereditary metabolic diseases of children. McGraw-Hill, New York 1996. [304]

Mann, D. M. A.: Molecular biology's impact on our understanding of ageing. BMJ 1997;315:1078–1081. [299]

Martin, J. B.: Molecular basis of the neurodegenerative disorders. N. Engl. J. Med. 1999;340:1970–1980. [288]

Masuhr, K. F., M. Neumann: Neurologie. Hippokrates, Stuttgart, 1996. [293]

Matthes, A., H. Schneble: Epilepsien. Georg Thieme Verlag, Stuttgart, New York, 1992. [193, 195, 197, 199]

McDonald, W. I., A. Compston, G. Edan, D. Goodkin, H.-P. Hartung, F. D. Lublin, H. F. McFarland, D. W. Paty, C. H. Polman, S. C. Reingold, M. Sandberg-Wollheim, W. Sibley, A. Thompson, S. van der Noort, B. Y. Weinshenker, J. S. Wolinsky: Recommended diagnostic criteria for multiple sclerosis: guidelines from the International Panel on the Diagnosis of Multiple Sclerosis. Ann.Neurol. 2001;50:121–127. [375]

McNamara, A. M., D. R. P. Guay: Update on drugs that may cause or exacerbate myasthenia gravis. Consult. Pharm. 1997;12:155–164. [403]

Medical Research Council: Aids to the examination of the peripheral nervous system. HMSO, London, 1976. [52]

Mendell, J. R.: Charcot–Marie–Tooth neuropathies and related disorders. Semin. Neurol. 1998;18:41–47. [396]

Montagna, P., P. Gambetti, P. Cortelli, A. Lugaresi: Familial and sporadic fatal insomnia. Lancet Neurology 2003;2:167–176. [114, 252, 280]

Moore, P. M., L. H. Calabrese: Neurologic manifestations of systemic vasculitides. Semin. Neurol. 1994;14:300–306. [180]

Moore, P. M., B. Richardson: Neurology of the vasculitides and connective tissue diseases. J. Neurol. Neurosurg. Psychiatry 1998;65:10–22. [180, 181]

Mumenthaler, M., H. Mattle: Neurologie. Georg Thieme Verlag, Stuttgart, New York, 1997. [93, 173]

Mumenthaler, M.: Neurologische Differentialdiagnostik. Georg Thieme Verlag, Stuttgart, New York, 1997. [61, 131, 374]

Mumenthaler, M., H. Schliack, M. Stöhr (eds.): Läsionen peripherer Nerven und radikuläre Syndrome. Georg Thieme Verlag, Stuttgart, New York, 1998. [33–37, 47, 153, 318–323, 357, 392]

Netter, F. H.: Farbatlanten der Medizin. Band 6: Nervensystem II–Klinische Neurologie. Georg Thieme Verlag, Stuttgart, New York, 1989. [101, 155, 167, 209, 239]

Neville, B. G. R.: Epilepsy in childhood. BMJ 1997;315:924–930. [373]

Nieuwenhuys, R., J. Voogd, C. Van Huijzen: Das Zentralnervensystem des Menschen. Springer-Verlag, Berlin, Heidelberg, New York, 1991. [3, 15, 17, 23, 27, 31, 81, 141, 143, 145, 171, 211, 283]

Noseworthy, J. H., C. Lucchinetti, M. Rodriguez, B. G. Weinshenker: Multiple sclerosis. N. Engl. J. Med. 2000;343:938–952. [214]

Ogilvy, C. S., R. C. Heros: Spinal cord compression. In: Ropper, A. H. (ed.): Neurological and neurosurgical intensive care. Raven Press, New York, 1993. 437–451. [380]

Online Medelian Inheritance in Man (OMIM): National Center for Biotechnology Information. http://www3.ncbi.nlm.nih.gov/omim [280, 398]

Pallis, C., D. H. Harley: ABC of brainstem death. BMJ Publishing Group, London, 1996. [121]

Parsons, M.: A colour atlas of clinical neurology. Wolfe Publishing, London, 1993. [207, 237]

Patten, J.: Neurological differential diagnosis. Springer-Verlag, Berlin, Heidelberg, New York, 1996. [83, 91, 215]

Paty, D. W., D. L. Arnold: The lesions of multiple sclerosis. N. Engl. J. Med. 2002;346:199–200. [218]

Perkin, G. D., F. H. Hochberg, D. C. Miller: Atlas of clinical neurology. Wolfe Publishing, London, 1993. [67, 233]

Phillips, L. H., P. A. Melnick: Diagnosis of myasthenia gravis in the 1990s. Semin. Neurol. 1990;10:62–69. [404]

Platzer,W.: Pernkopf Anatomie. Urban & Schwarzenberg, München, Wien, Baltimore, 1987. [5, 21, 75]

Plum, F., J. B. Posner: The diagnosis of stupor and coma. F. A. Davis Co., Philadelphia, 1980. [119, 151]

Poeck, K., W. Hacke: Neurologie. Springer-Verlag, Berlin, Heidelberg, New York, 1998. [127]

Posner, J. B.: Neurologic complications of cancer. F. A. Davis, Philadelphia, 1995. [263, 285]

Prange, H., A. Bitsch (eds.): Infektionskrankheiten des Zentralnervensystems. Wissenschaftliche Verlagsgesellschaft, Stuttgart, 2001. [224–232]

Prusiner, S. B.: Neurodegenerative diseases and prions. N. Engl. J. Med. 2001;344:1516–1526. [252]

Ptacek, L. J., K. J. Johnson, R. C. Griggs: Genetics and physiology of the myotonic disorders. N. Engl. J. Med. 1993;328:482–489. [401]

Quagliarello, V. J., W. M. Scheld: Bacterial meningitis: pathogenesis, pathophysiology, and progress. N. Engl. J. Med. 1992;327:864–872. [225]

Quagliarello, V. J., W. M. Scheld: Treatment of bacterial meningitis. N. Engl. J. Med. 1997;336: 708–716. [375]

Qureshi, A. I., S. Tuhrim, J. P. Broderick, H. H. Batjer, H. Hondo, D. F. Hanley: Spontaneous intracerebral hemorrhage. N. Engl. J. Med. 2001;344:1450–1460. [176, 178]

Remmel, K. S., R. Bunyan, R. A. Brumback, G. G. Gascon, W. H. Olson: Handbook of symptom-oriented neurology. Mosby, St. Louis, 2002. [47, 277]

Resnick, N. M.: Geriatric medicine. In: Fauci, A. S., E. Braunwald, E. M. Isselbacher, J. D. Wilson, J. B. Martin, D. L. Kasper, S. L. Hauser, D. L. Longo (eds.): Harrison's Principles of internal medicine. McGraw-Hill, New York, St. Louis, San Francisco, Colorado Springs, Auckland, 1998. Chapter 9. [382]

Ricker, K.: Miller-Fisher-Syndrom. Pers. Mitteilung, 1985. [327]

Ropper, A. H. (ed.): Neurological and neurosurgical intensive care. Raven Press, New York, 1993. [151, 163]

Ropper, A. H.: Miller Fisher syndrome and other acute variants of Guillain Barré syndrome. Baillière's Clin. Neurol. 1994;3:95–106. [326, 328]

Rosenberg, R. N. (ed.): Atlas of clinical neurology. Butterworth-Heinemann, Boston, 1998. [287]

Rowland, L. P., N. A. Shneider: Amyotrophic lateral sclerosis. N. Engl. J. Med. 2001;344:1688–1700. [304]

Rudnik-Schöneborn, S., W. Mortier, K. Zerres: Spinale Muskelatrophien. In: Rieß, O., L. Schöls (eds.): Neurogenetik. Springer-Verlag, Berlin, Heidelberg, New York, 1998. 294–308. [385]

Sacco, R. L.: Extracranial carotid stenosis. N. Engl. J. Med. 2001;345:1113–1118. [168ff]

Sadler, T. W.: Medizinische Embryologie. Georg Thieme Verlag, Stuttgart, New York, 1998. [293]

Sartor, K. (eds.): Neuroradiologie. Georg Thieme Verlag, Stuttgart, New York, 2001. [380]

Schaumburg, H. H., A. R. Berger, P. K. Thomas: Disorders of peripheral nerves. F. A. Davis, Philadelphia, 1992. [331, 396]

Scientific Advisory Council of the Federal Chamber of Physicians (Germany): Richtlinien zur Feststellung des Hirntodes. Dt. Ärztebl. 1998;30:49–56. [364]

Schmidt, D.: Epilepsien und epileptische Anfälle. Georg Thieme Verlag, Stuttgart, New York, 1993. [197]

Schmidt, R. F., G. Thews (eds.): Physiologie des Menschen. Springer-Verlag, Berlin, Heidelberg, New York, 1995. [101, 105, 109, 141, 149, 151]

Schnider, A.: Verhaltensneurologie. Georg Thieme Verlag, Stuttgart, New York, 1997. [25, 129, 133, 135, 353]

Schöls, L.: Erkrankungen des peripheren Nervensystems. In: Rieß, O., L. Schöls (eds.): Neurogenetik. Springer-Verlag, Berlin, Heidelberg, New York, 1998. 315–332. [396]

Seddon,H.J.: Three types of nerve injury. Brain. 1943;66:237–288. [330]

Skoog, I., J. Marcusson, K. Blennow: It's getting better all the time. Lancet. 1998;352(Suppl. IV):4. [299]

Speckmann, E.-J., C. E. Elger: Introduction to the neurophysiological basis of the EEG and DC potentials. In: Niedermeyer, E., F. Lopes da Silva (eds.): Electroencephalography—basic principles, clinical applications, and related fields. Williams & Wilkins, Baltimore, 1993. 15–26. [198]

Stefan, H.: Epilepsien—Diagnose und Behandlung. VCH, Weinheim, 1991. [195]

Stöhr, M.: Iatrogene Nervenläsionen. Georg Thieme Verlag, Stuttgart, New York, 1996. [321, 323]

Tandan, R.: Disorders of the upper and lower motor neurons. In: Bradley, W. G., R. B. Daroff, G. M. Fenichel, C. D. Marsden (eds.): Neurology in clinical practice. Butterworth-Heinemann, Boston, Oxford, Singapore, Melbourne, Toronto, Munich, Tokyo, New Delhi, 1996. 1823–1852. [385]

Taylor, B. V., P. J. Dyck: Classification of the diabetic neuropathies. In: Dyck, P. J., P. K. Thomas (eds.): Diabetic neuropathy. W. B. Saunders, Philadelphia, 1999. 407–414. [395]

Teasdale, G. M.: Head injury. J. Neurol. Neurosurg. Psychiatry 1995;58:526–539. [267]

The Deep-Brain Stimulation for Parkinson's Disease Study Group: Deep-brain stimulation of the subthalamic nucleus or the pars interna of the globus pallidus in Parkinson's disease. N. Engl. J. Med. 2001;345:956–963. [212]

Toole, J. F., A. N. Patel: Cerebrovascular disorders. McGraw-Hill, New York, 1974. [169]

Victor,M., A. H. Ropper: Adams & Victor's principles of neurology. McGraw-Hill, New York, 2002. [60, 163]

Warlow, C. P., M. S. Dennis, J. van Gijn, G. J. Hankey, P. A. G. Sandercock, J. M. Bamford, J. M. Wardlaw: Stroke—a practical guide to management. Blackwell Science Ltd., Oxford, 2001. [166 ff]

White, R. J., M. A. Likavec: The diagnosis and initial management of head injury. N. Engl. J. Med. 1992;327:1507–1511. [270, 379]

Wijdicks, E. F. M.: Brain death. Lippincott Williams & Wilkins, Philadelphia 2001. [120, 365]

Zimmermann, M., H. O. Handwerker: Schmerz—Konzepte und ärztliches Handeln. Springer-Verlag, Berlin, Heidelberg, 1984. [109]

Index

A

Aachen aphasia test 124
Abasia 276
Abetalipoproteinemia 280, 281,
   300, 307, 332
Abiotrophy 296
Abscess
   brain 222, 226, 227
      diagnosis 226
      pathogenesis 226
   candida 248
   epidural 222
   tuberculous 232
Absidia 248
Abulia 122, 123
Acalculia 128, 129
Acanthocytes 300, 301
Acetazolamide 338
Acetylcholine 140, 152, 210
Acetylcholine receptor anti-
   body titer 404
Acetylcholinesterase inhibitors
   298, 342
Acid maltase deficiency 340,
   402
Acidosis 162
Acoustic meatus, external 100
Acoustic neuroma 258, 259,
   294
Acquired immunodeficiency
   syndrome (AIDS) 240
   cytomegalovirus and 244
   progressive multifocal
      leukoencephalopathy and
      244
Acrodermatitis chronica
   atrophicans 228
ACTH-secreting tumors 258
Acute demyelinating ence-
   phalomyelitis (ADEM) 234
Acute dystonic reactions 66,
   204, 205
Acute inflammatory demyeli-
   nating polyradiculo-
   neuropathy (AIDP) 395
Acute motor-axonal neuro-
   pathy (AMAN) 395
Acute motor-sensory axonal
   neuropathy (AMSAN) 395
Acyclovir 236, 238

Adaptation, olfactory 76
Adenohypophysis 142
Adenoma, pituitary 258, 259,
   377
Adie syndrome 92
Adrenal medulla 140
Adrenoleukodystrophy 307
Adrenomyeloneuropathy 332,
   384
Ageusia 78
Aging 296, 382
   degenerative changes 296
   disease and 296
Agnosia 132
   body-image 132
   finger 132
Agrammatism 124, 126
Agraphia 128, 129
   alexia with 128
   aphasic 128
   apraxic 128
   isolated 128
   spatial 128, 132
Agyria 381
AIDS *see* Acquired immuno-
   deficiency syndrome
Akathisia 66
Akinesia 206, 208
   Huntington disease 300
Akinetic mutism 120, 122,
   368
Albendazole 250
Alcohol
   intoxication 312, 313
   withdrawal syndrome 312,
      313
Alcoholism 312, 313, 366
   fetal alcohol syndrome 314
   late complications 314
Alexia 128
   agraphia and 128
   anterior 128
   central 128
   isolated 128
Alien hand syndrome 24, 302
Alkalosis 162
Alleles 288
Allodynia 316, 346
Alzheimer disease (AD) 136,
   296–298, 299, 366

agraphia 128
   pathogenesis 297–298
   risk factors 296
   symptoms and signs 297
   treatment 298
   see also Dementia
Amaurosis fugax 82, 168, 372
Amblyopia, tobacco–alcohol
   314
Amimia 362
Amnesia 134, 268, 365, 368
   anterograde 134
   examination 134
   retrograde 134
Amoxicillin 228
Amphetamine abuse 314
Amphotericin B 248
Ampullary crests 56
Amygdala 144
Amyloid precursor protein
   (APP) 297
Amyloid-Aß 297
Amyotrophic lateral sclerosis
   (ALS) 304, 386
   adult-onset 304
   bladder dysfunction and 371
   juvenile 304
   sporadic 304
Amyotrophy, neuralgic 321,
   328, 329
Anal incontinence 370
Anencephaly 292
Anesthesia 106
Aneurysm 178, 179
   fusiform 178
   rupture 176, 178, 179
      treatment 178
   saccular 178
   septic-embolic 178, 226
Angiitis
   cerebral 180
   von Heubner 230
Angiography 354
Angiomatosis
   cutaneous 294
   encephalofacial 294
Angiopathy, amyloid 178
Anhidrosis, generalized 152
Anisocoria 90
Annulus fibrosus 30

Index

Anomia 124
Anosmia 76
  partial 76
Anosognosia 132
Anterocollis 64
Antibiotics 224
  adverse effects 389
  myasthenia gravis aggravation 403
  see also specific drugs and infections
Anticholinergic agents 212
Anticipation 300
Anticoagulants, stroke management 174
Anticonvulsants 198
  myasthenia gravis aggravation 403
Antidepressants, adverse effects 389
Antiemetics, acute dystonic reaction 204
Antiepileptic drugs (AEDs) 198, 264
  laboratory tests 407
  myasthenia gravis aggravation 403
Antimicrobial therapy see Antibiotics
Antioxidants, neuroprotective therapy 212
Antiplatelet therapy, stroke 174
Anton syndrome 132
Anxiety, Parkinson disease and 206
Apallic syndrome 117, 120, 121
Aphasia 124, 126–127
  Alzheimer disease and 297
  amnestic (anomic) 126
  Broca's 126, 127
  conduction 126
  crossed 126
  global 126, 127
  subcortical 126
  test of 124
  transcortical 126, 127
    motor 126
    sensory 126
  Wernicke's 126, 127
Aphemia 124
Apnea test 364
Apo E gene 297
Apomorphine 212
Apraxia 128, 129
  Alzheimer disease and 297
  buccofacial 128

constructional 132
dressing 128, 129, 132
gait 128, 374
ideational 128
ideomotor 128, 129
lid-opening 128, 129, 362
limb 128
Apraxia-like syndromes 128
Aqueduct, cerebral (of Sylvius) 8
Arboviruses 376
Arch, aortic 148, 150
Archeocerebellum 54
Area
  Broca's 124
  postrema 140
  Wernicke's 124
Argyll–Robertson pupils 92, 230
Arousal disorders 116, 117
Arrhythmias, neurogenic 148
Arteriovenous malformations (AVMs) 178, 179
  hemorrhage treatment 178
Arteritis 226, 227
  Takayasu 180
  temporal 180
  see also Vasculitis
Artery(ies)
  age-related changes 382
  basilar 14–15
    occlusion 170, 171
  callosomarginal 12
  carotid 10–12
    common 10
      occlusion 168
    external 10
    internal 10–12
      infarction 168, 169
      occlusion 168
  central
    posterolateral 16
    posteromedial 16
  cerebellar
    infarction 170
    inferior
      anterior 14, 170
      posterior 14, 170, 171
    occlusion 170
    superior 14, 170
  cerebral
    anterior 12, 13
      infarction 168, 169
    middle 12, 13
      occlusion 168, 169
    posterior 16–17
      occlusion 170, 171

    pars circularis 16
    pars terminalis 16
  choroidal, anterior 10
    infarction 168
  communicating
    anterior 12
    posterior 10, 16
  frontobasal 12
  frontobasilar 12
  frontopolar 12
  insular 12
  lenticulostriate 12
    occlusion 168
  medullary 22
  meningeal 6
    middle 10
  occipital
    lateral 16
    medial 16
  ophthalmic 10
    occlusion 168
  paracentral 12
  parietal
    anterior 12
    posterior 12
  parieto-occipital 12
  pericallosal 12
  precuneal 12
  radicular, great (of Adamkiewicz) 22
    occlusion 282
  recurrent, of Heubner 12
  retinal, central 10
  segmental 22
  spinal 22, 23, 283
    anterior 14, 22
      syndrome of 282
    posterior 14, 22
      syndrome of 282
  subclavian
    occlusion 170
    subclavian steal 170
  sulcocommissural artery syndrome 282
  temporal 12
  thalmostriate 12
  vertebral 14–15
    extracranial 14
    intracranial 14
    occlusion 170
Arthralgia, postpolio syndrome 242
Articulation 130
  dysarthria 130
Aspergillus fumigatus (aspergillosis) 248, 249
Aspiration 102

Aspirin, adverse effects 389
Astasia 276
Asterixis 68, 69
Astrocytoma 256, 377
  anaplastic 260, 261, 377
  low-grade 256
  pilocytic 256, 377
Ataxia 107, 276, 374
  autosomal dominant cere-
    bellar (ADCA) 280
  episodic (EA) 280
  Friedreich (FA) 280, 281
  gait 276, 277
  idiopathic cerebellar (IDCA)
    276
  postural 276
  spinal (sensory) 276, 374
  spinocerebellar (SCA) 280,
    384
  truncal 276
Ataxia-telangiectasia 280, 295
Athetosis 383
Atlas 30
Atrophy
  age-related 382
  cerebellar 279
    alcoholism and 314
  cerebral
    alcoholism and 314
    Huntington disease 300
  muscular 49–52, 107, 281,
    287, 334, 406
    peripheral neuropathy and
      316
    poliomyelitis and 242, 243
    spinal (SMA) 385
    spinobulbar 385
  olivopontocerebellar 302
  optic nerve 158, 159
  temporal papillary 215
Attack(s)
  drop 204, 205, 374
  panic 202, 203
  transient ischemic (TIA) 166
    crescendo 166
Attention
  deficits 122, 123
    directed attention 122
    divided attention 122
  evaluation 353
Auditory evoked potentials
  (AEP) 218, 352
Auditory pathway 100, 101
Aura
  migraine 184, 185
  seizure 192
Automatism 124, 126

Autonomic dysfunction 48,
  371
  diabetic neuropathy 324
  multiple sclerosis 216, 217
  neurosyphilis 230
  Parkinson disease 208, 209
  peripheral neuropathies 316,
    390
Autonomic nervous system
  (ANS) 2, 140–141
  central portion 140, 141
    afferent connections 140
    efferent connections 140
    neurotransmitters 140
  enteric 154
  peripheral portion 140–141,
    144–146
    afferent connections 140
    efferent connections 140
    neurotransmitters 140–
      141
  spinal nuclei 140
Autotopagnosia 132
Axis 30
Axonopathy 316
Axonotmesis 330, 331
Axons 2
Azathioprine 180, 220, 342,
  344

B

Babinski sign 40, 49
Baclofen, adverse effects 389
Bacterial infections 226–233
  brain abscess 226, 227
  Lyme disease 228–229
  meningitis/meningo-
    encephalitis 226, 376
  neurosyphilis 230–231
  septic encephalopathy 226
  vasculitis 226
  ventriculitis 226, 227
  see also specific infections
Ballism 66, 383
Bannwarth syndrome 228
Bárány's pointing test 276
Baroreceptors 148
Basilar impression 292, 293
Bassen–Kornzweig syndrome
  300
Becker muscular dystrophy
  336, 337, 400
Behavioral changes 122–123,
  368
  brain tumors 254, 255
  Huntington disease 300

intracranial hypertension
  158, 159
multiple sclerosis 216, 217
normal-pressure hydro-
  cephalus 160
Parkinson disease 206–209
stroke 166
Behçet disease 180, 234
Benedict syndrome 70, 358
Benperidol 204
Benzodiazepines 198
Biopsy 354, 399
  sural nerve 391
"Black-curtain" phenomenon
  168
Bladder dysfunction 156, 371
  multiple sclerosis 216, 217,
    218
  normal-pressure hydro-
    cephalus and 160, 161
  Parkinson disease 208
Bladder function 156, 157
  tests of 218
    residual urine volume 218
    urodynamic electro-
      myography 218
Blepharospasm 64, 65, 362
Blindness, transient monocular
  168, 372
Blink reflex 96, 98
Blood pressure 143, 148, 367
  Parkinson disease and 208
  see also Hypertension; Hy-
    potension
Blood-brain barrier 8–10
  disruption of 224
  multiple sclerosis and 220
  passage of pathogens 224
Blood–CSF barrier 8–10
Body(ies)
  geniculate, lateral 80
  inclusion 52, 252, 344, 345
  Lafora 307
  Lewy 208, 210, 302
  para-aortic 150
Body image perception distur-
  bances 132
Body temperature see Thermo-
  regulation
Body-image agnosia 132
Bone windows 4
Borrelia burgdorferi 228–229
Bourneville–Pringle disease
  294, 295
Bovine spongiform ence-
  phalopathy (BSE) 252
Brachycephaly 381

Index

Index

Bradykinesia 206
Huntington disease 300
Bragard's sign 318
Brain 2
abscess 222, 226, 227
diagnosis 226
pathogenesis 226
blood–brain barrier 8–10
degenerative changes 296, 382
fore brain 2
hind brain 2
mid brain 2, 26
syndromes 70, 71, 358–359
traumatic brain injury (TBI) 266–271
complications 269, 270
evaluation 266
pathogenesis 270, 271
primary injury 266, 270
prognosis 268
secondary sequelae 268, 270
treatment 270
hospital 270
scene of accident 270, 271
types of 266
see also Brain tumors
Brain death 120
Brain stem 2, 3, 24, 26–27
encephalitis 222
hemorrhage 176
syndromes 70–71
Brain tumors 254–265
ACTH-secreting 258
aging and 296
benign 256–257
bladder dysfunction and 371
classification 264
grades of malignancy 377
growth hormone-secreting 258
incidence 264
infratentorial region 258
malignant 260–261
metastatic disease 262–263
treatment 265
severity 264, 377
supratentorial region 258
symptoms and signs 254–255
behavioral changes 254, 255
epileptic seizures 254
focal neurological signs 254, 255

headache 254, 255
intracranial hypertension 254
nausea, vertigo and malaise 254, 255
treatment 264–265
aftercare 265
grade I tumors 264
grade II tumors 264
grade III tumors 264–265
grade IV tumors 265
metastases 265
symptomatic treatment 264
see also specific tumors
Breathing 150, 151
disorders 150, 151
Brivudine 238
Broca's
aphasia 126, 127
area 124
Bromocriptine 212
Bromopride 204
Brown–Séquard syndrome 48
Brudzinski's sign 222
Bruxism 114
Bundle, medial fore brain 144
Bupidine 212
Burns 312
Burst fracture 380

C

Cabergoline 212
Calcium antagonists
acute dystonic reaction 204
adverse effects 389
Calcium balance 310
Calcium channel dysfunction 338, 398
Caloric testing 26
Calvaria 4
metastases 262
Canal
ear 100
infraorbital 4
semicircular 56
spinal 30, 31
vestibular 100
Canalolithiasis 58
Candida albicans (candidosis) 248, 249
Capsule, internal, hemorrhage 176
Carbamazepine 198, 264
Carcinoma
choroid plexus 377
meningitis and 262

Cardiomyopathy 397
Carnitine deficiency 340, 402
Carnitine palmitoyl transferase (CPT) deficiency 402
Carpal tunnel syndrome 322
Cataplexy 374
Cataract 382
myotonic 338
Cauda equina 2
syndrome 319
Causalgia 110
Cavernoma 178, 179
Cefotaxime 228
Ceftriaxone 226, 228
Central core disease 402
Central nervous system (CNS) 2
infections 222–225
clinical manifestations 222
course of 222
localization 222, 223
opportunistic infections 240
pathogenesis 224, 225
prophylaxis 224
treatment 224
see also specific infections
see also Brain; Spinal cord
Central pontine myelinolysis 310, 315
alcoholism and 314
Central salt-wasting syndrome 310
Cerebellitis, acute 238
Cerebellum 2, 24, 42, 54–55
diseases 276–281
acquired 278–279
atrophy 279
alcoholism and 314
diagnostic studies 276
hereditary 280–281
autosomal dominant 280
autosomal recessive 280
signs of dysfunction 276
topography of lesions 276
see also specific diseases
hemorrhage 176
Cerebral blood flow (CBF) 162
hemodynamic insufficiency 174
hypoperfusion 174
Cerebral cortex 24–25
Brodmann classification 24, 25
cytoarchitecture 24
functional areas 24
ischemia 148

motor 42
  primary 42
    lesions 46
  supplementary 42
  premotor area 42
  projection areas 24
Cerebral palsy, infantile 288–291, 381
  causes 288
  symptoms and signs 288
  treatment 290
Cerebral perfusion pressure (CPP) 162
Cerebral vascular resistance (CVR) 162
Cerebral ventricles 8, 9
Cerebritis 222, 226
Cerebrospinal fluid (CSF) 8–9
  blood–CSF barrier 8–10
  circulation 8, 9
    impaired 160, 161, 372
  intracranial hypotension and 160
  leak 269, 372, 379
  lymphoma and 260
  multiple sclerosis and 218
  pressure measurement 161
  viral meningoencephalitis and 234
  volume 162
Cervical syndrome 188, 189
  upper 188
Charcot joints 230
Chemodetectoma 258
Chemoreceptors 104, 150, 151
Chemotherapy 264–265
  adverse effects 389
Cheyne–Stokes respiration 118
Chiari malformation 292, 293
Chiasm, optic 80
  lesions 82
Chickenpox 238
  symptoms and signs 238
Chloride channel disease 398
Chlorprothixene 264
Cholinergic crisis 404
Chondrosarcoma 260
Chorda tympani lesions 78
Chordoma 258, 259
Chorea 66–67, 300, 383
  secondary 66
  Sydenham's 66
Choreoathetosis 66
Chromosomal anomalies 381
Chronic inflammatory demyelinating polyradiculoneuropathy (CIDP) 327, 328

Chronic paroxysmal hemicrania (CPH) 186, 190
Chronobiology 112
Chronopathology 112
Churg–Strauss syndrome 180, 344
Cidofovir 244
Cingulate gyrus lesions 122
Cinnarizine 204
Ciprofloxacin 226
Circadian rhythm 112, 113
  disturbances 114
Circle of Willis 10, 12, 13
Circulation 148–149
  anterior 10
  central nervous regulation 148
  cerebrospinal fluid 8, 9
    impaired 160, 161, 372
  posterior 10
Cistern(s) 8
  ambient 8
  cerebellomedullary (cisterna magna) 8
  cerebellopontine 8
  chiasmatic 8
  interpeduncular 8
  posterior 8
Claudication, spinal 282, 284, 285
Clindamycin/folinic acid 250
Clock/numbers test 136, 137
Cluster headache see Headache
Cocaine abuse 314
Cochlea 100, 101
Cognitive impairment
  Alzheimer disease 297
  Huntington disease 300
Colon 154
Column
  Clarke's 104
  vertebral 30
Coma 92, 118–119
  pupillary dilatation 92
  pupilloconstriction 92
  staging 118–119, 267
    brain stem reflexes 118
    Glasgow coma scale 378
    respiratory pattern abnormalities 118
    spontaneous movement 118
    stimuli 118
Comalike syndromes 120–121
  akinetic mutism 120, 122, 368
  locked-in syndrome 120, 121, 170, 359

persistent vegetative state 120
Commissure, anterior 144
Complex regional pain syndrome (CRPS) 110
Compliance 162
Compression
  fracture 380
  nerve injuries 330
Computed tomography (CT) 354
  brain tumors 260, 265
  head trauma and 266
  multiple sclerosis 218
Confabulation 134
Confusion 116, 117, 368
  Alzheimer disease 297
Connective tissue diseases 234
Consciousness 116–117
  acute disturbances 116–117
    arousal disorders 116, 117
    confusion 116, 117
    somnolence 116, 117
    stupor 116, 117
  assessment of 116
  content of 116
  head trauma and 266, 267
    assessment 379
  level of 116
  normal state of 116, 117
  psychogenic disturbances 120
  stroke and 166
  see also Coma
Constipation 370
  Parkinson disease 208
Continence 156
  see also Incontinence
Conus medullaris 2
Conversion disorders 138
Convulsions, neonatal 196
  see also Seizures
Coordination dysfunction 276
  multiple sclerosis 216, 217
Corneal reflex 26, 96
Corpus callosum 24
  agenesis 290
Cortex
  auditory 100, 101
    primary 100
    secondary 100
  entorhinal 144
  premotor, lesions 122
  somatosensory 108
  see also Cerebral cortex
Corticobasal degeneration (CBD) 302, 303

Corticosteroids 143, 264, 342, 344
  adverse effects 389
  multiple sclerosis treatment 220
Cortisol 367
Cough reflex 26
Coumarins, adverse effects 389
Craniocervical junction anomalies 292
Craniopharyngioma 258, 259, 377
  adamantinomatous 258
  papillary 258
  treatment 264
Craniostenosis 381
Cranium 4
  roof 4
  see also Skull
Creatine kinase elevation 397
Creutzfeldt–Jakob disease (CJD) 252, 253
Crisis
  cholinergic 404
  myasthenic 404
Critical illness myopathy (CIM) 347, 379
Critical illness polyneuropathy (CIP) 347, 379
Crow–Fukase syndrome 328
Cryptococcus neoformans (cryptococcosis) 248, 249
Cupulae 56
Cyanocobalamin 286
Cyclophosphamide 180, 220, 328
Cyst
  arachnoid 290, 291
  colloid 258, 259
  porencephalic 290
Cysticercosis 250, 251
Cytokines 220
Cytomegalovirus (CMV) 244–245
  pathogenesis 244
  symptoms and signs 244

D

Dandy–Walker malformation 292
Dantrolene 347
Death 120–121, 364
Debrancher deficiency 340
Decerebration syndrome 46, 47, 118, 158, 159

Decortication syndrome 46, 47, 118
Deep brain stimulation 212
Deficiency
  acid maltase 340, 402
  carnitine 340, 402
  carnitine palmitoyl transferase (CPT) 402
  debrancher 340
  folic acid 286
  muscle phosphorylase 402
  phosphofructokinase 402
  vitamin B1 312
  vitamin B12 286, 287
  vitamin E 280
Degeneration 382
  corticobasal (CBD) 302, 303
  panthothenate kinase-associated 307
  striatonigral (SND) 302
  subacute combined (SCD) 286, 287
Degenerative changes 296
  radicular syndromes and 392
  see also Neurodegenerative diseases
Deglutition 102, 103
  disturbances 102, 103
  mechanism 102
  nerve pathways 102, 103
Dehydration 372
Dejerine–Sottas disease 332
Delirium 116, 368
  tremens 312
Dementia 136–137
  alcoholic 314, 366
  bladder dysfunction and 371
  classification 366
  diagnosis 136
    differential 383
  dialysis 310
  examination 136
  frontotemporal (FTD) 298, 299
  Parkinson disease and 208
  thalamic 116
  vascular 298, 299, 366
    multi-infarct 298
    strategic infarct 298
  with Lewy bodies 208, 302
  see also Alzheimer disease
Demyelination 220
Dens fracture 380
Depersonalization 202
Depression 366
  cortical spreading 184

differential diagnosis 383
  Parkinson disease and 206
Derealization 202
Dermatomes 32–36
Dermatomyositis 344, 345, 406
Developmental anomalies 288, 381
Diabetes mellitus 324, 325
Diabetic
  ketoacidosis 308
  neuropathy 324, 325, 395
    diagnosis 324
    symptoms and signs 324
    treatment 324
  pandysautonomia 395
Dialysis encephalopathy 310, 311
Diaphragma sellae 6
Diarrhea 370
Diencephalon 2
Diffuse Lewy body disease (DLB) 302
Diploë 4
Diplopia 86
  multiple sclerosis 214
Disconnection syndrome 24, 128
Disequilibrium syndrome 310
Disk(s)
  intervertebral 30
    herniation 318, 319, 392
  optic 80
Dislocation
  atlantoaxial 380
  fracture 380
Disorientation 132–133
  right–left 132
"Doll's eye" phenomenon 26, 302, 303
  coma and 118
Dopamine 210
  age-related changes 382
  Parkinson disease and 210
Dopamine agonists 208, 212
  adverse effects 389
Dopaminergic agents 212
Doxycycline 228
Drooling 206, 207
Drop attacks 204, 205, 374
Drop metastasis 260, 262
Duchenne muscular dystrophy 52, 53, 336, 337, 400
Duplex sonography 353
Dura mater 6
  fistula 178, 282, 283
  injuries 266
  spinal 30

Dysarthria 124, 130, 166, 276, 365
Dysarthrophonia 206, 276
Dysdiadochokinesia 276, 277
Dysesthesia 106, 316
Parkinson disease and 208
Dysgeusia 78
Dyskinesia(s)
drug-induced 66
orofacial 66, 67
tardive 66
Dysmetria 276, 277
ocular 276
Dysosmia 76
Dysphagia 102, 166, 370, 397
causes 362
Dysphonia 130
Dysplasia 288
Dysraphism, spinal 292, 293, 381
Dyssomnia 114, 116
Dyssynergy 276
Dystonia 64–65, 383
action 6
acute dystonic reactions 66, 204, 205
arm 64
cervical 64, 65
classification 64
craniocervical 64, 65
dopa-responsive 64
idiopathic torsion 64
leg 64
multifocal 65
oromandibular 64, 362
Parkinson disease 208, 209
paroxysmal, autosomal dominant 64
spastic 64
task-specific 64
Dystrophinopathy 336, 398
Dystrophy
limb-girdle 336, 337, 400
myotonic 52, 338, 339, 400, 401
reflex sympathetic 110
see also Muscular dystrophies

E

Ecchymosis, retroauricular 267
ECG abnormalities, neurogenic 148
Echolalia 124
Edema
cerebral 162, 163, 224

cytotoxic 162
hydrocephalic 162–163
treatment 264
vasogenic 162
leg, Parkinson disease and 208
Edinger–Westphal nucleus 26, 90
Edrophonium chloride test 404
Ejaculatory dysfunction 156
Elastance 162
Electro-oculography 352
Electroencephalography 352
Electrogustometry 78
Electrolyte balance disorders 310, 311
Electromyography (EMG) 352
myasthenia gravis 404
needle 391, 399
stimulation 399
urodynamic 218
Electroneurography 352
Embolism 172, 173
infectious 226
paradoxical 262
Emery–Dreifuss muscular dystrophy 336, 337
Empyema, subdural 222
Encephalitis 222
brain stem 222
clinical manifestations 222
hemorrhagic necrotizing 236
Lyme disease and 228
toxoplasmosis and 250
viral 234, 376
herpes simplex 236
Encephalocele 292
Encephalomyelitis 222
acute demyelinating (ADEM) 234
Lyme 228
Encephalopathy 306–315
burns and 312
chronic 308
dialysis 310, 311
endocrine 310, 311
hepatic 308, 309, 387
HIV 240
hypoxic–ischemic 308, 309
iatrogenic 314, 315, 389
Lyme disease and 228
metabolic 386–387
acquired 308–312
hereditary 306–307
infancy 387
neonatal 386

mitochondrial 281
multiple organ failure and 312
paraneoplastic 312
portosystemic 308, 387
progressive myoclonic 68
septic 226, 227, 312, 313
diagnosis 226
spongiform 252–253
bovine (BSE) 252
Creutzfeldt–Jakob disease (CJD) 252, 253
genetic 252
infectious 252
subcortical arteriosclerotic (SAE) 298
substance abuse and 312, 313
trauma and 379
uremic 310, 311
Wernicke 312, 313
Endarterectomy 174
Endocarditis, bacterial 226
Endocrine
encephalopathy 310, 311
myopathy 347, 398
Endolymph 56
Endoneurium 2
Endophthalmitis, candida 248
Entacapone 212
Enteroviruses 376
Enuresis 114
Eosinophilic fasciitis 344
Ependyma 6
spinal 256
Ependymoma 256, 257, 377
anaplastic 260, 377
Epidural
abscess 222
hematoma 268, 270
space 6, 30
Epilepsy 192–199
acquired 198
acute epileptic reactions 196
age of onset 197
causes 198, 379
classification 196–197
epileptic syndromes 196
generalized 194, 196
genetic predisposition 198
location-related 196
myoclonus
progressive, with Lafora bodies 307
with ragged red fibers (MERRF) 403
pathophysiology 198, 199

Epilepsy
  prognosis 198, 373
  seizure types 192–195, 373
    generalized 193, 194–195, 197
    grand mal 194, 195, 199
    partial (focal) 192–194, 197
  status epilepticus 196
    grand mal 196
  treatment 198
    antiepileptic drugs 198
  unclassified 196
  see also Seizures
Epineurium 2, 30
Episodic
  ataxia (EA) 280
  headache
    cluster 186, 190
    tension 182, 190
  memory 134
  paralysis 338, 339, 401
  vertigo 58
Epithelium, olfactory 76
Erb palsy 318
Erectile dysfunction 156
Erythema chronicum migrans 228, 229
Esophagus 154
Essential tremor 62, 357
Estradiol 367
Ethosuximide 198
Evoked potentials 352
  auditory (AEP) 218, 352
  motor (MEP) 218, 352
  somatosensory (SEP) 218, 352
  visual (VEP) 218, 219, 352
Examination 350–351
  see also specific conditions
Excitotoxicity 300
Executive functions 122
Exons 288
Expiration 150
Exteroceptors 104
Extinction phenomenon 132
Eye movements 84, 85
  convergence 90
  intracranial hypertension and 158
  reflex 84
  vergence movements 84
  voluntary 84

F

Fabry disease 307, 332
Factitious symptoms 138, 139
Falling 374
Falx
  cerebelli 6
  cerebri 6
Famcyclovir 238
Familial spastic paraplegia (FSP) 286, 287, 384
Fascicles 2
Fasciculations 50
Fasciculus
  arcuate 124
  cuneatus (lateral) 104
  gracilis (medial) 104
  longitudinal, medial 56, 84
Fasciitis, eosinophilic 344
Fatal familial insomnia 114, 280
Fatigue, multiple sclerosis 214
Felbamate 198
Festination 206
Fetal alcohol syndrome 314
Fever 152, 268
Fiber(s)
  commissural 24
  corticopontine 44
  parasympathetic 90, 140, 154, 156
  preganglionic 140
  sudoriparous 152
  sympathetic 90, 140, 154, 156
  taste 96
  "U fibers" 244
Fibromyalgia 52
Fibrosarcoma 260
Fila olfactoria 76
Filum terminale 2
  externum 30
  internum 30
Finger agnosia 132
Finger–finger test 276, 277
Finger–nose test 276
First aid 270, 271
Fistula, dural 178, 282, 283
Fits see Seizures
Fluconazole 248
Flucytosine 248
Fluid balance 143, 268, 367
  disorders 310
Flunarizine 204
Fluphenazine 204
Folic acid deficiency 286
Foramen(ina)

interventricular, of Monroe 8, 258
  of Luschka 8
  of Magendie 8
  vertebral 30
Forgetfulness 134
  benign senescent 134, 136
  see also Memory
Fornix 144, 145
Foscarnet 244
Fossa, cranial 4
  anterior 4
  middle 4
  posterior 4, 18
Fovea 80
Fracture
  skull 266
  vertebral 272, 380
    atlantoaxial dislocation 380
    bilateral axis arch 380
    burst 380
    compression 380
    dens 380
    dislocation 380
    Jefferson's 380
    stability 272, 273
Frey syndrome 362
Friedreich ataxia 280, 281
Fronto-orbital lesions 122
Fungal infections 180, 248–249
  aspergillosis 248, 249
  candidosis 248, 249
  cryptococcosis 248, 249
  mucormycosis 248, 249

G

Gabapentin 198
Gag reflex 26
Gait 60
  antalgic 60
  apraxia 128, 374
  ataxia 60, 61, 276–277
  cycle 60, 61
  disturbances 49, 60–61
    factitious 139
    intracranial hypertension 158
    neurosyphilis 230
    normal-pressure hydrocephalus 160, 161
    Parkinson disease 206, 207
  dystonic 60, 61
  spastic 60, 61
  steppage 60, 61
  waddling 60

Galactosemia 386
Galea aponeurotica 4
Gamma-aminobutyric acid (GABA) 140, 300
Gancyclovir 244
Gangliocytoma 377
Ganglioglioma 377
  anaplastic 377
Ganglioma, parasympathetic 258
Ganglion(a)
  basal 24, 42, 210, 211
    connections 210, 211
    hemorrhage 176
    Parkinson disease and 210, 211
  dorsal root 2
  spinal 2
  trigeminal
    central connections 94, 95
    peripheral connections 94, 95
    varicella-zoster and 238
Ganglioneuropathy 390
Ganglionitis 238
Gangliosidosis
  GM1 307, 387
  GM2 307
Ganser syndrome 138
Gastrointestinal function 154–155
  neurological causes of dysfunction 370
Gastroparesis 370
Gaucher disease 306, 307, 387
Gaze deviation
  contralateral 86
  skew 70, 89
Gaze palsy 88
  contralateral 86
  ipsilateral 86
  Parkinson disease 208
  progressive supranuclear palsy 303
Genetic predisposition
  epilepsy 198
  Parkinson disease 213
  spongiform encephalopathies 252
Genotype 288, 289
Germinoma 258, 377
Gerstmann syndrome 128
Gerstmann–Sträussler–Scheinker syndrome 280
Giant axon neuropathy 397
Gibberish, fluent 124

Gilles de la Tourette syndrome 68
Glasgow coma scale 378
Glatiramer acetate 220
Glioblastoma 260, 261, 265, 377
Glioma
  butterfly 260
  mixed 377
Gliomatosis cerebri 260
Globus
  hystericus 102
  pallidus 210
Glomeruli, olfactory 76
Glomus
  carotid 150
  tumor 377
Glutamate 140, 210
  antagonists 212
Glutamate decarboxylase 300
Glycerol 264
Glycogen storage disease 340
Goiter 311
Gonadotropins 143
Gordon reflex 40
Granulomatosis
  lymphomatoid 180
  Wegener 180
Growth hormones 143, 367
  GH-secreting tumors 258
Guillain–Barré syndrome 244, 326–327, 395
  clinical spectrum 395
  diagnosis 326, 396
  pathogenesis 326
  symptoms and signs 326
  treatment 326
Gustatory pathway 78
Gyrus(i)
  angular 124
  cingulate 144
  dentate 144
  postcentral 12
  precentral 12

H

Haemophilus influenzae 376
  chemoprophylaxis 226
  vaccination 226
Hair cells 100
Hallucinations
  olfactory 76
  Parkinson disease 208
Haloperidol 204
Hand grip test 369
Hangover 188

Hartnup disease 306
Head injury 267
  assessment criteria 379
  classification 267
  complications 269, 379
  see also Trauma
Head, zones of 110, 111
Headache 182–191, 373
  brain tumors and 254, 255
  cervical syndrome 188, 189
    upper 188
  chronic daily 182
    causes 373
  chronic paroxysmal hemicrania (CPH) 186, 190
  cluster 186, 187, 190
    chronic 186, 190
    episodic 186, 190
    pathogenesis 186
  combination 182
  diagnostic classification 191
  ice-pick 182
  intracranial hypertension and 158
  intracranial hypotension and 160
  migraine 184–185, 190, 373
    symptoms and signs 184
      aura 184, 185
      headache phase 184
      prodromal phase 184
      resolution phase 184
  nociceptive transmission 188, 189
  posttraumatic 270, 271
  prophylaxis 190
  sinus 186, 187
  substance-induced 188, 189
    acute 188
    rebound 188
  tension 182, 183
    chronic 182, 190, 373
    episodic 182, 190
    pathogenesis 182
  treatment 182, 190
  trigeminal neuralgia 186, 187, 190
    idiopathic 186
    pathogenesis 186
    symptomatic 186
  vascular processes and 166, 182, 183
    subarachnoid hemorrhage 176
Hearing 100–101
  age-related changes 382
  sound perception 100

Heart 148–149
Heel–knee–shin test 276
Heerfordt syndrome 362
Helicotrema 100
Hemangioblastoma 256, 257
Hemangioma 294
Hemangiopericytoma 377
Hematoma 268
    epidural 268, 270
    intracerebral 270
    intraparenchymal 268
    posttraumatic 267
    subarachnoid 268
    subdural 268, 270
        chronic 379
Hemianopsia 82
    heteronymous 82
    homonymous, altitudinal 82
Hemiballism 66–67
Hemicrania, chronic paroxys-
    mal (CPH) 186, 190
Hemineglect 132
Hemiparesis 47, 122
    contralateral 46, 158
Hemiplegia 122
    alternans 46
Hemodynamic abnormalities
    148, 174
Hemorrhage 166, 176–179
    intracerebral 166, 167, 176
        basal ganglia 176
        brain stem 176
        caudate 176
        cerebellar 176
        complications 176
        lobar 176
        massive hypertensive 178
        pathogenesis 178
        pontine 176
        putaminal 176
        thalamic 176
        treatment 178
    intraventricular 166, 176,
        177, 270
        complications 176
        symptoms and signs 176
    spinal 282
    subarachnoid 166, 176–177,
        270
        complications 176
        pathogenesis 178
        symptoms and signs 176
    treatment 178
    see also Stroke
Hepatic encephalopathy 308,
    309, 387
Hereditary diseases 288

diagnosis 288
inheritance 288, 289
mutations 288
phenotype 288
see also specific diseases
Hereditary hemorrhagic tel-
    angiectasia (HHT) 294
Hereditary motor–sensory
    neuropathy (HMSN) 332,
    333, 396
    type I 332, 333, 396
    type II 332, 396
    type III 332, 396
Hereditary neuropathy with
    pressure palsies (HNPP) 332,
    333
Hering–Breuer reflex 150
Herniation
    intervertebral disk 318, 319,
        392
    intracranial hypertension
        and 158, 159, 162
    subfalcine 162
    transtentorial 118, 158
Herpes labialis 236
Herpes simplex 236–237, 376
    pathogenesis 236
    symptoms and signs 236
    treatment 236
    type 1 (HSV-1) 236, 237
    type 2 (HSV-2) 236
Herpes zoster 180, 238, 239
    occipitocollaris 238
    ophthalmicus 238
    oticus 238
    sine herpete 238
    symptoms and signs 238
Hiccups 68
Hippocampus 144, 145
Histiocytoma, malignant
    fibrous 260
History taking 350
Holmes tremor 357
Homocystinuria 307
Hormones
    aglandotropic 142
    glandotropic 142
    growth 143
    thyroid 143
    see also specific hormones
Horner syndrome 48, 92, 152,
    318
    central 92
Hospital hopper 138
Human immunodeficiency
    virus (HIV) 240–241, 376
    antiretroviral therapy 240

pathogenesis 240, 241
primary infection 240
secondary complications
    240
symptoms and signs 240
Huntington 300
Huntington disease 66, 300,
    301
    inheritance 300
        anticipation 300
    pathogenesis 300
    symptoms and signs 300
    Westphal variant 300
Hydranencephaly 290, 381
Hydrocephalus 161–163, 290,
    291, 366, 379, 381
    acute 162, 290
    brain edema 162–163
    chronic 162
    communicating/malresorp-
        tive 162
    congenital 290
    external 162
    non-communicating/ob-
        structive 162, 258, 290
    normal-pressure 160, 161,
        162
    subarachnoid hemorrhage
        and 176
    symptoms and signs 290
    treatment 290
Hydrochlorothiazide 338
Hydrophobia 246, 247
Hydroxocobalamin 286
Hygroma, subdural 379
Hyperalgesia 316
Hyperammonemia 386
Hypercalcemia 310
Hypercapnia 308
Hypereosinophilia syndrome
    344
Hyperesthesia 316
Hyperglycemia 308, 324
    hyperosmolar nonketonic
        308
Hyperglycinemia, nonketonic
    386
Hyperhidrosis, Parkinson dis-
    ease and 208
Hyperkalemia 52, 338, 401
Hyperkinesia 383
Hypermetria 70
Hyperprolactinemia 258
Hypersomnia 114, 116
Hypertension 148
    intracerebral hemorrhage
        and 178

intracranial 158–160, 224, 268, 290
  causes 371
  treatment 264, 270
Hyperthermia
  central 152
  malignant 346–347
Hypertrophy, muscular 334, 338, 397
Hyperventilation syndrome 204, 205, 370
Hypervolemia 310
Hypesthesia 106
Hypocalcemia 310
Hypochondriacal disorder 138, 139
Hypogeusia 78
Hypoglycemia 308, 309, 324
  acute 308
  chronic 308
  subacute 308
Hypokalemia 52, 338
Hypokinesia 206
Hypomagnesemia 310
Hypometria 70
Hypomimia 206, 207, 362
Hypoperfusion 174
Hypophonia 206
Hyposmia 76
Hypotension 148, 268
  antiparkinsonian medications and 208
  idiopathic orthostatic 302
  intracranial 160–161
    causes 372
Hypothalamic–pituitary regulatory axis 367
Hypothalamus 24, 140, 142–143
  functions 142
    fluid balance 310
    thermoregulation 152
  neuroendocrine control 142, 143
  pain and 108
Hypothermia 152
Hypothyroidism 311
Hypoventilation 370
Hypovolemia 310
Hypoxia 268
  global cerebral 172
  hypoxic–ischemic encephalopathy 308, 309

I

Iatrogenic encephalopathy 314, 315, 389
Idiopathic
  cerebellar ataxia (IDCA) 276
  orthostatic hypotension 302
  Parkinson disease 302
  torsion dystonia 64
  trigeminal neuralgia 186
Immunization *see* Vaccination
Incisura, tentorial 6
Inclusion body myositis 52, 252, 344, 345
Incontinence
  fecal 216, 370
  urinary *see* Bladder dysfunction
Incus 100
Infantile cerebral palsy
  see Cerebral palsy
Infarction 172, 174
  anterior cerebral artery 168
  anterior choroidal artery 168
  border zone 168, 172, 173
  cerebellar arteries 170
  dementia and 298
    multi-infarct dementia 298
    strategic infarct dementia 298
  dorsolateral 170
  end zone 172, 173
  hemodynamic 172
  internal carotid artery 168, 169
    border zone 168
    territorial 168
  lacunar 168, 172
  low-flow 172
  paramedian 170
  pontine 170
  spinal
    central 282
    complete 282
  territorial 168, 172, 173, 224
    hemorrhagic conversion 172
  threshold 174
  types of 172
Infections *see* Central nervous system (CNS); *specific infections*
Inflammatory response 224
  multiple sclerosis 220
  tuberculous meningitis 232
Infundibulum 6

Inheritance 288, 289
  monogenic 288
  multifactorial 288
  polygenic 288
Innervation ratio 44
Insomnia 114
  fatal familial 114, 280
  psychogenic 114
Inspiration 150
Interoceptors 104
Intervertebral disks 30
Intestine
  colon 154
  pseudo-obstruction 370
  small 154
Intoxication 312, 313
Intracranial pressure (ICP) 158–163
  brain tumors and 254
  compliance 162
  elastance 162
  hypertension 158–160, 268, 290
    causes 371
    clinical features 158–160
    treatment 264, 270
  hypotension 160–161
    causes 372
    symptoms 160
  pathogenesis 162
Introns 288
Involution 296
Iodine–starch (Minor) test 152
Iris 90
Ischemia 166, 268
  cerebral 148
    delayed 176
    global 172
    hypoxic–ischemic encephalopathy 308, 309
    threshold 174
    transient ischemic attack (TIA) 166
    see also Stroke
Ischemic penumbra 174
Isocortex 24
Isoniazid 232
Itraconazole 248

J

Jaw jerk reflex 26
JC virus 244
Jefferson's fracture 380
Jet lag 114
Joints, Charcot 230
Jugum sphenoidale 4

K

Karnofsky scale 26, 378
Kearns–Sayre syndrome (KSS) 403
Keratoconjunctivitis 236
Kernig's sign 222
King–Denborough syndrome 347
Klippel–Feil syndrome 292, 293
Klumpke–Dejerine palsy 318
Korsakoff syndrome 76, 308, 312
Krabbe disease 307, 332, 387
Kufs disease 307
Kussmaul's respiration 118

L

Labyrinth 56
Lacrimation, test of 98
Lacunar state 172, 173
Lacunes 172, 298
Lambert–Eaton myasthenic syndrome (LEMS) 50, 52, 342, 343, 406
Lamotrigine 198
Lance–Adams syndrome 308
Language 124–125
    aphasia 124, 126–127
    model 124
Larynx, voice production 130
Lasègue's sign 318
Laterocollis 64
Lathyrism 286, 304, 384
Law of Bell and Magendie 30
Leigh disease 306
    maternally-inherited (MILS) 403
Lemniscus, trigeminal 94
Lennox–Gastaut syndrome 196, 198
Lens accommodation 90
Leprosy 328, 329
Leptomeninges 6
    metastases 262, 263
    treatment 265
Leukoaraiosis 298
Leukodystrophy
    globoid cell 387
    metachromatic 306, 307, 332, 333
Leukoencephalitis 234
Levetiracetam 198
Levodopa 208, 212
    adverse effects 389

Levomepromazine 264
Lewy bodies 208, 210, 302
Lhermitte's sign 48, 49, 214
Life expectancy 296
    active 296
Lifespan 296
Ligament, denticulate 30
Light reflex 90, 91
Light–near dissociation 92
Limb girdle dystrophy 336, 337, 400
Limbic system 80, 135, 144–145
    functions 144
    nerve pathways 144
    pain and 108
    structure 144, 145
    syndromes 368
Lipid metabolism disorders 332, 333
Lissencephaly 381
Listeria 376
Lisuride 212
Lobe
    frontal
        hemorrhage 176
        lesions 122
            left 122
            right 122
    occipital, hemorrhage 176
    parietal, hemorrhage 176
    temporal, hemorrhage 176
Locked-in syndrome 120, 121, 170, 359
LSD abuse 314
Lumbar puncture 2, 407
    intracranial hypotension and 160
    multiple sclerosis and 218, 219
Lungs 150
Lyme disease 228–229
    chronic 228
    clinical manifestations 228, 229
    diagnosis 228
    pathogenesis 228
    treatment 228
    Lymphadenosis benigna cutis 228
Lymphoma 180, 377, 385
    cerebral, primary 260, 261, 265
        ocular manifestations 260
    non-Hodgkin 260, 261

M

McLeod syndrome 300
Macroadenoma 258
Macrocephaly 290, 381
Macrographia 276
Macrophages 220
Maculae 56
    saccular 56
    utricular 56
Magnesium balance 310
Magnetic resonance imaging (MRI) 354
    brain tumors 260, 264–265
    multiple sclerosis 218, 219
Major histocompatibility complex (MHC) 220
Malaise, brain tumors and 254
Malaria, cerebral 250, 251
Malformations 288, 381
    Chiari 292, 293
    Dandy–Walker 292
Malignancy *see* Brain tumors; *specific tumors*
Malignant hyperthermia 346–347
Malignant neuroleptic syndrome 208, 347
Malingering 138
Malleus 100
Mannitol 264
Maple syrup urine disease 386
Marcus–Gunn pupils 214
MDMA abuse 314
Mean arterial pressure (MAP) 162, 174
Mechanoreceptors 104, 150
Medulla, adrenal 140
Medulla oblongata 2, 26
    caudal 148
    lesions 70
    rostral 148
    syndromes 70, 73, 361
        dorsolateral 361
Medulloblastoma 260, 261, 265
Megalencephaly 381
Meige syndrome 64, 362
Melkersson–Rosenthal syndrome 362
Melperone 264
Membrane(s)
    arachnoid 6
        spinal 30
    basilar 100
    tympanic 100
Memory 134–135

declarative (explicit) 134, 135
disorders 134, 368
  Alzheimer disease 297
  head trauma and 269
  Parkinson disease 208
episodic 134
examination 134, 353
long-term 134
nondeclarative (implicit) 134, 135
semantic 134
short-term 134
Ménière's disease 58
Meningeosis, neoplastic 262
Meninges 6–7
Meningioma 256, 257, 377
  anaplastic 377
  extracranial 256
  familial 256
  treatment 264
Meningism 222
Meningitis 222, 268
  aseptic 234, 236, 242
    postinfectious 234
    postvaccinal 234
  asymptomatic 230
  bacterial 180, 226, 376
    borrelia-related (Lyme) 228
    tuberculous 232–233
      pathogenesis 232
      symptoms and signs 232, 233
      treatment 232
  Candida and 248
  carcinomatous 262
  chronic 232
  clinical manifestations 222
  Lyme disease and 228
  Mollaret 234
  neurosyphilis and 230, 231
  prophylaxis 226
  viral 234, 376
    pathogens 234
    poliovirus 242
Meningococcus 376
  vaccination 226
Meningoencephalitis 222
  arteritis and 226
  bacterial 226, 376
  Candida and 248
  cryptococcosis and 248
  neurosyphilis and 230
  prophylaxis 226
  treatment 224
    guidelines 375
  tuberculous 232

viral 234–235
  herpes zoster 238
  pathogens 234
Meningopolyradiculitis 230
Mental retardation 381
Mesencephalon 2, 26
Metachromatic leukodystrophy 306, 307, 332, 333
Metastatic disease 262–263
  cascade hypothesis 262
  drop metastasis 260, 262
  intracranial 262, 263, 265
  spinal 262, 263, 265
  treatment 265
Methotrexate 220
Methylprednisolone 220, 238
Metoclopramide 204
Mexiletine 338
Microadenoma 258
Microaneurysm 179
Microangiopathy 172
Microcephaly 381
Microglia 10
Micrographia 128, 206, 207
Micturition 156
Migraine 184–185, 373
  pathogenesis 184
  symptoms and signs 184
    aura 184, 185
    headache phase 184
    prodromal phase 184
    resolution phase 184
  treatment 190
Migration disorder 381
Miller–Fisher syndrome 327, 395
Mini-Mental Status Examination 136
Mini-syndrome test 136
Minor test 152
Miosis 90, 382
  unilateral 92
Mitochondrial disorders 288, 307, 398
  encephalopathy 281
  myopathy 52, 398, 403
Mitoxantrone 220
Möbius syndrome 362
Mollaret meningitis 234
Monoclonal gammopathy of undetermined significance (MGUS) 328
Mononeuritis multiplex 240
Mononeuropathy 50, 180, 316, 318, 322–323, 390, 394
  multiplex 316, 390
  see also Neuropathy

Monoparesis 46, 47
Monoradiculopathy 316, 318
  lumbar 318
Monto–Kelli doctrine 162
Motor end plate 2
  lesions 50
Motor evoked potentials (MEP) 218, 352
Motor function
  age-related changes 382
  Parkinson disease and 210
Motor neuron diseases 304–305, 384–386
  lower 50, 304, 385, 386
  treatment 304
  upper 46, 304, 384, 386
Motor unit 44
Movements
  mass 46
  periodic leg 114
  reflex 42
  respiratory 150, 151
  rhythmic 42
  spontaneous 50
    coma staging 118
  voluntary 42
  see also Dyskinesia(s);
    Dystonia; Eye movements;
    Tics; Tremor
Mucor (mucormycosis) 248
  rhinocerebral 248, 249
Multi-infarct dementia 298
Multifocal motor neuropathy (MMN) 328, 329
Multiple organ failure 312
Multiple sclerosis (MS) 214–221
  clinical manifestations 214–217, 218, 219
    autonomic dysfunction 216, 217, 371
    behavioral changes 216, 217
    fatigue 214
    incoordination 216, 217
    pain 214
    paresis 214
    paroxysmal phenomena 216, 217
    sensory disturbances 214, 215
    spasticity 214
    visual impairment 214, 215
  course of 214, 216
    benign 216
    chronic progressive 214
    malignant 216
    relapsing-remitting 214
  diagnostic criteria 375

Multiple sclerosis (MS)
  differential diagnosis 216
  laboratory tests 218
    bladder function 218
    cerebrospinal fluid exami-
      nation 218, 219
    evoked potentials 218
    neuroimaging 218, 219
  pathogenesis 218–221
    activation 220, 221
    antigen presentation and
      stimulation 220
    demyelination 220
    passage through blood–
      brain barrier 220
    scar formation 220
  prognosis 216
  rehabilitation 220
  relapse 214, 220
  remission 214
  treatment 220
    symptomatic therapy 220
Multiple system atrophy
  (MSA) 276, 302, 303
  bladder dysfunction and 371
Mumps virus 376
Münchhausen syndrome 138
  by proxy 138
Muscle phosphorylase deficiency 402
Muscle(s)
  atrophy 49–52, 107, 281, 287,
    334, 406
    peripheral neuropathy and
      316
    poliomyelitis and 242,
      243
    spinal (SMA) 385
    spinobulbar 385
  cramps 397
  detrusor 156
  expiratory, auxiliary 150,
    151
  facial, syndromes affecting
    362
  functional disorders 52
  hypertrophy 334, 338, 397
  levator palpebrae superioris
    90
  pain 52
    see also Myalgia
  respiratory 150
    auxiliary 150
  segment-indicating 32, 357
  spasms 334
  stiffness 52, 334
  tarsal, superior 90

tone 276
  weakness 334, 374, 397, 405
  see also Myopathy
Muscular dystrophies 336–337,
  398, 400
  Becker 336, 337, 400
  diagnosis 336
  Duchenne 52, 53, 336, 337,
    400
  Emery–Dreifuss 336, 337
  facioscapulohumeral 337,
    400
  pathogenesis 336, 337
  symptoms and signs 336
  treatment 336
  see also Dystrophy
Mutation 288
  chromosome 288
  gene 288
  genome 288
  germ-line 288
  somatic 288
Myalgia 52, 334, 346, 397
  causes 346
  toxic 405
Myasthenia gravis 52, 342–
  343, 406
  aggravating drugs 403
  crises 404
  diagnosis 342
    ancillary tests 404
  pathogenesis 342
  symptoms and signs 342
  treatment 342
Mycobacterium
  leprae 328
  tuberculosis 232, 376
Mycosis, opportunistic systemic 248
  see also Fungal infections
Mydriasis 90
  unilateral 92
Myelin sheath 2
  lesions, multiple sclerosis
    220
Myelinolysis, central pontine
  310, 315
  alcoholism and 314
Myelinopathy 316
Myelitis 222, 282
  clinical manifestations 222
  Lyme disease and 228
  treatment 286
  viral 282, 376
    herpes simplex 236
    herpes zoster 238
Myelography 354

Myelomeningoradiculitis,
  tuberculous 232
Myelopathy 282–287
  acute 282–283
  cervical 284, 285
  chronic 48, 284–284
  diagnostic studies 286
  hereditary 186
  HIV 240
  subacute 284–285
    subacute combined degene-
      ration (SCD) 286, 287
  toxic 286, 287
  treatment 286
Myoclonus 66–69, 383
  epilepsy with ragged red
    fibers (MERRF) 403
  essential 68
  myoclonic encephalopathies
    68
  physiological 68
  progressive myoclonus
    epilepsy with Lafora bo-
      dies 307
  sleep 68, 114
  symptomatic 68
Myokymia 50
Myopathy 50–52, 334–347,
  397–405
  carnitine deficiency 304, 402
  causes 334
  centronuclear 402
  congenital 52, 340, 341, 398,
    402
  critical illness (CIM) 347, 379
  diagnosis 334, 399
  endocrine 347, 398
  episodic paralyses 338, 339
  hereditary 398
  inflammatory 344, 398
  malignant hyperthermia
    346–347
  metabolic 340, 341, 402
  mitochondrial 52, 340, 341,
    398, 403
  myalgia 346
  myasthenic syndromes 342–
    343
  myotonias 338, 339, 401
  nemaline 402
  paraneoplastic syndromes
    347
  primary 52
  rhabdomyolysis 346
  secondary 52
  symptoms and signs 334
  toxic 398, 405

neuromuscular syndromes 347, 398
see also Muscular dystrophies
Myopathy, encephalopathy, lactic acidosis and strokelike episodes (MELAS) 403
Myositis 52, 344–345
diagnosis 344
inclusion body 52, 252, 344, 345
infectious 344
Lyme disease and 228
ossificans 379
pathogenesis 344
syndromes 344
toxoplasmosis and 250
treatment 344
viral 52
Myotomes 32, 33
Myotonia 338, 339, 401, 405
action 338
congenital 52, 338, 339
Becker 401
Thomsen 401
fluctuans 401
paradoxical 338
pathogenesis 338
percussion 338
symptoms and signs 338
treatment 338
Myotonic dystrophy 52, 338, 339, 400, 401

N

Nacrolepsy 114
Nasal cavity 4
Natalizumab 220
Nausea
brain tumors and 254, 255
intracranial hypertension and 158, 159
Near response 90
Neck stiffness, meningitis and 222, 223
Necrosis 174
focal 224
Needle electromyography 391, 399
Neocerebellum 54
Neologisms 124, 126
Nerve injuries 330, 331
pathogenesis 330
compression 330
crushing injuries 330
transection 330

Nerve palsy
abducens 86, 87
facial 96, 98, 99
Lyme disease 228, 229
oculomotor 86, 87, 92, 158
trochlear 86, 87
complete 86, 87
incomplete 86
Nerve roots
dorsal 2
spinal 30
root filaments 30
trauma 272
avulsion 330
ventral 2
spinal 30
Nerve(s)
abducens, palsy 86, 87
alveolar
inferior 94
superior 94
auriculotemporal 94
axillary 35
mononeuropathy 322, 394
buccal 94
cochlear 100
cranial 2, 6, 28–29, 356
herpes zoster and 238
motor cranial nerve nuclei 130
nerve pathways 26, 28
see also specific nerves
cutaneous, lateral, of the thigh 37
mononeuropathy 323, 394
ethmoid
anterior 94
posterior 94
facial 96–99
functional systems 96
lesions 98–99
examination 98
palsy 96, 98, 99
nerve pathways 96
femoral 37
mononeuropathy 323, 394
frontal 94
gluteal, mononeuropathy 323
infraorbital 94
lacrimal 94
lingual 94
mandibular 94
maxillary 94
median 35
mononeuropathy 322, 394
meningeal 94

mental 94
musculocutaneous 35
nasociliary 94
obturator, mononeuropathy 323
oculomotor, palsy 86, 87, 92, 158, 325
olfactory 2
ophthalmic 94
optic 2, 372
atrophy 158, 159
peripheral 2
peroneal 37
mononeuropathy 323, 394
phrenic 150
radial 35
mononeuropathy 322, 394
sciatic 37
mononeuropathy 394
spinal 2, 31, 32, 150
supraorbital 94
supratrochlear 94
sural, biopsy 391
thoracic, long, mononeuropathy 322, 394
tibial 37
mononeuropathy 323, 394
trigeminal 6, 76, 94–95
dysfunction 98
mesencephalic nucleus 94
motor nucleus 94
principal sensory nucleus 94
spinal nucleus 94
trochlear, palsy 86, 87
ulnar 35
mononeuropathy 322, 394
vagus 6, 154
zygomatic 94
Neural tube defects 292, 293
Neuralgia 363
postherpetic 238
trigeminal 186, 187, 190
idiopathic 186
multiple sclerosis 214
pathogenesis 186
symptomatic 186
Neuralgic amyotrophy 321, 328, 329
Neurapraxia 330, 331
Neurites, Lewy 210
Neuritic plaques (NPs) 297
Neuritis
optic, multiple sclerosis 214, 218
retrobulbar 214
toxoplasmosis and 250

Neuroacanthocytosis 300, 301
Neuroblastoma 377
Neuroborreliosis 228–229
  chronic 228
  clinical manifestations 228, 229
  diagnosis 228
  pathogenesis 228
  treatment 228
Neurocranium 4
Neurocybernetic prosthesis (NCP) 198
Neurocysticercosis 250, 251
Neurodegenerative diseases 296–305
  aging 296
    degenerative changes and 296
    disease and 296
  see also specific diseases
Neurofibrillary tangles (NFTs) 297
Neurofibroma 294, 295
Neurofibromatosis 294, 295
  symptoms and signs 294
  type 1 (NF1) 294
  type 2 (NF2) 258, 294
Neurography 391, 399
Neurohypophysis 142
Neuroimaging 353–354, 391, 399
  brain tumors 254, 264–265
  multiple sclerosis 218, 219
  myasthenia gravis 404
Neuroleptics, adverse effects 389, 403
  acute dystonic reaction 204
  malignant neuroleptic syndrome 208
Neuroma, acoustic 258, 259, 294
Neuromodulators, autonomic nervous system 140–141
Neuromuscular junction 2
  lesions 50, 347, 398
    paraneoplastic syndromes 406
    postpolio syndrome and 242
Neuromyotonia 52, 406
Neuronal ceroid lipofuscinosis 307
Neuronopathy 316, 390, 406
Neurons
  medium spiny-type 210

spinal
  parasympathetic 140
  sympathetic 140
Neuropathy
  acquired 317, 390
  acute motor-axonal (AMAN) 395
  acute motor-sensory axonal (AMSAN) 395
  amyloid 333
  diagnosis 316, 391
  giant axon 397
  hereditary 317, 390
  peripheral 316–333
    diabetic 324, 325
    hereditary 332–333
      metabolic 332, 333
      nonmetabolic 332, 333
    infectious origin 328
    inflammatory poly-neuropathies 326–329
    mononeuropathies 318, 322–323, 390, 394
    multifocal motor (MMN) 328, 329
    nerve injuries 330–331
      pathogenesis 330
    plexopathy 318
    radicular lesions 318, 320
    uremic 324
    vasculitic 328, 329
  small fiber 316
  symptoms and signs 316
    autonomic 316
    motor dysfunction 316
    sensory dysfunction 316
  syndromes 316–317, 390
  tomaculous 332
Neuropeptides, pain reception and 108
Neuroprotective therapy 212
Neurosyphilis 230–231
  clinical manifestations 230, 231
    early meningitis 230, 231
    progressive paralysis 230, 231
    tabes dorsalis 230, 231
  meningovascular 230
  pathogenesis 230
  treatment 230
Neurotmesis 330, 331
Neurotransmitters
  autonomic nervous system 140–141
  pain reception and 108
  Parkinson disease and 210

Neurotuberculosis 232
Niemann–Pick disease 306, 307, 387
Nightmares 114
Ninhydrin test 152
Nociception 108
  see also Pain
Nodes of Ranvier 2
Nonneurological disorders 138–139
Norepinephrine 140, 382
Notch, tentorial 6
Nucleus(i)
  ambiguus 102, 148
  caudate 210
  cochlear
    anterior 100
    posterior 100
  cuneatus 104
  detrusor 156
  Edinger–Westphal 26, 90
  gracilis 104
  lentiform 210
  motor cranial nerve 130
  oculomotor 90
  Onuf's 156
  Perlia's 90
  pulposus 30
  red 24
  respiratory group
    dorsal 150
    ventral 150
  solitary tract 148
  subthalamic 24, 210
  tractus solitarius 102
  ventral posterolateral (VPL) 104
  vestibular 26, 56
Nystagmus 70, 86, 88–89
  congenital 88
  end-position 88
  examination 88
  gaze-evoked 88, 89, 276, 277
  gaze-paretic 88
  jerk 88
  multiple sclerosis 214, 215
  optokinetic 84, 88
  pathological 88
  physiological 88
  positional 70, 88
  see-saw 70
  spontaneous 88, 89
  vestibular
    central 88, 89
    peripheral 88, 89

O

Obstructive sleep apnea 114
Occlusion 172
    basilar artery 170, 171
    brachiocephalic trunk 168
    carotid artery
        common 168
        internal 168
    cerebellar arteries 170, 171
    cerebral artery
        middle 168, 169
        posterior 170, 171
    lenticulostriate artery 168
    ophthalmic artery 168
    subclavian artery 170
Ocular deviation 70
Oculomotor disturbances
    86–88, 276
    examination 86
    internuclear disturbances
        86
    peripheral disturbances 86
    stroke and 166
    supranuclear disturbances
        86
Oculomotor function 84–85
Odynophagia 102
Olfaction 76–77
    disturbances 76
    tests of 76
Olfactory pathway 76
Oligoastrocytoma 256, 377
    anaplastic 377
Oligodendroglioma 256, 377
    anaplastic 260, 261, 377
One-and-a-half syndrome 86
Onuf's nucleus 156
Ophthalmoplegia
    chronic progressive external
        (CPEO) 403
    internuclear 86, 87, 214
Ophthalmoscopy 80
Opiate abuse 314
Oppenheim reflex 40
Opportunistic infections 240
    fungal 248–249
        aspergillosis 248, 249
        candidosis 248, 249
        cryptococcosis 248, 249
        mucormycosis 248, 249
Orbit 4, 372
Organ(s)
    circumventricular 140
    of Corti 100
    subfornical 140
Organum vasculosum 140

Orientation evaluation 353
Orthostasis test 369
Osler–Weber–Rendu disease
    294
Osmoregulation 310
Ossicles, auditory 100
Overlap syndrome 344
Oxcarbazepine 198
Oxidative stress 212

P

Pachygyria 381
Pachymeninges 6
Pain 108–111
    classification of 363
    complex regional pain syn-
        drome (CRPS) 110
    diabetic neuropathy and 324
    dysesthesia 106
    facial, atypical 373
    multiple sclerosis 214
    myelopathies 282
    nerve pathways 104, 109
    neurosyphilis 230
    Parkinson disease 208, 209
    pathogenesis 108
    persistent somatoform pain
        disorder 138, 139
    processing 108, 109
        neurotransmitter/neu-
            ropeptide role 108
    pseudoradicular 32
    radicular 32
    reception 108
    referred 108, 110, 363
        headache 188, 189
    sensitization
        central 108
        peripheral 108
    transmission 108
    treatment 264, 324
    types of 108, 109, 363
        central 363
        chronic 363
        deafferentation 363
        neuropathic 108, 363
        nociceptive 108, 363
        phantom limb 363
        psychogenic 363
        radicular 363
        somatic 108, 363
        visceral 108, 110
    zones of Head 110, 111
    see also Myalgia
Paleocerebellum 54
Pallidotomy 212

Palsy
    cerebral, infantile 288–291,
        381
        causes 288
        symptoms and signs 288
        treatment 290
    Erb 318
    Klumpke–Dejerine 318
    progressive supranuclear
        (PSP) 208, 302, 303
    pseudobulbar 362
    see also Nerve palsy
Pancoast tumor 262
Panic disorder 202, 203
Papez circuit 144
Papilledema 158, 159, 160
    brain tumors and 254, 255
    chronic 158, 159
    meningitis and 222
Papilloma, choroid plexus 256,
    257, 377
Paraganglioma 258
    sympathetic 258
Paragrammatism 124, 126
Paralysis
    central 46–49
        upper motor neuron
            (UMN) lesions 46
    crossed 46, 47, 70
    episodic 338, 339, 401
        diagnosis 338
        pathogenesis 338
        prophylaxis 338
        symptoms and signs 338
        treatment 338
    peripheral 50–53
    poliomyelitis and 242, 243
    progressive, neurosyphilis
        and 230, 231
    spinal, familial spastic 286,
        287
Paramyotonia
    cold-induced 52
    congenita 338, 339, 401
Paraneoplastic syndromes 312,
    347, 388
    neuromuscular 406
Paraparesis 46
    tropical spastic 384
Paraphasia 126
    phonemic 124
    semantic 124
Paraplegia
    familial spastic (FSP) 286,
        287, 384
    in flexion 214
    spinal cord trauma and 274

Parapraxia 128
Paraproteinemic poly-
  neuropathy 328, 329, 406
Parasomnias 114
Parasympathetic nervous
  system 90, 140, 147, 148, 154
Paresis
  crossed 47
  ipsilateral 46
  Lyme disease and 228, 229
  multiple sclerosis 214
  peripheral 47
Paresthesia 106, 316
  multiple sclerosis 214
  spinal artery syndrome 282
Parinaud syndrome 70, 92, 358
Parkinson disease 62, 206–213
  agraphia 128
  autonomic dysfunction 208,
    209
    bladder disorders 208, 371
    blood pressure changes
      208
    constipation 208
    hyperhidrosis 208
    leg edema 208
    seborrhea 208
    sexual dysfunction 208
    sleep disorders 208, 209
  behavioral changes 206–209
    anxiety 206
    dementia 208
    depression 206
    hallucinations 208
  cardinal manifestations 206,
    207
    akinesia 206
    bradykinesia 206
    hypokinesia 206
    postural instability 206,
      207
    rigidity 206, 207
    tremor 206, 207
  dystonia 208, 209
  genetics of 213
  idiopathic 302
  pathogenesis 210–211
    basal ganglia 210, 211
    connections 210, 211
    motor function 210
    neurotransmitters 210
  sensory manifestations 208
    dysesthesias 208
    pain 208, 209
  treatment 212–213
    deep brain stimulation 212
    neuroprotective 212

  stereotactic neurosurgical
    procedures 212
  symptomatic 212
  transplant surgery 212
  visual disturbances 208
Parkinsonism 374, 383
  atypical 302–303
Parosmia 76
Paroxysmal depolarization
  shift 198
Pathway(s)
  auditory 100, 101
  cranial nerves 26–28
  deglutition 102, 103
  direct 210
  facial nerve 96
  gustatory 78
  indirect 210
  limbic system 144
  olfactory 76
  pain 104, 109
  pupillomotor 90
  somatosensory 104
  visual 80–81
Peduncle, cerebellar
  inferior 54
  lesions 358
  middle 54
  superior 54
Pelizaeus–Merzbacher disease
  387
Penicillin 230
Peregrinating patient 138
Pergolide 212
Pericranium 4, 6
Perineurium 2, 30
Peripheral nervous system
  (PNS) 2, 3
Peristalsis 154
Peritonitis 226
Perlia's nucleus 90
Perphenazine 204
Perseveration 126
Persistent somatoform pain
  disorder 138, 139
Persistent vegetative state 120,
  121
Personality 122
Phakomatoses 294–295, 381
Phencyclidine (PCP) abuse 314
Phenobarbital 198
Phenomenon
  black-curtain 168
  doll's-eye 26, 302, 303
    coma and 118
  extinction 132
  rebound 276, 277

Uhthoff's 214
Phenotype 288, 289
Phenylketonuria 306
Phenytoin 198, 264
Pheochromocytoma 258
Phonation 130
  dysphonia 130
Phosphofructokinase defi-
  ciency 402
Photoreceptors 104
Physical examination 350–351
Pia mater 6
  spinal 30
Pick disease 298, 299
Pineal region tumors 258, 259
Pineoblastoma 258, 377
Pineocytoma 258, 377
  "Pisa" syndrome 65, 66
Pituitary gland 6
  anterior lobe 142
  hypothalamic–pituitary reg-
    ulatory axis 367
  posterior lobe 142
  Sheehan's postpartum
    necrosis 258
  stalk 6
  tumors
    adenoma 258, 259, 377
    metastases 262
    treatment 264
Plasmodium falciparum (cerebral malaria) 250, 251
Platybasia 292, 293
Plexopathy 50, 318, 321
Plexus(es) 32–36
  brachial 32, 34, 318
    infraclavicular region 318
    Pancoast tumor 262
    plexopathy 318, 321, 393
    supraclavicular region 318
    trauma 272, 330
  cervical 32, 35
  cervicobrachial 34
  choroid 6, 8
    carcinoma 377
    papilloma 256, 257, 377
  coccygeal 32
  ganglionic, submucous 154
  lumbar 32, 36
  lumbosacral 36
    plexopathy 318, 321, 393
  myenteric 154
  pterygoid 20
  sacral 32
    lesions 318
  vertebral venous
    external 22
    internal 22

Pneumococcus 376
vaccination 226
POEMS syndrome 328
Poliomyelitis 242–243
bulbar 242
encephalitic form 242
major 242
paralytic 242
preparalytic 242
minor (abortive) 242
pathogenesis 242, 243
postpolio syndrome 242, 243, 385
prevention 242
spinal form 242
symptoms and signs 242
Poliovirus 242
Polyarteritis nodosa 180
Polymyalgia rheumatica 52
Polymyositis 52, 240, 344, 345, 405, 406
Polyneuropathy 50, 316
critical illness (CIP) 347, 379
diabetic (DPN) 324, 325, 395
diagnosis 324
symptoms and signs 324
treatment 324
distal symmetric 324, 325
focal 316
hereditary, genetic features 396
hypoglycemic 395
inflammatory 326–329
paraproteinemic 328, 329, 406
sensorimotor 406
small-fiber 395
see also Neuropathy
Polyradiculitis 236
Polyradiculoneuropathy 228, 406
acute inflammatory demy-elinating (AIDP) 395
chronic inflammatory demy-elinating (CIDP) 327, 328
HIV and 240
Polyradiculopathy 316
lumbosacral 244, 395
Pons 2, 6
hemorrhage 176
infarction 170
lesions 70
syndromes 70–72, 359–360
Pontocerebellum 54, 55
Porencephaly 290, 291, 381
Porphyria 332, 333
Postpolio syndrome 242, 243, 385

Posttraumatic syndrome 379
Posture 60, 61
disturbances 106, 276
Parkinson disease and 206, 207
test 276, 277
Pramipexol 212
Praziquantel 250
Predelirium 312
Presbycusis 382
Presbyopia 382
Presenilin genes 297–298
Primary complex 232
Primary lateral sclerosis 384
Primidone 198
Primitive neuroectodermal tumor (PNET) 260, 261, 265, 377
Prion protein (PrP) 252, 253
PRNP gene 252
Progesterone 367
Progressive multifocal leukoencephalopathy (PMS) 244–245
diagnosis 244
pathogenesis 244
symptoms and signs 244
Progressive supranuclear palsy (PSP) 208, 302, 303
Prolactin 367
Prolactinoma 258
Proprioception evaluation 106
Prosencephalon 2, 3
Prosody 124
Protein X 252
Pseudo-lupus erythematosus 405
Pseudodementia 297
Pseudoinsomnia 114
Pseudoradicular syndromes 318, 320, 392
causes 320
Pseudoseizures 200
Pseudotumor cerebri 160
Pseudounipolar cells 2
Pterion 4
Pupillary dysfunction 92–93
examination 92
swinging flashlight test 92
parasympathetic denerva-tion 92, 93
sympathetic denervation 92, 93
Pupillomotor function 90–91
pupilloconstriction 90
Pupil(s) 90–92
Argyll–Robertson 92, 230

Marcus–Gunn 214
pinpoint 92
tonic 92
Putamen 210
Pyramid, medullary 46
Pyrazinamide 232
Pyridostigmine bromide 342
Pyrimethamine/sulfadiazine 250

Q

Quadrantanopsia 82
Quadriparesis 46
Quadriplegia, spinal cord trauma and 274
Quantitative sudomotor axon reflex test (QSART) 152

R

Rabies 246–247
hyperexcitability stage 246, 247
paralytic stage 246
pathogenesis 246, 247
prodromal stage 246
prophylaxis 246
sylvatic 246
symptoms and signs 246
urban 246
Radiation, optic 80
Radiculitis 236, 238
Radiculopathy 316, 318, 320, 390
causes 320, 392
Radiography 354
Radiotherapy 264–265
adverse effects 389
Ramsay–Hunt syndrome 238
Raymond–Céstan syndrome 360
Reactions
acute dystonic 66, 204, 205
acute epileptic 196
Reading 124, 125
alexia 128
Rebound phenomenon 276, 277
Receptor(s) 2, 104
baroreceptors 148
chemoreceptors 104, 150, 151
cutaneous 104
exteroceptors 104
interoceptors 104
mechanoreceptors 104, 150

Index

Receptor(s)
  olfactory 76
  photoreceptors 104
  thermoreceptors 104, 152
Reflex(es) 26, 40–42
  abnormalities 46, 50
  acoustic 26, 96
  age-related changes 382
  blink 96, 98
  coma staging 118
  corneal 26, 96
  cough 26
  cutivisceral 110, 111
  extrinsic 40, 42
  flexor 40
  Gordon 40
  Hering–Breuer 150
  intrinsic 40, 42
  light 90, 91
  masseter (jaw jerk) 26
  oculocephalic 26
  Oppenheim 40
  optokinetic 84
  orbicularis oculi 96
  orbicularis oris 96
  palmomental 96
  pathological 40, 46
  pharyngeal (gag) 26
  pupillary light 26
  reflex arc 40
  reflex response 40
  snout 96
  stapedius 98
  startle 68
  sucking 96
  trigeminal autonomic reflex
    circuit 184
  vasodilatory axon 110, 111
  vestibulo-ocular (VOR) 26,
    84
    coma and 118
  viscerocutaneous 110, 111
  visceromotor 110, 111
  viscerovisceral 110
  visual blink 96
Refsum disease 332
Renal failure 310
Respiration 150–151
  auxiliary muscles 150, 151
  Cheyne–Stokes 118
  costal 150
  diaphragmatic 150
  disorders 150, 151, 370
    stroke and 166
  Kussmaul's 118
  respiratory movements 150,
    151

rhythm 150
Respiratory test 369
Restless legs syndrome (RLS)
  114
Reticular formation 26
  medullary 26
  mid brain 26
  pain and 108
  pontine 26
    paramedian 84
Retina 80
  lesions 372
Retrocollis 64
Rhabdomyolysis 346, 406
Rhabdomyosarcoma 260
Rhizopus 248
Rhombencephalon 2
Rhythm
  circadian 112, 113
    disturbances 114
  respiration 150
Rifampicin 226, 232
Rigidity 206, 207
  cogwheel 206, 207
Riluzole 304
Romberg sign 276
Ropinirol 212
Ross syndrome 92

S

Saccades 84
  abnormal 70, 276, 277
Saccule 56
Sacrum 30
Salivation, test of 98
Sarcoglycanopathy 398
Sarcoidosis 234
Sarcoma
  cerebral, primary 260
  meningeal 260
Scala
  tympani 100
  vestibuli 100
Scalp 4, 7
  injuries 266
Scaphocephaly 381
Scar formation, multiple
  sclerosis 220
Schellong's test (orthostasis)
  369
Schizencephaly 381
Schwann cells 2
Schwannoma 258, 377
Sclerosis
  amyotrophic lateral (ALS)
    304, 386

primary lateral 384
tuberous (TSC) 294, 295
see also Multiple sclerosis
Scotoma 82, 83
  central 82, 215
  homonymous
    bilateral 82
    unilateral 82
  junction 82
Scrapie 252
Seborrhea, Parkinson disease
  and 208
Segawa syndrome 64
Segment-indicating muscles
  32, 357
Seizures
  epileptic
    brain injury and 268
    brain tumors and 254, 264
    generalized 193, 194–195,
      197
      absence 194, 195
      atonic 194
      grand mal 194, 195, 199
      myoclonic 194
      tonic-clonic 194, 195
    isolated nonrecurring 196
    partial (focal) 192–194,
      197
      complex 192, 193, 194
      secondary generaliza-
        tion 192
      simple 192, 193, 194
    pathophysiology 198, 199
    postictal period 192
    status epilepticus 196
      grand mal 196
    stroke and 166
    tuberous sclerosis and 294
    types of 192–195
  nonepileptic 200–205
    acute dystonic reaction 66,
      204, 205
    drop attacks 204, 205
    hyperventilation syn-
      drome (tetany) 204, 205
    panic attacks 202, 203
    pseudoseizures 200
    psychogenic 200, 202, 203
      postictal phase 202
      premonitory signs 202
      semiology 202
    simulated 202
    syncope 200–201
    tonic spasms 204, 205
Selegiline 212
Senescence 296

Sensation 104–105
  epicritic 104
  protopathic 104
  somatic 104
  superficial 106
Sensory disturbances 106–107
  age-related 382
  examination 106
  interpretation 106
  location 106, 316, 317
  peripheral neuropathies 316, 318, 390
  radicular 107
  stroke and 166
Sensory receptors see Receptors
Sepsis 312, 313, 347
  candida 248
  see also Bacterial infections
Sexual behaviour disturbances 368
Sexual function 156
  multiple sclerosis and 216
  Parkinson disease and 208
Shingles see Herpes zoster
Shock, spinal 48, 274
Shulman disease 344
Shy–Drager syndrome 302
Sign(s)
  Babinski 40, 49
  Bragard's 318
  Brudzinski's 222
  Kernig's 222
  Lasègue's 318
  Lhermitte's 48, 49, 214
  Romberg 276
Sinus(es)
  carotid 10, 148
    massage 369
  paranasal 4
    ethmoid 4
    frontal 4
    maxillary 4
    sphenoid 4
  thrombosis 180, 181
    aseptic 180, 181
    etiology 180
    septic 180
    symptoms and signs 180
    treatment 180
  venous
    dural 6, 18
    thrombophlebitis 226, 227
Sinusitis 186
Skull 4–5
  base 4, 5
    metastases 262

syndromes 74–75
  fracture 266
Sleep 112–113, 363
  age changes 112, 113
  circadian rhythm 112, 113
    disturbances 114
  disorders 114–115
    neurogenic 114
    Parkinson disease 208, 209
    primary (dyssomnias) 114
      extrinsic 114
      intrinsic 114
      parasomnias 114
    psychogenic 114
    secondary 114
    systemic disease and 114
  non-rapid eye movement (NREM) 112, 363
  polygraphic recordings 112
  profile 112, 113
  rapid eye movement (REM) 112, 363
Smell 76–77
  age-related changes 382
  olfactory disturbances 76
  tests of 76
Sodium balance 310, 311
Sodium channel dysfunction 338, 398
Somatization disorder 138
Somatoform disorders 138
  persistent somatoform pain disorder 138, 139
Somatosensory evoked potentials (SEP) 218, 352
Somnambulism 114
Somnolence 116, 117
Sound perception 100
Space
  epidural 6, 30
  infratentorial 6
  subarachnoid 6, 8
    pathogen entry 224
    spinal 30
  subdural 6
  supratentorial 6
  Virchow–Robin 6
Space-occupying lesions, intracranial pressure and 162–163
Spasm
  multiple sclerosis and 214
  muscle 334
  right hemifacial 99
  tonic 204, 205
Spasmus nutans 88

Spasticity 46, 47
  multiple sclerosis 214
Spatial orientation disturbances 132–133
Spectral analysis 100, 101
Speech 130
  articulation 130
  disorders 124, 130
    dysarthria 124, 130, 276
    dysphonia 130
    neural basis of 130, 131
    voice production 130
Sphenoid bone 4
Spielmeyer–Vogt syndrome 307
Spina bifida 292, 293
Spinal automatisms 46
Spinal cord 2, 30–32
  blood supply 22–23
  claudication 282
  infarction
    central 282
    complete 282
  lesions 48, 275, 381
    bladder dysfunction and 371
    cervical 48
    lumbar 48
    sacral 48
    thoracic 48
    transection 48, 274, 282, 381
  trauma 274–275, 371
    acute stage (spinal shock) 274
    chronic stage–late sequelae 274
    closed 274
    open 274
    rehabilitation stage 274
    treatment 380
Spinal dysraphism 292, 293
Spinal muscular atrophy (SMA) 385
Spinal shock 48, 274
Spine 30–31
  hemorrhage 282
  metastases 262, 263
    treatment 265
  neoplasms 284, 285
  trauma 272–273, 380
    brachial plexus 272
    diagnosis 272
    nerve roots 272
    treatment 380
    vertebral fracture 272
    whiplash injury 272, 273, 380

Spinocerebellar ataxia (SCA) 280, 384
Spinocerebellum 54, 55
Spironolactone 338
Split-brain syndrome 24
Spondylolisthesis 392
Spondylosis deformans 392
Spongiform encephalopathies 252–253
  bovine 252
  Creutzfeldt-Jakob disease (CJD) 252, 253
  genetic 252
  infectious 252
Stapes 100
Staphylococcus 376
Startle reflex 68
Status epilepticus 196
  grand mal 196
Steele–Richardson–Olszewski syndrome 302
Stem cell transplantation, Parkinson disease 212
Stenosis
  craniostenosis 381
  spinal 392
    lumbar 284
Stomach 154
Strategic infarct dementia 298
Striatal foot 64
Striatonigral degeneration (SND) 302
Stroke 166–181
  bladder dysfunction and 371
  causes 167, 172
  hemorrhage 166, 176–179
    intracerebral 166, 176
      basal ganglia 176
      brain stem 176
      cerebellar 176
      lobar 176
      pathogenesis 178
    intraventricular 166, 176
      complications 176
      symptoms and signs 176
    subarachnoid 166, 176–177
      complications 176
      pathogenesis 178
      symptoms and signs 176
    treatment 178
  in evolution 166
  ischemia 166–175
    carotid artery territory 168
    pathophysiology 174, 175

hemodynamic insufficiency 174
  hypoperfusion 174
  prevention
    primary 174
    secondary 174
  risk factors 172
  treatment 174
    treatment window 174
  vertebrobasilar territory 170–171
  major 166
  minor 166
  sinus thrombosis 180, 181
    etiology 180
    symptoms and signs 180
    treatment 180
  symptoms and signs 166
Stupor 116, 117
Sturge–Weber disease 294, 295
Subacute combined degeneration (SCD) 286, 287
Subcortical arteriosclerotic encephalopathy (SAE) 298
Subdural
  empyema 222
  hematoma 268, 270
    chronic 379
  hygroma 379
  space 6
Subependymoma 256
Substance abuse 312, 314, 315
  see also Alcoholism
Substantia nigra 24, 210
Sucking reflex 96
Superoxide dismutase 1 (SOD1) 304
Suture(s) 4
  coronal 4
  lambdoid 4
  sagittal 4
Swallowing *see* Deglutition; Dysphagia
Sweating
  disturbances 152
  sweat gland innervation 152, 153
Swinging flashlight test 92
Sympathetic nervous system 90, 140, 147, 148, 154
Sympathetic skin response (SSR) 152
Symptoms
  nature of 350
  onset 350
  severity of 350

time course 350
see also specific conditions
Synchondroses 4
Syncope 200–201
  causes 374
  neurocardiogenic 148
Syndrome(s)
  acquired immunodeficiency (AIDS) 240
  Adie 92
  alcohol withdrawal 312, 313
  alien hand 24, 302
  anterior horn 48, 50
  anterior spinal artery 48
  Anton 132
  apallic 117, 120, 121
  apraxia-like 128
  Bannwarth 228
  Bassen–Kornzweig 300
  Benedict 70, 358
  brain stem 70–71
  Brown–Séquard 48
  carpal tunnel 322
  cauda equina 319
  cavernous sinus 75
  central cord 48
  central salt-wasting 310
  cervical 188, 189
    upper 188
  chiasm 75
  Churg–Strauss 180, 344
  clivus 75
  comalike 120–121
  complex regional pain syndrome (CRPS) 110
  conus medullaris 48
  Crow–Fukase 328
  decerebration 46, 47, 118, 158, 159
  decortication 46, 47, 118
  disconnection 24, 128
  disequilibrium 310
  encephalitic 222
  epileptic 196
  fetal alcohol 314
  Frey 362
  frontal lobe 122
    lateralized 122
    nonlateralized 122
  Ganser 138
  Gerstmann 128
  Gerstmann–Sträussler–Scheinker 280
  Gilles de la Tourette 68
  Guillain–Barré 244, 326–327, 395–396
  Heerfordt 362

herniation 158, 162
Horner 48, 92, 152, 318
  central 92
hypereosinophilia 344
hyperventilation 204, 205
Kearns–Sayre 403
King–Denborough 347
Klippel–Feil 292, 293
Korsakoff 76, 308, 312
lacunar 359
Lambert–Eaton 50, 52, 342, 343, 406
Lance–Adams 308
Lennox–Gastaut 196, 198
limbic 368
locked-in 120, 121, 170, 359
McLeod 300
malignant neuroleptic 208, 347
medullary 70, 73, 361
  dorsolateral 361
Meige 64, 362
Melkersson–Rosenthal 362
meningitic 222, 234
mid brain 70, 71, 358–359
Miller–Fisher 327, 395
Möbius 362
Münchhausen 138
myelitic 222
myopathy 397
myositis 344
neuropathy 316–317, 390
  of inappropriate ADH secretion (SIADH) 310
olfactory nerve 75
one-and-a-half 86
orbital apex 75
overlap 344
paraneoplastic 312, 347, 388
  neuromuscular 406
parasagittal cortical 46
Parinaud 70, 92, 358
Parkinsonian, atypical 302–303
"Pisa" 65, 66
POEMS 328
pontine 70–72, 359–360
  lateral pontomedullary 70
postanoxic 308
  delayed 308
posterior column 48
posterior cord 48
posterior horn 48
postpolio 242, 243, 385
posttraumatic 379
postviral fatigue 52
pseudoradicular 318, 320, 392

radicular 50, 392
Ramsay–Hunt 238
Raymond–Céstan 360
restless legs (RLS) 114
Ross 92
Segawa 64
Shy–Drager 302
skull base 74–75
sphenoid wing 75
Spielmeyer–Vogt 307
spinal artery
  anterior 282
  posterior 282
spinal cord transection 274
split-brain 24
Steele–Richardson–Olszewski 302
Sturge–Weber 294, 295
sulcocommisural artery 282
tethered cord 292, 293
top of the basilar 70, 359
transverse cord 180, 232, 380, 381
  sensory 214
Vogt–Koyanagi–Harada 234
Wallenberg 70, 170, 361
Weber 70, 358
Wernicke–Korsakoff 312, 314
West 196
Zellweger 386
Synkinesia 46, 99, 362
Syphilis 180
  latent 230
  see also Neurosyphilis
Syringomyelia 107, 284, 285
System
  craniosacral 140
  dioptric 80
  epicritic/lemniscal 104
  limbic 80, 135, 144–145
    functions 144
    nerve pathways 144
    pain and 108
    structure 144, 145
    syndromes 368
  protopathic 104
  reticular activating (RAS) 116
  spinocerebellar 104
  thoracolumbar 140, 152
  trigeminovascular 184, 185

T

T lymphocytes, multiple sclerosis and 220
Tabes dorsalis 230, 231

Taenia solium (neurocysticercosis) 250, 251
Takayasu arteritis 180
Tangier disease 332
Tapeworm infection 250, 251
Taste 78–79
  age-related changes 382
  disturbances 78
  tests of 78
Taste buds 78
Tay–Sachs disease 387
Tela choroidea 6
Telangiectasia 280, 281, 294, 295
  hereditary hemorrhagic (HHT) 294
Telencephalon 2
Temperature *see* Thermoregulation
Temporal arteritis 180
Temporomandibular joint 4
Tension headache *see* Headache
Tentorium cerebelli 6
Testosterone 367
Test(s)
  Aachen aphasia 124
  apnea 364
  Bárány's pointing 276
  caloric 26
  confrontation test 82, 83
  edrophonium chloride 404
  finger–finger 276, 277
  finger–nose 276
  hand grip 369
  heel–knee–shin 276
  iodine–starch (Minor) test 152
  lacrimation 98
  neurophysiological 352
  neuropsychological 352–353
  ninhydrin test 152
  olfaction 76
  posture 276, 277
  quantitative sudomotor axon reflex test (QSART) 152
  red vision test 82
  respiratory 369
  salivation 98
  Schellong's (orthostasis) 369
  Schirmer test 98
  smell 76
  swinging flashlight test 92
  sympathetic skin response (SSR) 152
  taste 78
  Wada 126

Tetany 204
Tethered cord syndrome 292, 293
Thalamus 24
  hemorrhage 176
  pain and 108
Thermoreceptors 104, 152
Thermoregulation 152–153
  disturbances 152
  neural control 152
Thiamin deficiency 312
Thromboembolism, infectious 226
Thrombophlebitis, bacterial 226, 227
Thrombosis 172, 173
  prophylaxis 264
  see also Occlusion
Thyroid hormones 143
Tiagabine 198
Tic douloureux 186
Tics 68–69, 362, 383
Tobacco–alcohol amblyopia 314
Toe-walking 60
Tonotopicity 100, 101
Top of the basilar syndrome 70, 359
Topiramate 198
Torcular Herophili 18
Torticollis 64
Toxoplasma gondii (toxoplasmosis) 250, 251
  bradyzoites 250
  congenital 250
  oocysts 250
  tachyzoites 250
Tract(s)
  corticobulbar 44
  corticonuclear 96
  corticopontine 44
  corticospinal
    anterior 44
    lateral 44
  motor 44
  pyramidal 44, 45
  reticulospinal 44
  rubrospinal 44
  spinocerebellar 104
  spinothalamic
    anterior 104
    lateral 104
    posterior 104
  trigeminocortical 94
  vestibulospinal 44
Transcranial Doppler (TCD) 353

Transient ischemic attack (TIA) 166
  crescendo 166
Transient monocular blindness 168, 372
Transmissible spongiform encephalopathies (TSEs) 252–253
  Creutzfeldt–Jakob disease (CJD) 252, 253
Transverse cord syndrome 180, 232, 380, 381
  sensory 214
Trauma 266–275, 366
  multiorgan 266
  spinal 272–273
    brachial plexus 272
    diagnosis 272
    nerve roots 272
    treatment 380
    vertebral fracture 272
    whiplash injury 272, 273, 380
  spinal cord 274–275
    acute stage (spinal shock) 274
    chronic stage–late sequelae 274
    rehabilitation stage 274
    treatment 380
  traumatic brain injury (TBI) 266–271
    complications 269, 270
    evaluation 266
    pathogenesis 270, 271
    primary injury 266, 270
    prognosis 268
    secondary sequelae 268, 270
    treatment 270
      hospital 270
      scene of accident 270, 271
    types of 266
Tremor 62–63
  action 62, 63
  cerebellar 357
  essential 62, 357
  genesis of 62
  Holmes 357
  intention 62, 63, 276
  kinetic 62, 63
  palatal 357
  Parkinson disease and 206, 207, 357
  physiological 357
  polyneuropathic 357

  postural 62
  psychogenic 357
  rest 62, 63
  task-specific 62
  types of 63, 357
Treponema pallidum 230
Triflupromazine 204
Triiodothyronine 367
Tropical spastic paraparesis 384
Trunk
  brachiocephalic 10, 148
    occlusion 168
  lumbar sympathetic, lesions 318
Tuberculoma 232, 233
Tuberculosis 180
  organ 232
  reactivated 232
  spinal 232
Tuberculous meningitis 232–233
  diagnosis 232
  pathogenesis 232
  symptoms and signs 232, 233
  treatment 232
Tuberous sclerosis (TSC) 294, 295
Tumors
  Pancoast 262
  paraneoplastic encephalopathy 312
  primitive neuroectodermal (PNET) 260, 261, 265, 377
  spinal 284, 285
  see also Brain tumors; specific tumors
Turicephaly 381

U

Uhthoff's phenomenon 214
Ulegyria 381
Ultrasonography 353
  duplex sonography 353
  transcranial Doppler (TCD) 353
Uremia 310, 311
Uremic
  encephalopathy 310, 311
  neuropathy 324
Urinary tract infection, multiple sclerosis 216
Utricle 56

V

Vaccination
  Haemophilus influenzae 226
  Lyme disease 228
  meningococcus 226
  Pneumococcus 226
  poliomyelitis 242
  rabies 246
Valacyclovir 238
Valproic acid 198
Valsalva maneuver (VM) 369
Varicella-zoster 238–239
  complications 238, 239
  ganglionic latency phase 238
  immunocompromised
    patients 238
  pathogenesis 238, 239
  symptoms and signs 238, 239
  treatment 238
  viral reactivation 238
Vascular reserve 174
Vasculitic neuropathy 328, 329
Vasculitides
  primary 180
  secondary 180
Vasculitis
  bacterial 180, 226
  cerebral 180, 181
    causes 180
    differential diagnosis 216
    immune 181
    Lyme disease and 228
    primary 180
    secondary 180
    symptoms and signs 180
    treatment 180
  CMV 244
  neurosyphilis and 230
Vasospasm 176
Vein(s)
  azygos 22
  basal (of Rosenthal) 18
  bridging 18
  central 18
  cerebral 18–19
    deep 10, 18
    great (of Galen) 18
    inferior 18
    internal 18
    superficial 10, 18
      middle 18
    superior 18
    thrombophlebitis 226
  cervical 20
    deep 20, 22
  cortical 18

cranial 20
diploic 18
emissary 18
facial 20
hemiazygos 22
iliac, common 22
intercostal, posterior 22
jugular
  external 20
  internal 20
lumbar 22
occipital 18, 20
radicular 22
retromandibular 20
sacral
  lateral 22
  medial 22
spinal 22, 23
  anterior 22
  lateral 22
  posterior 22
vertebral 20, 22
Vena cava, superior 22
Ventriculitis 222, 226, 227
Ventriculomegaly, long-standing overt (LOVA) 290
Vertebrae 30
  cervical 30
  coccygeal 30
  fracture 272, 380
    burst 380
    compression 380
    dens 380
    dislocation 380
    Jefferson's 380
    stability 272, 273
  lumbar 30
  thoracic 30
Vertebral column 30
Vertigo 58–59
  benign paroxysmal posi-
    tional 58, 59
  brain tumors and 254, 255
  episodic 58
  nonvestibular 58, 59
  physiological 58
  vestibular
    central 58
    peripheral 58
Vestibular system 56–57
  disorder 374
Vestibulocerebellum 54–56
Villi, arachnoid 8
Viral infections 234–247, 376,
  385
  cytomegalovirus (CMV) 244–
    245

herpes simplex 236–237
human immunodeficiency
  virus (HIV) 240–241
meningoencephalitis 234–
  235
pathogens 234
poliomyelitis 242–243
progressive multifocal
  leukoencephalopathy
  (PMS) 244–245
rabies 246–247
varicella-zoster 238–239
see also specific infections
Virchow–Robin space 6
Viremia
  primary 238
  secondary 238
Viscerocranium 4, 5
Vision
  color 80
    disturbances 80
  intracranial hypertension
    and 158
  stereoscopic 80
Visual disturbances
  color vision 80
  multiple sclerosis 214, 215
  Parkinson disease 208
  stroke and 166
  see also Visual field
Visual evoked potentials (VEP)
  218, 219, 352
Visual field 80
  binocular 80
  confrontation test 82, 83
  defects 82–83
    chiasmatic lesions 82
    perichiasmatic lesions 82
    retrochiasmatic lesions
      82
  monocular 80
  red vision test 82
Visual pathway 80–81
Vitamin B1 deficiency 312
Vitamin B12 deficiency 286,
  287
Vitamin E deficiency 280
Vogt–Koyanagi–Harada syn-
  drome 234
Voice production 130
  timbre 130
  volume 130
  whisper 130
  see also Speech
Volume regulation 310
Vomiting 370
  brain tumors and 254, 255

Vomiting
  intracranial hypertension
    and 158
    von Heubner angiitis 230
    von Hippel–Lindau disease
      294, 295
  hemangioblastoma and 256
  symptoms and signs 294
    von Recklinghausen dis-
      ease 294

W

Wada test 126
Wakefulness 116
  see also Consciousness
Wallenberg syndrome 70, 170,
  361

Water balance *see* Fluid
  balance
Watershed zones 22, 168
Weber syndrome 70, 358
Wegener granulomatosis 180
Wernicke–Korsakoff syndrome
  312, 314
Wernicke's
  aphasia 126, 127
  area 124
  encephalopathy 312, 313
West syndrome 196
Whiplash injury 272, 273
  severity classification 272
  symptoms and signs 272
  treatment 380
Whisper 130

White-matter lesions (WMLs)
  298
Wilson disease 208, 307
Writer's cramp 64, 65
Writing 124
  agraphia 128, 129

X

Xanthoastrocytoma, pleomorphic 256, 377

Z

Zellweger syndrome 386
Zones, of Head 110, 111